STAPLING IN SURGERY

Stapling in Surgery

FELICIEN M. STEICHEN, M.D.

Director of Surgery
Lenox Hill Hospital,
Professor of Surgery
New York Medical College
New York, New York

MARK M. RAVITCH, M.D.

Surgeon-in-Chief
Montefiore Hospital,
Professor of Surgery
University of Pittsburgh
School of Medicine
Pittsburgh, Pennsylvania

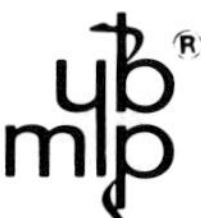

YEAR BOOK MEDICAL PUBLISHERS, INC.

CHICAGO • LONDON

Reprinted, July 1985

Library of Congress Cataloging in Publication Data

Steichen, Felicien M.
    Stapling in surgery.

    Includes index.
    1. Staplers (Surgery)   I. Ravitch, Mark M., 1910–
II. Title. [DNLM: 1. Surgical staplers.   2. Surgical
staplers—Atlases.   3. Suture technics—Instrumentation.
4. Suture technics—Instrumentation—Atlases.   WO 166
S818s]
RD73.S75S74   1983   617′.9178   83-10625
ISBN 0-8151-7108-0

Contents

Preface

THE AUTHORS have been involved in the development, experimental evaluation, and clinical use of staples in surgery for what, at the time of publication, will be a quarter of a century of collaboration.

In that period, what was taken for a gimmicky novelty has come to be a standard of the surgeon's instrumentarium. We have contemplated this book for a decade, and have had it in preparation now for several years, its completion being periodically delayed by the development of new instruments and the appearance of new clinical and experimental reports. The literature on stapling now is enormous. In our account of the development of stapling, we have tried to stay in the mainstream, as we understand it, of the development of the instruments and techniques as we utilize them today. Some of the illustrations and citations illustrate avenues of development that were abandoned and may yet be resurrected. A complete discussion of all such instruments would require a forbiddingly huge catalogue. By the same token, in this large literature, we have had to be selective in our citations. All papers referred to have been read in the original. To any whose instruments or papers are not referred to at all, or dealt with only briefly, we can only plead the exigencies of time and the intention to produce a book of a size to be read and used. It was our prediction from the first that the ingenuity of our surgical colleagues would result in techniques of use of the instruments and indications for their utilization not envisaged by us. In these pages appear many of the illustrations of such innovations, testimony to the imagination and ingenuity of surgeons around the world.

FELICIEN M. STEICHEN, M.D.

MARK M. RAVITCH, M.D.

Acknowledgments

WE ARE HAPPY TO ACKNOWLEDGE the friendly interest and cooperation in Russia of the directors and staff of the Scientific Research Institute for Experimental Surgical Apparatus and Instruments, particularly Drs. M.G. Ananiev, S.I. Babkin, and A.M. Geselevich, and of the surgeons in other hospitals and clinics—particularly Dr. N.M. Amosov of Kiev, in whose hands we first saw the instruments used, and, in Moscow, Dr. Pavel Androsov and Dr. Yu Ya Gritsman. The directors of the National Institutes of Health, in Bethesda, at the time expressed no interest in the development of an institute modeled along the lines of that in Moscow and suggested the Research Grant approach. Most of the experimental work here reported was made possible by such grant support, for which we are grateful. The experimental work and the clinical application of stapling instruments were enhanced by the support and encouragement of our colleagues on the house and attending staffs of the Baltimore City and Johns Hopkins Hospitals, the University of Chicago Hospitals, the Lincoln Hospital in the Bronx, the Montefiore and Veterans Administration Hospitals in Pittsburgh, the Lenox Hill Hospital in New York, and indeed of many clinics and places of learning on five continents. We owe the illustrations of our techniques in this volume, for the most part specially drawn for the purpose, to the generous support of the United States Surgical Corporation and the superb artistry of Mr. Bill Baker. It is a pleasure to express our gratitude to him for his always willing cooperation. To our secretaries, Janet Daniels, Lieselotte Gleich, and Mary Beth Madalinsky, and to Ruth Jacobson, Editorial Assistant, we express our gratitude and appreciation for their intelligence and perfectionistic labors, and amazement at their tolerance with our chronic need to revise and update. Mrs. Jacobson and Mrs. Madalinsky typed, retyped, and typed again. To Mrs. Jacobson we are particularly indebted for her indefatigable and obsessive insistence on accuracy and the efficient system she set up for insuring it.

PART I

The Instruments, Their History, Use and Effects

CHAPTER I

History of Mechanical Devices and Instruments for Suturing

IT WAS NOT UNTIL LATE in the nineteenth century, as will be shown in greater detail in Chapter III, that surgeons began to be confident of their ability to close wounds in the bowel and to perform intestinal anastomoses. From the earliest days of abdominal surgery, mechanical devices of varied kinds have been used as aids to intestinal suture. We here consider essentially only those instruments that, in fact, united intestinal wound edges. We have omitted consideration of the large variety of cylindrical templates, which served only as aids to suturing, although experimentation in this area continues up to the present (Hopcroft, 1968, 1972).

Felix-Nicholas Denans, at the February 24, 1826, meeting of the Société Royale de Médecine de Marseilles (Denans, 1827, 1837–38), demonstrated a dog on whom he had, ten days before, performed an end-to-end ileoileostomy with an ingenious apparatus. A second dog, operated on by the same method sometime earlier, was found at sacrifice to have a perfectly healed end-to-end anastomosis. Denans' apparatus was designed to combine the advantages of approximating the serous surfaces of the recurved, inverted ends of divided bowel, with stenting of the anastomosis by a hollow metal cylinder; he had devices both of pewter and of silver. The technique consisted of placing into the lumen of each bowel end a short cylinder, over the outer end of which the bowel end could be inverted. The inverted bowel ends then were pushed over the stenting, third hollow metal cylinder and brought into tight contact. Necrosis of the inverted bowel ends was produced by compression by the inner cylinder against the two ferrules. Initially, the two rings or ferrules were held together by a complicated suture (Fig I–1*A,B*). A later model provided a third, longer inner cylinder with a longitudinal split and overlapping margins, so that, on insertion, the cylinder could be compressed with a special forceps (Fig I–1*C*). After satisfactory placement of this cylinder into the ferrules carrying the inverted bowel ends, and tight approximation of the bowel over the spring-like inner cylinder, the latter was released and provided the necessary compression of the bowel ends.The serosal surfaces of the inverted bowel ends becoming adherent to each other, the inverted margins sloughed and the cylinders were released and passed in the stool. Denans noted in his first experiment that the ferrules were eliminated with the bowel movement on the seventeenth postoperative day. The dog had been eating a regular diet and had shown no signs of obstruction. The second dog was offered a small bone in a piece of bread and passed the ferrules at the end of eight days. Denans did not provide drawings of the device in his publications, but he did send a sample of his instruments to the Royal Academy of Medicine of Paris for its May 15, 1836 session (Denans, 1837–38; Amat, 1895). Illustrations of the various models, as well as of the techniques of their use were provided by Samuel D. Gross (1843), A. Nélaton (1857), Charles-Emmanuel Sédillot (1865–66), Gustave Gaujot and Emile Spillmann (1867–72), and R. von Frey (1895).

Professor Lallemand (1826) of Montpellier was present at the February 24, 1826 meeting of the Société de Médecine de Marseilles and was asked to give his opinion about Denans' original device. He stated that the instrument was acceptable in patients with recent traumatic wounds of the bowel, but that its use in cases with intestinal gangrene, due to strangulated hernia, seemed dangerous to him.

After Denans had presented his work, a committee was named to examine the dog that had evacuated stent and ferrules on the twelfth day. Gillet, the committee chairman, reported (March 25, 1826) that they had found minor adhesions of the bowel to the abdominal wall and the greater omentum. The circular anastomotic scar was quite solid and healing had occurred serosa-to-serosa. Later on, Denans abandoned the suture to hold the rings together and replaced the cylindrical stent with a spring-like stent. It was this second model that was sent by him to Paris in 1836 and that Sédillot illustrated in his textbook, giving no indications as to experimental or clinical use (Fig I–1C).

Charles Phillips of Liège (1834–35), while describing an apparatus developed by J.Z. Amussat, in which a ferrule of elder wood was used, mentioned the fact that Denans had further modified the inner ferrule through ''a circular row of springs similar to those used as clasps for ladies' bracelets.'' This made it easier to insert the inner ferrule and expand it against the proximal and distal ferrules, compressing the inverted bowel ends.

Jean Marc Bourgery, Claude Bernard, and N.H. Jacob (1866–71), in their extensive work on surgical anatomy and operative technique, mention the fact that P. Guersent had successfully used the Denans apparatus ''sur le vivant,'' i.e., a human. They suggested substituting hardened gelatin for Denans' metal ferrules. Jean Baptiste Lucien Baudens (Baudens, 1836; Nélaton, 1857) proposed that two matched cylinders be made, one of rubber and the other of metal. One bowel end was inverted over the rubber ring in the same fashion as in Denans' procedure, while the metal ring was placed inside the opposite bowel lumen without invagination of the bowel edges. The end containing the metal ring then was inserted into the end containing the elastic rubber ring, which held and compressed the inserted segment, without need for the third, stenting ferrule.

Antoine Lembert (1826) had emphasized the importance of inversion of the bowel and serosa-to-serosa approximation in anastomoses performed with needle and suture—silk or catgut. He referred in the course of his paper to the little book published by Benjamin Travers (1812), surely Astley Cooper's most distinguished disciple. Like almost everyone else who has quoted Travers, Lembert missed or ignored Travers' point that if the sutures were placed properly, everting anastomoses of bowel would heal. Lembert's insistence on serosa-to-serosa apposition of the bowel has been one of the unchallenged verities of intestinal anastomosis until fairly recently.

Also in 1826, and without, at least, any references to the publications of Travers, Lembert, or Denans, J.H.F. Henroz in Liège (1826) presented in his doctoral thesis the use of articulated rings containing alternating pins and holes. The rings were placed outside the bowel and a flange of either end everted. The opposing pins and holes were matched, the two rings snapped together, and an end-to-end anastomosis thus was completed (Fig I–2), the rings remaining permanently in place. This everting anastomosis succeeded in Henroz' animal experiments.

A.P.A. Pimenta of Oporto has described an ingenious stapling instrument for end-to-end bowel anastomoses (1980, 1981, 1981, 1982). In its simplest analysis, it is a sophisticated application of stapling (Fig I–3) to the principle evolved in 1826 by Henroz (see Fig I–2). The mechanism for driving in the staples is that of the suspended staple-driving-fin housing forced down by heavy pliers as used by Nakayama (see Fig I–15A) for his gastric stapler. There is no evidence that Pimenta knew of the devices of Henroz and Nakayama. He reported successful laboratory and clinical experience in esophago-gastric and colorectal anastomoses.

INTRALUMINAL DEVICES FOR COMPRESSION CLOSURE OF LINEAR BOWEL LACERATIONS—INVERTING

J. Bobrick of Berlin (Bobrick, 1850; von Frey, 1895) recommended the use of gutter-shaped sections of lead or silver, placed inside the bowel for closure of longitudinal wounds (Fig I–4A). The edges of the wound were invaginated into the gutter and the borders of the gutter were compressed from without. The wound edges then would heal on the outside and necrose on the inside of the lumen, with elimination of the lead or silver gutter through the intestinal tract. This procedure was used only experimentally.

A return to the concept of Bobrick was presented much later by the suggestion of J.L. Faure and Suarez (1895; Faure, 1895) for the use of clips in the management of longitudinal intestinal wounds (Fig I–4B). Except for the use of this technique in one dog, the method never gained any acceptance at a time (1895) when more sophisticated manual and mechanical suture methods already were available.

Jules Emile Péan (1869, 1869) presented yet another somewhat complicated method for the closure of longitudinal wounds. He used "serre fines," fine clips with a spring (Fig I–4C), held open and placed inside the bowel with a special slender, rod-like applicator. As the applicator—passed through a separate stab wound—released the clips, these caught the entire thickness of the inverted bowel edges from within the bowel lumen. The spring mechanism securely held the individual clips. This method never achieved any practical value.

NEEDLE-ARMED ANASTOMOSING BLOCKS AND CYLINDERS—INVERTING

Laurent Jean Baptiste Béranger-Féraud, Chief Physician to the French Navy and physician to His Highness Prince Napoléon, described (Béranger-Féraud, 1869, 1869, 1870) the use of two delicate blocks of cork 6 mm in thickness to secure an inverting closure of longitudinal bowel wounds (Fig I–5A). Fine needles driven through the width of the plates produced the appearance of two little combs. The cork plates were inserted in the bowel, on either side of the inverted bowel edges, and pressed against each other, driving the needles through the thickness of the two inverted lips and into the opposed cork plates. As the wound margins compressed between the plates sloughed, and the bowel healed external to this, the plates came loose and were eliminated with the feces. The account does not discuss experimental or clinical applications. Bonnier (Amat, 1895), working at the Val-de-Grâce Military Hospital in 1869, used the same principle for end-to-end inverting anastomoses over cylinders of cork mounted on metal rings (Fig I–5B). Fine hooked pins in the cylinder ends locked into the cork of the opposing cylinders fixing the inverted bowel.

For longitudinal wounds, Bonnier used rods made of boxwood or ebony, covered with cork and carrying the same hooked pins. Bonnier used his device only on cadaver intestines. Charles Amat used the Bonnier instrument with success in dog experiments. Bonnier entered the "Administrative Career" early in his life and, according to Amat, published his work in a small brochure, in 1885, at a time when he was "Préfet de l'Aveyron" (Amat, 1895). (The préfet, in the Provinces, represents the central Paris government, a function in the process of being modified by the present government of Mr. Francois Mittérand.)

INTERNAL, ABSORBABLE, SUTURED RINGS AND BUTTONS

We have not considered the tubular stents, made of various materials, that were used merely to facilitate intestinal suturing. However, the decalcified bone plates of Senn (1889) and the catgut rings of Abbe (1889, 1889) fall more genuinely in the class of anastomotic devices.

Senn's bone plates, decalcified in hydrochloric acid, were thin, wafer-like disks (Fig I–6*A*) with a central opening to maintain patency and four perforations to which sutures were affixed. For side-to-side anastomosis, a plate was slipped into each of the loops to be anastomosed and the sutures on both sides brought through the bowel wall and tied together, providing firm coaptation. Four Lembert sutures reinforced the anastomosis.

In the so-frequent way of independent and simultaneous explorations in widely separated laboratories, Rudolph Matas and Paul Michinard had been working in New Orleans on catgut rings and were at the point of publication when Abbe's article appeared (Cohn, 1960). Abbe (1889) of New York, finding the bone rings difficult to obtain on demand, devised rings of heavy catgut (Fig I–6*B*), which could be fashioned at the operating table and used in the same way. "On endeavoring to obtain larger plates from Dr. Senn's instrument-maker, I found it took many days to prepare them, and that the largest scarcely made more of an opening than the smallest, while the disposition to warp and not coaptate so well seems to increase as the plate is made larger. It occurred to me that a ring might be composed of the heaviest catgut, quite as absorbable and as firm as the softened bone. It can be made in a few minutes of any desired size, as shown in the cut, and thus are obviated the serious delays of sending to cities or special instrument-makers for the bone plate."

The techniques of Senn and of Abbe had a brief vogue in the United States and abroad, but were shortly replaced by the Murphy button.

Willy Sachs, Assistant in the Surgical Clinic of Bern—which is to say, Kocher's clinic—made a decalcified bone button that he used experimentally in rabbits (Fig I–6*C*). He placed only a few interrupted sutures. The rabbits lived up to 14 days. Two died of ileus because the buttons were so large. He proposed modifications in size and shape for gastroenterostomy and cholecystenterostomy.

In the April 16, 1892 issue of *The Lancet* appeared a paper by H. Littlewood, F.R.C.S., Hon. Assistant Surgeon to the General Infirmary at Leeds. Operating on a patient with complete obstruction by a tumor in the hepatic flexure (Moynihan, the resident surgical officer, was his assistant), Littlewood successfully utilized Senn's decalcified bone plates. Mr. Mayo Robson was in the operating room. Littlewood was able to say that, at that time, only four successful cases had been operated on in this manner, two of them by Senn. Littlewood was encouraged to have made for him a decalcified bone tube to fit into the two plates, obviating the need for the sutures in Senn's plates, in essence producing a three-piece, absorbable Murphy button! (Fig I–6*D*.) It is of more than passing interest that Littlewood concluded by saying, "In a very interesting paper by Dr. Halsted of Baltimore a method of lateral apposition by sutures is described. He insists very strongly on the importance of including some of the submucous layer of the intestinal wall in these and all suturing operations of the intestine. I am sure it is very important to recognise this observation, but cannot help thinking the bone plates will have the advantage over any method of suturing, owing to their simplicity and the time saved in using them."

In the April, 1893 *British Medical Journal,* Mayo Robson, like Sachs, expressed admiration for Senn: "The principle of lateral anastomosis by means of decalcified bone plates, invented by Dr. Senn, is now recognised as a most valuable surgical procedure, both in intestinal and in stomach surgery. The following method of employing a decalcified bone tube, shaped like a cotton bobbin, is brought forward as another means of accomplishing the anastomosis" (Fig I–6*E*). He reported its successful use in two cases. He did not mention the paper by Sachs and made no mention of Littlewood, who clearly had had the idea. It is of interest that Mayo Robson was present at Littlewood's operation in March, 1891 and might well have heard Littlewood speculate on having a bone button made. Mayo Robson's button was not decalcified. Murphy's dog experiments were begun in June, 1892. Mayo Robson's paper was delivered before the British Medical Association in July, 1892. The dates of his operations are not given.

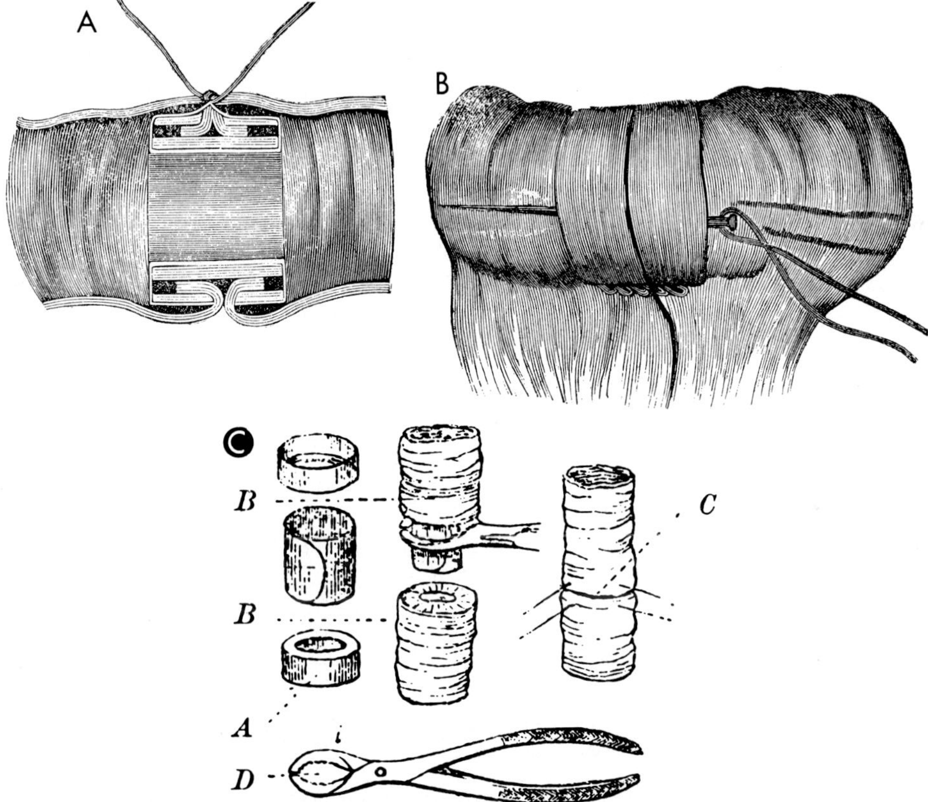

Fig I–1.—Denans' Cylindrical Stent-and-Ferrules Technique, 1827. The bowel ends were inverted over the two shorter ferrules. The cylinder, slightly smaller in diameter, was inserted into the two ends and the serosal surfaces of the recurved bowel ends abutted against each other. The cylinder compressed the inverted flanges until they necrosed and separated, allowing the apparatus to be passed. Denans seems not to have left any illustration of his device, which underwent several modifications. **A, B,** Samuel D. Gross (1843), in the book on the technique of intestinal suture, on which he set so much store, showed, in this illustration, methods of passing the suture to hold the Denans rings in place. **C,** illustration from Sédillot, 1865, of the second Denans model presented, with a letter from Denans, to the Paris Royal Academy of Medicine at its May 15, 1836 meeting. The principal modification is that the cylindrical stent actually is a rolled sheet of metal. The diameter is decreased by the forceps, the cylinder is inserted in the two ends and allowed to expand, holding the assembled apparatus and compressing the bowel ends. Widely spaced interrupted sutures tacking the bowel ends together complete the procedure.

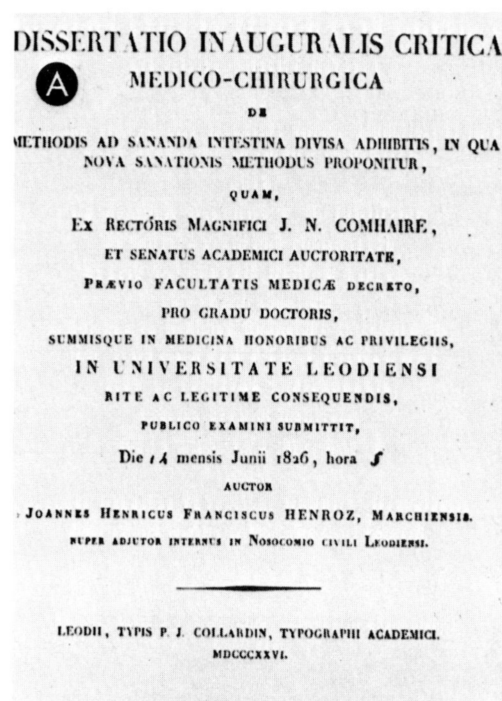

DISSERTATIO INAUGURALIS CRITICA

A MEDICO-CHIRURGICA

DE

METHODIS AD SANANDA INTESTINA DIVISA ADHIBITIS, IN QUA NOVA SANATIONIS METHODUS PROPONITUR,

QUAM,

EX RECTÓRIS MAGNIFICI J. N. COMHAIRE,

ET SENATUS ACADEMICI AUCTORITATE,

PRÆVIO FACULTATIS MEDICÆ DECRETO,

PRO GRADU DOCTORIS,

SUMMISQUE IN MEDICINA HONORIBUS AC PRIVILEGIIS,

IN UNIVERSITATE LEODIENSI

RITE AC LEGITIME CONSEQUENDIS,

PUBLICO EXAMINI SUBMITTIT,

Die 14 mensis Junii 1826, hora 5

AUCTOR

JOANNES HENRICUS FRANCISCUS HENROZ, MARCHIENSIS.

NUPER ADJUTOR INTERNUS IN NOSOCOMIO CIVILI LEODIENSI.

LEODII, TYPIS P. J. COLLARDIN, TYPOGRAPHI ACADEMICI.
MDCCCXXVI.

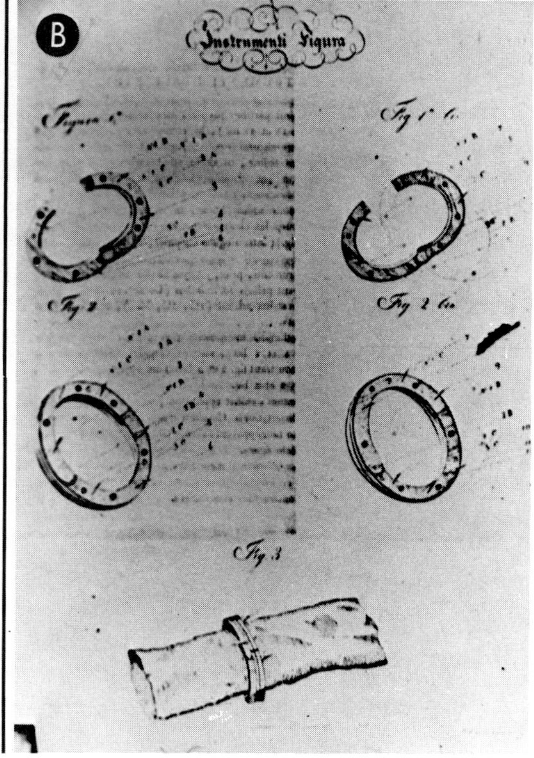

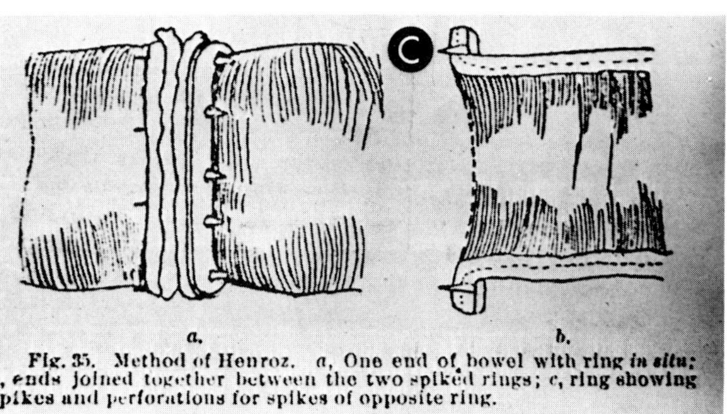

Fig. 35. Method of Henroz. a, One end of bowel with ring in situ; b, ends joined together between the two spiked rings; c, ring showing spikes and perforations for spikes of opposite ring.

Fig I–2.—Everting end-to-end anastomosis of Henroz, 1826. **A,** title page of his doctoral dissertation at Liège (1826). **B,** Henroz' illustration showing the two articulated metal rings of alternating pins and holes. The rings were slipped over the divided bowel, which was everted on the pins and the two halves then snapped together, producing a rapid, everting, circular anastomosis. The rings were left in place. Henroz reported several successes in dogs (see Fig I–3 for a modern update of this principle). **C,** Nicholas Senn (1893) provided illustrations of Henroz' technique but, airily ignoring the fact that Henroz had, in fact, reported that his method had succeeded, said, ". . . union was effected with the mucous membrane turned outward, consequently it must have proved a failure even in experiments on the lower animals."

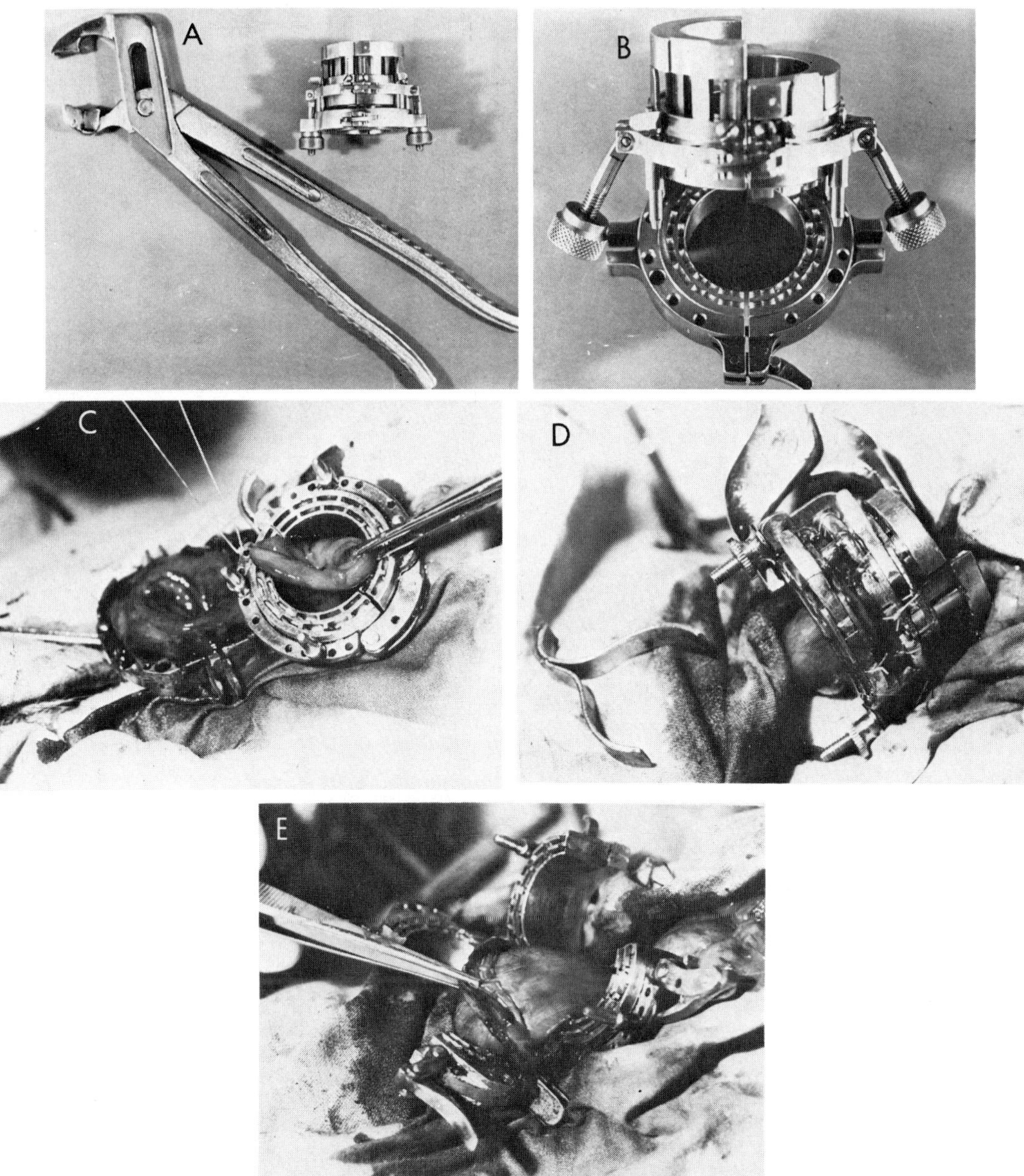

Fig I–3.—Pimenta's stapler for everting end-to-end bowel anastomoses, 1980. **A,** the two articulated rings hinge on each other. The upper contains two staggered rows of hand-loaded staples and the lower contains the anvil recesses. **B.** In the half of the cartridge on the left can be seen the slender staple drivers. A pins-and-holes arrangement matches the two halves accurately. At either side is the locking mechanism. **C,** the bowel ends are pulled through the rings, everted, and sutured to the holes in the outer ring. **D,** the two rings have been matched and the approximating screws tightened. Comparison with **B** shows how far the staple drivers have been pushed down by the compression forceps. **E,** the finished everting anastomosis. The rings are opened and removed. The everting anastomosis, aided by articulated rings is, of course, a throwback to Henroz more than 150 years earlier (Fig I–2) and the use of massive clamps to press down half of the staple-driving fins at a time was described by Nakayama some 30 years earlier (Fig I–15A). Pimenta reports 12 animal anastomoses—esophagogastric, small bowel, and large bowel, with a single death, from pneumonia (Pimenta, 1981) and seven patients—three esophagogastrectomies and four colocolostomies with no complications. The anastomoses required 15 minutes (Pimenta, Cardosa, and Rodrigues, 1980). (From A.P.A. Pimenta, V. Cardosa, J.S. Rodrigues, *Ann. Chir.,* 1981, used by permission.)

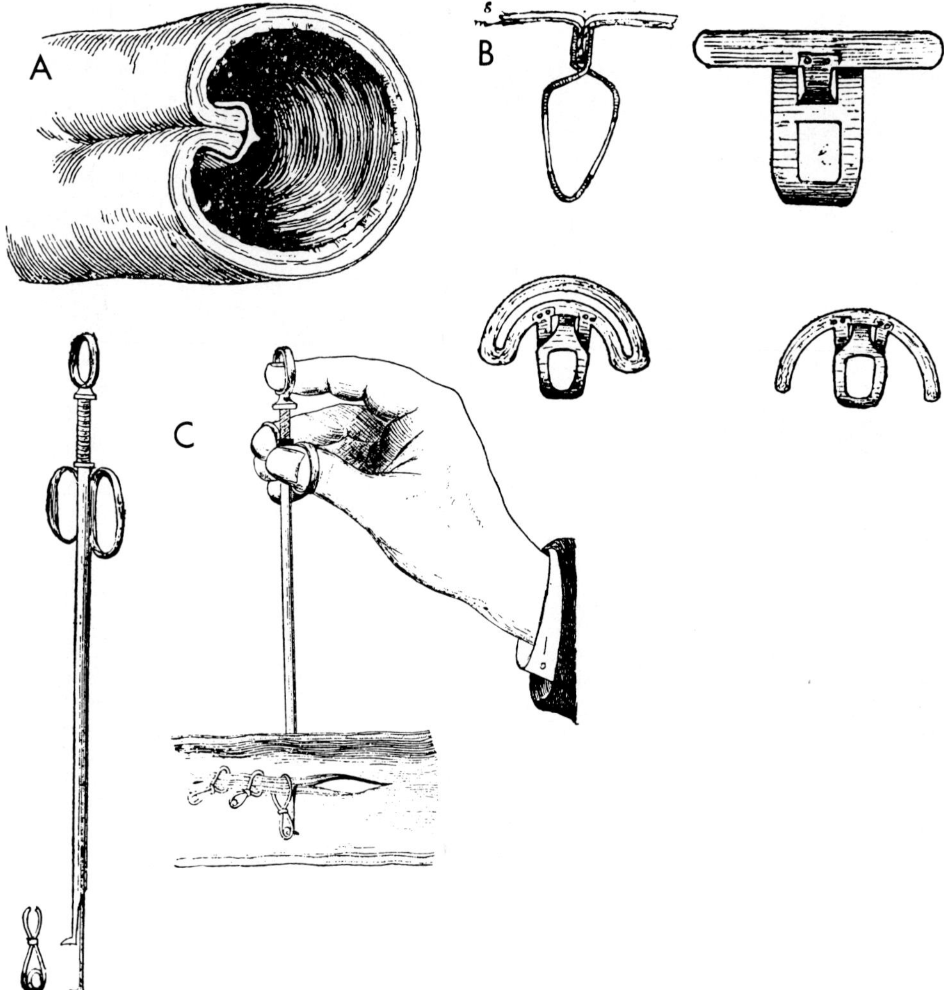

Fig I–4.—Intraluminal devices for compression closure of linear bowel lacerations. **A,** Bobrick's internal clip for closing longitudinal intestinal wounds, 1850. As is so often the case, the original publication contained no illustration, and this illustration is reproduced from von Frey (1895). Bobrick of Berlin suggested the use of a gutter-shaped segment of lead or silver for the closure of longitudinal intestinal wounds. The edges of the wound were to be invaginated into the gutter placed intraluminally, and the borders of the malleable gutter compressed from without. It was expected that the serosal surfaces would seal on the outside while the invaginated edges necrosed and permitted the discharge of the lead or silver device. Neither Bobrick nor von Frey mentioned clinical use of the technique. **B,** method of J.L. Faure and Suarez, 1895. Curved or straight clips were placed inside the bowel lumen while the edges of the linear opening in the bowel were invaginated between the arms of the clips, held open by pressure through the bowel wall. Release of the spring permitted closure of the clip and eventual necrosis of the bowel and passage of the clip. They reported experience with a single dog, abandoned their attempts, and, according to Terrier, returned to sutured anastomoses. (From J.L. Faure and Suarez, 1895.) **C,** individual internal clips of Péan, 1869. Péan's fine spring clips, which he called "serre-fines," were placed with a special slender applicator inserted through a separate stab wound, the clips seizing the inverted wound edges to produce an inverted closure of the original laceration, as seen in drawing on the right. The stab wound for insertion of the applicator then was closed manually. Péan made no mention of actual use of the instruments and subsequent comments like that of Gaujot, "The delicate nature of the technique required must preclude its popular acceptance," suggest that it had little success. (From J.E. Péan, 1869.)

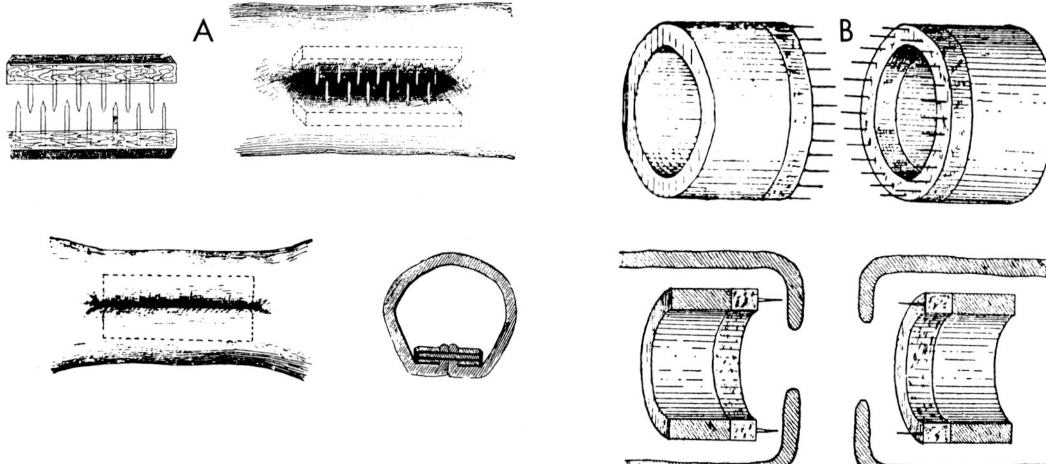

Fig I–5.—Needle-armed anastomosing blocks and cylinders—inverting. **A,** the internal, cork-block, and needle technique of Béranger-Féraud, 1869. For the closure of longitudinal wounds, appropriately sized blocks of cork were fitted with ordinary needles, placed through the width of the cork plates so as to form two little combs. The combs were placed inside the bowel through the wound that was to be closed, the bowel edges pulled over the protruding needle points and the cork plates approximated, the needles penetrating both thicknesses of the bowel wound into the opposite cork plate. As in the case of Bobrick's lead or silver gutter, it was expected that the compression would be firm enough to produce necrosis of the inverted bowel edges and passage of the cork-needle ensemble. No suggestion is made that either animal or clinical experience preceded the publication. (From L.J.B. Béranger-Féraud, 1869.) **B,** Bonnier's internally placed cork and needle stents for inverting end-to-end anastomoses, 1885. The technique is reminiscent of Henroz' articulated pins-and-holes device for everting anastomoses and of the Béranger-Féraud cork-and-pins technique for closing longitudinal wounds of the bowel. Bonnier, who did not picture his device, had tried the technique only on cadavers when he was at the military hospital of Val-de-Grâce. Charles Amat (1895) reported success in end-to-end anastomoses in dogs with Bonnier's device. Bonnier is said to have published a "petite brochure" in 1885, but Terrier in 1898 could not find it and our efforts have been similarly unavailing. (From C. Amat, 1895.)

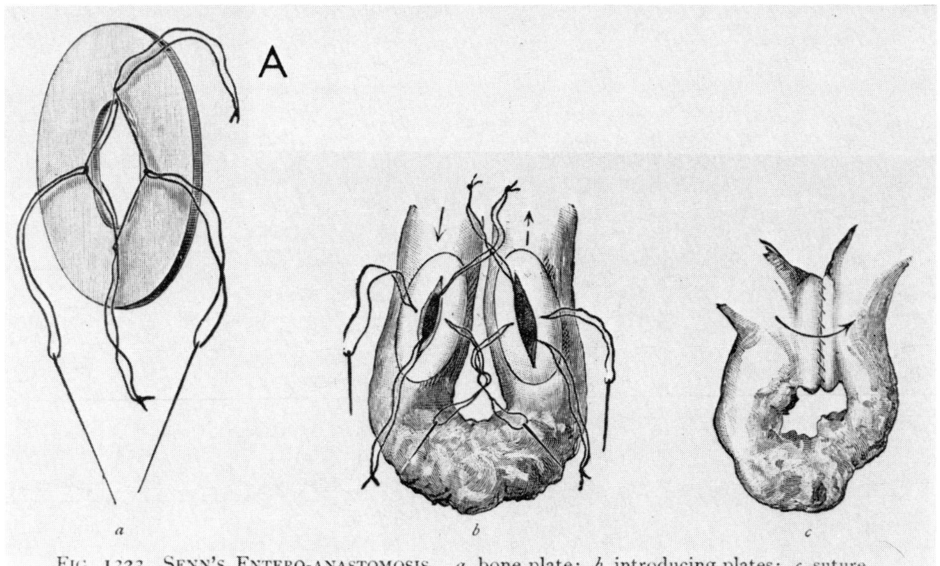

Fig. 1323. Senn's Entero-anastomosis. *a*, bone plate; *b*, introducing plates; *c*, suture
Bone plates fitting upon each other

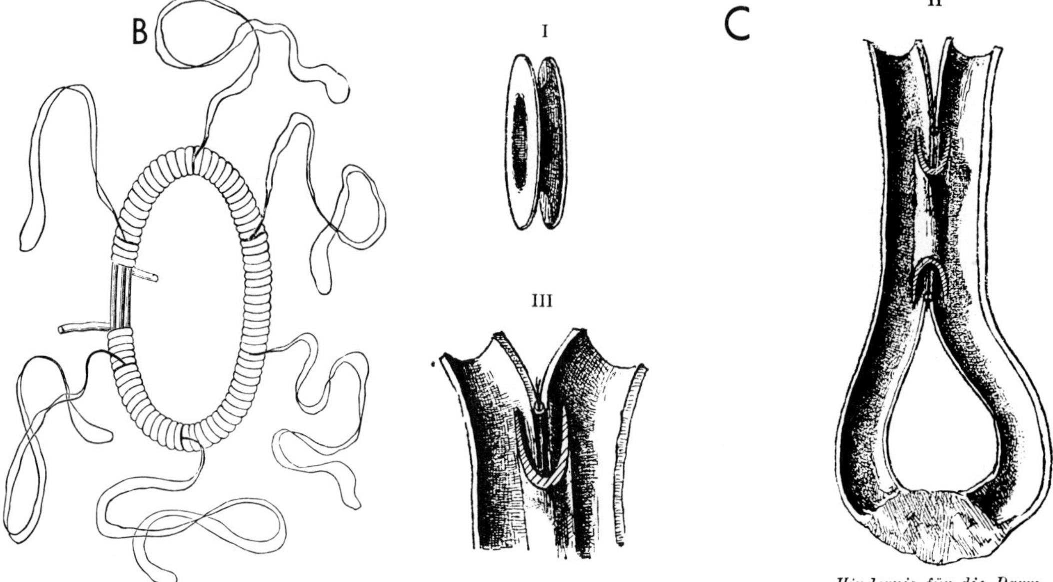

Die Verhältnisse sind nach einem Präparat, das vom Kaninchen gewonnen
wurde, dargestellt.
II zeigt den Knopf (längs geschnitten) in der definitiven Lage.
III soll nur die Lage der Serosanaht deutlicher machen. Die Rinne rings um
den Knopf ist zu breit gezeichnet im Verhältnis zur Darmwanddicke.

Fig I–6.—Internal, absorbable, suture rings and buttons. **A,** Senn's plates of decalcified bone, 1889. The thin plates of decalcified bone are slipped into incisions on either side of the lesion to be bypassed, the sutures in the ring brought through the bowel wall and tied, providing a firm approximation. The serosal surfaces around the anastomotic site are united by a few ordinary sutures. The plate disintegrates and is passed. The plates, manufactured commercially, were in wide use for a few years in America and abroad for entero-enterostomies and gastroenterostomies. (From Fr. von Esmarch and E. Kowalzig, 1901.) **B,** Abbe's catgut rings, 1889. (From R. Abbe, *New York Medical Journal,* 1889.) **C,** Sachs' decalcified bone button, 1890. (From W. Sachs, 1890.)

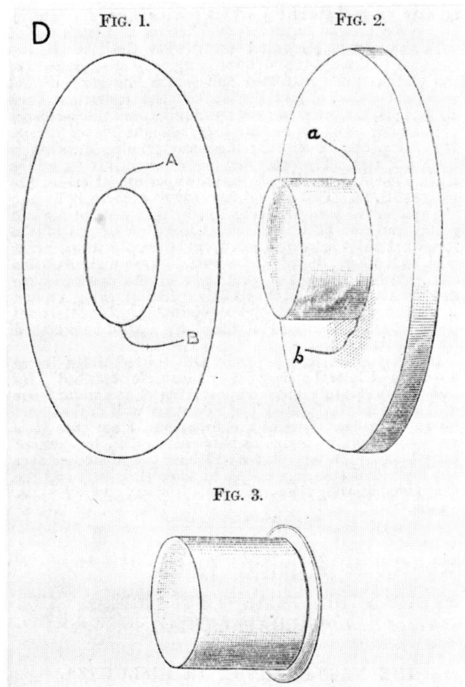

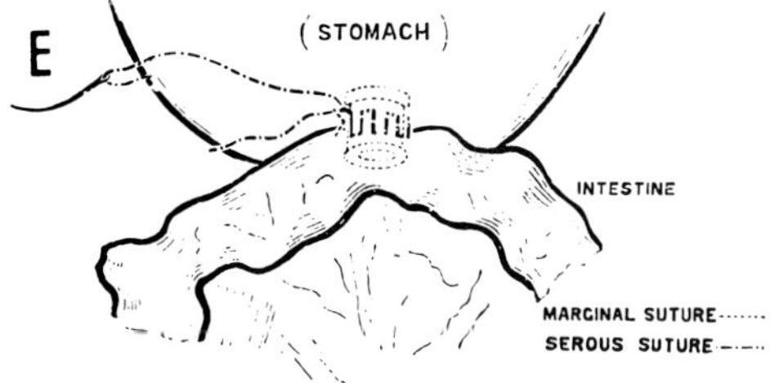

Fig. 4.—Showing the marginal suture tied and the anterior half circle of the serous suture completed.

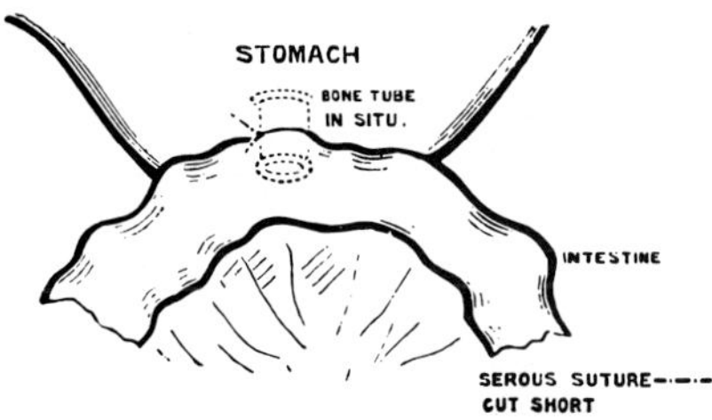

Fig. 5.—Showing the bone tube *in situ* and the serous suture completed, the ends being left long to show where the knot has been tied.

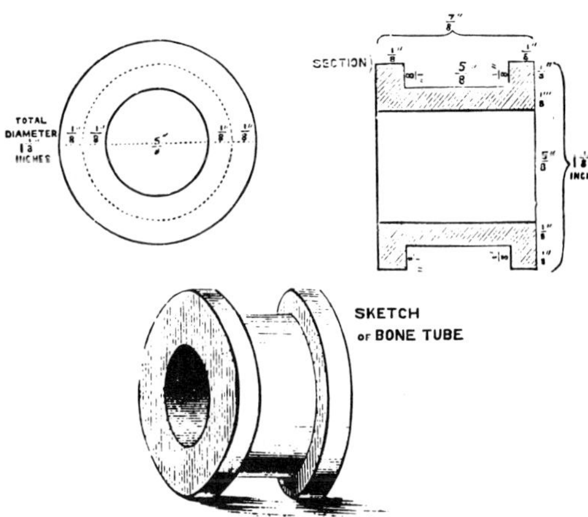

Fig. 6.—Diagram to show shape and measurements of tube.

Fig I–6 (cont.).—D, Littlewood's modification of Senn's bone plates, essentially a three-piece absorbable Murphy button! (From H. Littlewood, 1892.) **E,** Mayo Robson's bone bobbins, 1893. (From A.W. Mayo Robson, 1893.)

The contribution by John B. Murphy of Chicago, the Murphy button introduced in 1892, initially for the performance of cholecystoduodenal anastomoses (Murphy, 1892, 1893–94, 1894, 1894–95, 1894–95, 1895, 1895), was by all odds the single most useful implanted anastomotic device (Fig I–7), although Denans' and Bonnier's simple apparati had the priority of principle. Murphy made no historical references in his initial paper except with respect to cholecystoduodenostomy, commenting only that anastomoses by all previous methods often failed for a variety of reasons, which he listed disparagingly. Specifically, he did not refer to Senn, Sachs, and Littlewood, whose devices seem to present a continuum in the development of a button. Murphy's button came when Halsted (1887) already had demonstrated the safety of proper intestinal suture, but Murphy's button and its modifications were at once accepted the world over as the quickest and safest method of intestinal anastomosis. It was so referred to by the great surgeons of the day, and, although it began to fall into disuse after the turn of the century, continued to be used commonly for a decade or more thereafter. Thus, W.L. Rodman, in his 1900 Presidential Address before the American Surgical Association (Ravitch, 1981), discussing the technique of gastroenterostomy, "Where the element of shock is presumably to be an important one, gastro-enterostomy by one of the quicker methods—the Murphy button preferably—should be chosen."

Murphy's button consisted of two metal mushrooms with hollow stems that telescoped into each other, the mushroom cap of each end being secured in the bowel by a pursestring suture around the hollow stem. The stems were telescoped, compressing the mushroom caps together and, with them, the pursestringed bowel, the compression being augmented by an internal spring. The lumen of the bowel remained open by virtue of the channel through the caps and stems. Compression necrosis of the edges of bowel included between the two halves of the button allowed the button to be passed, by which time healing was secure. This button was widely used throughout the world and reports of its use came from the great surgical figures of the day. Advantages and disadvantages as well as complications were analyzed by Terrier (1894), Chaput (1893, 1894, 1895), Meyer (1894), Villard (1894, 1894), Zielewicz (1894), Marwedel (1895), Brentano (1896), Czerny (1896), and Terrier and Baudouin (1898).

Ⓐ Medical Record

A Weekly Journal of Medicine and Surgery

Vol. 42, No. 24.
Whole No. 1153.

NEW YORK, DECEMBER 10, 1892.

$5.00 Per Annum.
Single Copies, 10c.

Original Articles.

CHOLECYSTO - INTESTINAL, GASTRO - INTES-
TINAL, ENTERO-INTESTINAL ANASTOMO-
SIS, AND APPROXIMATION WITHOUT SUT-
URES. (ORIGINAL RESEARCH.)*

BY J. B. MURPHY, M.D.,

CHICAGO, ILL.,

PROFESSOR OF CLINICAL SURGERY, COLLEGE OF PHYSICIANS AND SURGEONS, CHICA-
GO; PROFESSOR OF SURGERY, POST-GRADUATE MEDICAL SCHOOL AND HOSPITAL;
ATTENDING SURGEON TO, AND PRESIDENT OF, THE MEDICAL STAFF OF COOK
COUNTY HOSPITAL; ATTENDING SURGEON TO ALEXIAN BROTHERS' HOSPITAL;
VICE-PRESIDENT OF NATIONAL ASSOCIATION OF RAILWAY SURGEONS, ETC.

MR. PRESIDENT AND GENTLEMEN : Intestinal surgery oc-
cupies a very advanced place in the category of great
surgical questions of the present day. Medical literature
teems with reports of successful cases operated on, and
not a few of the disasters are also placed on record. All
over the world investigators are trying to solve the many
perplexing problems that accident and disease of the gastro-intestinal tract present to them for consideration.
That this subject has had such exhaustive consideration
during the last decade, and that it is still a theme for
spirited controversy and discussion, carries with it the
implication that many vital points are yet unsettled and
need further investigation, experimental and clinical.
The results of experiments on lower animals have been
conducive to great improvement, both in principle and
technique of treatment of intestinal lesions in the human
subject. Fair results are obtained in the treatment of
bullet wounds of the intestines at present. At least an
effort is made by the surgeon to repair the injury.

The question above all others on which the profession
is divided is, " What are the best means and methods
of producing agglutination of surfaces and preventing
subsequent contraction at the point of adhesion ? " If
means can be devised—1, to hold the surfaces in contact ; 2, while in contact, to produce a speedy and permanent adhesion of the surfaces ; 3, to keep an opening
sufficiently large for the free passage of intestinal contents ; 4, to produce, as a result, a cicatrix that will not
contract to any great extent, and by the contraction produce complete or partial obstruction—we will have overcome the great barriers that still remain between us and
ideal success in intestinal surgery.

The marvellous ingenuity displayed in plans devised
for intestinal approximation and anastomosis is worthy of
the greatest success, and that success would have been
realized were it not that some of the following complications occurred : " The suture was imperfectly applied ;
the bowel sloughed through at line of suture ; the induced invagination increased after the operation until
complete obstruction was produced ; openings in the bone-
plates and disks were not in apposition ; the ends of the
bone-plates caused pressure, atrophy, and perforation ;
the catgut sutures were too rapidly absorbed ; lastly, and
with appalling frequency, prolonged operation produced
fatal shock," and many other well-known obstacles, not
necessary to mention here, intervened

To overcome these obstacles and thus lessen the risk
to the life of the patient, I have devised a mechanical
means to dispense with the need of sutures, the necessity
of invagination, the possibility of non-apposition, the

*Read before the Mississippi Valley Medical Association, October
15, 1892.

sloughing through of disks, the digestion of the catgut,
the almost insurmountable difficulties of technique of operation, the prolonged and fatal exposure of the abdominal contents, and the protracted anæsthesia. How much
I have accomplished by my labor I desire you to be the
judges, after I have demonstrated to you the results of
my experiments, and performed for you a gastro-enterostomy and an end-to-end approximation of intestine by
means of the device I here present to you, to be known
as the Anastomosis Button.

The buttons are made in three sizes. A button consists of two small circular bowls (Fig. 1); size No. 2
measures as follows : Diameter, 23 mm. ; depth, 8 mm.
There is "sweated" into a circular opening, 12 mm. in
diameter, at the bottom of one bowl, a cylinder 15 mm. in
length, with female screw thread on its entire inner surface.
The cylinder extends perpendicularly from bottom of
bowl. There is an opening in the male bowl in which is
"sweated" a similar and smaller cylinder of a size to
easily slip into the female cylinder. There are two brass
springs soldered on either side of the inner surface of the

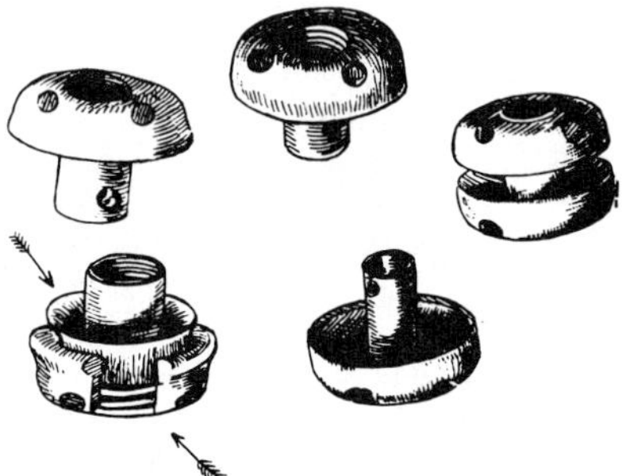

FIG. 1.—Appearance of Button with and without Spring-cup Attachment.

lower end of the male cylinder, which extend almost to
the top, where small points of them protrude through
openings in the cylinder ; these points are designed to
catch the screw-thread, when the male cylinder is pressed
into the female cylinder, and thus hold the bowls together at any point desired. To separate them again they
are simply unscrewed. A small brass ring, with a thin
though not cutting edge, to which is attached a wire spring,
is placed in the male bowl and retained in position, projecting one-eighth of an inch above the edge of the bowl.
This is held up by the wire spring, and is there for the
purpose of keeping up continuous pressure until the entire tissue between the edges of the bowls is cut off.
This spring attachment is absolutely necessary only when
the stomach is operated on. There are four openings, 5
mm. in diameter, in the side of each bowl, for the purpose of drainage. By this, it will be seen, we have two
hemispherical bodies held together by invaginating cylinders (Fig. 1). These hemispheres of the button are inserted in slits or ends of the viscera to be operated on.
A running thread is placed around the slit in the viscus, so that when it is tied it will draw the cut edges
within the clasp of the bowl. A similar running thread

Fig I–7.—The Murphy button. **A,** title page, Murphy's presentation, October 15, 1892 before the
Mississippi Valley Medical Association. His figure shows his buttons, which were essentially like two
mushrooms with hollow stems, the stems telescoping into one another, the through-and-through
opening permitting the passage of gas or feces. The necrosis of the bowel caught between the two
halves of the button allowed the button to be discharged and the lumen to be widely re-established.
Murphy's dog experiments on cholecystoenterostomy were performed in June, 1892, his gastroenterostomy experiments in July, 1892. (From J.B. Murphy, 1892.)

(continued)

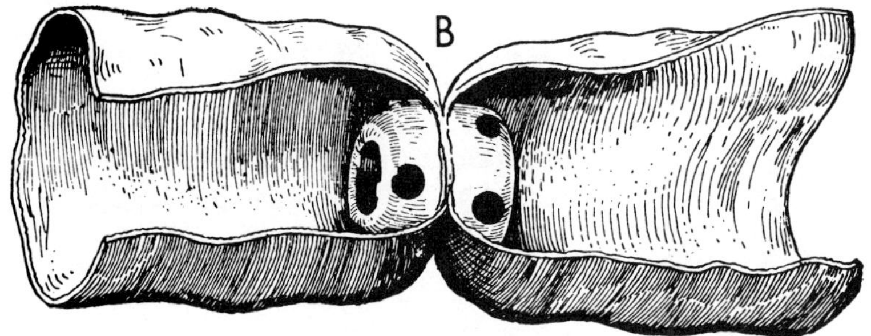

Section of end-to-end anastomosis by means of Murphy button.

cystostomy, an external biliary fistula which may of itself be a menace to life and require a second operation even more critical than the first, as is shown in the following reports of Courvoisier; also the difficulties and dangers of cholecystectomy.

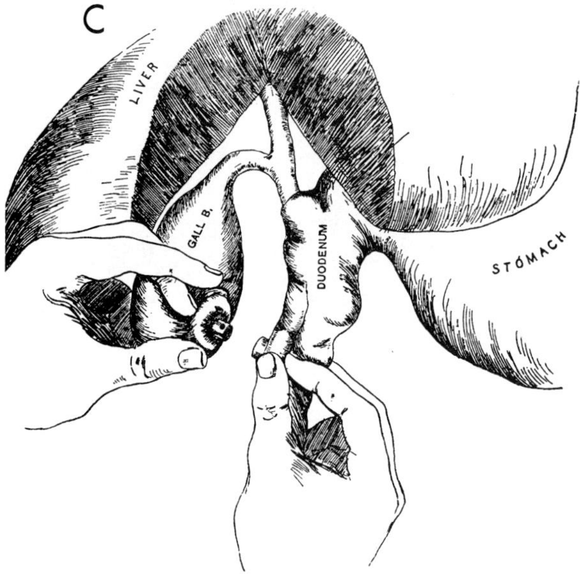

The effect of a permanent fistula of the gall bladder and constant escape of bile secreted, as frequently follows cholecystostomy, is different, depending, first, on the quantity of bile that escapes from the opening; and, second, what proportion is admitted into the intestinal tract. This fact has been lost sight of by many of the surgeons that have operated and had an external fistula remain and thus leads to the many differences of opinion on the gravity of biliary fistula. Where the fistula of the gall bladder only

Fig I–7 (cont.).—B, The cutaway section of the button in place shows the two bowel ends purse-stringed around the stems of the buttons and the buttons compressed against each other. The button was soon modified to have an internal ring that would be compressed upward by a coiled spring to make the production of necrosis of the bowel ends more certain. (From E. von Bergmann, P. von Bruns, J. von Mikulicz, et al., 1904.) **C,** Murphy's drawing of cholecystoduodenostomy with his button. He had begun performing this operation experimentally in dogs in June, 1892. This first clinical report is of three patients with jaundice and biliary lithiasis. All three survived cholecystoduodenostomy with the button. (From J.B. Murphy, 1892.)

Adalbert Ramaugé (1893, 1893), Professor of Surgery at the School of Medicine at Buenos Aires, described an elegant button of his own (Fig I–8*A,B*). In his original publication, he states that "on the tenth of December, 1892, Professor Murphy of Chicago issued his first publication on an anastomotic button of his own invention in the *Medical Record* of New York, and a few days after that, the twentieth of January, 1893, the last day for reception by the South American Medical Congress of work in its various sections, I presented an apparatus for synthesis of the lower intestine by the name of 'enteroplexo.' " Murphy had, in fact, presented his button to the Chicago Medical Society on the nineteenth of October, 1892. In his 1902 paper, Ramaugé says, ascribing to Denans the inspiration for mechanical anastomosing devices, "The seminal idea of Denans was our inspiration, and, by a curious coincidence the idea of a mechanical intestinal synthesis arose simultaneously in both Americas." He goes on to quote from the delightful comments of "el Profesor Jeannel" of France, who said, "I believe I know how to sew, yet I side with the 'boutonnistes.' The ranks of the 'suturistes' include only the prestidigitators of our profession. But I beg these skilled men to consider that they are the exception, that they cannot have a monopoly of intestinal surgery. . . . Is it to be denied that for the average surgeon it is easier to apply an anastomotic button, than to suture an anastomosis? And friends, when the suturists point to the failures of the buttons, have they forgotten their own failures? Who would dare to say that suturing has not had and will not have more victims than the buttons?"

In point of fact, the great surgeons of the day, for the most part, were "boutonnistes" and considered the button a great advance. To be sure, it permitted relatively unskilled surgeons to perform an anastomosis, and, given the transportation facilities of the day and the general level of surgical expertise, this was a great advantage, and in this country the Murphy button continued to be used well into the twentieth century.

Ramaugé's rings (see Fig I–8*A,B*) were flat and slender, leaving an extremely large lumen. The bowel ends were wrapped over these and the two rings joined by appropriate catches providing the compression required for healing.

Ramaugé (1902) presented a modification (Fig I–8*C*) of his apparatus in which each half was represented by an outer ring, connected to a smaller central ring by spiral arms. The outer or peripheral rings were armed with flexible spikes over which the bowel ends were invaginated and impaled. When the halves were approximated and held tightly by the central rings that were joined by the appropriate catches, the slender spikes collapsed, thus allowing for a safe end-to-end inverting "enteroplexie." Ramaugé used his button, produced by the firm of Collin in Paris, both experimentally and clinically. But even in his own country it never gained the recognition accorded the Murphy button.

Modifications of the Murphy button, or its technique of application, were presented in succeeding years by numerous surgeons. Among them in the United States were Benjamin Brabson Cates of Knoxville (1894), who used essentially a smaller Murphy button; Robert Fulton Weir of New York (1898), who reported the creation of a Murphy button for gastroenterostomy with little wings on the female portion placed in the jejunum (Fig I–8*D*), thus preventing the button from falling back into the stomach on completion of the anastomosis, a problem that had been troublesome; Jacob Frank of Chicago (1896, 1897, 1897), who presented a greatly simplified method, an internal elastic rubber tube, to keep the two mushrooms—made of decalcified bone—compressed together (Fig I–8*E,F*).

The principle of elastic compression was also adopted by R. Martin Gil of Malaga (1897, 1897), who used two saucer-shaped buttons of chemically softened ivory held together by elastic bands. The bowel ends were maintained in position by inverting pursestring sutures (Fig I–8*G*). The instrument was used for ileocolostomy and gastroenterostomy in dogs.

In France, Etienne Destot of Lyon (1894), like Ramaugé, eliminated the need for pursestring sutures by the use of alternating spikes and tubes over which the bowel ends were inverted, thus creating a combination of the Murphy and Bonnier instruments (Fig I–8*H*); Eugène Villard of Lyon (1895), to engage the two halves, provided a groove in the female half, into which the spring-like tongues of the male half were engaged (Fig I–8*I*); Jaboulay, A. Poncet, and E. Villard are reported to have used this instrument for gastroenterostomy, with two deaths and two successes; the instrument maker R. Mathieu, in 1895 (Terrier and Baudouin, 1898), presented a model similar to the American one, except that the spring was attached to the female part of the instrument, which could be completely disassembled (Fig I–8*J*). Derocque of Rouen (1897, 1897) described the use of a button in which the male half had tooth-like serrations. Murphy had a forceps-like device that locked around the stem of his button to hold it while the button was being inserted into the bowel and the pursestring suture tied. Derocque's instrument is quite different. The two limbs of the instrument were inserted through the two ends of the divided bowel. When his ''bouton entérotome'' was closed, the cutting male half punched out the disk of bowel from the two thicknesses of intestine, and when the instrument was disengaged, the two locking rings maintained the apposition of the anastomosed limbs. The two open ends then were closed manually (Fig I–8*K*). Although Derocque described the construction of his apparatus (Fig I–8*L*) in great detail, clinical use of the instrument never was initiated because of the complexity of the instrument, the fact that it produced a side-to-side anastomosis and the bowel ends still had to be sutured manually. The possibility of a blind loop was not recognized at that time. One of us (MMR) was shown in November, 1981, the handmade prototype of a stapler newly patented by a surgeon, which operated on the principle of Derocque's apparatus.

In Germany, two instrument makers, H. Windler of Berlin (1912) and Dröll of Mannheim (the supplier of Vincenz Czerny in Heidelberg), in 1895, produced buttons based on the general principles of the American model (Czerny, 1896). Windler supplied a hollow tube that could be used to separate the two halves of his button.

At the XXV Congress of the German Society of Surgery, in 1896, Czerny said that manual anastomoses, silk or catgut, one-layer or two-layer, were time-consuming and difficult. Of Murphy's button he said, ''The Murphy button is still not the final solution of the problem of intestinal suture, but is a powerful step toward it, and deserves to be carefully investigated.'' He set his pupil, Marwedel to work using the Murphy button in animal experiments. Marwedel achieved excellent results with three anastomoses, a side-to-side enteroenterostomy, an end-to-end enteroenterostomy, and a gastroenterostomy. In the last, the button did not pass, but all anastomoses were smooth and firm and free from adhesions. Czerny reported 11 patients in whom he had used the button— with three deaths, two in patients with gangrenous strangulated hernias and one in whom there was found a perforation of the bowel near the button.

In Italy, Eugenio Garbarini of Milano (1896) created two modifications of the Murphy button, one for side-to-side and one for end-to-end anastomosis. In Garbarini's buttons, compression was achieved by a locking system of lugs and grooves. If the button was thought to be improperly assembled, it could be removed by turning the lugs of the male half to match longitudinal slots interrupting the grooves in the female half. Traction on both halves then permitted disassembly. C. Garampazzi, of the Ospedale Maggiore di Novara (1897), created a button that could break down into four component parts once the anastomosis was healed (Fig I–8*M*). Each half was made of aluminum, and the four articulating parts were held together by a circular catgut tie. As the catgut was resorbed, the button disassembled and was eliminated with the feces. His initial report documented successful animal use and two clinical cases. Achille Boari (1897, 1897) created buttons by mounting ivory cups on central cylinders of metal. As the ivory was resorbed, expulsion of the remaining cylinders was facilitated. In a second model, he used ivory for the entire button and in experiments on dogs, limiting the use to gastroenterostomy, the button (Fig I–8*N*) was completely digested in ten to 12 days.

In Romania, E. Juvara, of Bucharest (1896) devised a button with large perforations of both cups (Fig I–8*O*). The female half had circular grooves and the cylinder of the male half was divided into eight longitudinal bands with their ends bent outward to hold the button in place. The bowel was fixed over each half with a circular tie and not a pursestring suture. Thomas Jonnesco (1896, 1896) presented a modification of the technique of the Murphy button for gastroenterostomy. Special clamps were introduced, through separate stab wounds in the stomach and jejunum and out through the purse-stringed gastric and jejunal openings used for the anastomosis, to seize the two buttons. The button halves were matched with the instrument, then manually locked and the two stab wounds closed by suture (Fig I–8*P,Q,R*). That this rather clumsy technique was even entertained by a surgeon as experienced as Jonnesco suggests, as do some of the other techniques, that by Murphy's original technique, the maintenance of the button during placement of the pursestrings was not altogether free from difficulty. Jonnesco used this technique in 20 gastroenterostomies on the dog with excellent results and indicated that he had used it for gastroenterostomy in man. However, Terrier notes that this technique was not attractive to surgeons in view of its complexity and the need for two additional stab wounds.

Boerema of Amsterdam (1954) described his plastic apparatus, which, as he said, had the same principle as the Murphy button, composed of two locking plastic "half-eggs" for esophagojejunostomy after total gastrectomy (Fig I–8*S,T,U*). A string passed down the esophagus and fixed to the device allowed it to be retrieved in 12 days when the inverted esophageal and jejunal flanges had necrosed through. Although his text suggests considerable satisfactory experience, no numbers are given.

In 1970, he (Boerema, Klopper, and Holscher) applied the same instrument to the problem of esophageal varices, commenting that, "To obviate leakage the authors have employed their button-anastomosis technique," not commenting further on his gastrectomy experience. In patients with varices, the two plastic half-eggs, on a flexible rod, were placed in the esophagus through a gastrotomy and the esophagus strongly ligated on the rod between the two cups, which then were compressed by the introducing instrument. The plastic anastomosing button was withdrawn through the mouth after 12 days by a thread attached to it at the time of operation. Taking all comers for the procedure, there was no recurrent bleeding up to two years and eight months after operation in their 34 patients, but 12 died in the hospital within two months of operation. No statement is made as to any leaks or strictures. This is, of course, the technique that has since been successfully adapted to the PKS and EEA[TM] staplers.

Actually, Vosschulte of Giessen (1957) had reported use of this principle. Through a gastrotomy, he inserted into the esophagus a hollow, bullet-shaped, tripartite cylinder, the three sections being held by a catgut tie. The cylinder was secured in place by a tight circumferential ligature that was buried by a row of sutures. Clinical results were good.

The experiments of M.A. Verschuyl of Utrecht (1965) actually partake of the use of a device as a temporary prosthesis to facilitate the anastomosis, in his case sutureless, with methyl-2-cyano-acrylate. This category of device we have, in general, excluded from our discussion, but Verschuyl's temporary gelatin prosthesis is of interest in that it was designed as a Murphy button.

Prioton of Montpellier (1973) reported his experience since 1968, using actual Murphy buttons for control of esophageal varices with a ligature inverting the undivided esophagus between the halves of the button inserted from below through a gastrotomy. In 20 patients, 14 bleeding actively, he had eight deaths, none from bleeding. There was a single and fatal perforation, as a result of an attempt to pass a stomach tube. Three stenoses required dilatation and one required operation.

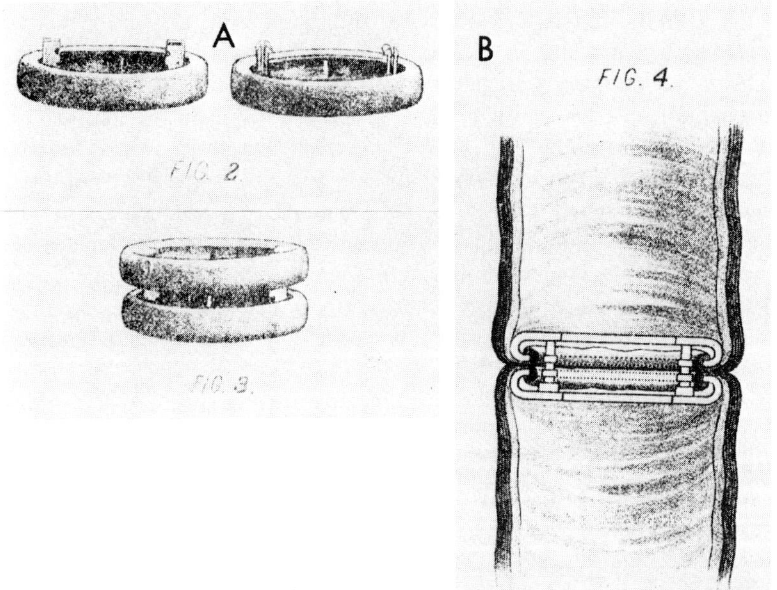

Fig I–8.—Modifications of the Murphy button. The ingenuity and the simplicity and the success of the Murphy button led to its wide use throughout the surgical world and the immediate development of multiple modifications. **A** and **B,** Adalbert Ramaugé of Argentina was at some pains to state that his work was independent of Murphy's despite the very close temporal association of his first work and of Murphy's. Ramaugé's first model consisted of slender, flat rings that engaged each other by catching devices that served also to hold the bowel ends inverted into the rings, obviating the need for pursestrings. The snap mechanism maintained the degree of compression required for ultimate necrosis of the inverted bowel wall and the slender construction of the rings permitted a large lumen in the interval. (From A. Ramaugé, 1893.)

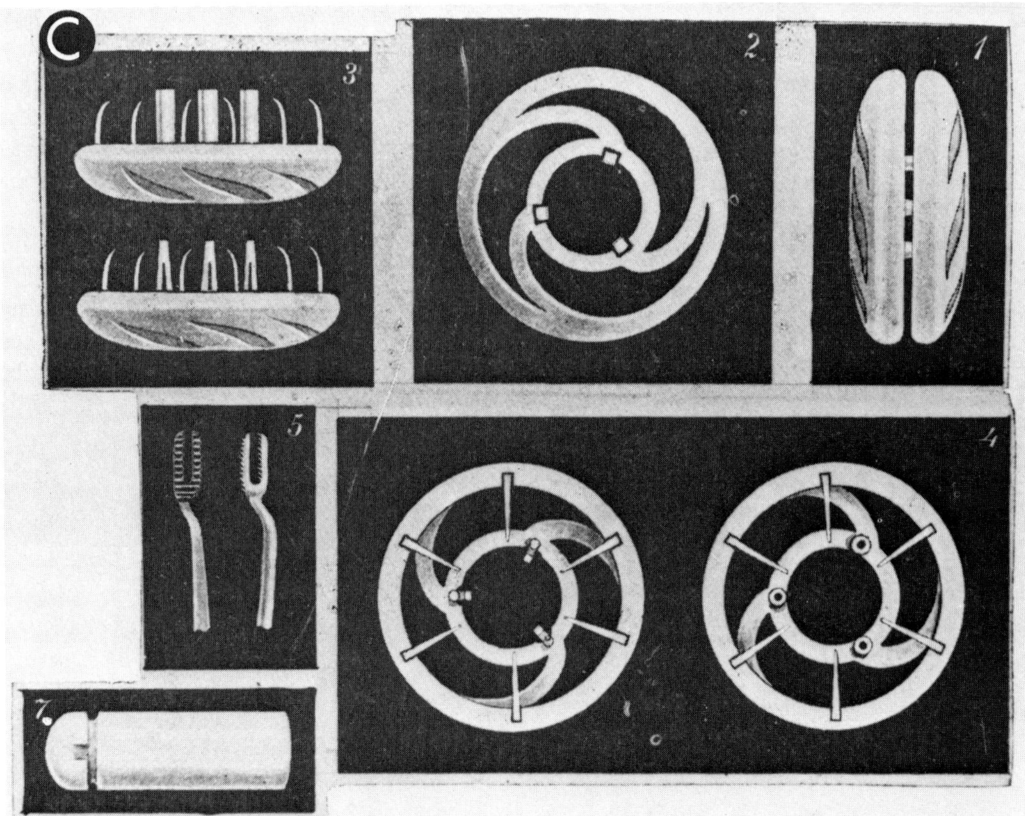

Fig I–8 (cont.).—C, later Ramaugé model. The pins on the outer rings serve to retain the inverted bowel and are fine enough to be compressed as the instrument is closed. (From A. Ramaugé, 1902.)

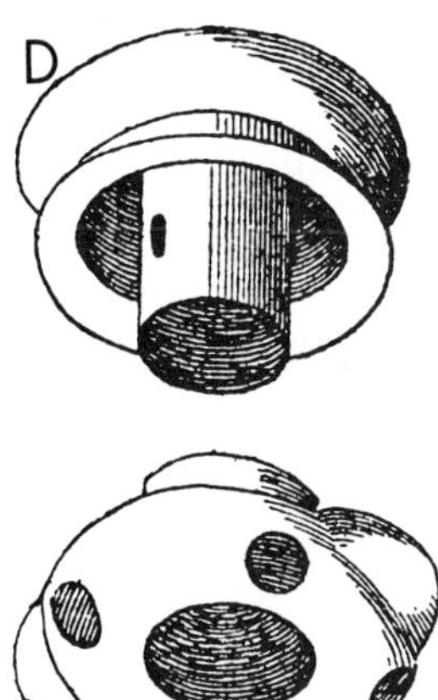

Fig I–8 (cont.).—D, modification of R.F. Weir of New York, 1898. Weir's gastroenterostomy button had wings for the female (jejunal) end to prevent the button from falling into the stomach after the flanges had necrosed away, a sometimes annoying problem with the Murphy button gastroenterostomy. (From R.F. Weir, 1898.)

(continued)

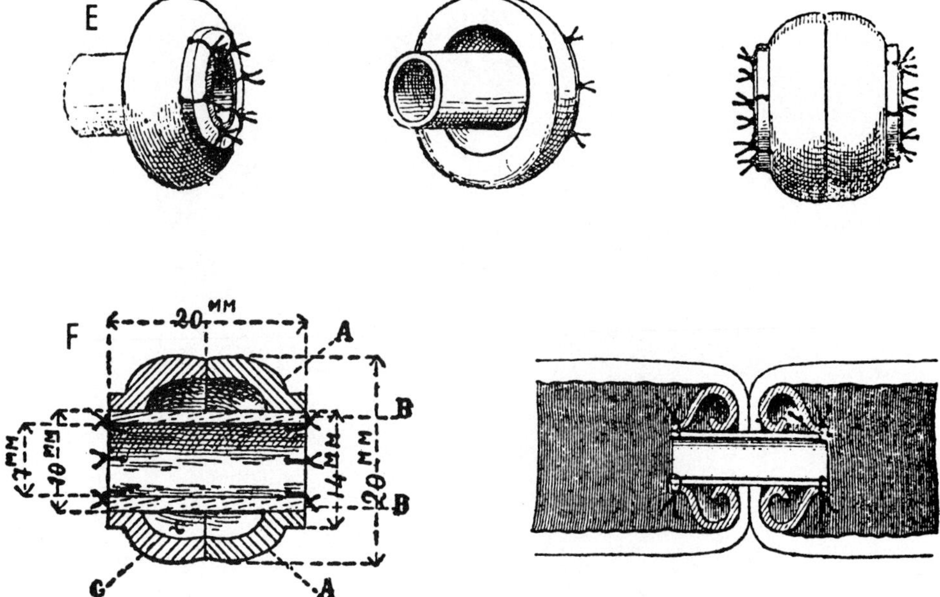

Fig I–8 (cont.).—**E** and **F,** composite bone and red rubber tubing button of J. Frank of Chicago (1897). Frank used his button on 20 animals, but still was waiting to use it on humans at the time of his publication. He had his buttons made by Schorse and Company of Milwaukee, Wisconsin. Apparently H. Windler of Berlin made the same instrument. (From J. Frank, 1897.)

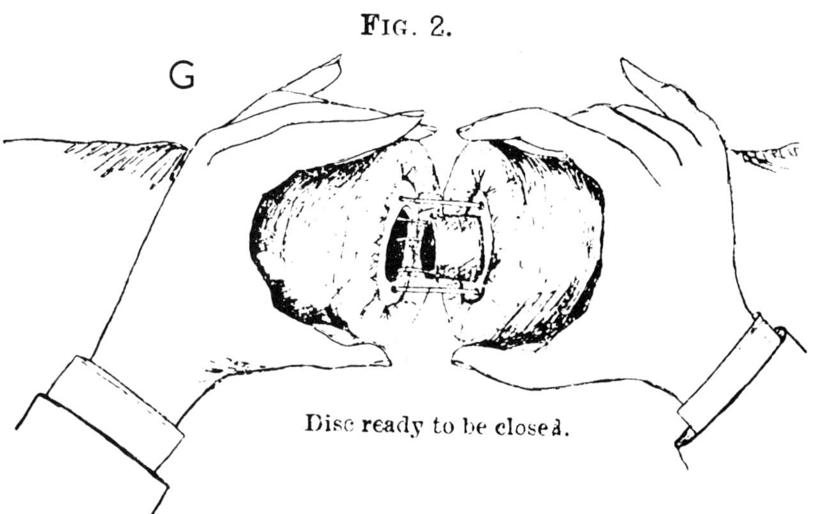

Fig I–8 (cont.).—**G,** technique of R. Martin Gil, 1897, of Malaga. Gil's saucer-shaped, acid-softened ivory buttons were held together with elastic bands (From R. Martin Gil, 1897.)

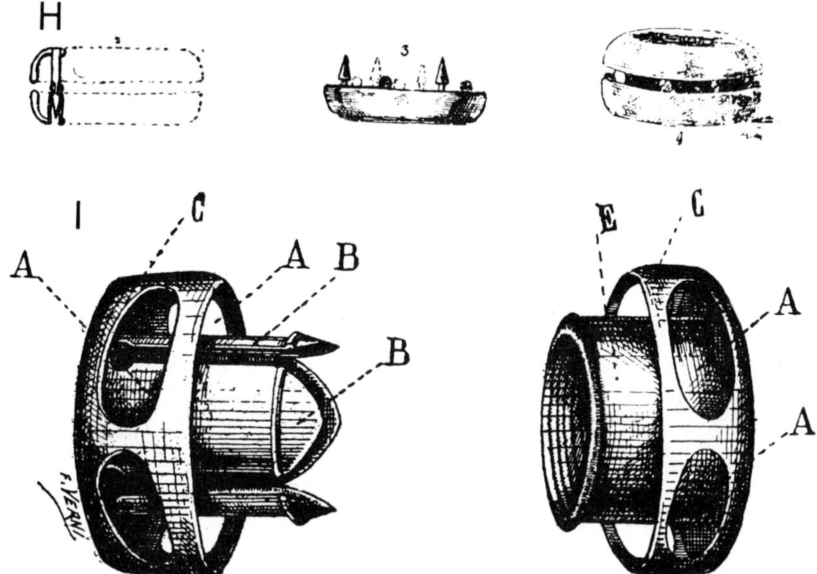

Fig. 1. — Bouton anastomotique modifie.

A. Fenêtres latérales.
B. Languettes ressorts de la pièce mâle.
C. Anneau périphérique.
E. Cylindre central de la pièce femelle.

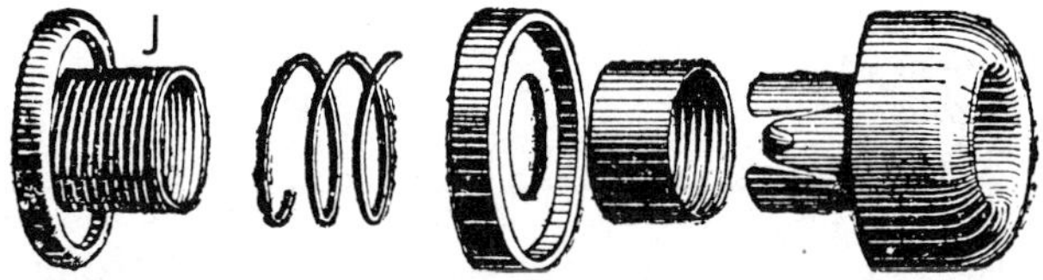

Fig I–8 (cont.).—H, Modification of E. Destot, 1894. (From E. Destot, 1894.) **I,** fenestrated button of E. Villard, 1895. (From E. Villard, 1895.) **J,** spring-loaded compression in button of R. Mathieu, 1895. (From F. Terrier and M. Baudouin, 1898.)

(continued)

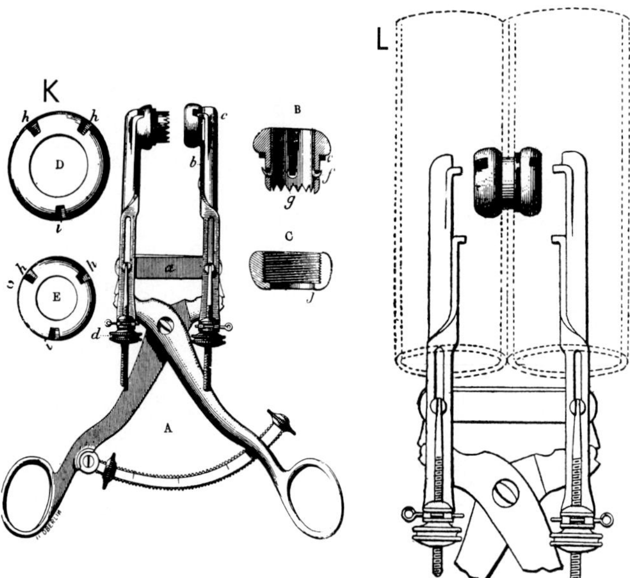

Fig I–8 (cont.).—**K** and **L,** side-to-side anastomotic device of P. Derocque of Rouen, 1897. The toothed button, clamped in place by the forceps, cut out a disc of the adjoining walls of the bowel. The open ends were closed by manual sutures. (From P. Derocque, 1897.)

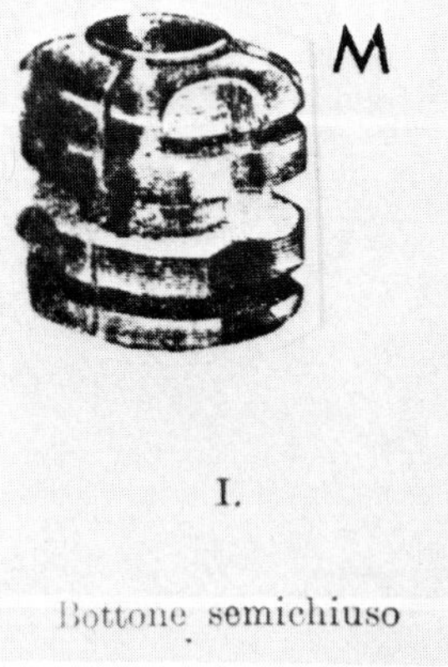

Fig I–8 (cont.).—**M,** C. Garampazzi's 1897 four-part button, held by a catgut ring and falling apart in the lumen when catgut dissolved. (From C. Garampazzi, 1897.)

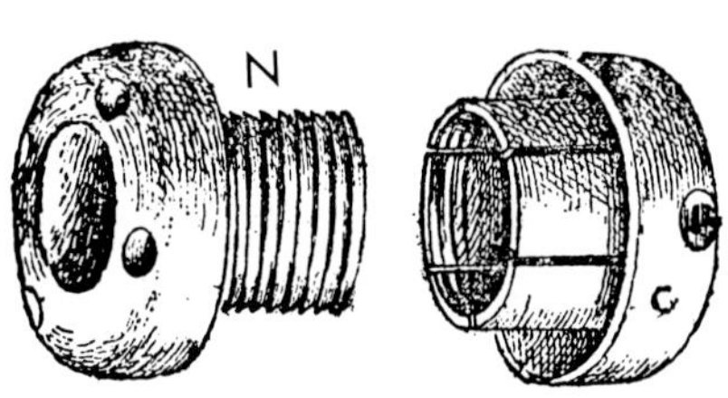

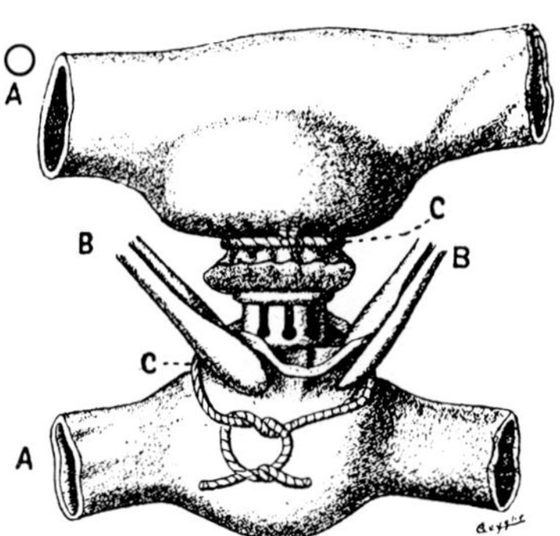

Fig I–8 (cont.).—N, model of A. Boari, 1897. In this second model, he reproduced the entire Murphy button in ivory. (From A. Boari, 1897.)

O, E. Juvara of Bucharest, 1896, showing a ligature instead of a pursestring suture. (From E. Juvara, 1896.)

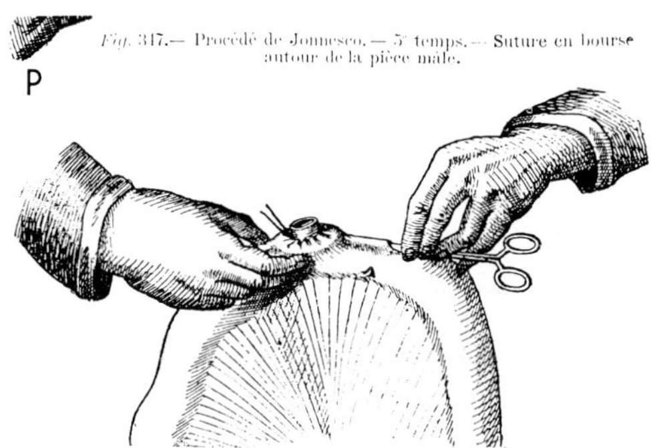

(*Fig.* 3{3). et l'engage dans l'intestin par la boutonnière qu'on vient de créer. A 3 centimètres, en deçà ou au delà, on fait

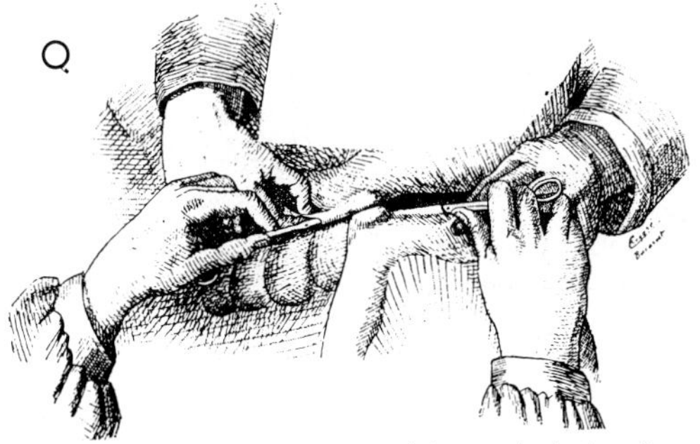

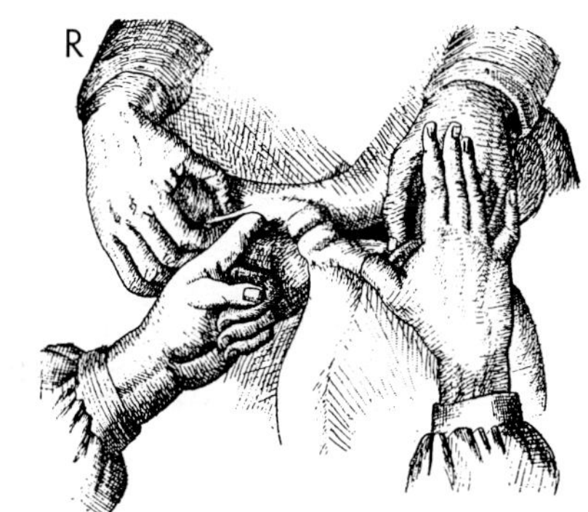

Fig I–8 (cont.).—P, Q, and **R,** the technique of Jonnesco, 1896. (From F. Terrier and M. Baudouin, 1898, who, in fact, as was done in other cases, reproduced the illustrations of the original author.)

(continued)

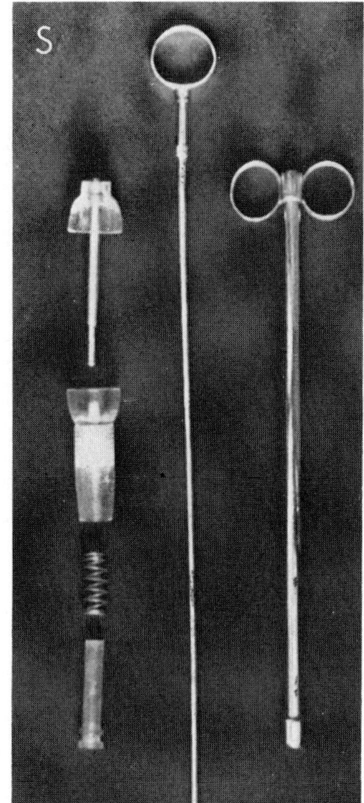

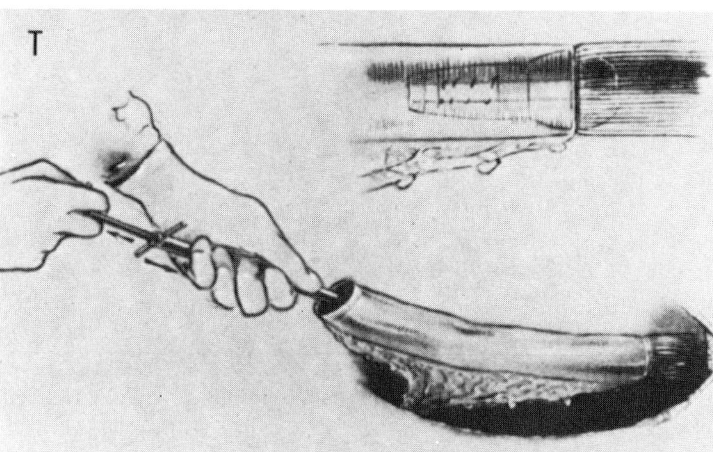

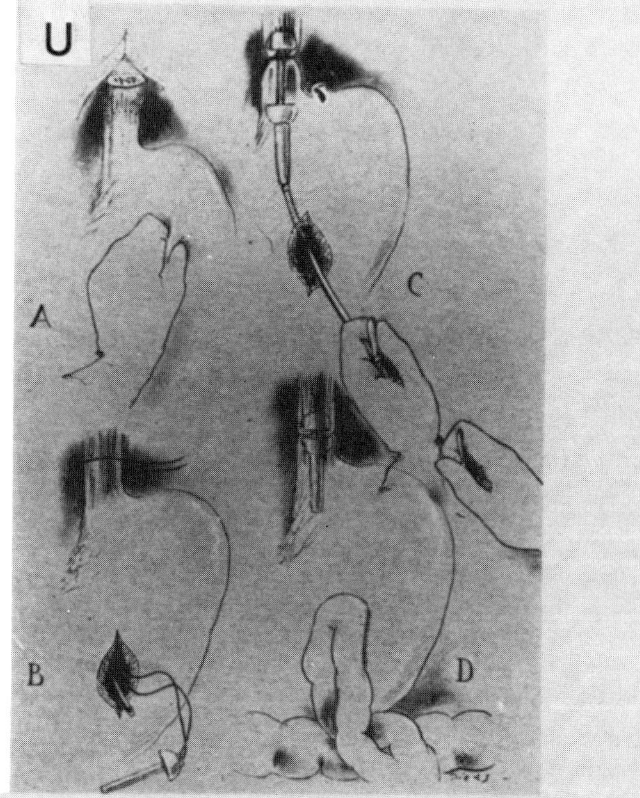

Fig. 3. *A*, Transverse incision through peritoneum on the esophagus in the hiatus. *B*, Vagotomy in the hiatus. Nylon string around the esophagus. Upper half of the button being pulled into the esophagus. *C*, Esophagus tied off on the button. Second half applied. *D*, Button closed. Segment of the esophagus caught between the two halves. Gastroenterostomy and anastomosis performed according to the method described by Braun.

Fig I–8 (cont.).—S, T, and **U,** Boerema's plastic buttons for esophageal reconstruction and for esophageal varices. Boerema described this as a modification of the Murphy button (Boerema, 1954.) (From I. Boerema, P.J. Klopper, and A.A. Holscher, *Surgery,* 1970, used by permission.)

ENDORECTAL ANASTOMOTIC DEVICES

Even after the ordinary manually sutured anastomosis was well established and regularly successful in most situations in the stomach and bowel, it was recognized that anastomosis of the colon to the rectum in the pelvis presented a special problem. William S. Halsted (1910) presented before the American Surgical Association one of a number of techniques with which he was to experiment over the next decade in an attempt to solve the special problem of rectosigmoid anastomosis by one or another "bulkhead" technique. His final paper on the subject was published in 1922, the year of his death (Halsted, 1922). The pursestring-closed ends of the colon and rectum were sutured together. To restore intestinal continuity through the closed ends, an assistant passed through the anus a sheathed knife, which the surgeon then guided through the joined ends of colon and rectum, following this with dilators from below. It is not clear whether the method (Fig I–9A,B) was ever tested clinically. In the light of current instrumentation (the EEA^{TM}), it is interesting that Halsted said in his 1910 paper, "To eliminate this diaphragm [of the abutted pursestring-closed ends of colon and rectum], I devised a sharp-edged punch, with the idea of introducing it at a higher point in the bowel through a lateral opening, slipping it down to the diaphragm and pressing it through this obstruction and into a cork introduced per anum, to withdraw both cork and punch by means of a thread attached to the former. This method was not tested." It will be recognized that this is the principle involved in low rectal anastomoses when the EEA^{TM} is inserted from above, as preferred by Nance (1979) and others.

The recurrence of the perception and application of principles, often in combination, in anastomotic devices—surely without awareness of the preceding experiences—is seen in the device of Sugarbaker (Fig I–9C). Sugarbaker (1951) described a new device that he had utilized for rectocolic anastomoses. It involved the Murphy button principle with the pins-and-holes retention mechanism, which Henroz had described in 1826 (for his everting anastomosis), and which Bonnier, in 1885, used in the ends of cork, metal, and ebony ferrules devised before Murphy. A number of the Murphy button variants utilized this principle. A hollow stem, threaded at its upper end and long enough to protrude from the rectum, compressed the two Murphy button analogues together. Compression was increased on the third and sixth days, on the principle of the Dupuytren spur crusher (Dupuytren, 1828; Ravitch, 1979). The inverted flanges necrosed and the instrument came loose and could be withdrawn by the tenth day. Sugarbaker reported in detail eight such operations, with one anastomotic leak, and indicated that he had performed still others (Sugarbaker, 1964; Exon and Sugarbaker, 1978).

A simpler version of this instrument was presented by Hallenbeck, Judd, and David (1963) (Fig I–9D). In the single patient operated on, the end of the tube protruding from the rectum was connected to tubing for discharge of feces and gas and the instrument came away in five days without complication. They made no reference to Sugarbaker's 1951 paper. A refined and sophisticated version of this concept, introduced some two years later by Brummelkamp (1965) with his Retroresector (Fig I–9E,F), included a novel method to insure the excision of the tumor with safe margins.

Jansen and colleagues from Utrecht (Jansen, Becker, Brummelkamp, Keeman, and Klopper, 1981; Jansen, Brummelkamp, Davies, Klopper, and Keeman, 1981) (Fig I–9G) have proposed a still further modification of this principle. The ends of rectum and colon are inverted over metal rings containing powerful magnets. The bowel ends are held by pins in the metal rings. An applicator passed per rectum guides the two ends together. The magnetic compression of the inverted ends causes the flanges of bowel to necrose. The magnets pass in seven to 12 days. In 11 sigmoid resections and nine low anterior resections there was one suture line dehiscence, requiring reoperation, one small dehiscence with an infected hematoma, and one death of myocardial infarction. In all other patients, "primary intestinal healing was demonstrated roentgenologically and sigmoidoscopically."

Ton (Ton, Boelens, and Gallas, 1973), noting that Boerema had tried his button in the rectum and had abandoned that use, assumed that the problem lay in the extremely small central channel of the Boerema button, adequate for saliva but not for feces. Ton's button (Fig I–9*H,I,J*) consisted of two slender metal rings mounted on central telescoping tubes by a single slender flying buttress. The rings were approximated by tautening a heavy rubber band inside the central channel, one end of it fastened distally, the other end drawn up and caught in the central channel by fine teeth. To draw up the rubber strand, a separate proximal colotomy was required. The device thus utilized the elastic traction principle of the Murphy button variants of Frank (see Fig I–8*E,F*) and of Martin Gil (see Fig I–8*G*) but required an additional colotomy. In 13 patients there were two suture line dehiscences, one fatal. It occurs to one that if the device were inserted with its ends reversed, it might be possible in low anastomoses to draw the rubber traction strand tight from below, within the lumen, obviating the need for the colotomy.

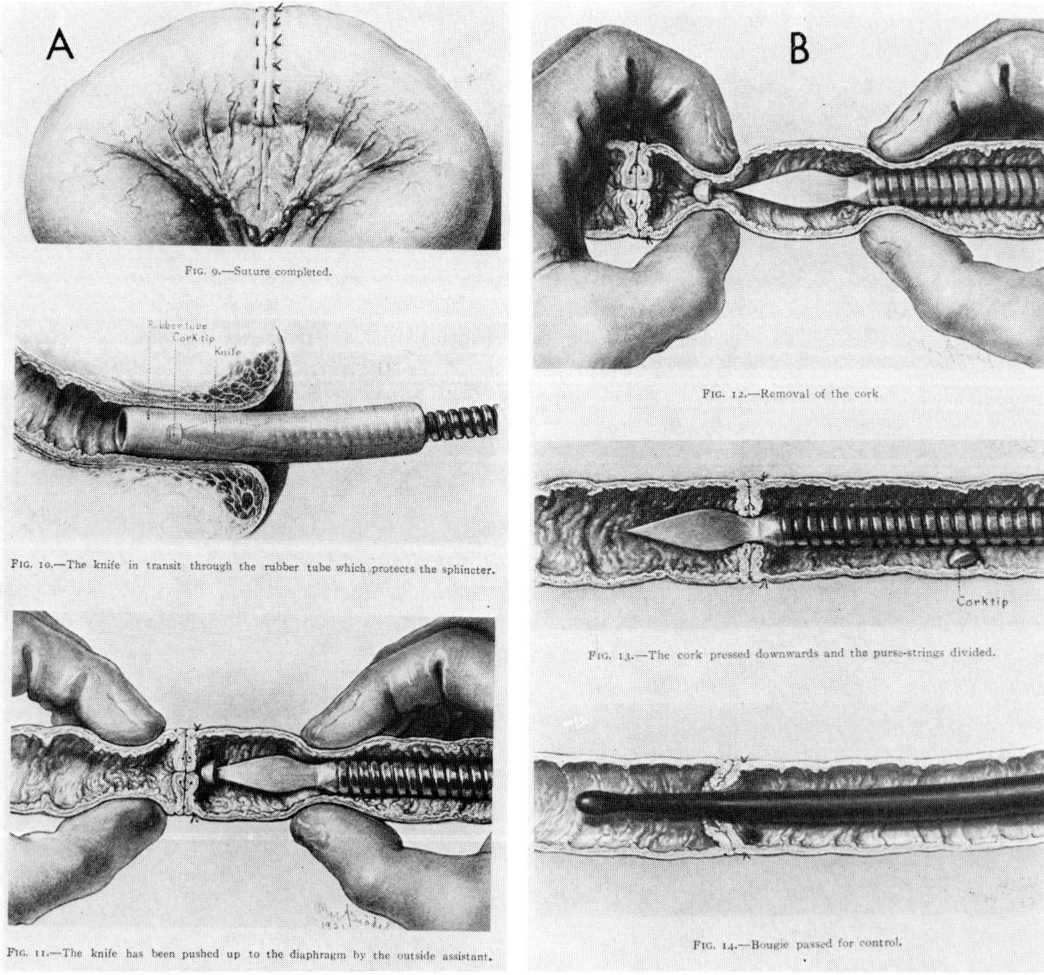

FIG. 9.—Suture completed.

FIG. 10.—The knife in transit through the rubber tube which protects the sphincter.

FIG. 11.—The knife has been pushed up to the diaphragm by the outside assistant.

FIG. 12.—Removal of the cork.

FIG. 13.—The cork pressed downwards and the purse-strings divided.

FIG. 14.—Bougie passed for control.

Fig I–9.—See legend on facing page.

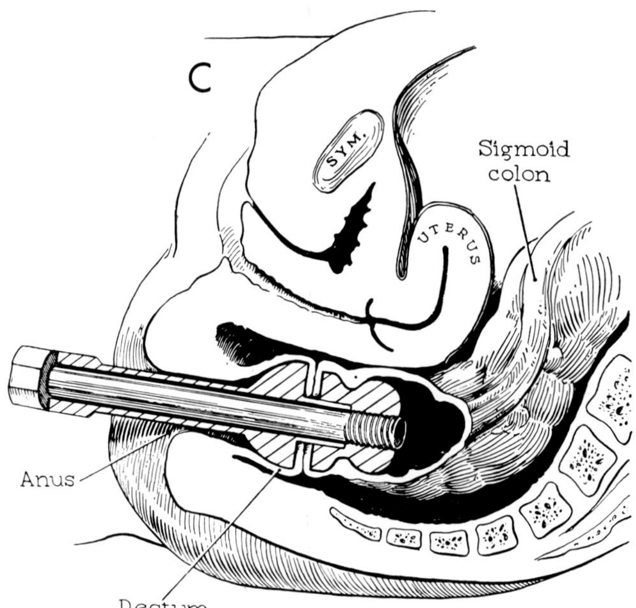

Fig I–9 (cont.).—C, colorectal anastomosis technique of
E. Sugarbaker, 1951. (From E.D. Sugarbaker and
H.M. Wiley, *SG&O,* 1951, used by permission.)

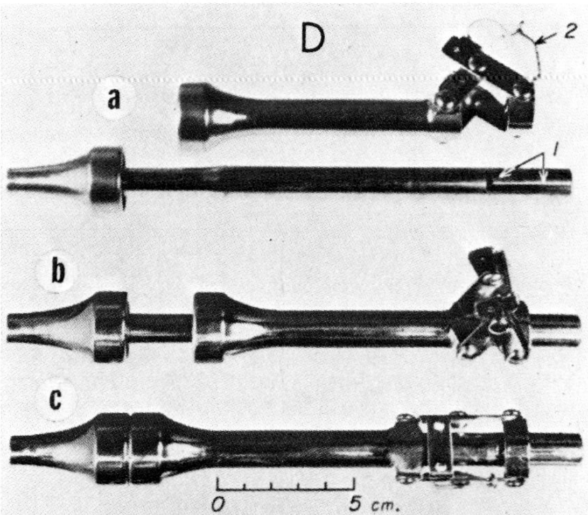

Fig I–9.—Endorectal anastomotic devices. **A** and **B,** aseptic bulkhead anastomosis of W.S. Halsted for colorectal anastomosis (1922). The specimen has been resected and the two pursestringed ends united. The double diaphragm is perforated from below. (From W.S. Halsted, Annals of Surgery, 1922.) *(continued)*

Fig I–9 (cont.).—D, colorectal anastomosis instrument of Hallenbeck, Judd, and David, from the Mayo Clinic, 1963. The device was a more elegantly constructed instrument on the principle of Sugarbaker and Wiley (1951). (From G.A. Hallenbeck, E.S. Judd, and C. David, *Diseases of the Colon and Rectum,* 1963, used by permission.)

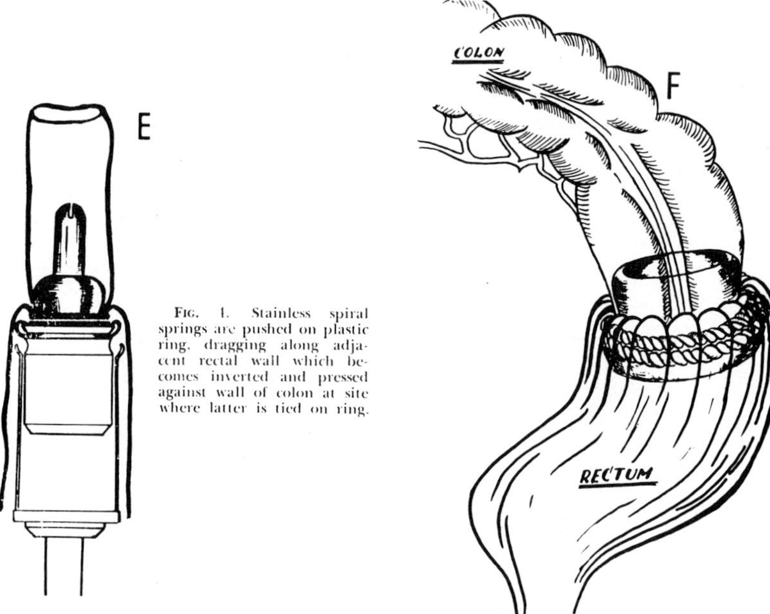

Fig I–9 (cont.).—E and **F,** lower rectal anastomosis technique of R. Brummelkamp, 1965. (From R. Brummelkamp, *Diseases of the Colon and Rectum,* 1965, used by permission.)

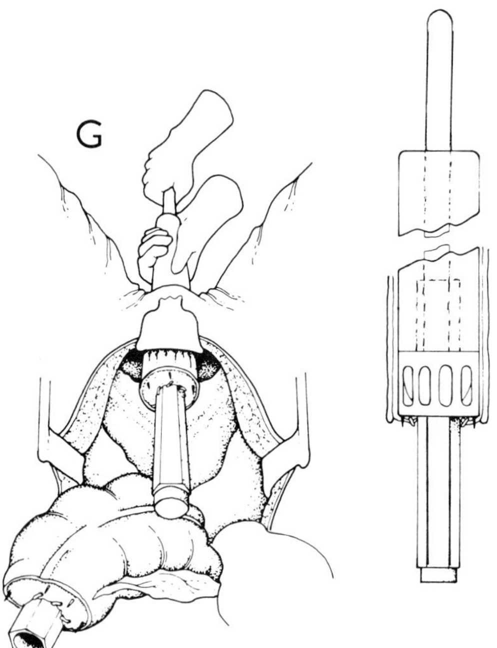

Fig I–9 (cont.).—G, Jansen's magnetic rings for rectal anastomosis. (From A. Jansen, W.H. Brummelkamp, G.A.G. Davies, P.J. Klopper, and J.N. Keeman, *SG&O,* 1981, used by permission.)

(continued)

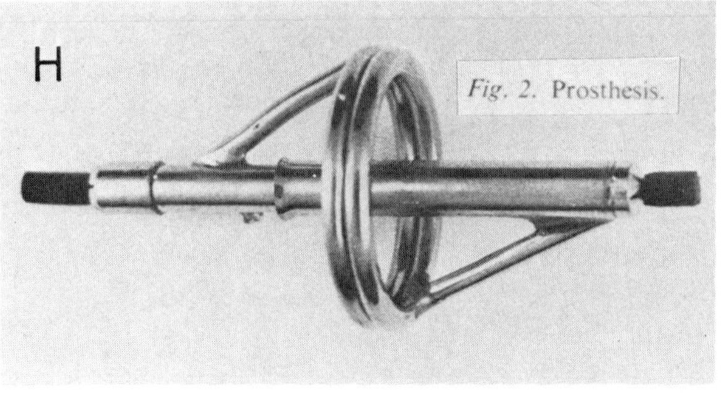

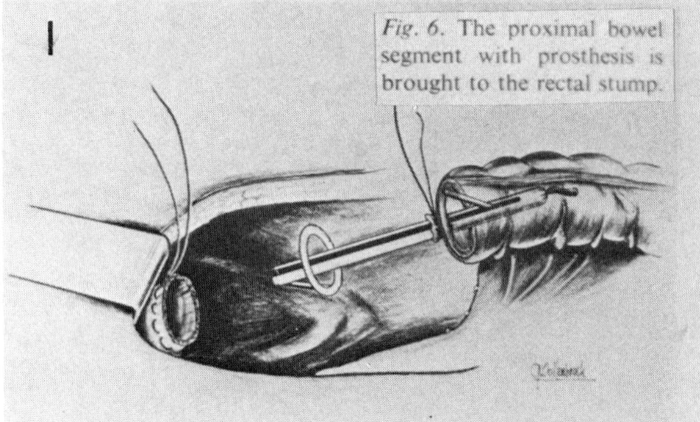

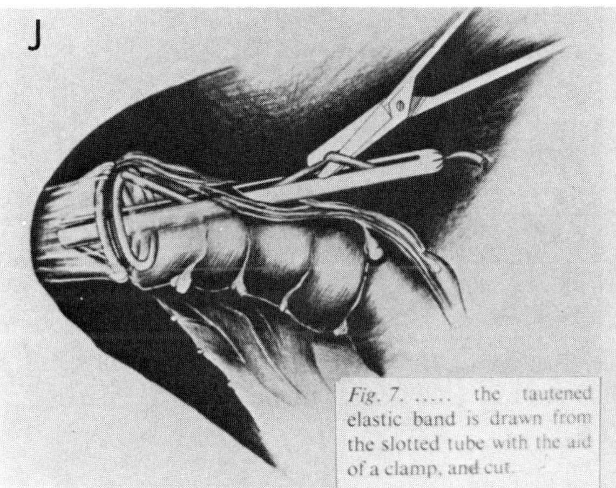

Fig I–9 (cont.).—H, I, and **J,** Ton's modification of Boerema's button for rectal anastomoses (Hengelo, The Netherlands, 1973). **H,** Ton's rings, with central telescoping stems mounted on flying buttresses. The rubber strand is threaded through the central cylinder and grasped by fine teeth in the lower end. **I,** the two rings are inserted in the pursestringed bowel ends. **J,** the upper (right-hand) end of the tube is exposed through a proximal colotomy, the heavy rubber band drawn taut, approximating the rings. Fine teeth in the central channel fix the rubber band in its tautened position and the enterotomy is closed. It seems apparent that in really low anastomoses, if the device were reversed, the rubber band could be tautened from below without need for the colotomy. (From J.G. Ton, W.C. Boelens, and Gallas, *Archivum Chirurgicum Neerlandicum,* 1973, used by permission.)

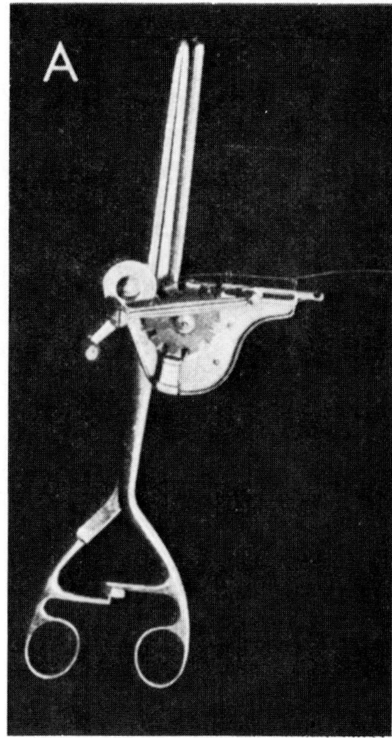
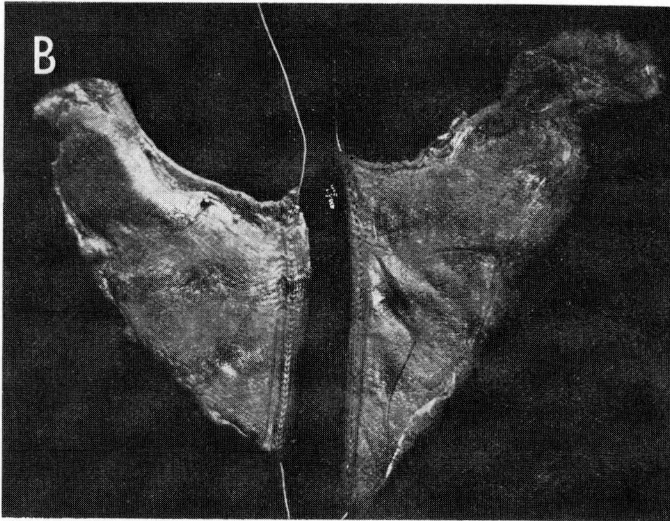

Fig I–10.—A and **B,** sewing machine of Florian Hahn, 1910. Hahn adapted a small sewing apparatus to a compression clamp. Turning the little crank produced a running sewing machine suture that was left long at the end and threaded into a needle for inversion by a continuous manual suture. The one-half page account gave no experimental or clinical data. (From F. Hahn, 1910.)

A true mechanical sewing instrument, using needle and thread, was presented by Florian Hahn (1910) of Nürnberg at the 39th German Congress of Surgery. This instrument (Fig I–10) closed stomach or large bowel at the site of transection, mucosa-to-mucosa. The small hand-driven sewing machine was attached to an arm on the clamp that closed the bowel, and placed a sewing machine stitch through-and-through the cut end. The clamps then having been removed, the end of the thread, left long for the purpose, was used to invert the cut end. Hahn (1911) made a further report on his instrument, announcing that the firm of M. Schaerer of Berne, Switzerland had undertaken to produce an improved version of the original and was ready to provide this new instrument to surgeons. The literature of the era does not suggest that Hahn's instrument was widely used.

STAPLING INSTRUMENTS

Mechanical suture instruments using staples originated with the work of Humer Hültl (1909) of Budapest, who, in 1908, at the Second Congress of the Hungarian Surgical Society, presented an instrument for use in distal gastrectomy (Fig I–11*A–D*). The instrument was heavy (3.5 kg—von Petz 1924) and assembly of its various parts was difficult and time-consuming. However, it did place two double rows of fine steel wire staples, quite similar to those used today, so the stomach or duodenum could be transected, leaving a double row of staples on either side of the section. The staples closed in the B shape, which has been the standard staple closure ever since. It is of interest that the internal mechanism for driving the staples home is, in fact, that which 50 years later was used by the Russians in their gastrointestinal anastomotic instrument, the NZhKA (Svinkin, 1964). The first staple instrument was the result of the combined efforts of Hültl, the surgical innovator, his brother—an engineer (Grausman, vide infra), and Victor Fischer, the talented manufacturer of surgical instruments. Robicsek (1980) has provided considerable background on the association of Fischer and Hültl. Humer (the Hungarian for ''Fidelius'') Hültl was Chief Surgeon of St. Stephen's Hospital and of St. Rokus Hospital in Budapest, the institution in which Semmelweis once worked and taught. A leading surgeon of his time, Hültl, considered an elegant and skillful operator, was a renowned teacher, attracting visitors to his clinic. He was an innovator in surgical teaching and reasoning, colorful, perhaps even eccentric, spoke fluent English, German, and French, and possessed an encyclopedic knowledge of the surgical literature. He believed strongly in asepsis. The wards and operating rooms in which he worked were impeccably clean. He used tincture of iodine for skin preparation and was the first in Hungary to use face masks and sterile gloves (like Mikulicz, first of cotton and later of rubber).

Hültl had a special concern for the risk of contamination of the peritoneum by gastric and intestinal contents, and took great care to isolate the operative field with laparotomy pads and towels, a procedure that he called "the wallpapering of the viscera." He was led by this concern to envision an instrument that would seal off the viscus before its division by placing a row or rows of metal staples through the walls of the stomach or bowel to eliminate the possibility of spillage. In 1907, Hültl charged Victor Fischer with the creation of a mechanical suture instrument that would "one, shorten the duration of the operation as much as possible; two, close the stomach and duodenum in the simplest but most reliable way; three, allow for resection of the whole viscus in a clean manner, whereas hitherto the hands of the operator had come in contact with the infected thread." Fischer responded to the challenge, became a daily visitor to the operating room, and presented Hültl with the stapler in 1908. Two sizes of the instrument were available, with staple lines 11 cm in length for gastric closure and 7 cm in length for the pylorus.

The massive Hültl instrument had two long jaws, one containing the slots for the insertion of the four rows of round cross-section steel wire staples and the other containing the curved depressions—anvils—for forming the staples. The jaws of the clamp, having been locked on the viscus, the turning of a crank, much like that of an old-fashioned coffee grinder, advanced a bar, which as it moved forward drove the staples in sequentially. The instrument being removed, the viscus then was transected between the two middle rows of staples, leaving on either side of the divided viscus a double-stapled, through-and-through, mucosa-to-mucosa closure. Hültl used this only for temporary closure to prevent soiling, and always inverted the stapled ends with conventional sutures.

He used the new instrument for the first time on May 9, 1908. The details of this operation, as well as those of 83 conventionally performed gastric resections done in the previous three-year span, were presented by Lajos Adam, Hültl's assistant, at the Second Annual Meeting of the Hungarian Surgical Society (1908), some 20 days after the stapling instrument had been successfully used for the first time. In his report, Adam stated that of all the gastric resections, ten of them for carcinoma of the stomach, "the last one is especially interesting because we used for the first time the stapling machine constructed by the engineer Fischer, according to ideas of Professor Hültl. The sutures held beautifully and after dividing the stomach, we had nothing else left to do but to cover the suture line with Lembert peritoneal sutures. After that we performed an antecolic gastro-jejunostomy. The duration of the operation was 40 minutes. The patient did well and was ambulatory on the third postoperative day." Adam gave a second report (1909) in the *Yearbook of the Royal Hungarian Surgical Society,* in which he presented one of his own patients, a 33-year-old woman operated on for cancer of the stomach. In that year, Hültl had successfully operated on 21 patients using his stapling instrument.

Until relatively recently, the principle of stapling of the gastrointestinal tract was best known to surgeons in the von Petz instrument, which was presented on September 21, 1921, at the Eighth Annual Meeting of the Hungarian Surgical Society (von Petz, 1924, 1927). The von Petz instrument (Fig I–12A–D), which derived from the Hültl stapler, was produced by Jetter and Scheerer Company in Tüttlingen, Württemberg. Aladar von Petz had had considerable experience with the Fischer-Hültl instrument and also with the "sewing machine" of Florian Hahn. von Petz' instrument was considerably lighter and simpler than Hültl's. It consisted essentially of a giant Payr clamp. The two rows of staples were inserted in one jaw and formed by the anvil grooves in the other. As in the Hültl instrument, a bar was driven forward to drive in the staples sequentially. The activating mechanism was a wheel, which actually probably was not an improvement over the Hültl crank. von Petz at that time was a young assistant at the Second Surgical Clinic directed by Professor Kuzmik at the University of Budapest. It had been expected that there would be a heated debate between Hültl and von Petz. According to Robicsek's charming account (1980), Hültl arrived before the presentation, sat down next to the nervous von Petz and asked for his instrument. Trying out the instrument on his own leather spectacle case, he inspected the suture line carefully and said, "It is better!" He congratulated von Petz and left the room. The Fischer-Hültl stapler, which underwent some modifications over the 20 years, was last manufactured in 1928. In retrospect, it seems to us that Hültl's gracious yielding to the younger man may have been more generous than appropriate, since the use of fine wire staples and double staggered rows initiated by Hültl has prevailed over the single Indian file row of flat German silver wire utilized by von Petz. To Hültl also goes the credit for having clearly recognized the need to use an instrument that functions in two steps—first, to compress and hold the tissues and, second, to drive in the staples. The need for the legs of the staples to perforate both walls of the viscus, strike the anvil, and recurve into the tissues to form a B staple closure, first recognized by Hültl and Fischer, has been an accepted principle of every stapling instrument since theirs. Both Hültl's and von Petz' instruments were considered to deliver a necrosing compression, the closure was considered only temporary, and always was inverted by manually placed sutures.

M.E. Jascalevich (1967) modified von Petz' stapler so as to have three rows of staples, the double, staggered row on the patient side and a single row on the specimen side of the gastric transection, the double row having nevertheless to be inverted, but preventing annoying bleeding. In a later paper (1972), he reported his instrument modified, like Nakayama's (see Fig I–15A), with a slot between the two proximal and one distal rows of staples, through which a knife blade was pulled. He now believed that with two rows of staples in the gastric stump, it was not necessary to invert these. There were no leaks. Jascalevich closed the duodenal stump with the TA^{TM} instrument, performed the anastomosis with the GIA^{TM} instrument and closed the GIA^{TM} opening manually.

Although von Petz' instrument gained wider reputation and was in longer use, Hültl's instrument was fairly well known for a time. Dr. Roland Grausman of New York, who had trained with Hültl in 1923, brought a Hültl stapler to the United States and used it here (Grausman, v.i.). His instrument, already modified (see Fig I–11D) from the initial prototype, and now in the possession of the New York Academy of Medicine, we have utilized in operations on dogs, using modern staples. It was a pleasure to find in our correspondence a charming letter from Doctor Grausman, which we reproduce for its historical interest, with respect to Hültl, and because of its sidelight on the training of American surgeons in that day.

8 Briny Avenue
Pompano Beach, Fla.
January 27, 1975

Dear Doctor Ravitch:

Your letter finally reached me here. First it went to Nantucket, where we spend the summers, then to my old office address (I have been retired for the last three years), then to my home address in N.Y.C., and finally here where I will remain until the end of March.

Needless to say, Doctor Hültl, Humer, meant a great deal to me—as a man of great character, inspiring teacher and mentor.

I graduated from P & S Columbia, Class of 1921, then spent two years as an intern at Mt. Sinai Hospital. At that time it was usual and important before starting practice to travel and gain European experience. As I recall, late one afternoon Dr. Emanuel Libman [the distinguished internist] called me to meet him at his office at six o'clock. That was not just a request but a command. I arrived on time wondering what had gone wrong. First he asked me to cross-index a card for a new book, then he placed a record on his victrola asking me to identify the composition on the record. Fortunately I gave the correct answer. We then departed for his favorite restaurant, Buchler's at 62nd Street and Lexington. On our way back after dinner he said that he had heard that I was anxious to further my knowledge of surgery and study in Europe. He told me that he had confidence in me and wanted me to go abroad. With that he handed me a check for $2,000 to be returned at a later date with or without interest in order to help someone else. I was astonished and thrilled but refused the money as I had that much in my savings account for this purpose. He told me that Leon Ginzburg was working with an outstanding surgeon in Budapest, with Professor Hültl. I wrote the Professor, gave him my qualifications. I received a cable, "come". I left the States immediately and upon arrival in Budapest rented a room at the Pajor Sanitarium where the Professor did all of his private operations. The following morning at eight o'clock I was at his office in St. Rokus Hospital (similar to our city hospitals). We conversed in German. I liked him at once. He was direct, magnetic and charming. He first asked if I had come to teach him American methods of surgery. No, I had come to learn Hungarian methods. When do I wish to operate? he asked. When he thought I was capable, I replied. That may be never, he said. Well, if that is the case it was better to know now, I said. The Professor told me to report at 7:30 the next morning, I had come to learn.

The following morning I was told to observe their methods and techniques, also learn the names of the surgical instruments. The daily schedule was St. Rokus, 7:30 to lunchtime, Pajor Sanitarium at 1:00 p.m. where the Professor had his own operating room and staff.

In order not to become "homesick" I worked in the anatomical department from four to six in the afternoon. After three weeks of this, a young doctor asked if he could dissect with me. I was delighted of course. We proceeded to do various operations together on the cadaver. I did not learn until later that he reported back to the Professor as to my knowledge and ability. One morning I was surprised to find my name posted to perform a thyroidectomy. From then on I was delegated to perform different operations.

Professor Hültl was a great teacher and technician. He used individual silk sutures and after each stitch he threw the needle and holder out of the field of operation, to be washed and resterilized. He used thirty to forty in each operation.

The Hültl stomach sewing machine was a "Brain Child" of a great surgeon and a great engineer, his brother. It was first demonstrated in 1911 at a European surgical meeting. I was amazed and thrilled with its speed and helpfulness. I had never seen anything like it. I used it with success but could not get other N.Y. doctors to use the instrument. The machine was heavy but sewed with four lines of metal clips. von Petz was one of the Professor's assistants who went to Berlin to live and there modified the machine making it lighter with two lines of suture clips. With the lighter machine, there were more instances of hemorrhage and leakage. The line of clips was always inverted with individual silk sutures. Seldom did one see any infection although only cotton gloves were used. (Following the Second World War [sic] they did not have rubber gloves.)

I was in Budapest for six months when the Professor became ill with a severe nasal hemorrhage. I wrote him a letter wishing a speedy recovery and offering to be a blood donor. Some weeks later I had dinner with him and during our conversation, he told me he was touched by my offer of blood. No one in his family had done so. He then told me why he became interested in teaching young American surgeons. Right after World War I, an American Red Cross officer came to see him from Vienna offering to help him in any way. The Professor promptly asked for food, clothing and medicine for the children in the pediatric wards. His requests were forthcoming in a few days. In his words, these wards were changed from "hell and inferno" to "paradise and bliss". Right then and there he made up his mind that if any young American doctor wished to study with him he would adopt him as his "son" and teach him as much as possible to repay that debt. I was one of the lucky ones. Needless to say, I could go on and on.

I am certain that you can obtain information from Leon Ginzburg, former Surgeon-in-Chief at Beth Israel Hospital in New York City. Also Dr. Stephen Rosenak whose office is on Park Avenue around 90th Street, 1100 approximately. He was born in Hungary and worked in the Professor's clinic before coming to the States.

I returned to Budapest to visit the Professor in 1928 and again on my wedding trip in 1932. In 1928 he asked me to scrub up with him to assist him with a gallbladder operation. While we were scrubbing up he discussed the case with me giving me all the details of the condition of the patient. When we were ready to operate he turned to the ampitheater, removed his gloves and announced that his American son would perform the operation.

His technique in the O.R. was outstanding especially considering that after the first World War they had very little in the way of supplies. The procedure was to remove the outer garments, don a rubber apron and scrub arms and hands with soap and water for twenty minutes. This was followed by an antiseptic, a solution of alcohol and weak iodine. Long sterile cotton gowns and cotton caps and masks were put on. Rubber gloves were impossible to obtain so sterile cotton gloves were used. Sterile bandages were used to keep the cuff of the gown and top of gloves in place.

The Professor's technique was superior. Infections were rare. His surgical skill was acclaimed throughout Hungary, Austria, Italy and neighboring countries. He was appointed surgeon to the King and Queen. Royalty came from near and far to consult with him. He was a brilliant man and read and wrote extensively. He spoke several languages fluently.

I hope this will be of help to you, . . .

Willy Meyer published a brief paper in the *Zentralblatt für Chirurgie* (1913), saying that having used Jianu's greater-curvature gastric tube brought up antethoracically as in the first of his multiple-stage esophagectomy and reconstruction procedures, it occurred to him that the tube might be made sufficiently long, if nourished by the left gastroep-iploic artery, to reach the proximal esophagus and could be brought up through the thoracotomy at the time of operation. He said that in his animal experiments Hültl's staple suturing instrument served admirably for the longitudinal division and suture of the stomach required in construction of the tube. In the following year in the *J.A.M.A.* (Meyer 1914) (see Fig I–11*F*), Meyer said that he now had attempted the procedure in three patients, in the first with manual sutures, and then "in Cases 2 and 3, I tried Hültl's wire stitching instrument. All three patients made a good recovery."

Meyer (1915), speaking before the American Surgical Association, twice referred to using the Hültl instrument in gastrectomy, in one case merely stating, "On dividing the stomach, which had an unusually distended cardiac pouch, with Hueltl's large wire-stitching instrument. . .", suggesting that the instrument was known to his audience.

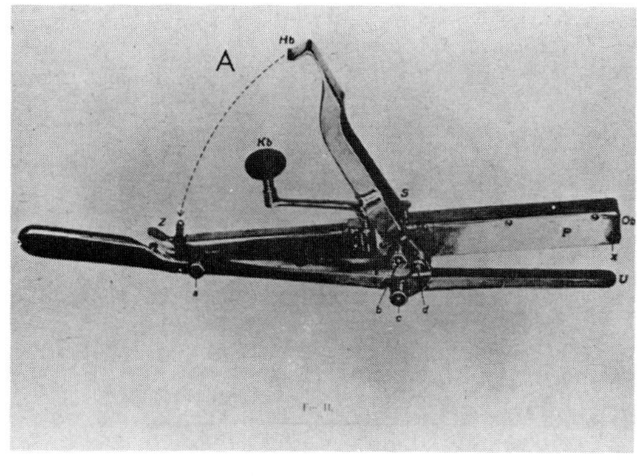

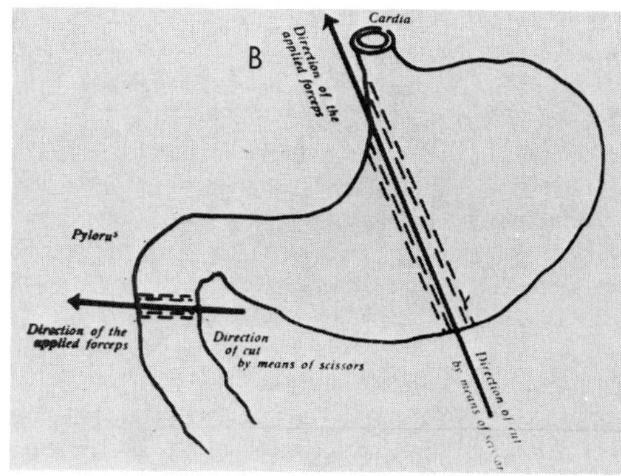

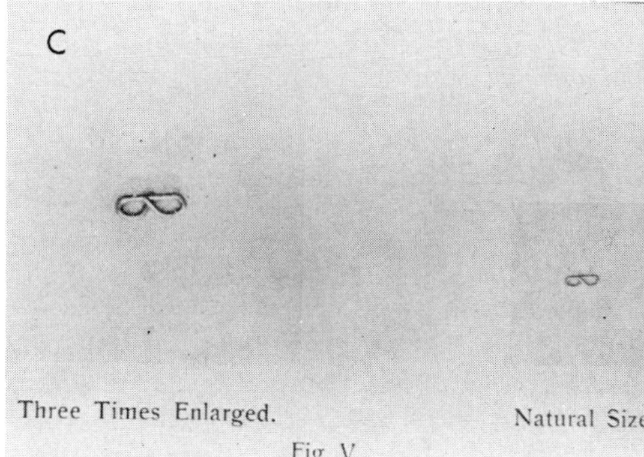

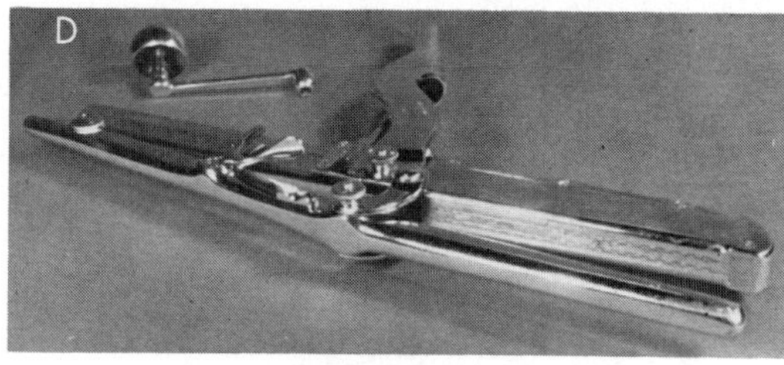

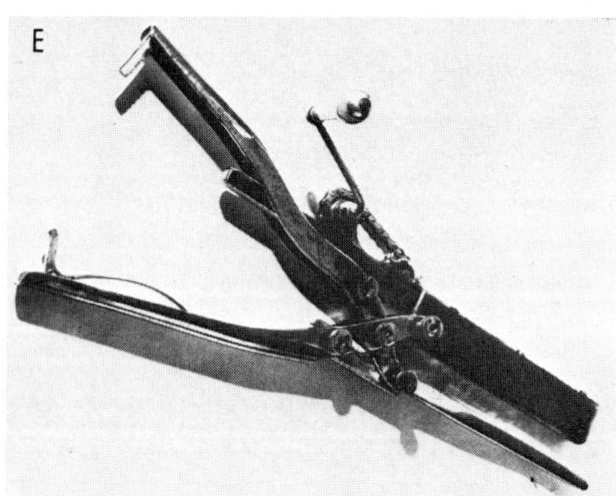

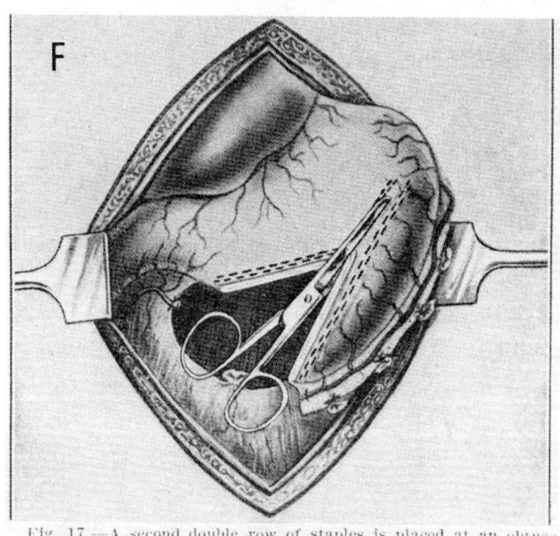

Fig. 17.—A second double row of staples is placed at an obtuse angle with Hültl's second (smaller) instrument beyond the turn of the left inferior epiploic artery; scissors traverse the dry, crushed center portion between the inner rows.

Fig I–11.—The first stapling instrument—Humer Hültl, 1908. **A,** as in all of the stapling instruments, the instrument was first closed, producing the required degree of compression, and the staples then driven through the fixed tissues. Turning the crank advanced a rod that drove the staples in sequentially. **B,** the instrument utilized fine wire staples and placed four staggered rows, permitting the operator to divide the viscus, leaving two rows on either side. Nevertheless, the closure always was inverted by manual sutures. **C,** the staples closed in the B shape, which has been standard ever since. (**A, B,** and **C** taken from the original brochure, in English, supplied by the manufacturer.) **D,** photograph of the model brought to this country by Dr. Roland Grausman and presented by him to the New York Academy of Medicine. The instrument, on loan to us from the Academy, was found to be in perfect working order. Hand-loaded with fine wire staples provided by the U.S. Surgical Corporation, it performed satisfactorily in experimental animals. **E,** Hültl instrument, early model. Dr. C. Kieninger of Tübingen kindly obtained for us (July, 1979) this photo from Dr. Imre Littman of Budapest. The instrument, in the Semmelweis museum in Budapest, is thought to be the only survivor in Hungary of the 50 instruments said to have been manufactured. This, presumably early, model shows a chain and sprocket drive instead of the direct drive of the later models. **F,** greater-curvature reversed gastric (Beck-Jianu) tube with the Hültl instrument. Willy Meyer, before the American Medical Association, reported two such operations, mentioning the Hültl instrument in a way suggesting that it was well known to his audience. In this paper he pictures the gastric tube brought antethoracically. (**F** from W. Meyer, 1914.)

Dieser Nähapparat, welcher die Dimensionen der gewöhnlichen Payr'schen Magenquetschzange mit Exzenterhebelschluß nur wenig überschreitet, besteht

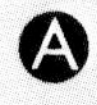
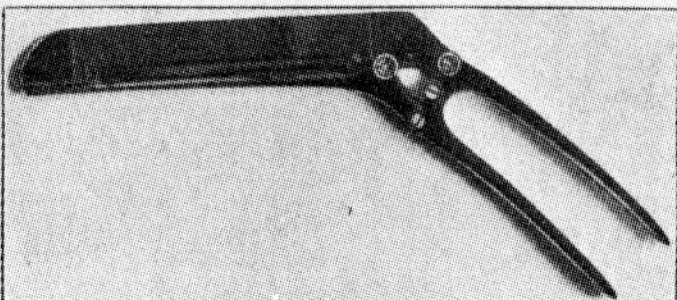

Fig. 1.
Nähapparat geschlossen.

aus einem unbiegsamen oberen (Fig. 3 A) und aus einem harten, jedoch elastischen unteren Quetscharm (B), welche beide mittels eines Exzenterhebelschlusses nahezu als Parallelzange wirken. Bei der Schließung der Zange berühren sich erst die Spitzen der Quetscharme und die Quetschwirkung verteilt sich von hier aus gleichmäßig in der Richtung des Verschlusses. In dem etwas breiteren oberen Quetscharm (A) ist die Nähkonstruktion untergebracht, die vor dem Gebrauch mit den feinen U-förmigen Neusiberklammerchen mittels Pinzette und Füllstift gefüllt wird (Fig. 4).

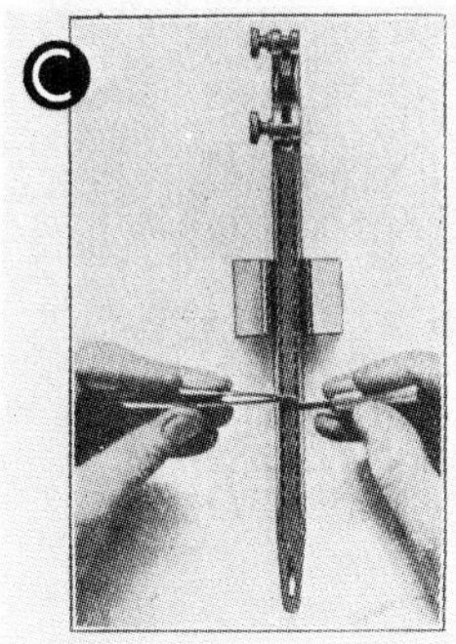

Fig. 4.
Obere Zangenbranche auf Fixateur ruhend, die beiden Reihen der Klammeröffnungen werden mit den feinen U-förmigen Klammerchen mittels Pinzette und Füllstift gefüllt.

Wird die Drehkurbel in der Uhrzeigerrichtung gedreht, so kommt die Triebstange (6) in Bewegung und bringt das Daumenrad (7) in Tätigkeit. Dieses rückt zwischen den Rippen (4) vorwärts und schiebt inzwischen die U-förmigen Schieberplättchen gegen die untere Branche des Instruments. Wurden in die Klammeröffnungen (3) Drahtklammerchen eingesetzt, so werden sie bei dieser Bewegung des Daumenrades aus der oberen Branche herausgedrängt, und hatten wir den

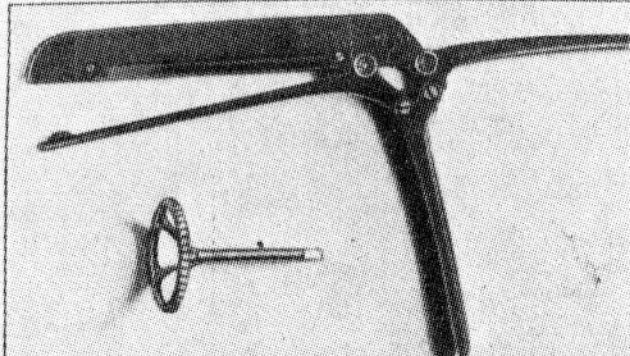

Fig. 2.
Geöffneter Nähapparat mit Drehkurbel.

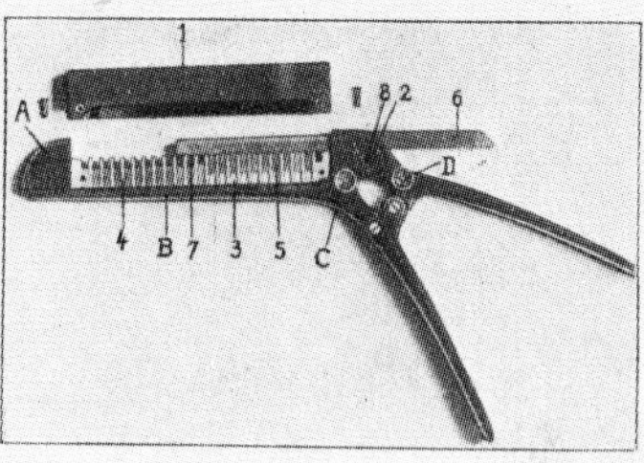

Fig. 3.
Mechanik des Nähapparates.

Magen oder den Darm in die Quetsche gefaßt, so durchdringen die Spitzen der Klammerchen beide Wände des gequetschten Organs und werden auf den gegenüberstehenden Einkerbungen der Branche B -förmig umgebogen.

Fig I–12.—Stapler of Aladar von Petz, 1924. **A, B,** and **C,** reproductions from von Petz' original publication. Note that he describes his clamp as being of the dimensions of an ordinary Payr clamp, which it does, in fact, resemble. His *Figure 2* shows a large upper jaw in which the staples are inserted manually, the slender lower jaw grooved with anvils to form the B-shaped staples, and the wheel used to advance the rod (6 in von Petz' *Fig 3*) that drives in the staple pushers. The two rows of staples are loaded by hand as in von Petz' *Figure 4*. The stomach was to be divided with scissors, leaving a single row of staples on either side, to be inverted by sutures. *(continued)*

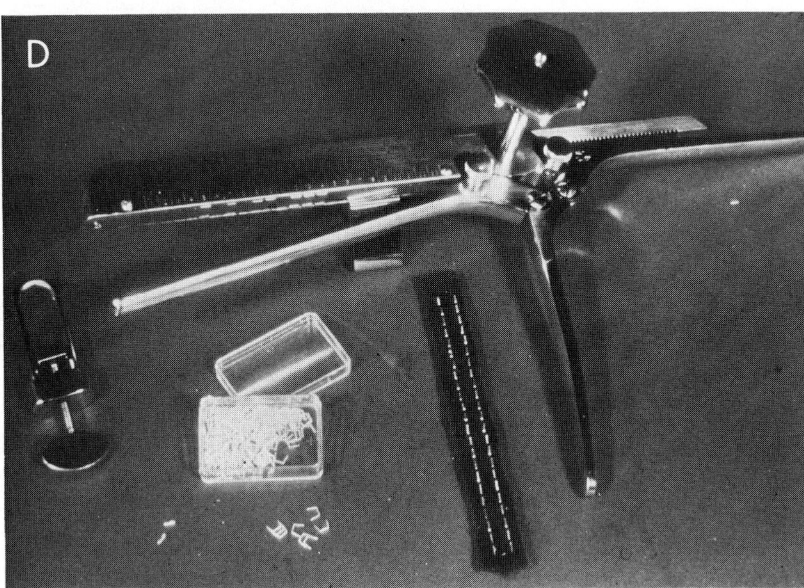

Fig I–12 (cont.).—D, late model of the von Petz clamp shown with the coarse, flat German silver staples, the two Indian-file rows of staples applied to a sheet of felt, and on the left the screw clamp to secure the nose of the instrument. The instrument shown now is in the collection of the Smithsonian Institution. For almost three decades, stapling in surgery meant the von Petz clamp.

Stefan Sándor (1936), another Hungarian and a student of Hültl's, presented a new stapling instrument, lighter and mechanically much simpler than Hültl's. Like Friedrich's instrument (v.i.), all of the staples were driven in simultaneously rather than sequentially as in Hültl's. In addition, in a compromise between von Petz' Indian file staple line and Hültl's double staggered rows of staples, Sándor's instrument placed the staples obliquely to the axis of the staple line. Sándor, like Friedrich, continued to use the heavy, flat German silver wire staples of von Petz. He said that he had given some thought to using interchangeable cartridges but found that this would have complicated his instrument unacceptably (Fig I–13*A,B*).

Tomoda (1937, 1937), at the Kyushu University of Japan, presented his stapling instrument, in fact a simpler and improved version of the von Petz instrument. In addition to a lighter construction, the transmission of the activating mechanism was mechanically much simpler. For the first time, there was a provision for varying the degree of compression of the staples to provide for some adaptation to variable tissue thickness (Fig I–14). The staples closed in a somewhat open B, which may not have been critical, since the cut end of the stomach or bowel was oversewn.

Komei Nakayama (1954), in Japan, further simplified von Petz' instrument by removing the wheel and the advancing bar. The staples were loaded into slots in the jaws of the Payr-like clamp, the instrument closed, and the staples driven home with a huge pair of pliers, which pressed down the housings holding the staple drivers. There were two such housings for the whole suture line (Fig I–15*A*), a principle much later incorporated in Pimenta's everting, end-to-end anastomotic stapler (see Fig I–3).

A shorter (one staple driver housing) and a longer (three housings), curved version for the creation of reversed gastric tubes were presented by Uchiyama, Tokunaga, and Kajisa (1962) (Fig I–15*B*).

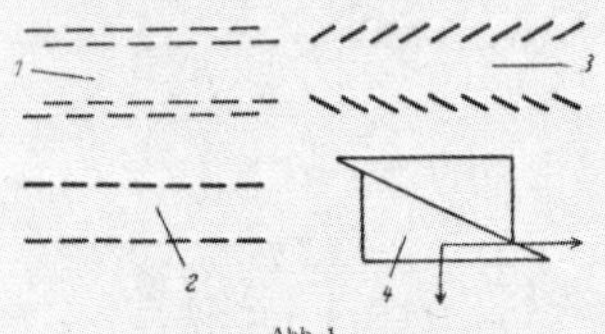

nehmen viel Wärme in sich auf. Hültl macht darauf in seiner vor 26 Jahren veröffentlichten Mitteilung aufmerksam und empfiehlt die sorgfältige Abkühlung des Instrumentes mit sterilem kalten Wasser. Trotzdem ereignete sich mir einmal, daß der Magen zwischen den heißen Zangebacken des Instrumentes nicht bloß gequetscht und genäht, sondern zugleich auch gekocht wurde. Das Resultat war eine eitrige Peritonitis und ich fand einen bescheidenen Trost in den bei der Obduktion nachgewiesenen Karzinommetastasen für den technischen Fehler.

Bei der Anfertigung der ersten Hültl'schen Apparate konnte man den Gedanken nicht loswerden, eine Nähmaschine müsse Räder besitzen. Diese Prachtstücke der Präzisionsmechanik stellten Monstra von über 5 kg Gewicht dar. Die Firma Peter Fischer sorgte bereits im Jahre 1911 für die Vereinfachung des Apparates. Immerhin entstand dabei ein noch immer viel zu schweres, kompliziertes Instrument, welches über 100 auseinander zu nehmende Bestandteile hatte. Die Reinigung und Zusammenstellung des Instrumentes bedeutete eine heikle, beinahe 2 Stunden beanspruchende Arbeit. Nehmen wir noch die hohen Herstellungs- und Verkaufspreise hinzu, so kann es uns nicht wundernehmen, daß das Instrument keine Verbreitung fand, obwohl einige Stücke selbst nach Japan und Amerika verkauft wurden. Indessen wurde das mechanische Problem durch dieses Instrument vollkommen gelöst. Die Präzisität und Festigkeit der Ausführung dieser Apparate erhellt daraus, daß die im Jahre 1911 besorgten Exemplare im Instrumentarium unseres Krankenhauses heute noch in tadellosem Zustande sind. Die Hültl'sche doppelte Nahtreihe ist die beste und verläßlichste (Abb. 1, 1). Dieses Modell von Hültl wurde unter völliger Beibehaltung des mechanischen Prinzips der Kraftübertragung durch Zahnrad und Zahnstange 13 Jahre nachher von Aladar v. Petz in einer überaus gelungenen und geistreichen Weise vereinfacht. v. Petz berichtete über seine ersten Versuche im September 1921 in der Sitzung der Gesellschaft ungarischer Chirurgen, sein Instrument wurde in seiner gegenwärtigen Form 1923 patentiert in Deutschland, wo es auch erzeugt wird. Diesem Instrument verdankt die Naht mit Metallklammern ihre Verbreitung in weiteren Kreisen. Das Wesentlichste in der v. Petz'schen Neuerung erblicke ich meinerseits in der Anwendung der aus Metallpfättchen von 1 mm Breite und 0,2 mm Dicke geformten Klammern an Stelle der Hültl'schen aus 0,4 mm dicken Draht bestehenden Klammern. Jene eignen sich zur Naht besser und bewirken eine größere Festigkeit der einreihigen v. Petz'schen Naht (Abb. 1, 2).

Abb. 1

1 Klammerreihe nach Hültl, *2* Klammerreihe nach v. Petz, *3* Klammerreihe nach Sándor, *4* Schema der Kraftübertragung durch Keilverschiebung

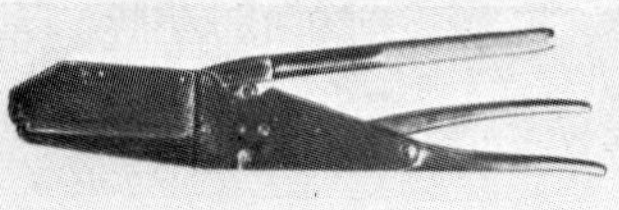

Abb. 2. Nähinstrument geschlossen

In der Bestrebung, das Instrument leicht zu machen, ist man meines Erachtens etwas zu weit gegangen. Dadurch erscheint es für seine Aufgabe als Quetschzange zu schwach gebaut. Auf diesen Umstand scheint es hinzuweisen, daß die erzeugende Firma sich veranlaßt fühlte, die Modifikation nach Koegel herauszubringen, welche viel massiver ist und einen kräftigen, parallelen Verschluß besitzt. Die ähnlichen Konstruktionen der letzten Jahre, wie z. B. die von Neuffer-Ullrich, stellen ebenfalls massive, kräftige, gut quetschende Instrumente dar.

Es gelang mir nach jahrzehntelangen Versuchen und Enttäuschungen im Jahre 1933 die Konstruktion eines Instrumentes, welches bei gutem Quetscheffekt alle Klammern auf einen Druck hin gleichzeitig, schräg zur Nahtlinie in fest schließender Reihe einlegt (Abbildung 1, 3). Ich ließ dieses Instrument, da es sich in der Anwendung sehr gut bewährte, im Juli 1933 patentieren. Als Ziel schwebte mir dabei die Konstruktion eines möglichst vereinfachten, aber kräftigen und zuverlässig funktionierenden Apparates vor, der leicht auseinandergelegt, gereinigt und gepflegt werden kann. Die Kraftübertragung wird durch einen beweglichen Keil geleistet, welcher an einem befestigten Keil entlanggleitet. Der gleitende Keil wird bei waagerechter Bewegung auch in die senkrechte Richtung ausgelenkt (Abb. 1, 4) und schiebt einen kammförmigen Bestandteil vor sich, dessen Zähne wiederum die eingelegten v. Petz'schen Metallplattenklammern aus dem Apparat herausdrücken. (Abb. 3 u. 4.) Durch die schräg gestellten Klammern wird aus dem gequetschten Gewebe ein Streifen vernäht, welcher genau die Breite der Hültl'schen Doppelnaht hat. Diese wasser- und luftdicht angelegte Naht darf als zuverlässig gelten. Auseinandergenommen besteht mein Instrument aus sechs Schrauben und acht Bestandteilen, welche so massiv sind, daß Bruch oder Abnützung kaum vorkommen kann, wenngleich auch die Bestandteile leicht ersetzt werden können. Die Armierung der Klammern beansprucht 5 Minuten, die Auskochung etwa 10 Minuten. So viel Zeit hat man wohl selbst im »Großbetrieb« zwischen zwei Magenresektionen! Es erschien mir daher auch nicht notwendig, das Instrument mit einem vertauschbaren Klammermagazin zu komplizieren. Die Erzeugung und Einführung in den Handel brachte Schwierigkeiten mit sich, die mich zwangen, davon Abstand zu nehmen. Auf Anregung meines ehemaligen Chefs und Meisters, Prof. Hültl,

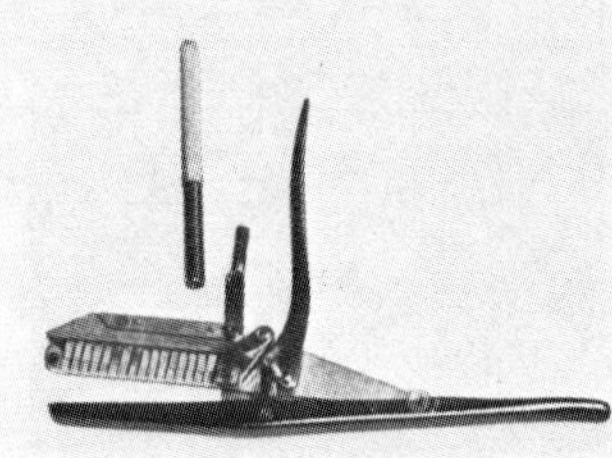

Abb. 3. Nähinstrument offen, Deckplatte entfernt

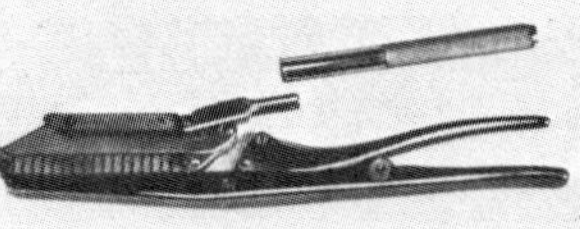

Abb. 4. Nähinstrument nach vollendeter Naht, Deckplatte entfernt

Fig I-13.—Stefan Sándor, 1936. Sándor's illustrations show a compact instrument with three handles. The lower two close the jaws of the clamp. Pressing down on the upper handle now drives in the staples. Sándor acknowledged the instruments of Hültl and von Petz, adding the obliquity of the staples and the simplicity of action, a significant advance over the crank and wheel mechanism of their instruments. The illustrations (**A** and **B**) show successively the staple suture lines of the Hültl, von Petz, and Sándor instruments, the instrument closed, the instrument opened with the housing cover removed, revealing the staple-driving fins, and the instrument closed with the housing cover still removed. Note in his *Abb. 1* (**A**), the sliding triangles that, activated by the handle, pressed down the fins and drove in the staples. Sándor, acknowledging Hültl as his former chief and master, who encouraged him to have his new instruments manufactured, nevertheless said of Hültl's instrument that it weighed over 5 kg, had over 100 separate parts to assemble, and that cleaning and assembly took nearly two hours of assiduous work. He considered adding a replaceable magazine to his own instrument but thought that unnecessary in an instrument so easily cleaned and loaded. The machine was fabricated and sold by Peter Fischer of Budapest, who had made Hültl's instrument. Sándor refers to a number of cases of clinical use. (From S. Sándor, 1936.)

Um die nachteiligen Eigenschaften beseitigen zu können, ist es zunächst erforderlich, sie vom praktischen Standpunkt aus genau zu erforschen.

1) Im Spitzenteil eines oberen Quetscharmes befindet sich bei dem Petz'schen Apparat ein Rad, welches den wichtigsten Teil des ganzen Nahtmechanismus darstellt. Da sich dieser Spitzenteil des Quetscharmes an der Nahtführung nicht beteiligt und obendrein ziemlich lang ist, so wirkt er besonders bei der Einführung des Apparates in schmale Räume äußerst störend und stellt einen nicht auszunützenden Teil dar, so z. B. bei der Durchtrennung des Pylorus oder des Duodenum, die stark verwachsen sind und daher nur ungenügend präpariert und mobilisiert werden können, ferner bei der Durchtrennung des Magens, oben an der kleinen Kurvatur, besonders in der Nähe der Cardia, weiter bei Resektionen des Colon transv. oder desc., dessen Mobilisierung wegen der starken Verwachsung nur beschränkt möglich ist.

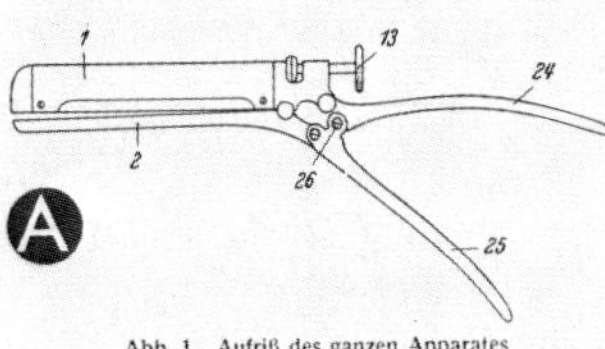

Abb. 1. Aufriß des ganzen Apparates

Diese Nachteile des Petz'schen Apparates sind infolge seines grundsätzlichen Aufbaues von vornherein nicht vermeidbar.

2) Bei dem Petz'schen Apparat wirkt stets die bestimmte (stets maximale) Quetschkraft völlig auf die Klammer und das Gewebe, ganz unabhängig davon, welche Dicke das zu nähende Gewebe hat. Bei dem Apparat ist also die Stärke der Quetschkraft und damit der Nahtkraft nicht regelbar, so daß bei der Herstellung einer Naht in dünnem Gewebe (z. B. im Dünndarm), leicht eine kleine Lücke

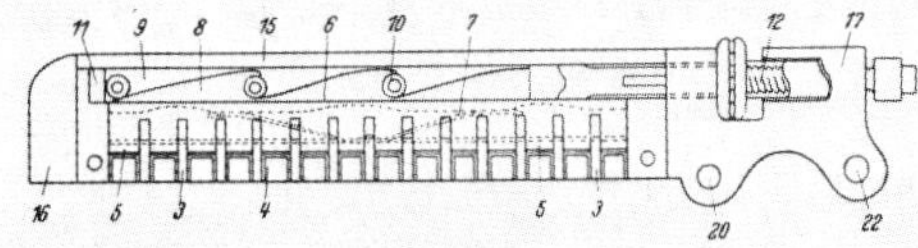

Abb. 2. Oberer Quetscharm in teilweise geschnittener Ansicht

zwischen einem Klammerchen und dem Gewebe im geklammerten Zustande entstehen kann. Eine solche Lücke kann aber leicht die Ursache einer Blutung des Resektionsstumpfes infolge ungenügender Quetschkraft sein.

3) Der obere Quetscharm ist sehr breit, wodurch die Handhabung des ganzen Apparates erheblich erschwert ist.

Infolge der beabsichtigten Eigenschaften und des bestimmten Aufbaues kann man jedoch die Breite des Quetscharmes bei dem Petz'schen Apparat nicht verringern.

4) Die Neufüllung des Nähapparates dauert unnötig lange, weil man mit dem Füllstift in jeder Klammeröffnung das Schieberplättchen zurückschieben muß.

In den nachfolgenden Darlegungen soll das Grundprinzip der Nähvorrichtung und des Nähvorganges in dem neuen Apparat mathematisch eingehend erklärt werden.

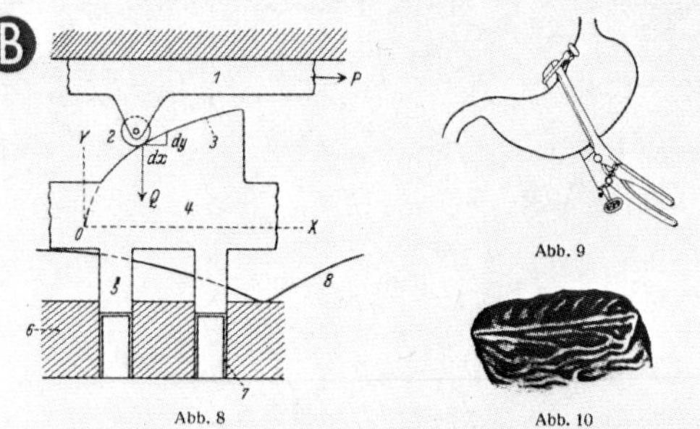

Abb. 8

Abb. 9

Abb. 10

In der Abb. 8 zeigt Y die Richtung der Bewegung der Klammer und X die zu der Bewegungsrichtung der Klammer rechtwinklige Richtung. Zieht man die Triebstange 1 in der Richtung X, so preßt das Gleitkügelchen 2 infolge seiner Gleitbewegung entlang der Ebene 3 des Fortsatzes 4 in der Richtung —Y nach unten. Für diese Preßwirkung nach unten bilden die Teile 5 und 6 die Ableitungen. Der Reibungswiderstand zwischen 5 und 6 ist dabei sehr gering, weil die Teile sehr genau ineinanderpassend ausgebildet sind.

Fig I–14.—A and **B,** M. Tomoda, 1937. Although the instrument appears superficially like the von Petz, its mechanism was in fact radically different. The wheel at the end made the instrument easier to operate. As it was turned, the shaft was pulled back, the three small wheels, *15,* each simultaneously riding up on a cam, *4,* to which the bar holding the staple-driving fins was attached, simultaneously driving in all the staples with a few turns of the wheel. The degree to which the driving wheel was tightened allowed some difference in the tightness of stapling for thicker or thinner tissues. The staples are shown to close again in a **B** (i.e., in the form of a **B**). He reported (1937) a successful gastrectomy experience in nine patients with his stapler, starting in 1935. (From M. Tomoda, 1937.)

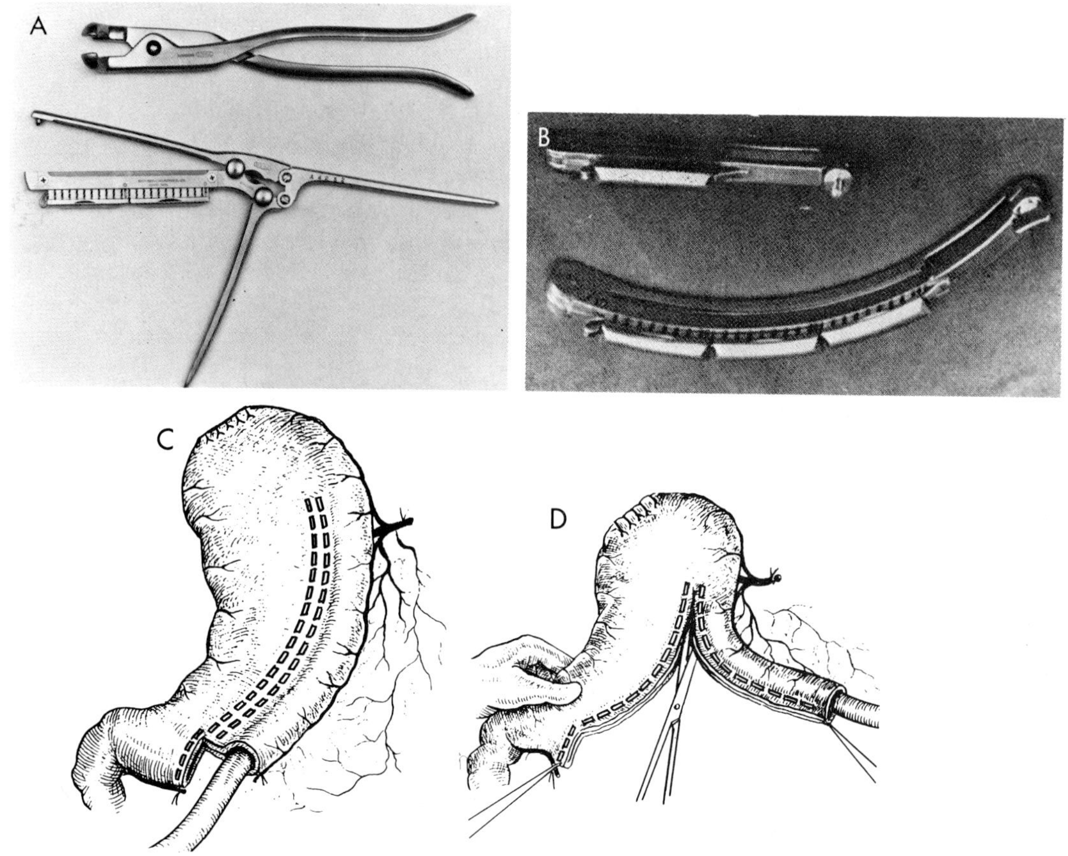

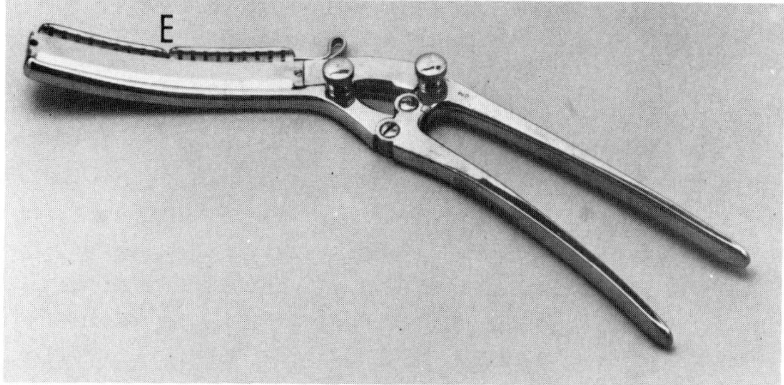

Fig I–15.—Japanese modifications of von Petz instruments. **A,** K. Nakayama's instrument (1954). Nakayama simplified the von Petz instrument, still utilizing two rows of B-shaped German silver staples. The staples were loaded in the instrument jaw, the jaws closed, and the two staple-driving units, seen hanging down from the jaw, pressed down by the massive pliers. (See also Pimenta's 1980 instrument, Fig I–3.) Perhaps the most attractive feature of this simple instrument is the slot in the slender upper jaw—not visible in the photograph— which permits scalpel division of the tissues between the two staple lines while the clamp still holds the viscus firmly. (Photograph courtesy of Dr. H. Akiyama.) **B– E,** H. Uchiyama, 1962. This modification of the Nakayama clamp, devised for the creation of greater-curvature gastric tubes in various models, has one or three of the pusher bar units to drive in the staples by compression with massive pliers, and is supplied with or without handles. (**B–D** From H. Uchiyama, T. Tokunaga, and T. Kajisa, *Annals of Surgery,* 1962, used by permission of the publisher.) The model shown with handles

Fig I–15 (cont.).—(E)—essentially a curved Nakayama instrument—was presented to M.M.R. by Dr. H.J. Heimlich. (Photograph courtesy of the Smithsonian Institution.)

H. von Seeman (1934) described a quite simple stapler (Fig I–16) specifically for transsacral amputation of the rectum, which he pictures, but useful he thought also for stomach and bowel. He had demonstrated his instrument at a meeting of the Munich Surgical Society, before the report of Friedrich's instrument. Perhaps because, unlike all other staplers, tissue apposition and staple driving were not separate steps, this instrument does not seem to have been taken up.

Friedrich of Ulm (1934) contributed an instrument that represented a substantial advance over the Hültl and von Petz instruments. Friedrich continued to use the coarse, flat wire, German silver staples of von Petz, but the configuration of the instrument was changed entirely (Fig I–17A,B). The two jaws slid down against each other with a compression of the handles. The release of a catch allowed a second compression of the handles to drive in the staples in two parallel, Indian-file rows. The staples closed in the now-familiar B shape. Another major advance in the instrument was the provision of removable cartridges that could be preloaded, permitting repeated use of the instrument in a single operation, which was not practical with the von Petz or Hültl instruments because of the time involved in reloading. The closure still was considered merely a temporary hemostatic seal, and always inverted by conventional sutures. The instrument seems not to have been widely used, but the exemplar we have used in the laboratory, and which now is at the Smithsonian Institution, was used by Dr. Dallas Phemister at the University of Chicago. W. Heneage Ogilvie of Guy's Hospital, writing in the *British Medical Journal* (1935) on gastrectomy, pictures the use of Friedrich's instrument, saying,

"The Petz sewing clamp, which crushes the line of intended section and then inserts a double row of tiny metal clips across the crushed line, has made such suture a job of the greatest simplicity. The original Petz clamp was a cumbersome instrument, and had to be reloaded between each application. The latest form, which has been made by Heinrich C. Ulrich of Ulm to the suggestions of Neuffer in Professor Friedrich's clinic, is much simpler, and carries the clips in separate magazines, so that it can be used for several suture lines in succession. In physiological gastrectomy the pyloric section is finished with one application of the clamp and a row of Lembert sutures. The Finsterer anastomosis is done by closing the whole cut surface with the clamp and reinforcing the right half of this line with a double row of Lembert sutures: the left half remains closed and clean while the first line of the anastomosis is being sewn, and is only opened up for the haemostatic suture. Further time is saved because the cut surfaces of that part of the stomach which is to be removed are securely closed against leakage.''

An elegant and versatile instrument was presented in Vienna by Hans von Brücke of Innsbruck (1935). In contrast to all the previous stapling instruments, von Brücke's allowed for the repeated individual placement of single staples (Fig I–18A,B). The staples are loaded on a bar with a square cross-section, much as in a paper stapler, and held against the mechanism by a spring. Each squeeze of the handles compressed the tissues and drove in a staple. The illustration (Fig I–18B) shows the staples closing the bowel on the patient's side of an intestinal resection and then, as with all previous stapling instruments, the suture inversion of the staple closure. In the illustrated case, the inversion of the stapled end is with pursestring sutures. He did not mention the number of the staples in a load or their character. He made reference to clinical use in stomach, small bowel, and colon, and showed x-rays of a gastrectomy in which the staples are visible three months after operation. The configuration of the closed staples is not known to us. The von Brücke instrument obviously is the precursor of a Russian instrument for repetitive placement of individual staples from a magazine-loaded instrument (see Fig I–19F,G). Later, a similar instrument, but magazine loaded, with 15 staples, for placing single staples in bowel or blood vessel was presented in the United States by Cooper, Mallina, and Tolins (1967) (see Fig I–18*C-E*). A similar instrument was presented by Rygg, (Bertelsen and Rygg, 1967) (Fig I–18*F,G*), in Denmark, for placing a series of individual staples in manually apposed everted blood vessel edges. The cartridge holds ten staples each in its own plastic case, but each case must be separately loaded in the staple-driving clamps. After abundant use in experimental animals, they reported, in patients, closure of 52 transverse femoral arteriotomies, 28 femoral or iliac patch grafts, 60 staplings of intima after endarterectomy, all without hemorrhage or thrombosis (see Fig I–18*G* "*5, 6, and 7*"). Neither the Cooper nor the Rygg instrument gained acceptance. Samuels (1955) and Vogelfanger and Beattie (1958), all from Canada, used a technique of applying singly what were essentially miniature Michel clips to flanges of everted vessels.

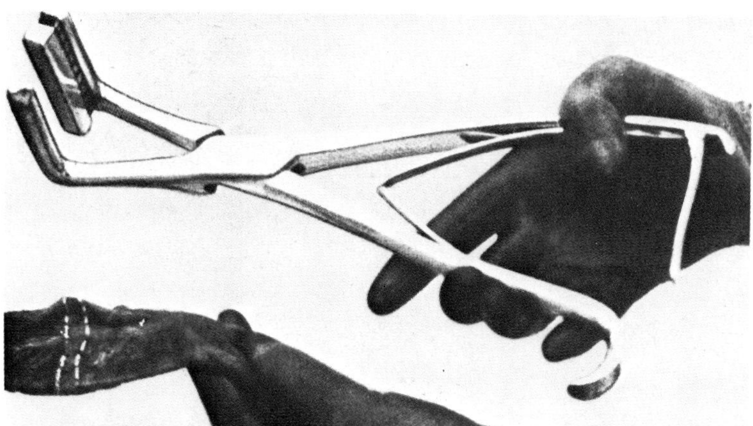

Fig I–16.—von Seeman's (1934) stapling clamp for closure of rectum or bowel. von Seeman's simple instrument, which he said he presented at the Munich Surgical Society before Friedrich's publication appeared (Fig I–17A), seems to have a floating hand-loaded staple cartridge. Unlike all of the other stapling instruments, von Seeman's operated with a single compression of the clamp, which approximated the tissues as simultaneously increasing pressure on the clamp drove the staple-driving fins, in the upper jaw, down through the floating staple magazine to complete the closure. The illustration indicates the same coarse German silver staples used by von Petz and Friedrich. The two rows of staples are sufficiently separated to permit division of the tissues between them. (From H. von Seeman, 1934.)

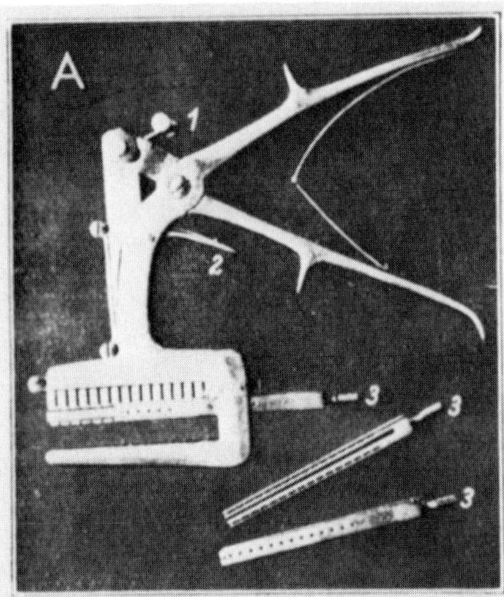

Abb. 1. Letztes Modell. Die Klammer-
kammer ist, um sie sichtbar zu machen,
nur zur Hälfte eingeschoben. Neben dem
Apparat 2 Reserveklammerkammern. Hin-
sichtlich der Hebel 1 und 2 siehe die Be-
schreibung der Anwendungsweise

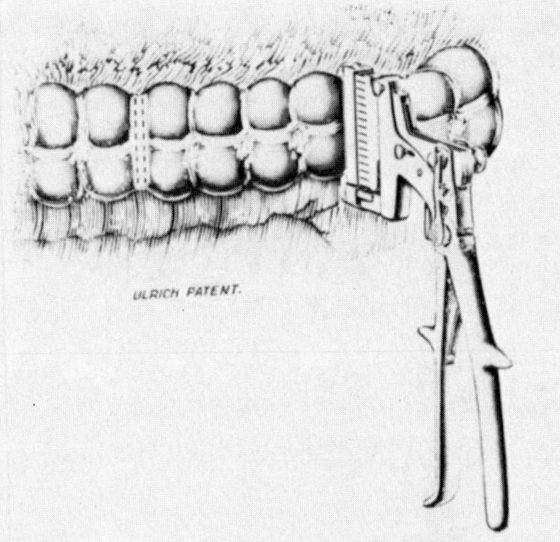

Abb. 2 zeigt die Anwendung des Apparates
am Dickdarm

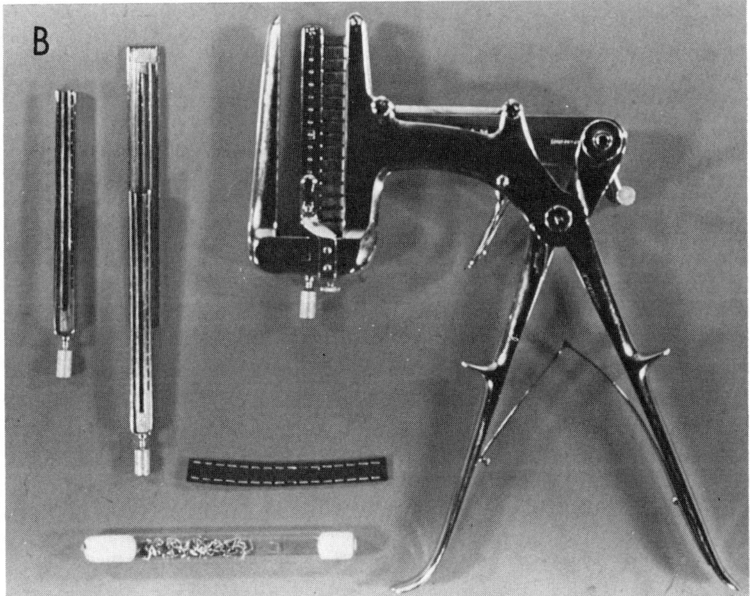

Fig I–17.—Gastrointestinal stapler of H. Friedrich, 1934. **A,** reproduction from Friedrich's publication referring to his "latest model." Interchangeable cartridges could be preloaded, permitting repeated use of the instrument in a single operation. A squeeze of the handles closed the jaws of the instrument, the release *(1)* being thrown and the handles again squeezed, two rows of staples were driven in. The bowel then was to be divided manually. (From H. Friedrich, 1934.) **B,** model of the instrument owned by Dallas Phemister at the University of Chicago, and now at the Smithsonian Institution. Division of the bowel after stapling resulted in only a single staple line, which then was always manually inverted, but the operation of the instrument was infinitely simpler than that of the von Petz and Hültl instruments and the interchangeable cartridges represented a real advance.

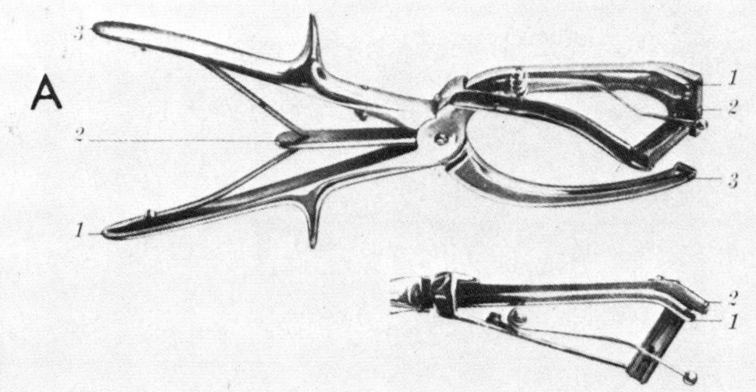

Abb. 1. Oben: Ansicht des Instrumentes von der Seite her. Unten: Ansicht der vorderen Hälfte des Instrumentes von oben gesehen. Einzelheiten siehe Text

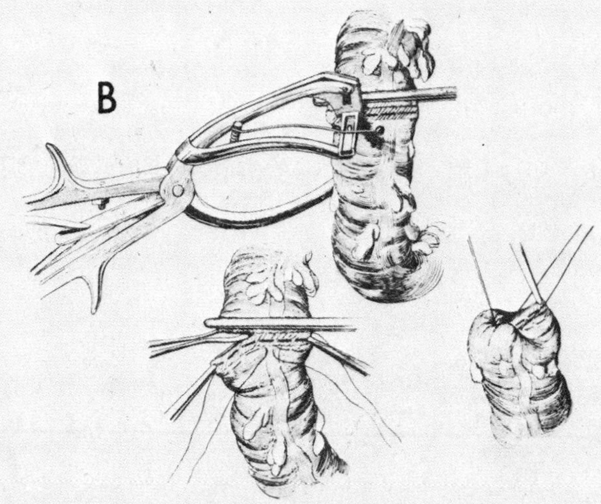

Abb. 2. Verwendung der Nähzange zur Dickdarmresektion. Oben: Darmquetsche liegt am wegfallenden Darmabschnitt. Anlegen der Metallklammern in einer Quetschfurche. Unten links: Zwei halbe Tabaksbeutelnähte sind angelegt, Durchtrennen des Darmes mit dem Glühbrenner. Unten rechts: Einstülpen der Klammernaht mit Hilfe der vorher angelegten halben Tabaksbeutelnähte

Fig I–18.—Instruments for placing individual staples. **A** and **B,** von Brücke, 1935. Instrument for serial placement of individual staples. (From H. von Brücke, 1935.)   *(continued)*

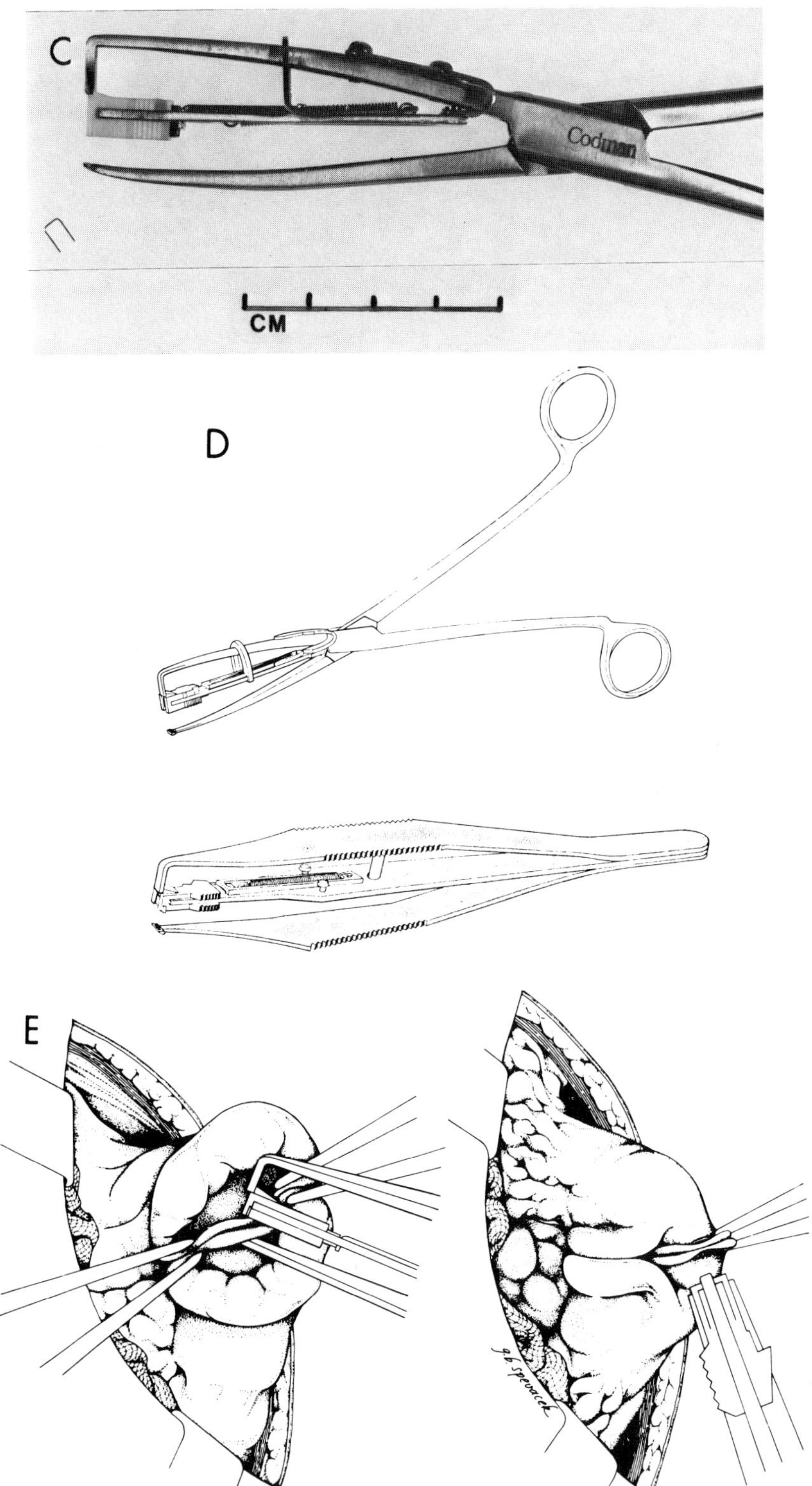

Fig I–18 C–E.—See legend on facing page.

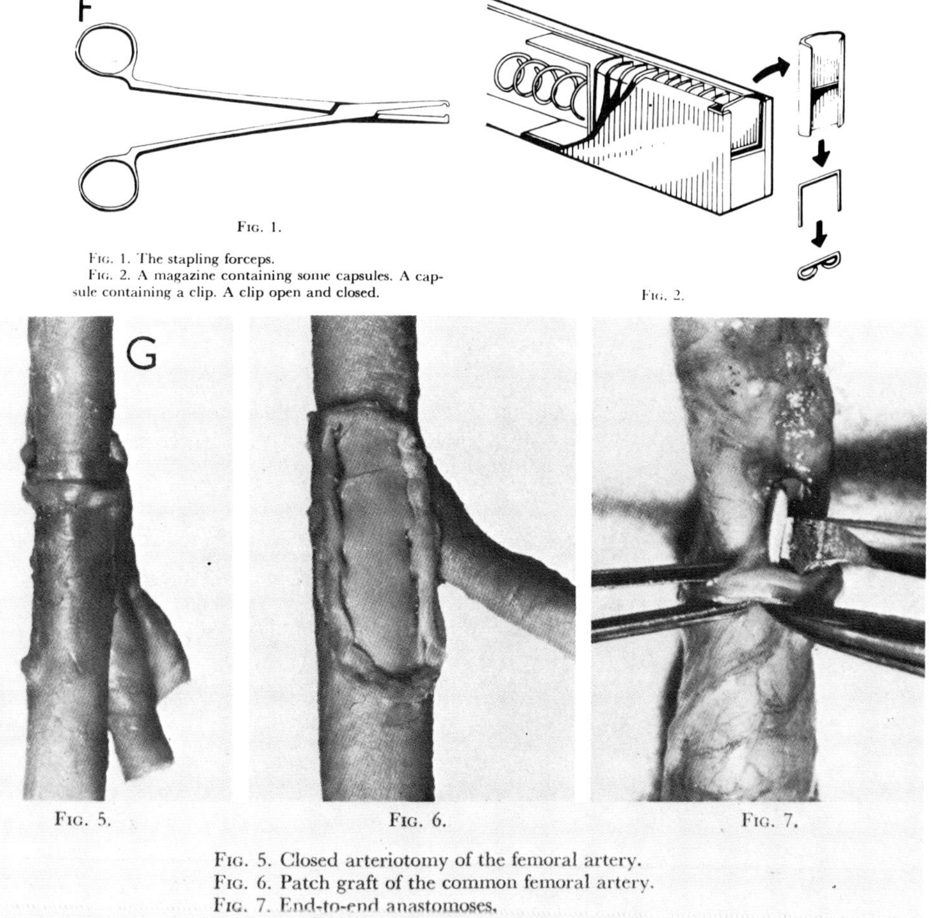

Fig. 1.

Fig. 1. The stapling forceps.
Fig. 2. A magazine containing some capsules. A capsule containing a clip. A clip open and closed.

Fig. 2.

Fig. 5.

Fig. 6.

Fig. 7.

Fig. 5. Closed arteriotomy of the femoral artery.
Fig. 6. Patch graft of the common femoral artery.
Fig. 7. End-to-end anastomoses.

Fig I–18 (cont.).—C–E, P. Cooper, R.F. Mallina, and S.H. Tolins, June, 1967. Instrument for repetitive placement of fine individual staples here shown creating by triangulation an inverting-everting anastomosis in small bowel, the posterior row inverting, the side rows everting. Experimentally, success was reported with its use in small and large bowel and in blood vessels. Note the tiny cartridge, holding 15 staples. (**D** and **E** from P. Cooper, R.F. Mallina, and S.H. Tolins, *American Journal of Surgery,* 1967, with permission.)

F and **G,** S. Bertelsen and I.H. Rygg, November, 1967—the instrument sold in Scandinavia as "Dr. Rygg's stapling device." (From S. Bertelsen and I.H. Rygg, *S.G.&O.,* 1967, used by permission.)

THE SOVIET RUSSIAN INSTRUMENTS

A major step in the development of stapling instruments was the undertaking, in Moscow at the Scientific Research Institute for Experimental Surgical Apparatus and Instruments, of a systematic program for the development of stapling instruments for every conceivable surgical application. Gudov's (1950) stapling instrument for vascular anastomoses appears to have been the first instrument described (Fig I–19*A,B*). There then developed an entire series of complicated vascular stapling instruments (Androsov, 1956, 1956, 1956). These produced mathematically perfect, circular, everting end-to-end or end-to-side anastomoses without any narrowing, the staples invisible from the lumen. The instruments have been sharply limited in their clinical application because they require essentially normal vessels and relatively long, free segments for eversion of the vessel ends. The beautifully engineered instruments are complicated, have many individual parts (see Fig I–19*A*), and their use requires a considerable number of steps. One can learn to sew a vascular anastomosis by hand more quickly than one can master the involved instruments, as we have shown in experiments with medical students. However, once the instrumental technique has been learned, it is faster and it does produce perfect vascular anastomoses. Instruments were also produced that permit end-to-side stapled vascular anastomoses (see Fig I–19*C–E*) (Androsov, 1962 or later). Somewhat simplified versions of these instruments were devised by Vogelfanger and associates in Canada (Vogelfanger and Beattie, 1958; Vogelfanger, Beattie, Brown, Devitt, Scobie, and Scobie, 1962), by the Japanese (Nakayama, Tamiya, Yamamoto, and Akimoto, 1962; Inokuchi and Kusaba, 1974), and in the United States by Mallina, Miller, Cooper, and Christie (1962), whose instrument (see Fig I–21) was a lightweight, direct modification of the Russian vascular stapler, but made undependable by its very lightness and simplification. We have not used the Russian vascular instruments clinically and some of the U.S. and Canadian instruments were used only experimentally by their authors.

Apart from the vascular instruments, an extremely broad range of Russian instruments was developed, which may be divided into several groups.

1. A magazine-loaded instrument for the repeated placement of individual staples as in the everted edges of blood vessels being anastomosed (Fig I–19*F,G*). The instrument is much like von Brücke's (see Fig I–18*A,B*), and we found it too heavy for convenient use. The Cooper and the Rygg instruments (see Fig I–18*C-G*) represent partially successful attempts to fashion more delicate instruments for the purpose. More recently, the Russians (Petrova, Rabinovich, Kapitanov, and Bogomolova, 1975) have developed a substantially more delicate stapler, the SB-2, in the shape of forceps with exchangeable magazines containing eight staples each. The round drum-shaped magazines are loaded manually. They tested it experimentally in applying a patch graft to the pulmonary artery in dogs and indicated its use in the serial application of staples to end-to-end and end-to-side vascular anastomoses.

2. Instruments for terminal or tangential linear closure (Androsov, 19)—bronchi, pulmonary vessels, auricular appendage, pulmonary parenchyma, and elements of the GI tract (Fig I–19*H–R*). The instruments resemble nesting Ls, the staple cartridge in the short leg of the inner L and the anvil in the short leg of the outer L. Metal cartridges were preloaded by hand with fine wire staples, originally of tantalum and then of a steel alloy. The instruments required to be partially disassembled to replace cartridges (Fig I–19*J*). For cleaning between operations, the entire instrument had to be taken apart. The staple-driving fins, on a rod inside the instrument, were delicate and subject to injury and the instruments suffered when dismantled for cleaning and then were reas-

sembled. Each instrument could accept only a cartridge with a single type of staple pattern. For each change in pattern of the staple line, another instrument was required. The jaws were approximated by turning a knurled knob and the staples driven in by squeezing handles. In the gastrointestinal tract, and sometimes in the lung parenchyma but not in the bronchus, it was considered essential to invert the stapled stump either manually or by one of the two entirely different instruments devised to accomplish this. A similar instrument with a slightly altered pattern of the staple line was manufactured for closing the atrial appendage or atrium, but we have found no need for this variation. The UKL—and American TA^{TM}—proved to be satisfactory for closing the atrium, as in pneumonectomy with intrapericardial resection of pulmonary veins. The paper by N.M. Amosov and K.K. Berezovsky of Kiev (1961) says that the UKL "was designed in 1957 at the Moscow Research Institute for Experimental Surgical Apparatus and Instruments by N.S. Gorkin and A.K. Strekopytov. . . ." The earliest paper we have found is, in fact, that of Androsov in 1955 (Androsov, Potekhina, Savchenko, Strekopytov, Thliakova, and Sheinber, 1955). The instrument was fully described though not yet named, and was used on the bronchus in three pneumonectomies. One complicated L-shaped instrument (UTL) with two sets of jaws (Fig I–19*L–P*) permitted one to place a double row of staggered staples across the stomach, release the distal jaw, and tuck back the stapled closure through the still-open proximal jaw, which then was closed and staples driven home, inverting the first closure. A quite different-appearing instrument (UKZh) devised especially for long suture lines (up to 10 cm) on the stomach, and dubbed by the Russians the "crocodile" (Fig I–19*S–V*), was used by some Russian surgeons (Androsov 19 , 1965, 1970) for the same purpose.

3. An instrument for the creation of side-to-side gastrointestinal anastomoses (Fig I–19*W–Z*). The Russian instrument (NZhKA) (Androsov 19 , Svinkin, 1964) consists of two limbs to be inserted into the lumina of the loops, the instrument halves then being mated and locked. In one limb there are two rows of hand-inserted staples separated by a slot for a knife, in the other the anvils. As the knife is pushed through, it serially drives in the staples on each side and divides the stapled tissue midway between the staple lines. The minute channels, for the delicate pushers that drive in the small staples, tend to become encrusted with coagulated protein, so that the operation of the instrument becomes stiffer and stiffer with each clinical use. Whereas the instrument initially can be activated with the thumb pushing the knife home, there is provided in addition a bar and fulcrum arrangement to drive the knife handle in step by step when, after repeated use, operation of the instrument becomes difficult. As well, with each use, the knife dulls. Ultimately, it is necessary for an expert mechanic to disassemble the instrument, clean and reassemble the tiny individual staple drivers, and adjust the instrument. The fine staples, as in all the Russian instruments, are loaded by hand before or during each operation. If there is any difficulty with the staple drivers, the services of an expert machinist are required to readjust them. The instrument delivers only two rows of staples, resulting in a single row of staples on each side of the division, so that this always was reinforced manually. The single opening, resulting from division of the stapled septum between the two openings made for insertion of the limbs of the instrument, was closed with a pursestring suture, which we modified to a Connell type suture (Ravitch and Rivarola, 1966), inserted with the GIA^{TM} limbs in place and tightened as the instrument is withdrawn. A special miniaturized anastomosing instrument of this kind has been made for use in the newborn.

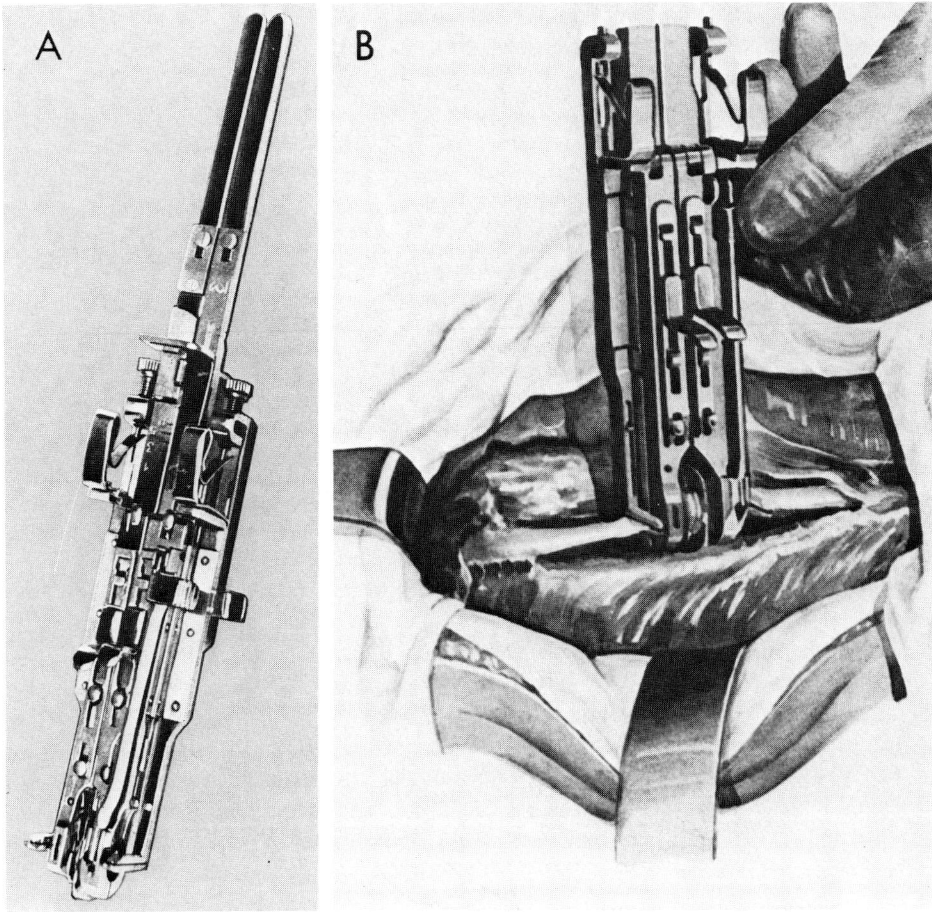

Fig I–19.—The Russian stapling instruments. Beginning with a vascular anastomotic instrument in 1950 (Gudov), the Russians at the Research Institute for Experimental Surgical Apparatus and Instruments in Moscow developed an extraordinary variety of stapling instruments for special purposes and in varying sizes. **A** and **B,** the end-to-end vascular anastomotic stapler ASTs. The two halves of the stapler are shown assembled, mated, and locked. The occluding vascular clamps on both sides are also part of the apparatus. In essence, split cartridge and anvil bushings are placed over the proximal and distal vessel ends, which are everted and held on the two bushings by bivalved ring clamps on the apparatus. With the instrument halves now mated and locked, the depression of a lever drives the staples from the cartridge bushing through the everted vessel ends and forms the staples on the anvils on the other bushing. The instrument then is disassembled, the bushings split apart and removed, leaving a perfect everting anastomosis. (From P.I. Androsov, 19).

C–E, instrument for end-to-side vascular anastomosis, as for portacaval shunt—USTs (Androsov, 1962 or later; Kukushkin, 1964). The U-shaped clamp occludes the vena cava and locks into the rest of the assembly. The portal vein is everted over the anvil bushing. The vena cava, held in the forks of the special clamp, is incised. The portal vein, everted on its bushing, is inserted through the incision in the vena cava, the edges of which are compressed, intima to intima against the portal vein. A bivalved staple cartridge is fitted around the vessels coapted over the anvil bushing, the staples driven in and the instrument removed. (Instrument photograph courtesy of the Smithsonian Institution.) (Instrument drawings from P.I. Androsov, 1962 or later.)

→

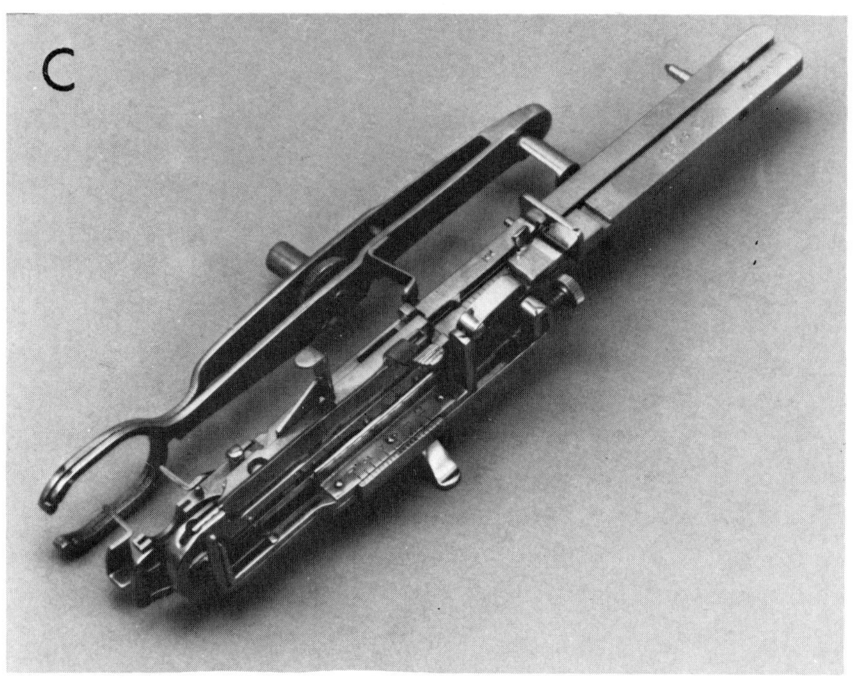

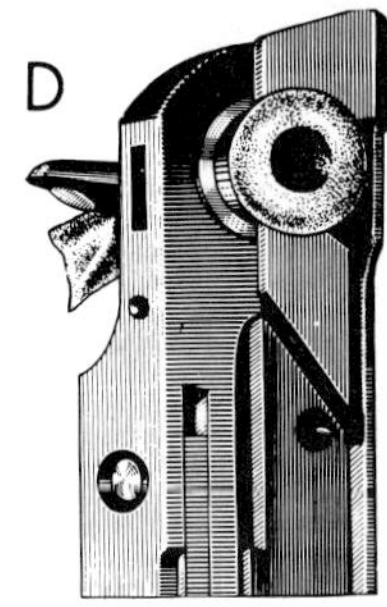

Fig. 56. Evertion of vessel to be connected onto bush

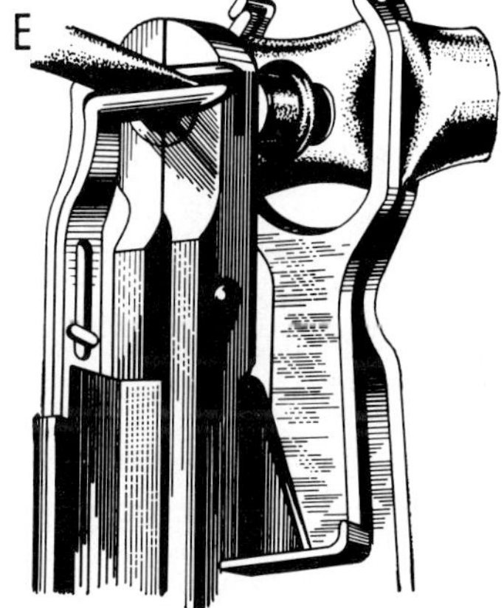

Fig. 58. Insertion of vessel to be connected into opening in principal vessel

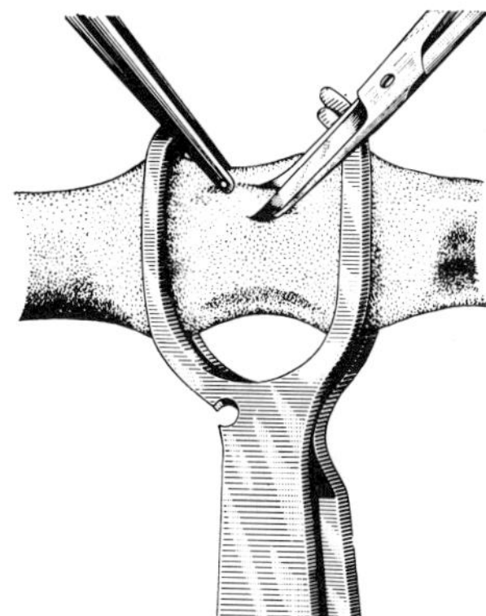

Fig. 57. Incision of opening in anterior vessel wall

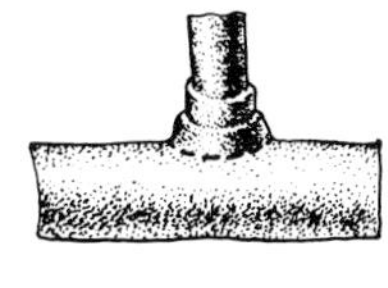

Fig. 59. Vessels sutured end-to-side

Fig I–19 C–E.—See legend on facing page.

(continued)

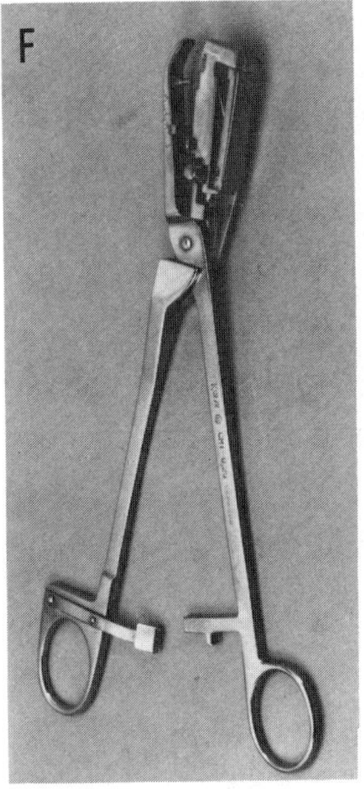

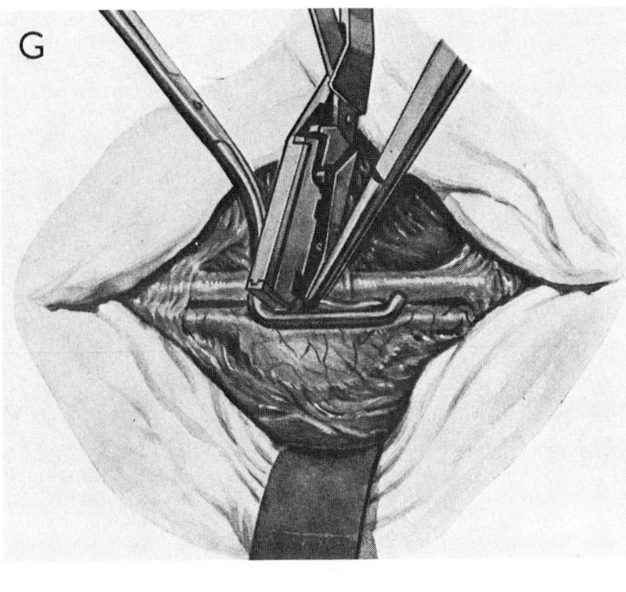

Fig I–19 (cont.).—**F** and **G,** instrument for repeated placement of individual staples from a magazine-loaded instrument—SMT. The instrument is reminiscent of von Brücke's 1935 device (Fig I–18**A,B**), and of the later Cooper (Fig I–18**C–E**) and Rygg (Fig I–18 **F,G,**) devices. It comes in varying sizes for application to a variety of tissues. In laboratory use, we found it rather coarse and cumbersome. (Operative drawing from P.I. Androsov, 19 . Instrument photograph courtesy of the Smithsonian Institution.)

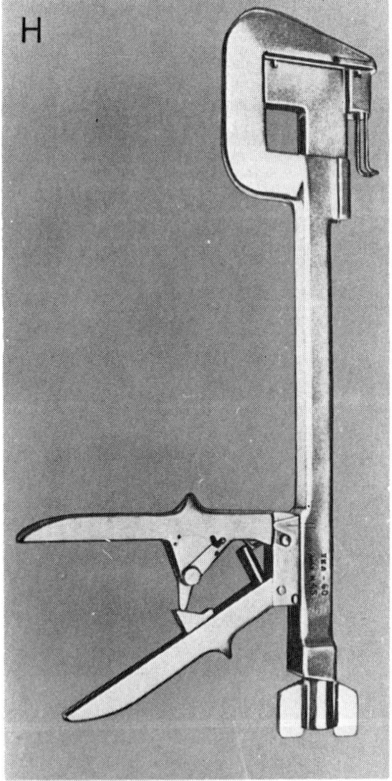

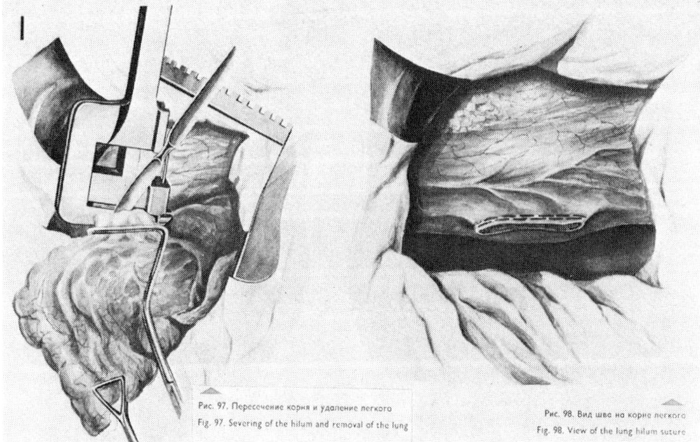

Fig I–19 (cont.).—**H** and **I,** the UKL instrument (Azina, 1956). This is the prototype of the double sliding-L type of instrument. The tissues are approximated by turning a wing nut or knurled nut. The tissue-retaining pin is visible. A squeeze of the jaws drives down a slender rod, in the handle, to which are attached the fine fins that push in each staple. This instrument delivers a double staggered row of staples and is widely used for a variety of purposes. It is shown here securing the entire pulmonary hilus—bronchus, veins, and pulmonary artery. (From P.I. Androsov, 19 .)

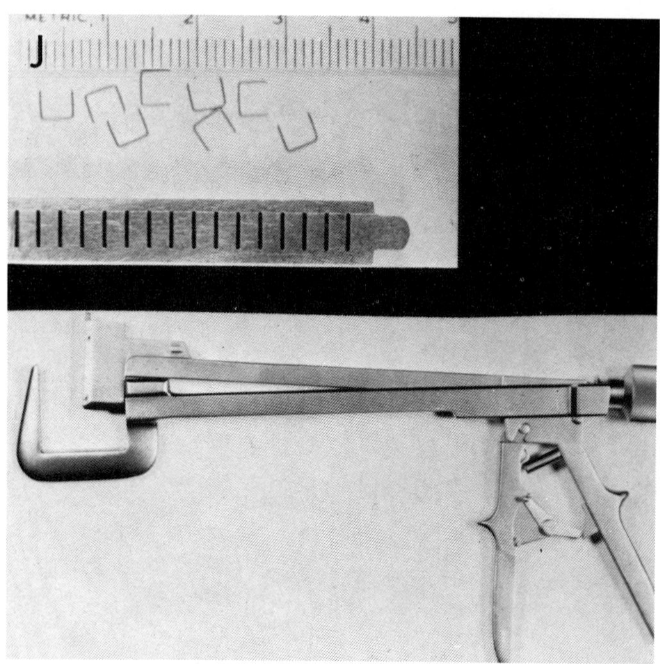

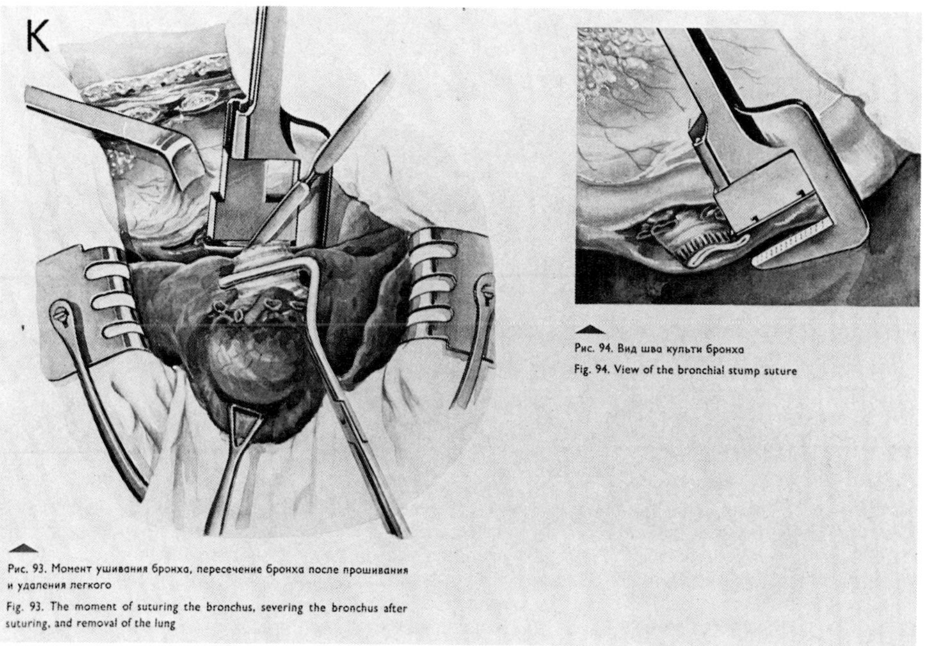

Fig I–19 (cont.).—J–K, the bronchial stapler—UKB (Androsov, Potekhina, Savchenko, Strekopytov, Thliakova, and Sheinber, 1955). In this case, the staples are aligned across the cartridge, in the long axis of the bronchus to produce less interference with the vascularity of the cut end. **J,** photograph of the instrument that we obtained in Leningrad in 1958 and began using in the laboratory and the clinic at that time. The instrument now is in the Smithsonian Institution. The Russian instruments of this general type had removable cartridges and, at that time, tantalum staples, subsequently replaced by stainless steel staples. The photograph shows the degree to which the instrument was required to be disassembled in order to exchange cartridges. The cartridges were steel and loaded by hand. From M.M. Ravitch, I.W. Brown, and G.F. Daviglus, *Surgery,* 1959, used by permission.) **K,** application to pneumonectomy. (From: P.I. Androsov, 19 .) Although we found the instrument satisfactory, the much more widely applicable UKL type instrument (Fig I–19**H,I**) placing a double staggered staple line, the staple bars parallel to the cut end of the bronchus, was just as satisfactory, and obviated the need for a special instrument for the bronchus.

(continued)

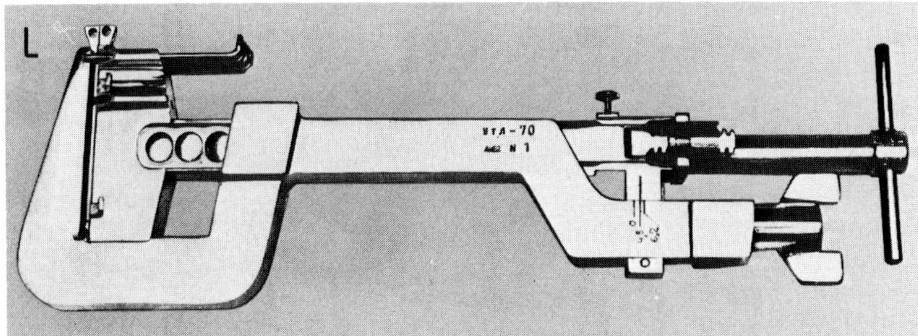

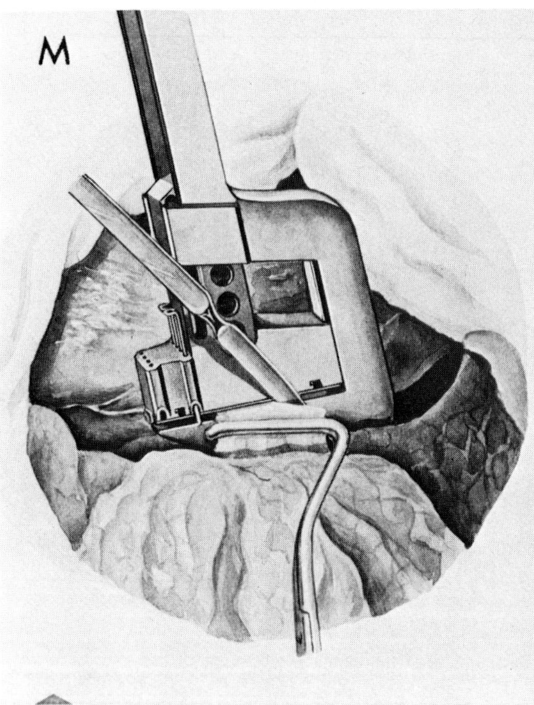

Рис. 106. Пересечение корня и удаление легкого

Fig. 106. Severing of the lung hilum and removal of the lung

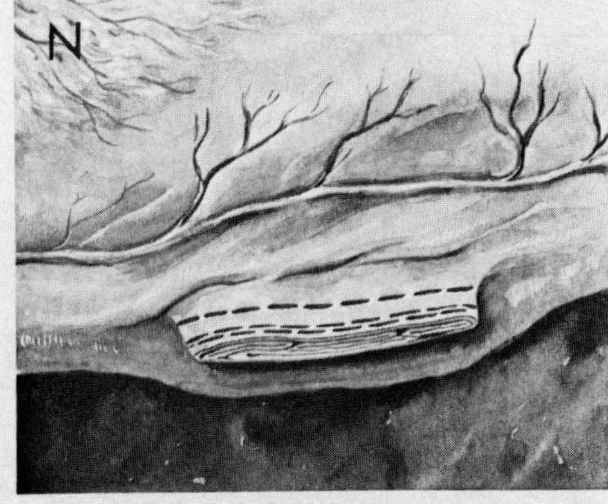

Рис. 107. Вид шва, наложенного аппаратом на корень легкого

Fig. 107. View of the suture applied to the lung hilum by the use of th apparatus

Fig I–19 (cont.).—L–P, the UTL-70 double-jawed instrument **(L),** designed for placing a single row of reinforcing staples behind the double staggered row as shown in the illustration of suture of the entire hilus in pneumonectomy (Fig I–19 **M,N.**)

Alternatively, as in gastric transection (Fig I–19 **O,P**), the one activation of the instrument drives in the double staggered suture line, then, with the distal upper jaw released, the stapled end is inverted and closure of the more proximal jaw drives in a single row of staples, inverting the double row. (From P.I. Androsov, 19 .) This worked quite well in practice and with a little experience we found it not difficult to perform, but the inversion of the stapled suture line of the portions of the intestinal tract, whether manually or by machine, proved in our experience to be quite unnecessary. →

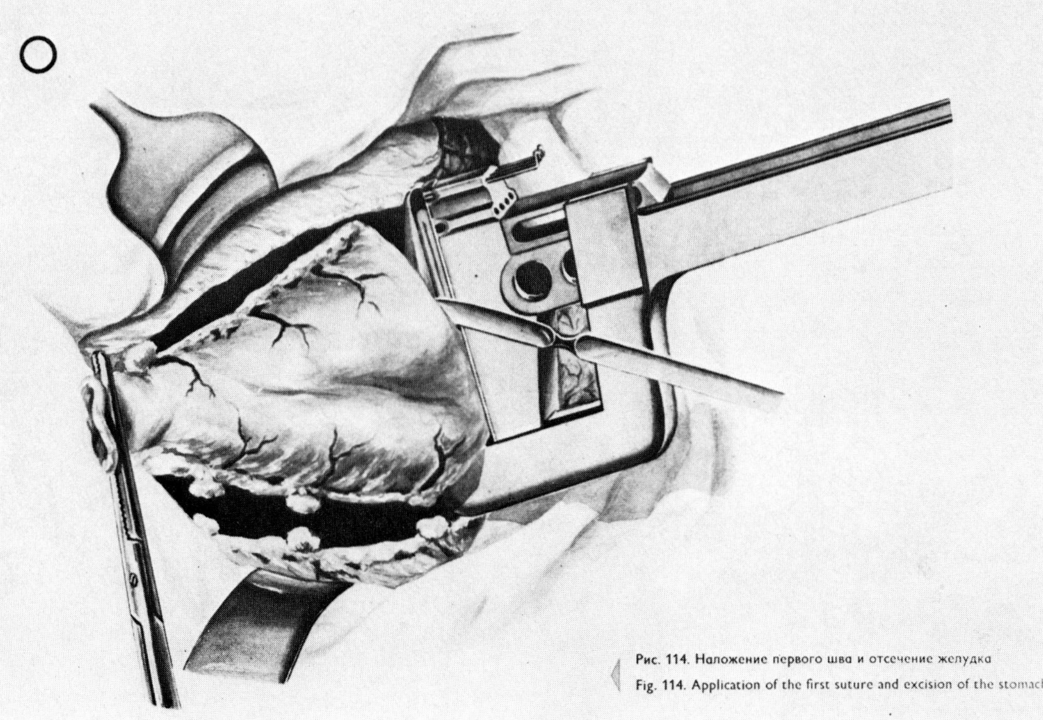

Рис. 114. Наложение первого шва и отсечение желудка
Fig. 114. Application of the first suture and excision of the stomach

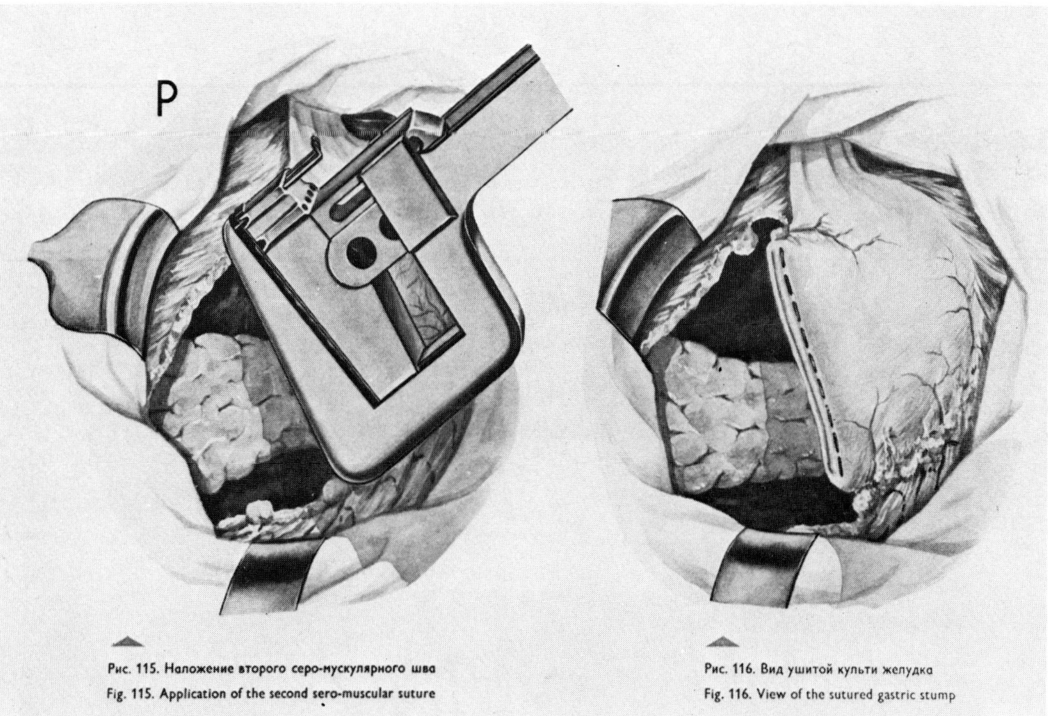

Рис. 115. Наложение второго серо-мускулярного шва
Fig. 115. Application of the second sero-muscular suture

Рис. 116. Вид ушитой культи желудка
Fig. 116. View of the sutured gastric stump

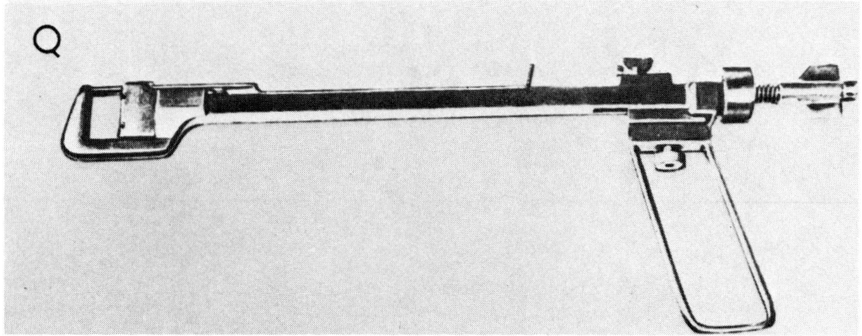

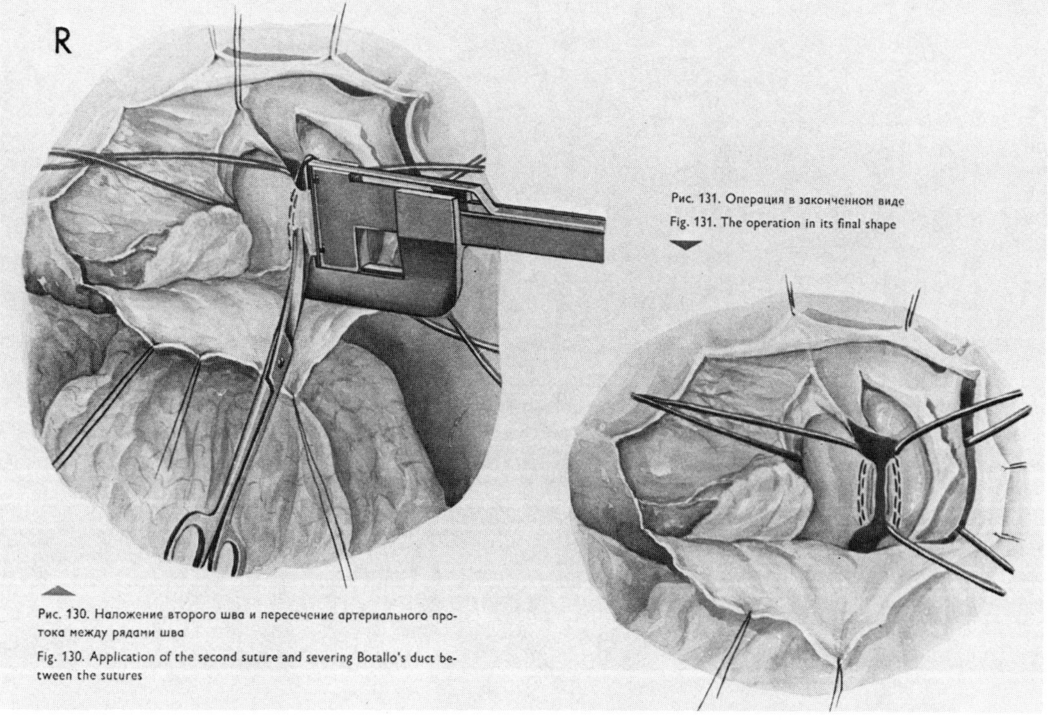

Рис. 131. Операция в законченном виде
Fig. 131. The operation in its final shape

Рис. 130. Наложение второго шва и пересечение артериального протока между рядами шва

Fig. 130. Application of the second suture and severing Botallo's duct between the sutures

Fig I–19 (cont.).—**Q** and **R,** instrument (UAP) for closure of the patent ductus. This extremely delicate instrument of the series was fine enough to be applied twice to the ductus arteriosus, which then could be divided between the two double rows of staples. (From P.I. Androsov, 19 .) There is abundant clinical experience with stapling of the patent ductus and the American TA 30™ stapler has been used to close Potts' aorticopulmonary anastomoses at the time of total correction of the tetralogy of Fallot (Leand, Bender, Martz, Crisler, Agnew, and Gott, 1971).   *(continued)*

←

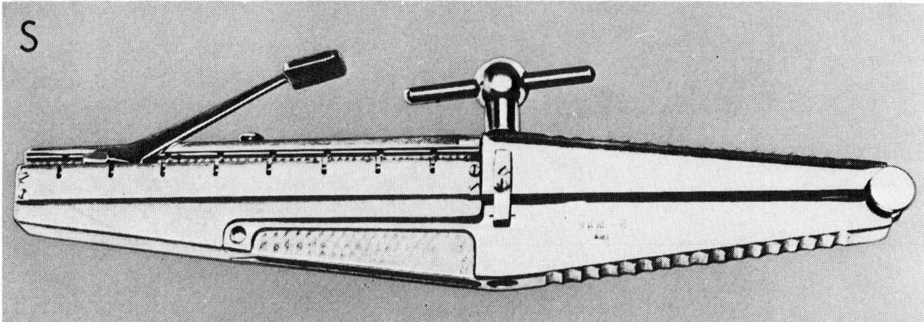

Fig I–19 (cont.).—S–V, instrument for gastric closure (UKZh) (Fig I-19**S**) this instrument (called by the Russians the "Crocodile") serves for closure of the stomach (Fig I–19**T**) with a double staggered row of staples, the closure then being inverted by a single row of staples. As with the UTL, the second, inverting, application of the staples is not through and through. When the distal jaws of the instrument are released, a special instrument (Fig I–19**U**) is used to displace the stapled end while the stomach still is held sufficiently by the proximal jaws so that the end is inverted and another row of staples driven in. Figure I–19**V** shows diagrammatically the nature of the closure and the appearance of the stomach. A single row of staples now is visible. (From P.I. Androsov, 19 .) →

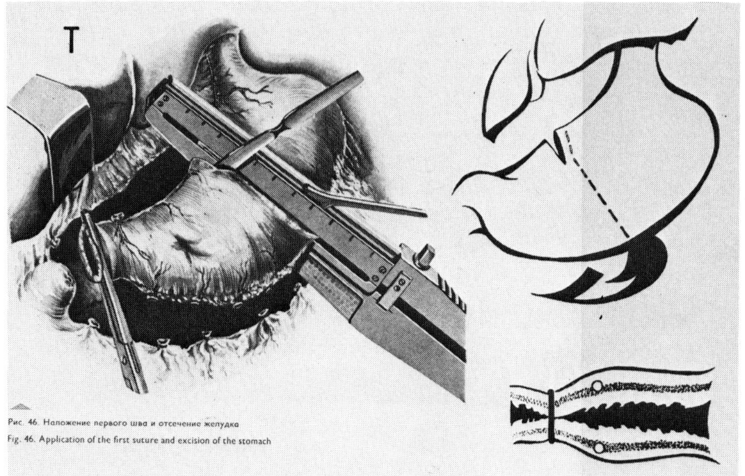

Рис. 46. Наложение первого шва и отсечение желудка
Fig. 46. Application of the first suture and excision of the stomach

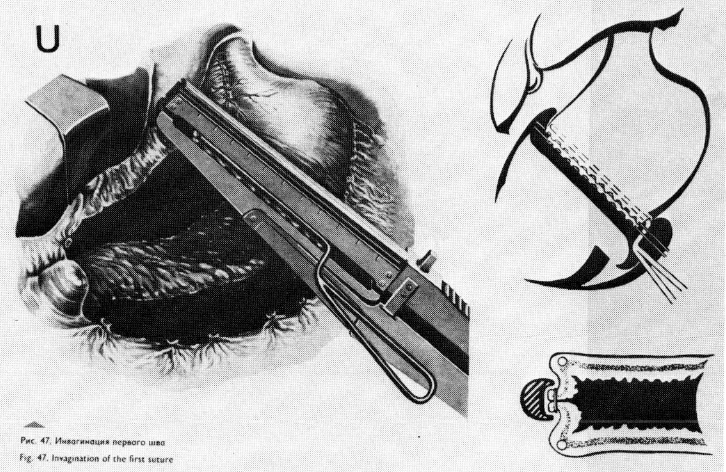

Рис. 47. Инвагинация первого шва
Fig. 47. Invagination of the first suture

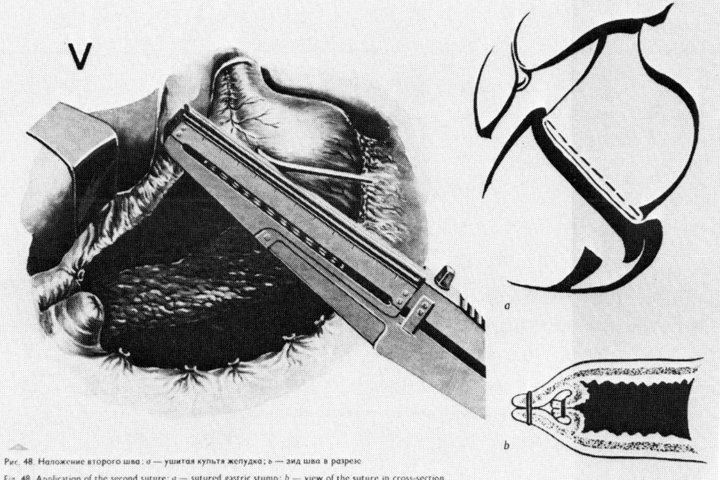

Рис. 48. Наложение второго шва: *a* — ушитая культя желудка; *в* — вид шва в разрезе
Fig. 48. Application of the second suture: *a* — sutured gastric stump; *b* — view of the suture in cross-section

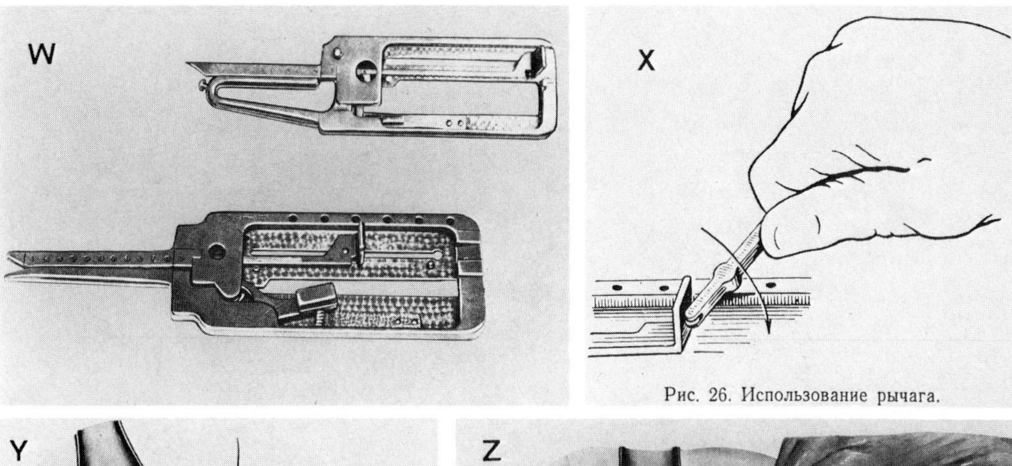

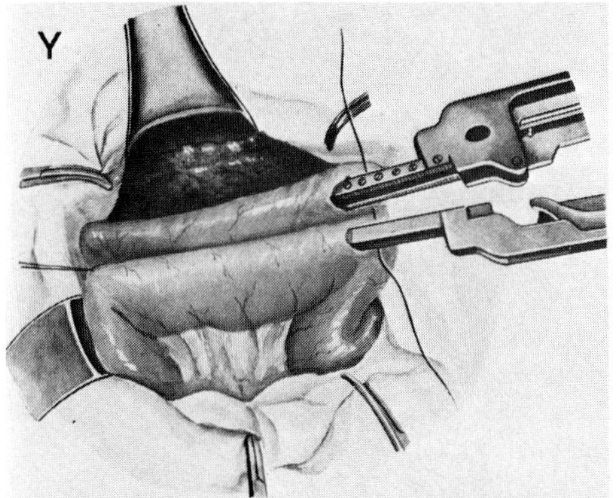

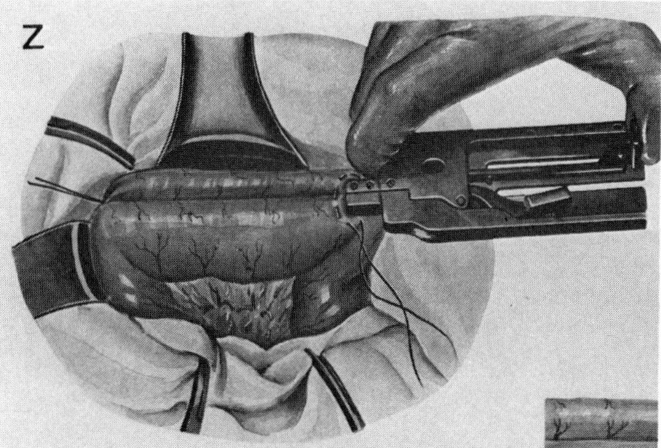

Fig I–19 (cont.).—W–Z, Side-to-side gastrointestinal anastomosing instrument (NZhKA) (Bobrov and Gritsman, 1960). The pediatric and adult models of the side-to-side intestinal anastomosing instrument **(W).** With the prongs of the instrument in the two lumina, and the instrument locked, a knife blade is advanced by pushing on the bar **(Y,Z).** The knife blade also drives in the staple pushers on either side of the knife. The little screws shown on the upper limb of the instrument are each separately set to insure the proper position of each staple-driving fin. With use, the instrument accumulates sufficient protein deposits in the fine interstices so that the knife-staple driver cannot be pressed home by hand. The holes in the upper edge of the frame of the instrument are made for a pin on the side of a bar that is sequentially advanced to lever the knife-pusher forward and even this may require considerable effort **(X).** (**W** is from P.I. Androsov, 1962 or later; **X** is from Yu Ya Gritsman, 1961. **Y** and **Z** are from B.S. Bobrov and Yu Ya Gritsman, 1960. (The Russian stapling instruments are continued in Fig I–20.)

4. Instrument for inverting, end-to-end, circular anastomoses in the gastrointestinal tract (PKS, SPTU, KS) (Androsov 19 , 1970) (Fig I–20*A–C*). In essence, this consists of a cylindrical sigmoidoscope-like shaft with a knurled knob at one end for advancing beyond the cylinder a nose cone that contains the anvils for the single row of staples, and just inside them a plastic cutting ring. The circular end of the barrel of the instrument is slotted for the manual insertion of a single row of staples, just within which is a circular knife. The nose cone and the cylinder are separated or approximated by turning the knurled knob. The pursestringed proximal and distal loops of bowel are drawn over the nose cone and over the end of the main cylinder. The pursestrings are tightened on the slender shaft and the nose cone and staple-bearing cylinder are brought together by turning the knurled knob. The staples then are formed in the tissues by squeezing the

handle. The same compression of the handle drives home the circular knife, which cuts through the two pursestring-closed ends of bowel, against the plastic cutting ring in the nose cone, leaving two doughnuts of tissue on the central spindle of the instrument.

Kalinina and Kriuchkova (1963), writing from the Scientific Research Institute for Experimental Surgical Apparatus and Instruments in Moscow, said that the problem of a stapling instrument for transabdominal use in reconstruction after gastrectomy had been faced at the Institute in 1958 and resolved by 1960. They reported animal experiments only, did not show photographs or diagrams of the instrument, and gave it no name.

In 1966, Kalinina said that instruments of this type were developed between 1961 and 1963, together with the engineers Babkin, Kasulin, and Gambashidze. She then described the cylindrical apparatus for rectal anastomosis called the KTs-28, similar to the PKS-25 instrument. Interesting in this connection is a diagram (see Fig IX–7) showing what are described as six variations out of 37 that they used in animals for performing rectal anastomoses with the tubular instrument, most of which have been independently rediscovered in the past two or three years by Auto Suture® users in the Western world.

Writing in 1967, Kalinina described, with Kasulin, the use of the PKS-25 in esophagojejunostomy and esophagogastrostomy, attributing the creation of the instrument to V.S. Kasulin, S.I. Babkin, T.V. Kalinina, G.V. Astafiev, A.N. Burtsev, M.G. Achalaya, and G.M. Tateshvili in 1960 (credit to Directors of the Institute, engineers, and surgeons). The first reference given is to Kalinina and Kriuchkova (1963).

A number of Russian surgeons (Kalinina, 1960; Kalinina, Babkin, Kasulin, and Astafiev, 1962; Goureieva and Rivkine, 1967) have used the PKS instrument or its variants at both ends of the gastrointestinal tract in most of the various ways one would think possible, and the instrument has been fairly widely used in Western Europe (Vankemmel, 1972; Gautier-Benoit, 1976; Beckers and Deldime, 1978; Goligher, 1979; Cady, Godfroy, Sibaud, and Mercadier, 1980).

In 1968, in the experimental laboratory (Ravitch, 1968), we found that assembly of the instrument and appropriate registration of staples and anvils presented some difficulties and had basic concern over the use of a single row of staples in these critical anastomoses but found that we could successfully perform extremely low rectal anastomoses in a series of dogs.

Figure I–20C shows the instrument used in our laboratory for low rectal anastomosis in a dog. Although a dozen consecutive dogs survived the operation, at extremely low levels, with no leaks or abscesses, in some there could be seen small mucosal defects in the healing suture line, and at that time we recommended manufacture of an instrument—with the preloaded, presterilized, disposable cartridges—providing a double staggered staple line and a curved shaft for easier use in the human rectum.

More recently, Chinese surgeons have become interested in the use of similar mechanical suture instruments that are handtooled in hospital centers and therefore often vary in construction details from hospital to hospital (see Fig I–22).

5. An instrument for end-to-end, stapled, everting anastomoses of bowel, the jaws of the instrument being applied externally. The united, everted lips then were inverted by ordinary sutures. The machine (SK) (Fig I–20D–G) is ingenious, but in the laboratory we found it difficult to use and insecure, the staple lines always requiring inversion by manually placed sutures.

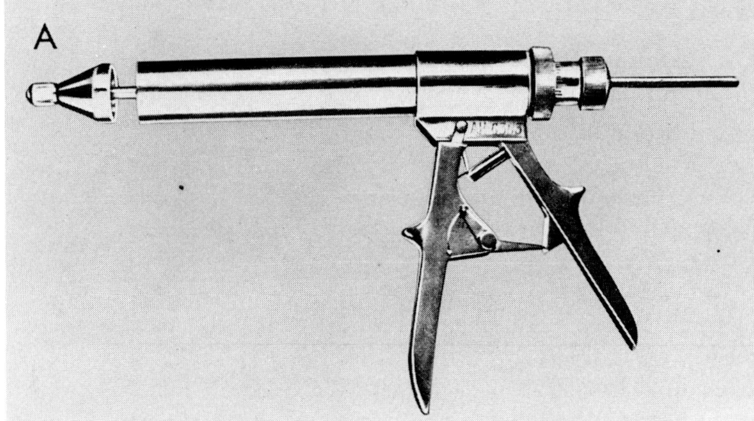
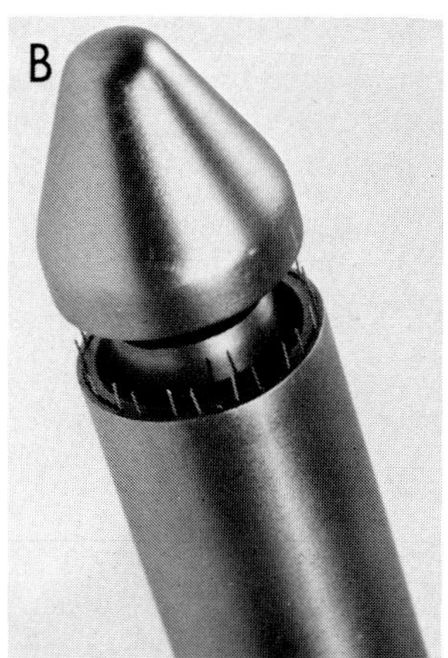
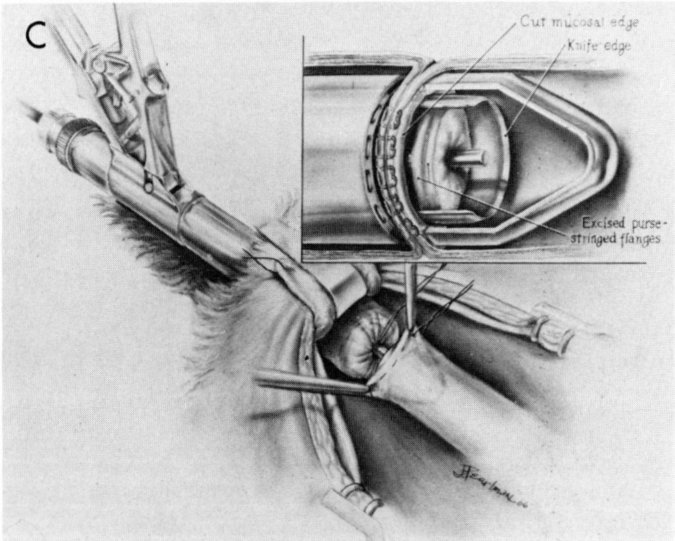

Fig I–20.—The Russian stapling instruments **(cont.).** Instrument for inverting end-to-end or end-to-side anastomoses of the gastrointestinal tract (KTs, PKS) (Kalinina, 1966; Kalinina and Kasulin, 1966). As with many of the Russian instruments, successive models frequently were produced either as improvements or to satisfy the special preferences of individual surgeons. **A,** the instrument resembles a sigmoidoscope whose obturator protrudes beyond the barrel. In the end of the cylinder is the housing for a single row of staples and just within that a circular knife. The staple-driving fins and the knife mounted on a central shaft are both driven down by a single squeeze of the handle. **B,** earlier Russian model without screw-cap tip for removal of the nose cone. The instrument is shown as having been fired with the gap open between barrel and nose cone; note the single ring of staples and the circular knife well within that ring. **C,** the PKS in use for a low rectal anastomosis in a dog—cutaway diagram of action of the instrument (Ravitch, 1968). By turning the knurled knob, the colon, pursestringed around the anvil containing nose cone, is drawn tightly against the rectum. A squeeze of the handle drives in the single row of staples. The circular knife, cutting against a plastic ring (not shown) in the nose cone, cuts out the pursestringed ends of the two segments of bowel, producing an end-to-end anastomosis with minimal inversion. (**A** and **B** are from P.I. Androsov, 19 .)   *(continued)*

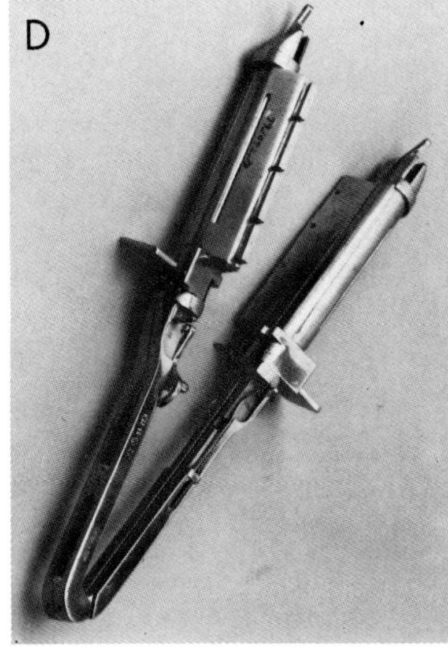

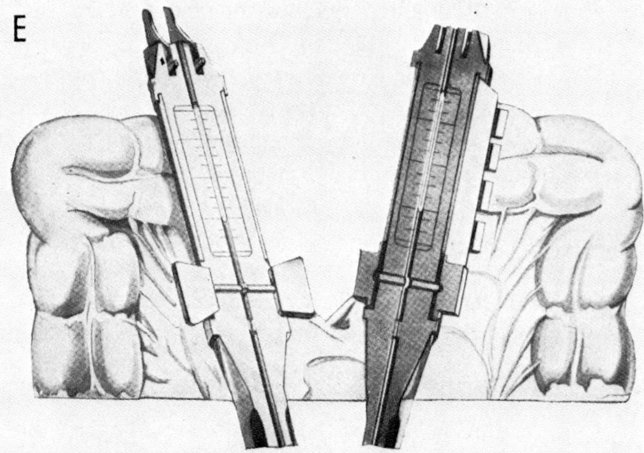

Fig. 117. Instrument halves with intestinal ends compressed in them prepared for being joined

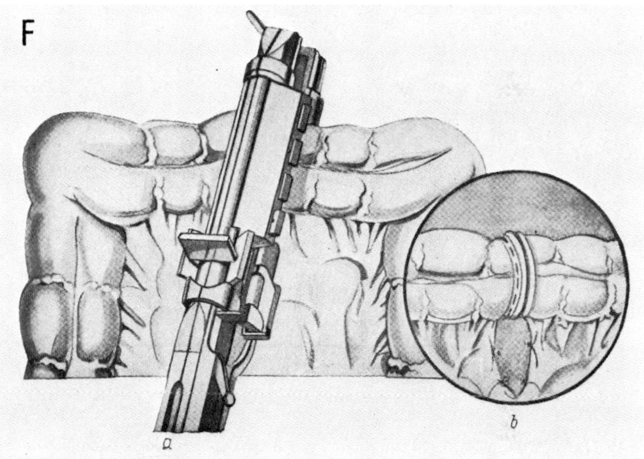

Fig. 118. (a) Instrument at suturing moment; (b) view of anastomosis

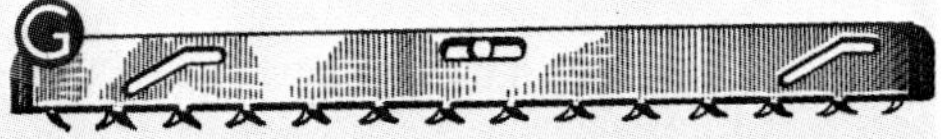

Fig. 114. Catches for fixation of sutured intestinal walls

Fig I–20 (cont.).—D–G, instrument for everted end-to-end anastomosis (SK) (Kalinina, 1958, 1961; Kalinina and Astafiev, 1957; Kalinina and Kriuchkova, 1958). **D,** the instrument (one half). **E,** there are two such hinged halves, which serve first as resection clamps. Fine hooks engage a partial thickness of the intestinal wall. **F,** with the two instrument halves locked together an ingenious mechanism permits the apposed upper and lower halves of the bowel circumferences to be held apart and stapled, mucosa-to-mucosa, the staples driven in by manual compression of the protruding lugs. The everting closure was inverted by sutures. We tested this instrument in the laboratory and in our hands it proved awkward and unsatisfactory. Androsov credits Kalinina with using it in 74 patients for end-to-end and end-to-side anastomoses, without comment on the results. **G,** detail of the retractable hooks that engage the outer coats of the bowel, separating the opposing bowel walls during manipulation of the instrument. (**D,** Courtesy of the Smithsonian Institution; **E–G** from P.I. Androsov, 1962 or later.)

(continued)
→

6. Two quite similar instruments were devised for clipping vessels in continuity (Ananiev, Antoshina, and Gritsman, 1957). One (ULAV) (Fig I–20*H*) was designed for ligature of the pulmonary vessels (Garin and Savchenko, 1955; Garin, 1956). A squeeze of the instrument, operated like a syringe, placed two tantalum staples, the most central one encircling and occluding the vessel, the more distal one closing in a B and perforating the vessel. A smaller model served for the cystic duct (Garin, Gritsman, and Tanich, 1957). Geselevitch and Gorkin (1961) said that the instrument had been abandoned. A similar-appearing instrument (Fig I–20*I,J*), for smaller, i.e., omental, mesenteric vessels ("instrument for ligature of vessels in deep cavities") placed two occluding staples, the vessel between them then having to be divided with scissors (Androsov, Babkin, Beliakov, Klemina, and Kriuchkova, 1957). We experimented with the latter instrument in the laboratory and found the instrument itself to be unsatisfactory and the ligations undependable. The American manufacturers charged with making this instrument, and at the same time adding a knife that would divide the doubly stapled tissues, solved the problem satisfactorily (Ravitch, Hirsch, and Noiles, 1972) (see Figs II–10 and II–11).

Fig I–20 (cont.).—**H–J,** instruments for ligature of vessels. **H,** stapler (ULAV) for ligation of pulmonary vessels applies a proximal encircling and occluding staple and, simultaneously, a distal transfixing staple. This instrument was briefly used clinically in the Soviet Union (Ananiev, Antoshina, and Gritsman, 1957), but Geselevitch himself, long the historian, champion and scientific publicist for the Soviet stapling instruments, stated (1961) ". . .they have not found appreciable use, as they proved poor timesavers in suturing blood vessels in the lungs.") **I,** instrument for ligation of vessels in deep cavities (Androsov, Babkin, Beliakov, Klemina, and Kriuchkova, 1957; Gritsman, 1961). The vessel-containing tissue is held in the hook of the instrument. Compression of the handle, as in operating a hand-held piston-syringe, closed a staple on either side (15 pairs are loaded on the bars on the sides). The metal bar on which the staples are loaded, and the spring mechanism for feeding the successive staples, are reminiscent of von Brücke's stapler (Fig I–18**A, B** (I–18A,B). **J,** the tissue between the staples, closed in a flat B, then is divided with scissors. Although there are a number of references in the Russian literature to the clinical use of this instrument (Androsov, Babkin, Beliakov, Klemina, and Kriuchkova, 1957) for mesenteric vessels, cystic duct ligation, etc., we found it awkward and unreliable in the laboratory and have the impression that it is not in much use abroad. In the early model pictured in the drawing, the magazine slides on the shaft. The mechanism, and the configuration of the closed staples in the American LDS™ surgical stapling instrument (Figs II–10 and II–11), are radically different and that instrument includes, as well, a knife dividing the tissues between the staples. (**H** is from A.M. Geselevitch and N.S. Gorkin, 1961; **I** is courtesy of the Smithsonian Institution; **J** is from M.G. Ananiev, N.V. Antoshina, and Yu Ya Gritsman, 1957.)

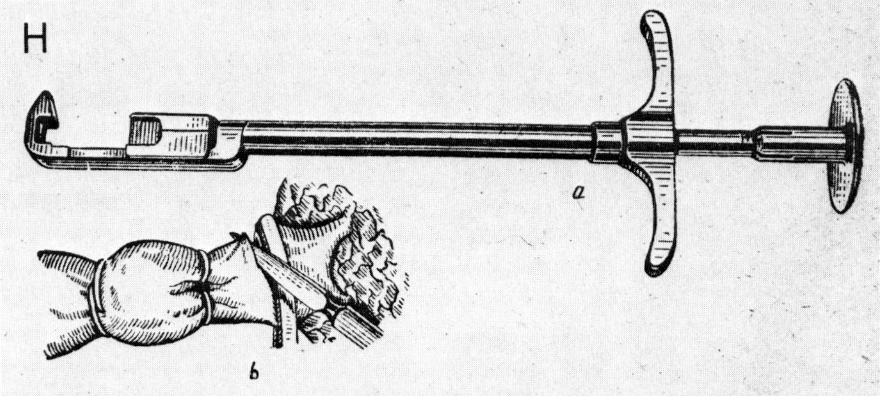

Fig. 32. Type УЛАВ ligature applicator for major blood vessels

a — general view; b — enveloping clip; c — suturing clip. The vessel is excised away from the B-shaped clip towards the periphery

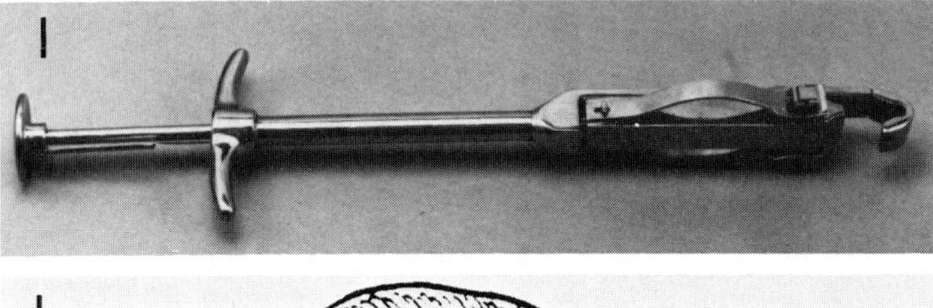

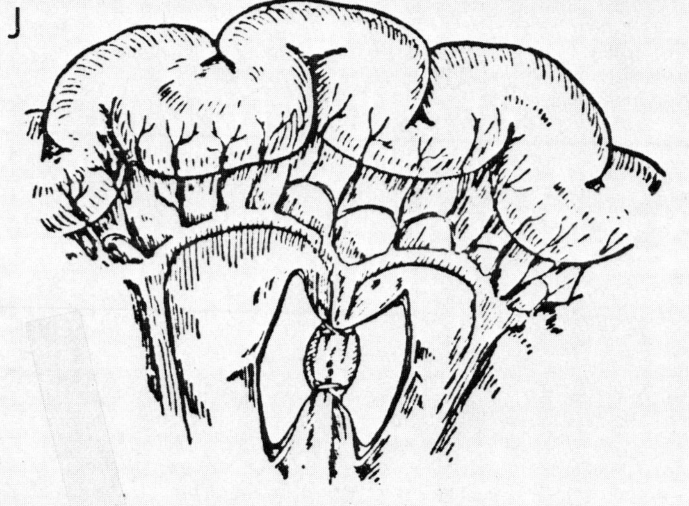

Рис. 12. Сосуды брыжейки тонкой кишки, перевязанные аппаратом.

Fig I–20 H-J. See legend on facing page.

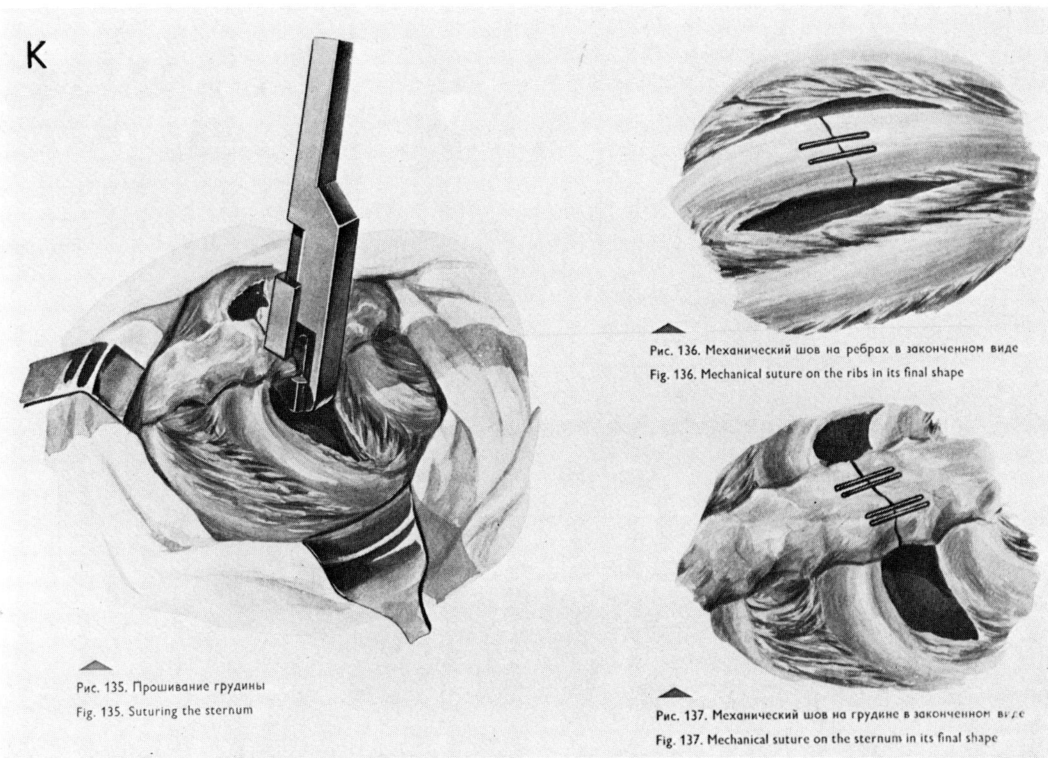

Рис. 135. Прошивание грудины
Fig. 135. Suturing the sternum

Рис. 136. Механический шов на рёбрах в законченном виде
Fig. 136. Mechanical suture on the ribs in its final shape

Рис. 137. Механический шов на грудине в законченном виде
Fig. 137. Mechanical suture on the sternum in its final shape

K, Russian stapler for sternum or ribs (SGR). Each loading of the instrument is with a parallel pair of heavy staples. We have not evaluated this instrument, which is suitable largely for the soft, flat bones of the chest wall. (From P.I. Androsov, 19 .)

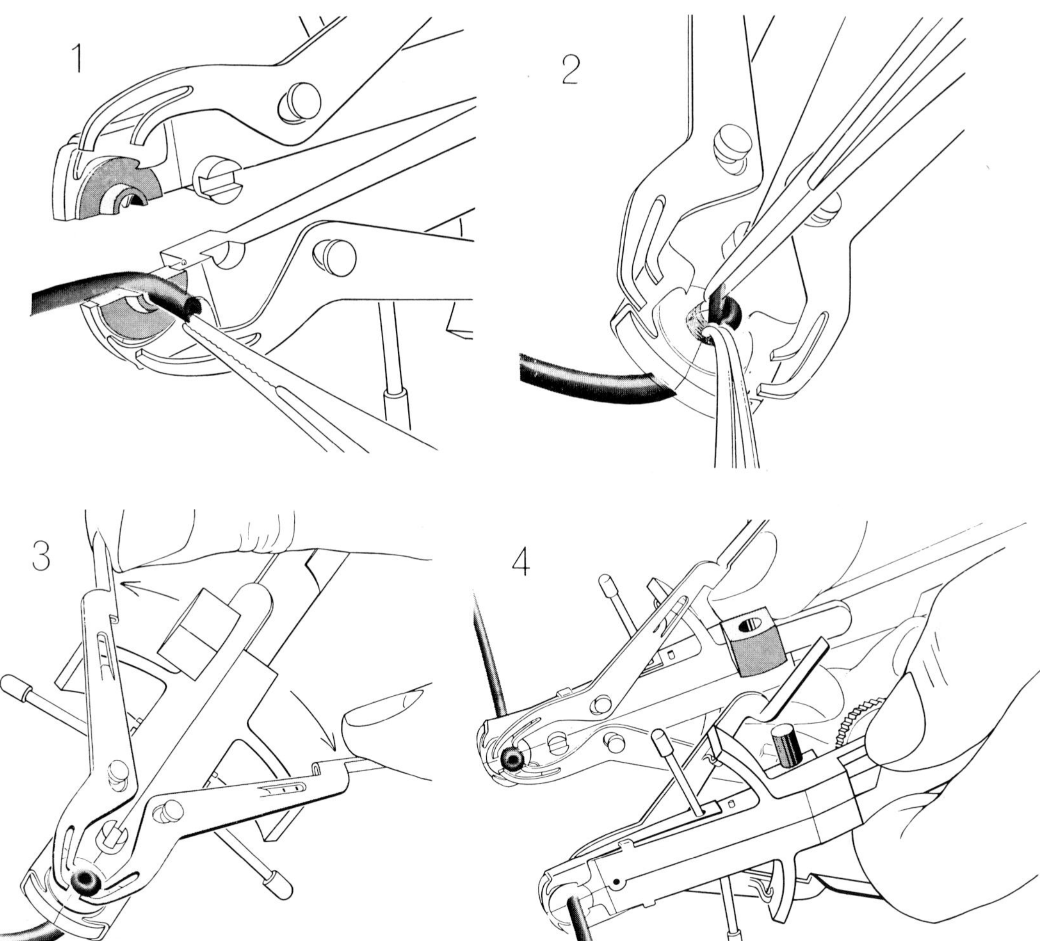

Fig I–21.—Vascular stapler (R.F. Mallina, T.R. Miller, P. Cooper, and S.G. Christie, 1962). Mallina's instrument, on precisely the principle of the Russian instrument, is simpler and somewhat lighter, but proved to be not as reliable. These are the clearest drawings we have seen illustrating the principle of the Russian vascular anastomosing instrument. The Russian instrument included, in addition, the vascular occluding clamps on each side, which locked into the anastomosing apparatus. (1) One end of a blood vessel is laid in the groove of the bushing half. (2) The other bushing half is locked over it and the vessel end is inverted to form a cuff around the bushing. (3) Holding clamps are closed on the cuff. (4) This procedure is repeated with the other end of the vessel, using the other half of the stapler. The two halves of the instrument then are joined by setting the coupling pin of one in the coupling socket of the other. The vessel ends having been brought firmly together by means of the adjustable screw (5 not reproduced). *(continued)*

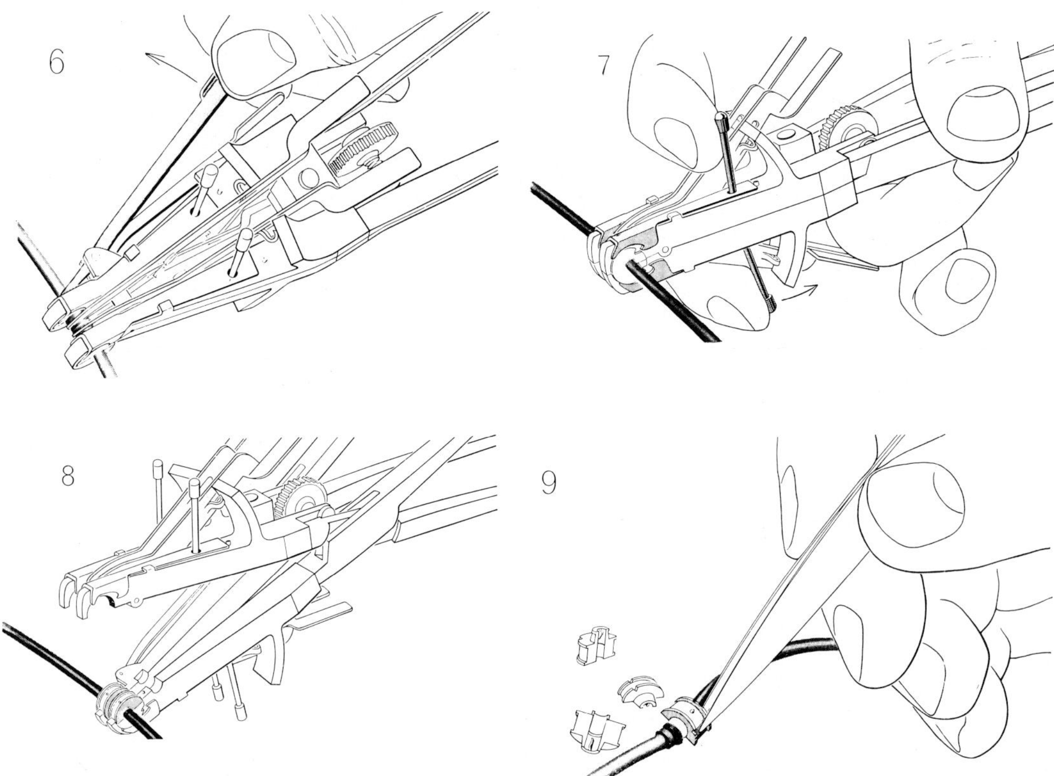

Fig I–21 (cont.).—(6) the staples are forced through the cuffs by the staple levers. (7) The bushings are released by pressing the bushing levers. (8) The instrument is opened and removed. (9) The bushing halves are picked from under the cuffs. (From R.F. Mallina, T.R. Miller, P. Cooper, and S.G. Christie, *Scientific American,* 1962, used by permission.)

ESOPHAGOGASTROSTOMIC ANASTOMOSIS INSTRUMENT

(A) Wu Wei-chi 吴维继, Chen Feng-tsai 陈凤才, Chou Hsin-kuan 周心官, Wei Lin-fa 魏林法, Liu Pao-wan 刘宝万 and Chang Ching-chen 张庆震

Kiangsu Hospital, Hsuyi, Kiangsu and Kiangsu Cancer Prevention and Treatment Institute, Kiangsu

ABSTRACT

A newly-designed surgical instrument for esophagogastrostomic anastomsis is fully described. It works on the principle of a "stapler". It had been tried on isolated pig organs for nearly a hundred times and experimental esophagogastrostomy on 16 dogs, before it was actually used clinically in 1975. It has been used clinically with success ever since and has been approved unanimously by noted surgeons as an effective new surgical instrument.

It is supperior to the conventional way of such operation by manual suture in achieving good exposure and relatively accurate apposition of the mucosal layers, and thus in reducing complications, such as leakage or stricture at the anastomosis site.

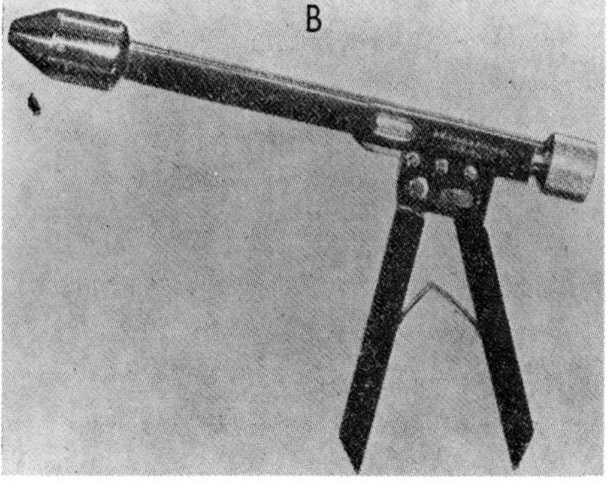

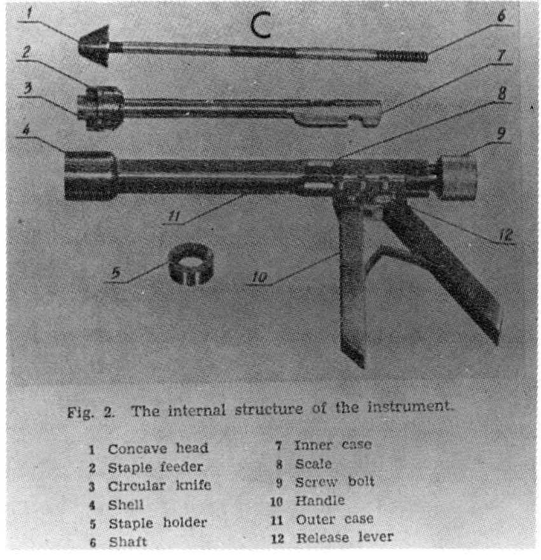

Fig. 2. The internal structure of the instrument.

1	Concave head	7	Inner case
2	Staple feeder	8	Scale
3	Circular knife	9	Screw bolt
4	Shell	10	Handle
5	Staple holder	11	Outer case
6	Shaft	12	Release lever

Fig I–22,A,B,C.—Chinese end-to-end anastomotic stapler. The high incidence of carcinoma of the esophagus in China has given surgeons in several centers (Wu Wei-chi, Chen Feng-tsai, Chou Hsin-kuan, Wei Lin-fa, Liu Pao-wan, and Chang Ching-chen, 1978; Wu Ying-K'ai and Huang Kuo-chun, 1979) ample opportunity to utilize a tubular anastomotic device that does not appear to differ significantly from the Russian model (to which no reference is made in the papers cited). (From Wu Wei-Chi, Chen Feng-tsai, Chou Hsin-kuan, Wei Lin-fa, Liu Pao-wan, and Chang Ching-chen, *Chinese Medical Journal,* 1978, permission requested.)

7. A considerable variety of instruments for special uses, for stapling ribs, sternum (Fig I–20*K*), fractured bones, for affixing corneal grafts, etc.

REFERENCES

Abbe R.: Complete obstruction of the colon successfully relieved by using Senn's plates. A proposed substitute of catgut rings. *N.Y. Med. J.* 49:314, 1889.

Abbe R.: Intestinal anastomosis. *The Medical News* (Phila.) 54:589, 1889.

Adam L.: Second Annual Meeting of the Hungarian Surgical Society, 1908.

Adam L.: *Yearbook of the Royal Hungarian Surgical Society,* 1909.

Amat C.: Les appareils à sutures: Les viroles de Denans; les pointes de Bonnier; les boutons de Murphy. *Arch. Med. Pharm.* Militaires, Paris XXV:273, 1895.

Amosov N.M., Berezovsky K.K.: Pulmonary resection with mechanical suture. *J. Thorac. Cardiovasc. Surg.* 41:325, 1961.

Ananiev M.G., Antoshina N.V., Gritsman Yu Ya: Apparatus for tissue suture with tantalum staples. *Eksp. Khirurg.* (Moskova) 2:28, 1957.

Androsov P.I.: *Atlas of Surgical Operations by Means of Suturing Instruments,* 2d edition. Moscow, V/O Medexport, Vneshtorgizdat, 19

Androsov P.I.: New method of surgical treatment of blood vessel lesions. *Arch. Surg.* 73:902, 1956.

Androsov P.I.: Operations in cases of aneurysms. Restoration of continuity of arteries by means of grafts, without isolating the aneurysmatic sac. *Arch. Surg.* 73:911, 1956.

Androsov P.I.: Blood supply of mobilized intestine used for an artificial esophagus. *Arch. Surg.* 73:917, 1956.

Androsov P.I.: *New Surgical Instruments and Their Clinical Use*. Moscow, V/O Medexport, 1962 or later.

Androsov P.I.: Apparat zum Vernähen des Magenstumpfes und die Erfahrung bei seiner Klinischen Anwendung. *Zentralbl. Chir*. 92:436, 1965.

Androsov P.I.: Experience in the application of the instrumental mechanical suture in surgery of the stomach and rectum. *Acta Chir. Scand*. 136:57, 1970.

Androsov P.I., Babkin S.I., Beliakov P.D., Klemina E.P., Kriuchkova G.S.: Apparat dlia mekhanicheskoi pereviazki sosudov (Apparatus for mechanical ligation of blood vessels). *Nov. Khir. Appar*. 1:86, 1957.

Androsov P.I., Potekhina L.A., Savchenko E.D., Strekopytov A.A., Thliakova L.S., Sheinber S.A.: A new method of suture of bronchial stump. *Khirurgia* 8:66, 1955.

Azina M.A.: Materials and evaluation in gastric resection (dissertation). Sverdlovsk, 1956.

Baudens J.B.L.: *Clinique des Plaies d'Armes a Feu*. Paris, J.B. Baillière, 1836, p. 318.

Beckers J., Deldime P.: À propos de 50 anastomoses colorectales basses par suture mécanique. *Acta Chir. Belg*. 77:327, 1978.

Béranger-Féraud L.J.B.: Nouveau procédé de suture de l'intestin. *Bull. l'Acad. Impériale Med*. Paris, 25 Decembre, XXXIV:1253, 1869.

Béranger-Féraud L.J.B.: Nouveau procédé de suture de l'intestin. *Gaz. Hôp. Civils et Militaires*, Paris, 1869, pp. 599–600.

Béranger-Féraud L.J.B.: A new method of applying intestinal sutures. *Lancet* 1:234, 1870; and *Allg. Wien. M. Ztg*. XV:233, 1870.

von Bergmann E., von Bruns P., von Mikulicz J., et al.: Surgery of the alimentary tract, in: *A System of Practical Surgery* IV:404–06, Lea Brothers and Co., New York and Philadelphia, 1904.

Bertelsen S., Rygg I.H.: A simple stapling device for vascular surgery. *Surg. Gynecol. Obstet*. 125:1087, 1967.

Boari A.: Modificazioni al metodo anastomotico di Murphy. Nota critico sperimentale. *Clin. Chir.*, Milano V:141, 1897.

Boari A.: Modificazioni al bottone anastomotico di Murphy. *Archivio ed Atti di Soc. Ital. di Chir. Roma* I:XLV, 1897.

Bobrick J.: Zur Technik der Darmnaht. *Allg. Mediz. Centr. Zeitung*. Berlin XIX:152, 1850.

Bobrov B.S., Gritsman Yu Ya: Particulars of use of the apparatus for side-to-side gastrointestinal anastomoses. Results of experimental studies, in *New Surgical Apparatus and Instruments and Experience with Their Use*. Moscow, 1960.

Boerema I.: The technique of our method of transabdominal total gastrectomy in cases of gastric cancer. *Arch. Chir. Neerl*. 6:95, 1954.

Boerema I., Klopper P.J., Holscher A.A.: Transabdominal ligation-resection of the esophagus in cases of bleeding esophageal varices. *Surgery* 67:409, 1970.

Bourgery J.M., Bernard C., Jacob N.H.: *Traité Complet de l'Anatomie de l'Homme, Comprenant l'Anatomie Chirurgicale et la Médecine Opératorie*. Paris, L. Guérin & Cie, 1866–71, Vol. VII, p. 110.

Brentano A.: Die bisherigen Erfahrungen mit dem "Murphy Knopf." *Berl. Klin. Wochenschr*. XXXIII:443, 1896.

von Brücke H.: Über ein neuartiges chirurgisches Nähinstrument. *Zentral. Chir*. 62:1684, 1935.

Brummelkamp R.: The rectoresector: A new instrument for resection of the rectum and colorectal anastomosis without sutures. *Dis. Colon Rectum* 8:49, 1965.

Cady J., Godfroy J., Sibaud O., Mercadier M.: La désunion anastomotique en chirurgie colique et rectale. Étude comparative des procédés de suture manuelle et mécanique à propos d'une serie de 149 résections. *Ann. Chir*. 34:350, 1980.

Cates B.B.: Some experiments upon the primae viae with report of a new method of enterorrhaphy: Its technique and result. *J.A.M.A*. 22:751, 1894.

Chaput H.: Conférence sur l'anastomose cholécysto-intestinale, gastro-intestinale, entéro-intestinale, et leur rapprochement sans sutures (Procédé de Murphy). *Rev. Chir.*, Paris, pp. 328–30, 1893.

Chaput H.: Recherches experimentales sur le Bouton de Murphy. *Bull. Mém. Soc. Chir.*, Paris XX:738, 1894.

Chaput H.: Avantages et inconvénients du Bouton de Murphy. *Belg. Méd.* (Gand-Haarlem) II:385, 1895.

Cohn I.: *Rudolph Matas. A Biography of One of the Great Pioneers in Surgery.* Garden City, N.Y., Doubleday & Co. 1960, p. 232.

Cooper P., Mallina R.F., Tolins S.H.: An automatic cartridge stapler. *Am. J. Surg.* 113:856, 1967.

Czerny V.: Ueber die Verwendung des Murphyknopfes als Ersatz für die Darmnaht. Verhandlungen der Deutsch. *Ges. Chir.*, Berlin, XXV Congress, 1896, p. 94.

Denans F-N.: Nouveau procédé pour la guérison des plaies des intestins. Recueil de la Société Royale de Médecine de Marseille [Séance du 24 fev. 1826, rédigé par M.P. Roux], Imprimerie d'Archard, Marseille, Tome I:127–31, 1827.

Denans F-N.: Lettre avec envoi d'un système de viroles qu'il propose en remplacement de la ligature pour la réunion des plaies transversales de l'intestin. Bulletin de l'Académie Royale de Médecine [Séance du 15 mai 1836, Rapporteur Emery], Paris, 1837–38, p. 719.

Derocque P.: De l'entérectomie avec rétablissement immédiat de la continuité de l'intestin. [Carré et Naud, n. 486.] Thèse de Doctorat, Paris, 1897.

Derocque P.: De la réunion de l'intestin par la méthode des sutures après entérectomie. *Presse Méd.*, Paris 5:206, 1897.

Destot E.: Sur une modification du Bouton de Murphy. *Arch. Provinciales Chir.*, Paris III:736, 1894.

Dupuytren G.: Mémoire sur une méthode nouvelle pour traiter les anus accidentels. *Mem. Acad. R. Méd.*, Paris, 1 Sec. de Med., 1828.

von Esmarch Fr., Kowalzig E. (edited by N. Senn): *Surgical Technic.* New York, The Macmillan Company, 1901, p. 709.

Exon C.S., Sugarbaker E.: Recto-colic anastomosis, a sutureless alternative to stapling. A 28-year experience with the Sugarbaker three-piece clamp. Exhibit ACS Congress, 1978.

Faure J.L.: Sur une méthode nouvelle d'oblitération des plaies de l'intestin. *Mercredi Méd.*, Paris VI:184, 1895.

Faure J.L., Suarez: Méthode nouvelle d'oblitération des plaies intestinales. *Bull. Soc. Anatomique Paris* LXX, IX:285, 1895.

Frank J.: A new contrivance for intestinal end to end anastomosis. *Med. Record,* New York 50:469, 1896.

Frank J.: Intestinal anastomosis. *J.A.M.A.* 28:1163, 1897.

Frank J.: Pathological histology of intestinal end to end approximation after the use of the Frank coupler. *Med. Record,* New York 52:403, 1897.

von Frey R.: Ueber die Technik der Darmnaht. Beitr. Z, *Klin. Chir.* 14:1, 1895.

Friedrich H.: Ein neuer Magen-Darm-Nähapparat. *Zentralbl. Chir.* 61:504, 1934.

Garampazzi C.: Un nuovo bottone (alla Murphy) scomponibile. *Riforma Med.*, Napoli, IV:27–31, 37–42, 50, 51, 1897.

Garbarini E.: Delle anastomosi intestinali col bottone di Murphy; contributo sperimentale. *Clin. Chir.*, Milano, IV:49, 1896.

Garin N.D.: Mekhanicheskaia pereviazka sosudov legkovo v klinike (Mechanical ligation of pulmonary vessels in clinical conditions). *Eksp. Khir.* 1(4):33, 1956.

Garin N.D., Gritsman Yu Ya, Tanich L.F.: Mekhanicheskaia pereviazka puzyrnovo protoka pri kholetsistektomii (mechanical ligation of the cystic duct in cholecystectomy). *Eksp. Khir.* 2 (6):21, 1957.

Garin N.D., Savchenko E.D.: Primenenie apparata dlia mekanicheskoi pereviazki sosudov kornia legkovo v eksperimente (Use of an apparatus for the mechanical ligation of the blood vessels of the radix pulmonis in experimental conditions). *Khirurgiia* No. 9:80, 1955.

Gaujot G., Spillmann E.: *Arsenal de la Chirurgie Contemporaine* II:609, 1867–72. [Figs. 1255,1256.] Paris, J.B. Baillière et Fils.

Gautier-Benoit C.: Anastomoses intestinales termino-terminales par suture mécanique. *Nouv. Presse Med.* 5:1639, 1976.

Geselevitch A.M., Gorkin N.S.: *New Instruments and Equipment for Chest Surgery.* Moscow, V/O Medexport, 1961.

Goligher J.C.: Use of circular stapling gun with peranal insertion of anorectal purse-string suture for construction of very low colorectal or colo-anal anastomoses. *Br. J. Surg.* 66:501, 1979.

Goureieva K.F., Rivkine V.L.: Expérience clinique de l'emploi de la suture mécanique pour les anastomoses colo et iléorectales. *Acta Chir. Belg.* 2:163, 1967.

Gritsman Yu Ya: *Tantalum Mechanical Sutures for Gastric Resection.* Moscow, Medgiz, 1961.

Gross S.D.: *An Experimental and Critical Inquiry Into the Nature and Treatment of Wounds of the Intestines.* Louisville, Prentice and Weissinger, 1843.

Gudov V.F.: A method for the application of vascular sutures by mechanical means. *Khirurgiia* 12:58, 1950.

Hahn F.: Nähapparat für Magen-und Dickdarmresektionen. 93-ter Congress, 4 ter Sitzungstag, *Dtsch. Gesellsch. Chir.*, April 2, 1910.

Hahn F.: Nähapparat für Magen-und Darmresektionen. *Muench. Med. Wochenschr.* p. 1919, September 5, 1911.

Hallenbeck G.A., Judd E.S., David C.: An instrument for colorectal anastomosis without sutures. *Dis. Colon Rectum* 4:98, 1963.

Halsted W.S.: Circular suture of the intestine—an experimental study. *Am. J. Med. Sci.* XCIV:436, 1887.

Halsted W.S.: End-to-end suture of the intestine by a bulkhead method. *Trans. Am. Surg. Assoc.* 28:256, 1910.

Halsted W.S.: Blind-end circular suture of the intestine, closed ends abutted and the double diaphragm punctured with a knife introduced per rectum. *Ann. Surg.* 75:356, 1922.

Henroz J.H.F.: Dissertatio Inauguralis Critica Medico-Chirurgica de Methodis ad Sananda Intestina Divisa Adhibitis, In Qua Nova Sanationis Methodus Proponitur. Universitate Leodiensi, June 1826. P.J. Collardin, Typographi Academici, 1826.

Hopcroft S.C.: An absorbable intestinal prosthesis for rapid intestinal anastomosis. *Exp. Med. Surg.* 26:9, 1968.

Hopcroft S.C.: The use of an absorbable prosthesis in intestinal colonic anastomosis. *Med. J. Aust.* 1:118, 1972.

Hültl H.: II Kongress der Ungarischen Gesellschaft für Chirurgie, Budapest, May 1908. *Pester Med.-Chir. Presse* 45:108–10, 121–22, 1909.

Inokuchi K., Kusaba A.: Alternative device for vascular stapling anastomosis. *J. Cardiovasc. Surg.* (Torino) 15:458, 1974.

Jansen A., Becker A.E., Brummelkamp W.H., Keeman J.N., Klopper P.J.: The importance of the apposition of the submucosal intestinal layers for primary wound healing of intestinal anastomosis. *Surg. Gynecol. Obstet.* 152:51, 1981.

Jansen A., Brummelkamp W.H., Davies G.A.G., Klopper P.J., Keeman J.N.: Clinical applications of magnetic rings in colorectal anastomosis. *Surg. Gynecol. Obstet.* 153:537, 1981.

Jascalevich M.E.: A new stapler for gastric operations. *Surgery* 62:1100, 1967.

Jascalevich M.E.: The gastrectomy operation revisited with automated suturing devices. *Arch. Surg.* 105:524, 1972.

Jonnesco T.: Modifications au bouton de Murphy. *Gaz. Hôp.,* Paris 69:1297, 1896.

Jonnesco T.: Un nouveau procédé pour l'application du bouton de Murphy. *Arch. Sci. Méd.* (de Bucarest), Paris I:45, 1896.

Juvara E.: Un nouveau modèle de bouton anastomotique intestinal avec une nouvelle technique. *Arch. Sci. Méd.* (de Bucarest), Paris I:253, 1896.

Kalinina T.V.: Apparat dlia sshivaniia kishok (Apparatus for suturing the intestine). *Nov. Khir. Arkh.* 2:115, 1958.

Kalinina T.V.: *Mechanical Sutures for Intestinal and Esophagointestinal Anastomoses.* Proceedings II Congress of Kazakstan Surgeons Alma-Ata, 1960.

Kalinina T.V.: Nalozhenie kishechnovo anastomoza konets v bok s pomoshch'iu apparata (Application of end-to-side intestinal anastomoses with the aid of an apparatus). *Vestn. Khir. Grekov* 86(5):131, 1961.

Kalinina T.V.: The use of mechanical suturing for the creation of anastomoses between the rectum and the small or large intestine. *Klin. Khir.* (Kiev) 10:56, 1966.

Kalinina T.V., Astafiev G.V.: Sshivanie kishok mekhanicheskim shvom (Anastomosis of the intestine with a mechanical suture). *Vestn. Khir. Grekov* 79(7):129, 1957.

Kalinina T.V., Babkin S.I., Kasulin V.S., Astafiev G.V.: Mechanical sutures for esophago-intestinal (gastric) anastomoses. *Clin. Surg.* (Moscow) 8:81, 1962.

Kalinina T.V., Kasulin V.S.: A modified PKS-25M apparatus. *Khirurg.* (Moskova) 42:141, 1966.

Kalinina T.V., Kasulin V.S.: Peculiarities of the PKS-25-M instrument for suturing the esophagus to the intestine or to the stomach. *Klin. Khir.* (Kiev) 5:86, 1967.

Kalinina T.V., Kriuchkova G.S.: K voprosu sshivaniia kishok tantalovymi skobkami (eksperimental'noe issledovanie) (On the problem of intestinal anastomosis with tantalum staples [experimental studies]). *Nov. Khir. Appar.* 2:13, 1958.

Kalinina T.V., Kriuchkova G.S.: Tantalovyi shov v pishchevodno-kishechnykh i pishchevodno-zheludochnykh anastomozakh. (Tantalum sutures in esophago-intestinal and esophagogastric anastomoses.) *Zdravookhr Beloruss* 9:13, 1963.

Kieninger G.: Personal communication, July 29, 1979.

Kukushkin L.E.: Apparatus for suture of blood vessels, in Ananev M.G., Geselevitch A.M.: Experience with *Clinical Use of New Surgical Apparatus and Instruments.* Moscow, Meditsina, 1964.

Lallemand C.F.: Receuil de la Société Royale de Médecine de Marseille 129–31, 1826.

Leand P.M., Bender H.W., Martz M.N., Crisler C., Agnew H.D., Gott V.L.: A simple method for closure of the Potts anastomosis with a mechanical stapler. *J. Thorac. Cardiovasc. Surg.* 62:285, 1971.

Lembert A.: Mémoire sur l'entéroraphie. *Rep. Gen. d'Anat. et de Physiol. Pathol.* II:101, 1826.

Littlewood H.: Ileo-sigmoidostomy (Senn's method) for intestinal obstruction due to malignant disease of the hepatic flexure of the colon. *Lancet,* pp. 864–66, April, 1892.

Mallina R.F., Miller T.R., Cooper P., Christie S.G.: Surgical stapling. *Sci. Am.* 207:48, 1962.

Martin Gil R.: Decalcified ivory discs for end to end and lateral anastomosis of the intestine. *Lancet* 2:522, 1897.

Martin Gil R.: Memoria solve discos de marfil descalcificado para les anastomosis y reunion de extremo con extremo del intestino. *An. r. Acad. de Med.,* Madrid XVII:48, 1897.

Marwedel G.: Ueber Enteroanastomose nebst experimentellen Beiträgen zur Frage des Murphyschen Darmknopfes. *Beitr. Klin. Chir.* XIII:605, 1895.

Mayo Robson A.W.: A method of performing intestinal anastomosis by means of decalcified bone bobbins. *Br. Med. J.,* pp. 688–89, April, 1893.

Meyer W.: Murphy's Knopf in der Chirurgie des Magen Darm-Kanales und der Gallenblase. *Zentralbl. Chir.* XXI:866, 1894.

Meyer W.: Ein Vorschlag bezüglich der Gastrostomie und Ösophagoplastik nach Jianu-Roepke. *Zentralbl. Chir.* XL:267, 1913.

Mcycr W.: Extrathoracic and intrathoracic csophagoplasty in connection with resection of the thoracic portion of the esophagus for carcinoma. *J.A.M.A.* 62:100, 1914.

Meyer W.: Resection of the cardia for carcinoma. *Trans. Am. Surg. Assoc.* 33:733, 1915.

Murphy J.B.: Cholecysto-intestinal, gastro-intestinal, entero-intestinal anastomosis, and approximation without sutures (original research). *Medical Record,* New York 42:665, 1892, and *Chicago Medical Record* XIII:803, 1892.

Murphy J.B.: Intestinal approximation: Its pathological histology of reunion, and statistical analysis. *Medical Record,* New York 65:650–63; 684–92; 721–22, 1894, and *Chicago Clinical Review* III:479–558, 1893–94.

Murphy J.B.: Intestinal approximation, with special reference to the use of the anastomosis button. *Lancet* 2:621, 1894.

Murphy J.B.: Remarks on intestinal anastomosis. *Trans. Am. Assoc. Obstet. Gynecol.* VII:384, 1894–95.

Murphy J.B.: An analysis of the cases operated with the Murphy button up to date. *Chicago Clinical Review* IV:248, 1894–95.

Murphy J.B.: Analysis of cases operated on with the aid of the Murphy button up to present time. *Medical News,* Philadelphia LXVI:141, 1895.

Murphy J.B.: Reports of one hundred and eleven additional cases operated upon with the anastomosis button. *Medical News,* Philadelphia, November 16 and 23, 1895.

Nakayama K.: Simplification of the Billroth I gastric resection. *Surgery* 35:837, 1954.

Nakayama K., Tamiya T., Yamamoto K., Akimoto S.: A simple new apparatus for small vessel anastomosis (free autograft of the sigmoid included). *Surgery* 52:918, 1962.

Nance F.C.: New techniques of gastrointestinal anastomoses with the EEA stapler. *Ann. Surg.* 189:587, 1979.

Nélaton A.: *Eléments de Pathologie Chirurgicale*. Paris, Germer Baillière, IV:144, 1857.

Ogilvie W.H.: Some points in the operation of gastrectomy. *Br. Med. J.*, pp. 457–62, March 9, 1935.

Péan J.E.: Note sur un nouveau mode d'occlusion des solutions de continuité de l'intestin. *Bull. Acad. Impériale Méd.*, Paris XXXIV:1236 (14 December) 1869.

Péan J.E.: Nouveau mode d'occlusion des solutions de continuité faites aux parois mêmes de l'intestin. *Gaz. Hôp. Civils et Militaires,* Paris, pp. 586–87, 1869.

Petrova N.P., Rabinovich J.J., Kapitanov N.N., Bogomolova O.R.: Employment of two new stapling devices (Models SB-2 and US-18) in experimental combined resections of the bronchus and pulmonary artery. *Ann. Thorac. Surg.* 19:67, 1975.

von Petz A.: Zur Technik der Magenresektion. Ein neuer Magen-Darmnähapparat. *Zentralbl. Chir.* 51:179, 1924.

von Petz A.: Aseptic technique of stomach resections. *Ann. Surg.* 86:388, 1927.

Phillips C.: New mode, by M. Amussat, of employing suture of the intestines. *Lancet,* pp. 202–04, 1834–35.

Pimenta A.P.A.: Personal communication, September 20, 1981.

Pimenta A.P.A., Cardoso V., Rodrigues J.S.: A mechanical suturing method for the gastrointestinal tract: Experimental and clinical experience with a new stapling instrument. 6th World Congress of the Collegium Internationale Chirurgiae Digestivae, Lisbon, Portugal, September, 1980.

Pimenta A.P.A., Cardoso V., Rodrigues, J.S.: Un nouvel instrument pour agrafage mécanique en chirurgie gastro-intestinale. Étude expérimentale préliminaire. *Ann. Chir.* 35:469, 1981.

Pimenta A.P.A., Cardoso V.M.B., Rodrigues J.S.: A mechanical suturing method for the gastrointestinal tract: Clinical experience with a new stapling instrument. *World J. Surg.* 6:786, 1982.

Prioton J-B.: La ligature de l'oesophage sur bouton de Murphy dans les hémorragies par rupture de varices oesophagiennes. *Ann. Chir.* 27:343, 1973.

Ramaugé A.: Entéroplexie. Considérations préliminaires. Mémoire presenté et couronné au concours de Médicine International Sud-Américain, pp. 5–32, 20 January, 1893.

Ramaugé A.: Enteroplexis. Consideraciones preliminares. Memoria presentada al jurado del concurso de Medicine International Sudamericano, pp. 7–41, Ed. Jacobo Peuser, 1893.

Ramaugé A.: Enteroplexo. *Rev. Soc. Méd. Argentina* 2:667, 1902.

Ravitch M.M.: Unpublished observations, 1968.

Ravitch M.M.: Dupuytren's invention of the Mikulicz enterotome with a note on eponyms. *Perspect. Biol. Med.* 22:170, 1979.

Ravitch M.M.: *A Century of Surgery*. Philadelphia, J.B. Lippincott Co. 1981, p. 239.

Ravitch M.M., Brown I.W., Daviglus G.F.: Experimental and clinical use of the Soviet bronchus stapling instrument. *Surgery* 46:97, 1959.

Ravitch M.M., Hirsch L.C., Noiles D.: A new instrument for simultaneous ligation and division of vessels, with a note on hemostasis by a gelatin sponge-staple combination. *Surgery* 71:732, 1972.

Ravitch M.M., Rivarola A.: Enteroanastomosis with an automatic instrument. *Surgery* 59:270, 1966.

Robicsek F.: The birth of the surgical stapler. *Surg. Gynecol. Obstet.* 150:579, 1980.

Sachs W.: Drei kleine Beiträge zur Darmchirurgie. *Zentralbl. Chir.* 17:753, 1890.

Samuels P.B.: Method of blood vessel anastomosis by means of metal clips. *Arch. Surg.* 70:29, 1955.

Sándor S.: Magen-Darmnaht mit Metallklammern nach Hültl und ein neues Nähinstrument. *Zentralbl. Chir.* 63:1334, 1936.

Sédillot C.E.: *Traité de Médecine Opératoire*, 3d ed. Paris, J.B. Baillière et Fils II:314, 1865–66.

von Seeman H.: Zur Operation des Mastdarmkrebses Eine Nähquetsche für die hohe sakrale Amputation. *Zentralbl. Chir.* 61:848, 1934.

Senn N.: *Intestinal Surgery*. Chicago, W.T. Keener, 1889.

Senn N.: Enterorrhaphy: Its history, technique and present status. *J.A.M.A.* 21:217, 1893.

Sugarbaker E.D.: Low anterior proctosigmoidectomy using an anastomotic instrument. *Am. J. Surg.* 108:64, 1964.

Sugarbaker E.D., Wiley H.M.: Rectocolic anastomosis. A simplified method. *Surg. Gynecol. Obstet.* 93:597, 1951.

Svinkin E.K.: Extension of the indications for the use of the suture instruments of the NZhKA, in *Experiences in the Clinical Use of New Surgical Apparatus and Instruments.* Moscow, Meditsina, 1964.

Terrier F.: Société de Chirurgie de Paris, Meetings of March 14, October 31, November 7, and November 14, 1894.

Terrier F., Baudouin M.: La suture intestinale, in *Histoire des Differents Procédés d'Entérorraphie.* Paris, Institut de Bibliographie Scientifique, 1898, pp. 44–368.

Tomoda M.: Ein neuer Magen-Darmnähapparat. *Zentralbl. Chir.* 64:1455, 1937.

Tomoda M.: Eine neue Modifikation der Magenresektionstechnik mit eigenem Magen-Darmnähapparat. *Zentralbl. Chir.* 64:1584, 1937.

Ton J.G., Boelens W.C., Gallas: Resection of the rectum with preservation of the anal sphincter. *Arch. Chir. Neerl.* XXV–II:179, 1973.

Travers B.: *An Inquiry Into the Process of Nature in Repairing Injuries of the Intestines.* London, Longman, 1812, pp. 128–35, 180–89.

Uchiyama H., Tokunaga T., Kajisa T.: Gastro-pseudo-esophagoplasty following total or subtotal mediastinal esophagectomy: Evaluation of antethoracic or presternal gastroesophageal reconstruction. *Ann. Surg.* 156:727, 1962.

Vankemmel M.: Anastomoses oeso-gastriques et oeso-jéjunales par agrafes métalliques à l'appareil PKS 25. *Lille Méd.* 17:850, 1972.

Verschuyl M.A.: Non-suture anastomosis of the small intestine. An experimental study. *Arch. Chir. Neerl.* XVII:95, 1965.

Villard E.: Note sur l'emploi du bouton anastomotique suivant la méthode de Murphy. *Lyon Méd.* LXXVII:491, 1894.

Villard E.: Recherches expérimentales sur les entérectomies par la méthode de Murphy. *Lyon Méd.* LXXVII:171, 1894.

Villard E.: De l'emploi d'un Bouton de Murphy modifié dans les interventions sur le tube digestif. *Gaz. Hebd. Med. Chir.*, Paris XXXII:137, 149, 163, 1895.

Vogelfanger I.J., Beattie W.G.: A concept of automation in vascular surgery: A preliminary report on a mechanical instrument for arterial anastomosis. *Can. J. Surg.* 1:262, 1958.

Vogelfanger I.J., Beattie W.G., Brown F.N., Devitt J.E., Scobie T.K., Scobie D.H.: The problem of small vessel anastomosis. *Surgery* 52:354, 1962.

Vosschulte K.: Place de la section par ligature de l'oesophage dans le traitement de l'hypertension portale. *Lyon Chir.* 53:519, 1957.

Weir R.F.: On the operation of gastro-enterostomy conjoined with entero-anastomosis. *Medical Record,* New York LIII:541, 1898.

Windler H.: Hauptkatalog 50, Chirurgie-instrumente, Krankenhaus Möbel, Bandagen, Apparate zur Orthopädie, etc., Berlin, 1912, p. 545.

Wu Wei-chi, Chen Feng-tsai, Chou Hsin-Kuan, Wei Lin-fa, Liu Pao-wan, Chang Ching-chen: Esophagogastrostomic anastomosis instrument. *Chin. Med. J.* 4:204, 1978.

Wu Ying-K'ai, Huang Kuo-chun: Chinese experience in the surgical treatment of carcinoma of the esophagus. *Ann. Surg.* 190:361, 1979.

Zielewicz I.: Der Murphysche "Anastomosis-Button." *Zentralbl. Chir.* XXI-n.43:1025, 1894.

CHAPTER II

American Mechanical Suture Instruments

Author's Note

In 1941, I had prepared myself for the final year of Residency in surgery by studying Frank Lahey's *Surgical Practice of the Lahey Clinic* and had been impressed by Lahey's use of the von Petz stapler in gastric surgery. My request to Alfred Blalock to purchase one of these instruments for the Johns Hopkins Hospital was met with the simple reply, "It's too expensive." Somewhat annoyed, I took to the Hunterian Laboratory an ordinary office paper stapler and, as Vivien Thomas remembers, had it boiled up for use in stapling bowel. The one-step slam-bang operation of such a stapler obviously was unacceptably traumatic, the moist heat-sterilized staples did not feed well, and I abandoned the experiment. In 1958, on a visit to the Soviet Union, I observed the brilliant use of the staple instruments in pulmonary surgery by N.M. Amosov in Kiev (Amosov, Berezovsky, Zabroda, 1958; Amosov and Berezovsky, 1961) and thereafter made the first of many visits to Moscow to the Scientific Research Institute for Experimental Surgical Apparatus and Instruments. Attempts to purchase instruments from the Institute or through various ministries to which I was directed were unavailing. In the end, chance conversation in a Leningrad café elicited the information that the instruments were manufactured in that city. I recalled what I had dimly wondered at—in a country where all surgery is performed in government hospitals—a sign over a store on the Nevsky Prospekt proclaiming it a store for surgical instruments and apparatus. It proved to be just that. The only stapling instrument on hand was the UKB bronchial stapler (see Fig I–19*J*), the staples at right angles to the staple line, thus in the long axis of the bronchus. Then and there I purchased it in its elegant wooden, velvet-lined box and a few days later was "checked out" on it at the Institute in Moscow. We began experimental and clinical evaluation at once on returning home (Ravitch, Brown, Daviglus, 1959; Ravitch, Steichen, Fishbein, Knowles, Weil, 1964). Shortly thereafter, we obtained a full range of the Russian instruments and began evaluating those in the laboratory and in the clinic (Ravitch, Lane, Cornell, Rivarola, McEnany, 1966; Ravitch and Rivarola, 1966; Ravitch, Rivarola, VanGrov, 1967; Ravitch, Canalis, Weinshelbaum, McCormick, 1967), moving then into the experimental and clinical use of the American instruments as they became available (Steichen, 1968; Steichen, Talbert, Ravitch, 1968; Steichen, 1971; Ravitch and Steichen, 1972; Steichen and Ravitch, 1973).—M.M.R.

THE SOVIET INSTRUMENTS were finished by hand, so their parts were not interchangeable. The staples had to be hand-loaded, although there were replaceable cartridges available for some of the instruments. In addition, those instruments that accepted a cartridge required partial disassembly to replace an expended cartridge (see Fig I–19*J*). Possibly the chief problem with the Russian instruments was the fact that the multiple fine moving parts were incorporated into the basic instrument, creating difficulties in cleaning and maintenance, and inviting breakage. Each instrument accepted only a single size of cartridge and with a single arrangement of staples so that in Russia one saw on the nurse's table at each operation a huge basket filled with a quite large variety of these instruments.

Beginning in the fall of 1958, at the laboratory of the Department of Surgery at the Baltimore City Hospitals, and continuing from 1966–69 in the laboratories of the Division of Pediatric Surgery at the University of Chicago, we studied the use and effectiveness of the Russian instruments. We studied first the L-shaped instruments, the use of one of which in Amosov's hands in Kiev had so impressed us when, with one application, he stapled the right main bronchus, pulmonary artery, and both pulmonary veins. We found to be of no consequence the multiple variant staple line patterns, which the Russians had devised specifically for bronchi, pulmonary vessels, left atrium, and bowel. The double staggered pattern of the UKL, the instrument that had so excited us, we found served well for the bronchus, for the pulmonary vessels (we never cared, esthetically, for stapling the hilum en masse and never evaluated that technique), for pulmonary parenchyma, for the atrium, and for transecting all segments of the gastrointestinal tract. We discuss in Chapter III studies of the healing of closures of the gastrointestinal tract performed with the Russian instruments.

Author's Note

In 1963, when I joined the faculty of the Albert Einstein College of Medicine as Associate Director of the Department of Surgery at the Lincoln Hospital, we devoted the laboratory largely to the study of stapling, with the active support of P.H. Weil, the Director of the Department. Much of this work was not published, since much of the experimental work done at the time was immediately applied clinically. The first result was the functional end-to-end anastomosis (Steichen 1968) with the GIA^{TM} stapler, to us still the workhorse of most small and large bowel anastomoses.

The first Hunt-Lawrence and Paulino pouches with staplers were made at Lincoln Hospital with Fernando Paulino in attendance.

We studied use of the GIA^{TM} surgical stapling instrument inserted from below and above to avoid any cul-de-sac at all in the Duhamel procedure.

The first clinical gastrectomy (June 6, 1967), and shortly thereafter the first pulmonary lobectomy, with the American instruments loaded with cartridges as they now are available, were done at Albert Einstein College and Lincoln Hospitals.

The triangulating, end-to-end bowel anastomosis was developed at the Lincoln laboratory by Turi Josefsen and Gershon Efron.

Esophageal coloplasty, using the stapling instruments, was developed in those days at the Lincoln and Van Etten Hospitals.

It was also then that we started to make permanent tube gastrostomies with the GIA^{TM} surgical stapling instrument and to transect and close bowel with the GIA^{TM} surgical stapling instrument.

Many of the other clinical applications of the instruments in routine use today were intensely studied in the laboratory before they were used on patients.—F.M.S.

It was the recommendation to the American manufacturers (United States Surgical Corporation, Norwalk, Conn.), who entered the field after two of the major manufacturers of sutures had made the decision not to get involved with staples, that exciting as the vascular instruments were they would require essentially total redesign for practical use, and that, unless organ transplantation became a major matter, instruments requiring considerable lengths of normal vessel, as the Russian instruments did, would not be widely used. On the other hand, the instruments of the UKL variety—the two nesting Ls with staple cartridge and anvil on the upper and lower short legs, respectively—had wide applicability. The instrument, in addition to being better balanced and lighter, should be provided with preloaded, presterilized, color-coded disposable cartridges. An instrument of a given size should be able to accept cartridges with various patterns of staple lines. The staple cartridge should be replaceable without partial disassembly of the instrument.

These desiderata were all met by the manufacturers and, in addition, a basic new principle was introduced by them—the fine moving parts, staple-driving fins and the knife blades—were incorporated in the disposable staple cartridge, leaving the basic instrument as a sturdy, relatively simple, trouble-free compression device. There was no Russian counterpart of the skin and fascia stapler, developed in the American series, and the Russian prototype of the ligating and dividing stapler was not a dependable instrument, nor did it contain a knife.

The American instruments are characterized, in addition, by a better balance than the Russian instruments, by modifications in shape—particularly the lower jaw of the instruments of the TA^{TM} series—facilitating their use. The knurled knob by which the jaws were opened or closed was replaced by the more practical wing nut. From the first, we insisted that the linear anastomotic instrument (GIA^{TM}) insert a double staggered row of staples instead of the single row of the Russian instrument. The same requirement was imposed and met for the circular end-to-end anastomosing instrument (EEA^{TM}). Most recently, the instruments made by the original American surgical stapler manufacturers (United States Surgical Corporation, Norwalk, Conn.) have become available as completely disposable units, incorporating a given basic instrument with its corresponding cartridge, all disposable after a single use. Perhaps understandably, since they are the newest instruments, despite the fact that they are totally disposable, these instruments variously embody significant changes in design and improvement in function. In the disposable instruments of the TA^{TM} series, a single lever approximates the jaws, eliminating the somewhat annoying need to screw down the jaws. And, in these instruments, the tissue-retention and jaw-aligning pin is part of the instrument and slips into place as the jaws are approximated by the lever. As this is being written, these various improvements have just been introduced into new steel Premium^{TM} TA instruments in which only a cartridge-anvil assembly is disposable. The Disposable GIA^{TM} instrument, and the Premium^{TM} model as well, have a mechanism for maintaining approximation of the jaws out to the tip and also produce a more hemostatic staple pattern. The Disposable EEA^{TM} surgical stapling instrument has a superior operating mechanism and the PSS^{TM} disposable skin stapler and LDS^{TM} vessel stapler are operated by puffs of gas released from an integral cartridge. Firms newly entering the field in the United States appear also to be opting for totally disposable instruments.

With the exception of the skin stapler, and of the ligating and dividing stapler in which the gathering and compression of the tissue, stapling, and division are one continuous operation effected by a single squeeze of the handle (and in the newest, totally disposable models by a puff of compressed gas released by fingertip pressure), the stapling instruments, following the principle first developed in the original Hültl instrument, operate in two stages. In the first step, the instrument jaws are approximated so as to coapt the tissues with the desired degree of compression and, in the second, the staples are driven through the fixed tissues, which are held immobile, so that the sharpened staples penetrate without tearing the tissues.

At the present writing, all the stapling instruments studied experimentally and utilized clinically by us are made by a single manufacturer (United States Surgical Corporation, Norwalk, Conn.), and these are the instruments described in the following pages. The intensive interest in stapling techniques, and their great surge in popularity among surgeons here and abroad in the past decade, currently are drawing the attention of suture manufacturers. Three other manufacturers have released skin staplers (see Fig II–14), and one manufacturer has a prototype end-to-end anastomotic instrument undergoing clinical trials (see Fig II–9). It is to be confidently expected that other manufacturers will present new instruments, possibly by modifications of the existing ones but conceivably by changes in basic principles. It is unequivocally certain that the existing instruments and the new instruments will find applications so far not yet envisaged.

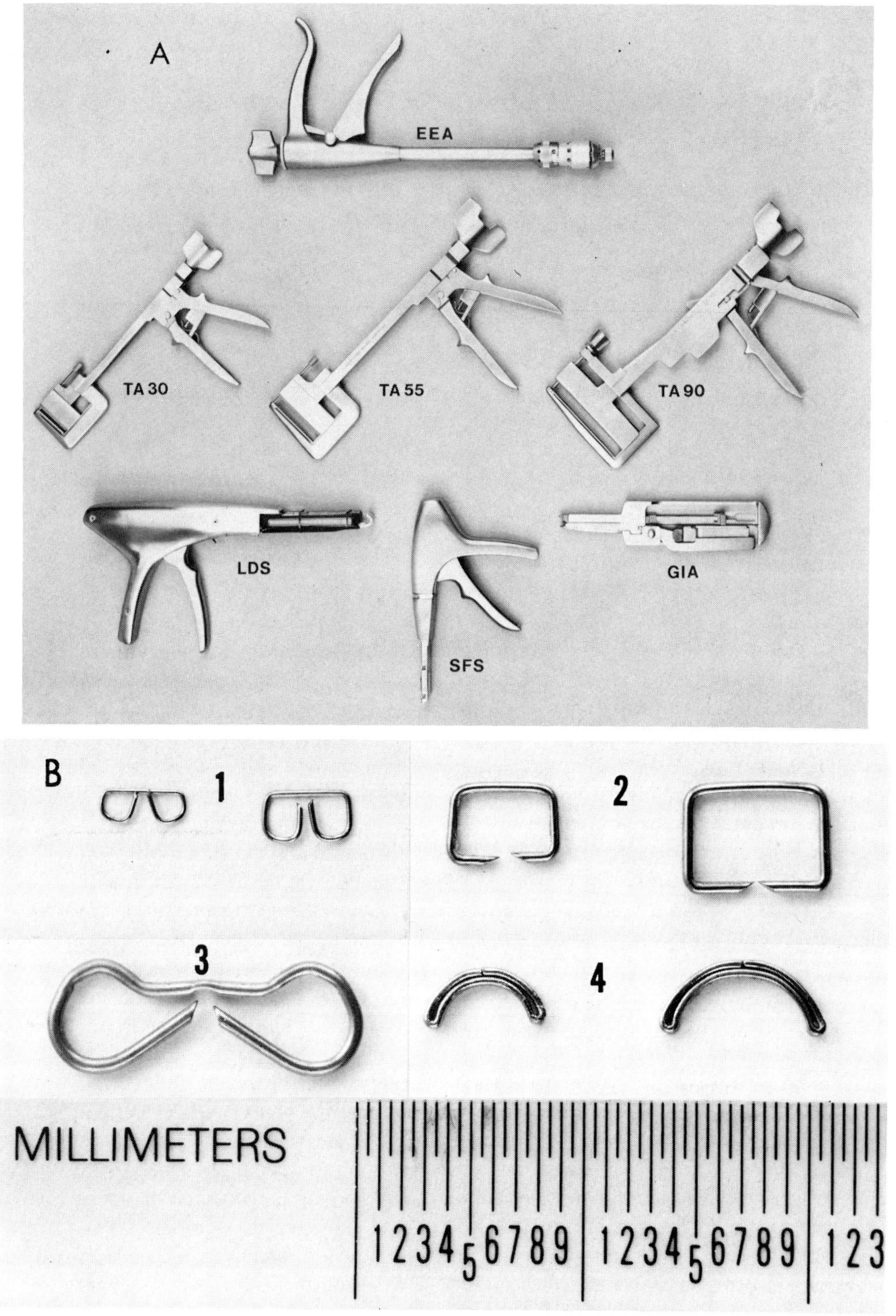

Fig II–1 A–B.—See legend on facing page.

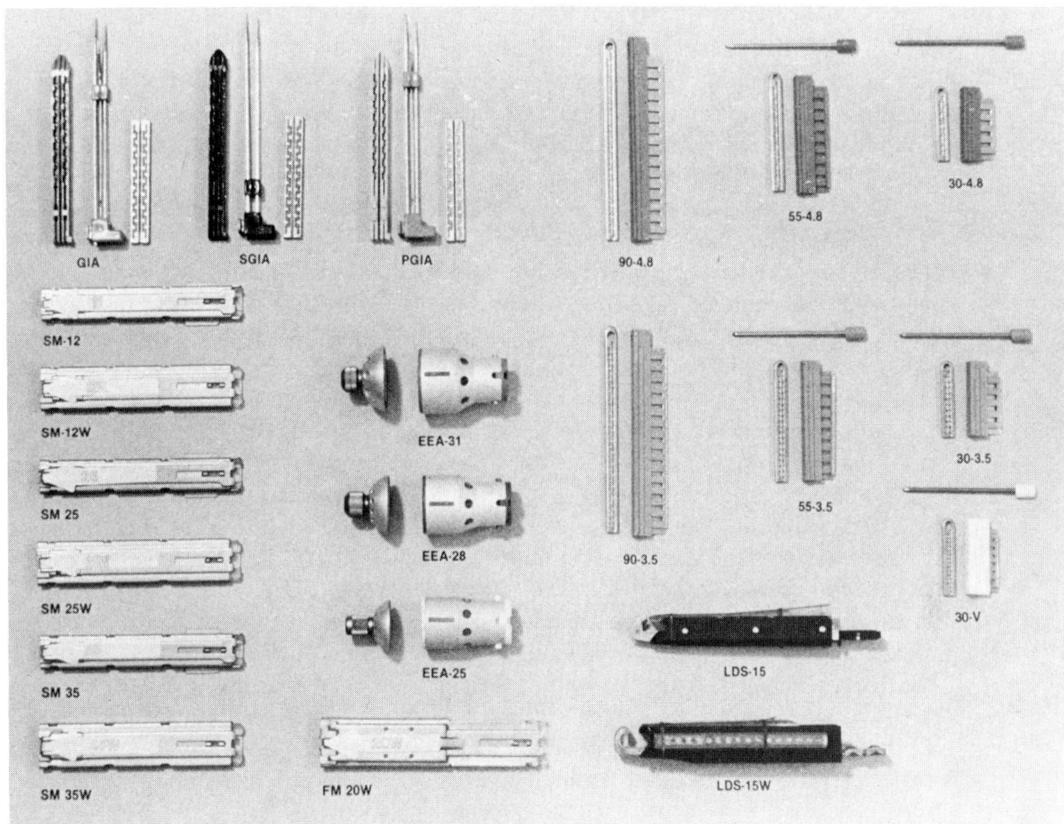

Fig II–2.—The varieties of disposable cartridges used for the several stapling instruments, varying in size of the staples, in the length or diameter of the staple row, or, for magazine-loaded instruments (SM™, FM™, SDS™), in the number of staples.

Fig II–1.—**A,** the original American-made stapling instruments, each loaded with disposable, presterilized, preloaded cartridges interchanged for repeated use during operation. The LDS™ instrument for double clipping and dividing of mesenteric or omental vessels and the SFS™ instrument for stapling skin or fascia are supplied with cartridges permitting multiple discharges before reloading. The others require reloading after each use. An early model of the SFS™ instrument in clinical use was powered by a replaceable CO_2 cartridge. **B,** staple configuration. *(1)* As in almost all the stapling instruments, beginning with Hültl's, the staples for suturing parenchymal organs begin in a squared-off U (as do the staples in *2* and *3*) and close in a B, which is nonstrangulating, non-necrosing, and permits vessels to pass through the staple loops. Shown formed are the staples of 3.5 and 4.8 mm leg lengths. *(2)* The removable skin staples of two sizes. By an ingenious mechanism, these do not require an anvil to complete their rectangular closure. *(3)* The staples for fascial suture are much heavier and require a different configuration to resist distraction of the sutured tissues. *(4)* The LDS™ staple, in two sizes, for securing of blood vessels, cystic duct, etc., is initially shaped in a rounded U and compresses to a flattened crescent, the vessel being securely held between the two layers of the formed crescent.

The instruments to be described below are a family of seven (Fig II–1): the TA 30[TM], the TA 55[TM], the TA 90[TM], GIA[TM], EEA[TM], LDS[TM], and the Skin and Fascia Stapler (Ravitch and Steichen, 1972; Ravitch, Hirsch, Noiles, 1972; Ravitch, 1978; Steichen and Ravitch, 1980). In all instances, the number attached to the designation of the instrument indicates in millimeters the length of the staple suture line (Fig II–2). The cartridge and staple specifications are to be found in Table II–1.

I. The TA[TM] instrument consists of two nesting Ls, whose long vertical limbs slide on each other, the short horizontal limbs forming the jaws. The upper jaw holds the disposable staple cartridge while the disposable metal anvil slips over the lower jaw. A pin dropped through the cartridge jaw into the anvil jaw insures alignment of cartridge and anvil during the compression, as well as preventing the tissues from escaping beyond the staple line. Turning the wing nut at the upper end of the instrument causes the Ls to slide on each other, approximating the short limbs. The tissues to be sutured thus are compressed within a minimally variable thickness, as indicated by two vernier lines on the vertical limbs, which indicate the area of compression within which the B of the staple will be properly formed. A squeeze of the activating handle drives the push rod contained within the long limb of the inner, cartridge-carrying, L. The rod ends in a bar that presses on the staple-driving fins in the cartridge, which in turn force the staples through the tissues. As these strike the curved recesses in the anvil, the staple ends are curved back into the tissues in the shape of a B. The entire row of staples is driven through and formed simultaneously. Each TA[TM] instrument has several specific uses. The three, combined, cover the field of terminal, or tangential, linear sutures required in pulmonary, gastrointestinal, and vascular surgery. The fine stainless steel staples used in all of these instruments are essentially nonreactive in the tissues and are provided in sterile, preloaded cartridges, color-coded to indicate the pattern and size of the staples.

TABLE II–1.—STAPLE SPECIFICATIONS FOR DISPOSABLE LOADING UNITS
(APPROXIMATIONS)

DISPOSABLE LOADING UNIT	WIRE DIAMETER	WIDTH × LENGTH	CLOSED HEIGHT
LDS[TM]-15/LDS[TM]-6 dlu	0.35 mm × 0.64 mm	5.8 mm × 5.2 mm	5.3 mm (width)
LDS[TM]-15W/LDS[TM] -6W dlu	0.35 mm × 0.64 mm	8.0 mm × 7.2 mm	7.3 mm (width)
TA 90[TM]-4.8 dlu	0.28 mm	4.0 mm × 4.8 mm	2.0 mm
TA 90[TM]-3.5 dlu	0.23 mm	4.0 mm × 3.5 mm	1.5 mm
TA 55[TM]-4.8 dlu	0.28 mm	4.0 mm × 4.8 mm	2.0 mm
TA 55[TM]-3.5 dlu	0.23 mm	4.0 mm × 3.5 mm	1.5 mm
TA 30[TM]-4.8 dlu	0.28 mm	4.0 mm × 4.8 mm	2.0 mm
TA 30[TM]-3.5 dlu	0.23 mm	4.0 mm × 3.5 mm	1.5 mm
TA 30[TM]-V dlu	0.21 mm	3.0 mm × 2.5 mm	1.0 mm
GIA[TM] dlu	0.20 mm	4.0 mm × 4.0 mm	1.75 mm
PGIA[TM] dlu	0.20 mm	4.0 mm × 3.0 mm	1.25 mm
SGIA[TM] dlu	0.20 mm	4.0 mm × 4.0 mm	1.75 mm
EEA[TM]-31 dlu	0.28 mm	4.0 mm × 4.8 mm	2.0 mm
EEA[TM]-28 dlu	0.28 mm	4.0 mm × 4.8 mm	2.0 mm
EEA[TM]-25 dlu	0.28 mm	4.0 mm × 4.8 mm	2.0 mm
EEA[TM]-21 dlu	0.28 mm	4.0 mm × 4.8 mm	2.0 mm
FM[TM]-20W dlu	0.7 mm	18.75 mm × 6.3 mm	4.75 mm
FM[TM]-25 dlu	0.56 mm	14.1 mm × 3.4 mm	4.7 mm
SM[TM]-12/SM[TM]-25/ SM[TM]-35	0.51 mm	10.2 mm × 2.4 mm	3.4 mm
SM[TM]-12W/SM[TM]25W/ SM[TM]-35W dlu	0.56 mm	14.1 mm × 3.25 mm	4.7 mm

dlu = disposable loading unit.

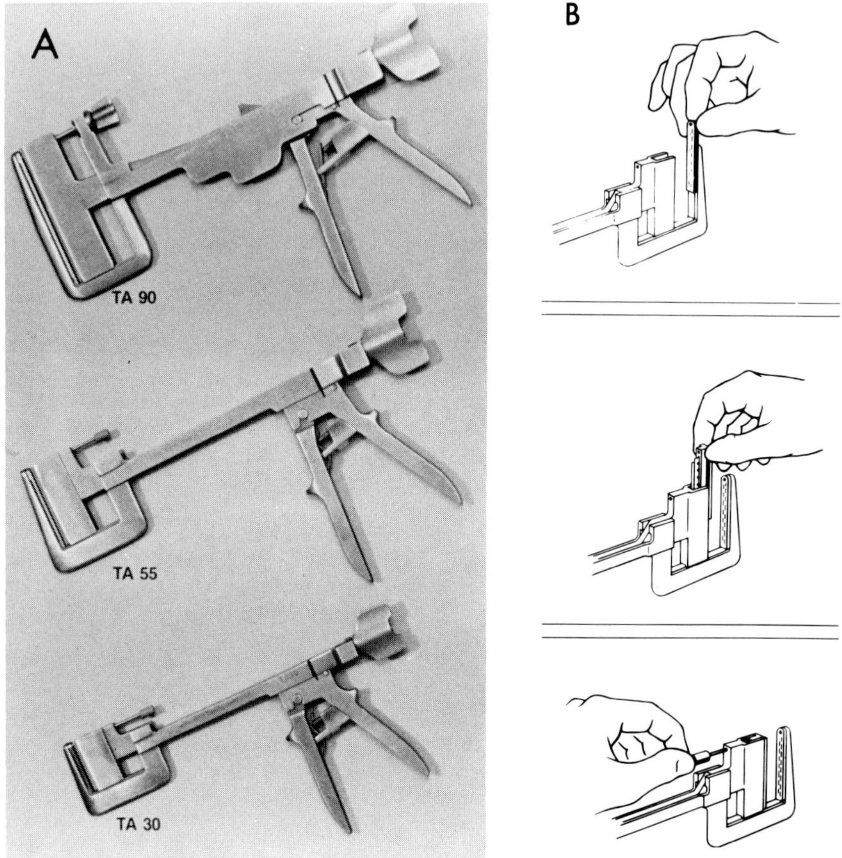

Fig II–3.—The instruments of the TA™ series. **A,** the steel stapling instruments of the TA™ series in the design in clinical use since 1967. The numbers 90, 55, and 30 refer to the length of the suture lines in millimeters. **B,** for each use, the metal shoe containing the anvil grooves is placed on the lower jaw and the plastic staple cartridge is slipped into the upper jaw and the retaining pin inserted. Turning the wing nut approximates the jaws, vernier markings on the shafts indicating the range within which the staples are properly formed. A squeeze of the handle fires the staples.   *(cont.)*

For the TA 55™ and the TA 90™ instruments, two sizes of staples are available, with legs of 3.5 mm or 4.8 mm, to provide for tissue of varied thickness. The thickness of the cartridges permits tissue stapled with the 3.5 mm staples to be compressed to 1.5 mm and with the 4.8 mm to 2.0 mm.

As this is being written, totally disposable equivalents of each of these instruments (Fig II–3D) have become available. The specifications in some, the mode of action in others, the principle of activation in still others are different from those of the steel instruments. The description of the new, totally disposable devices in all instances here follows after the description of the heretofore standard stainless steel instruments with disposable cartridges. With the exception of the GIA™ instrument, there has been no change in staple size or configuration of staple line, and the experience with the standard instruments quoted in subsequent chapters can be expected to be at least equaled with the totally disposable instrument. To the degree that the disposable instruments are superior because of improved design, and safer because always correctly assembled and loaded, results with them may be expected to be superior.

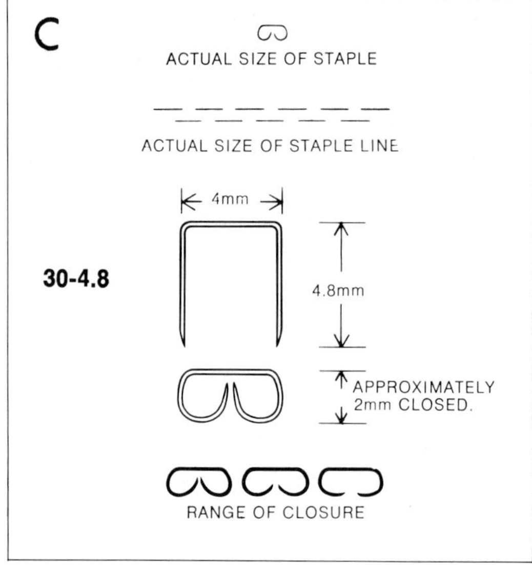

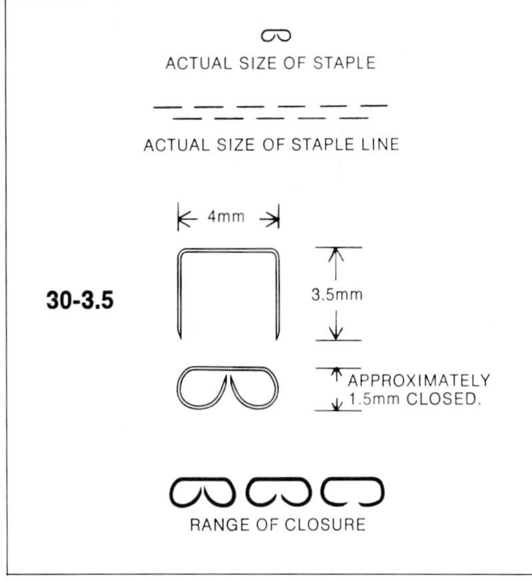

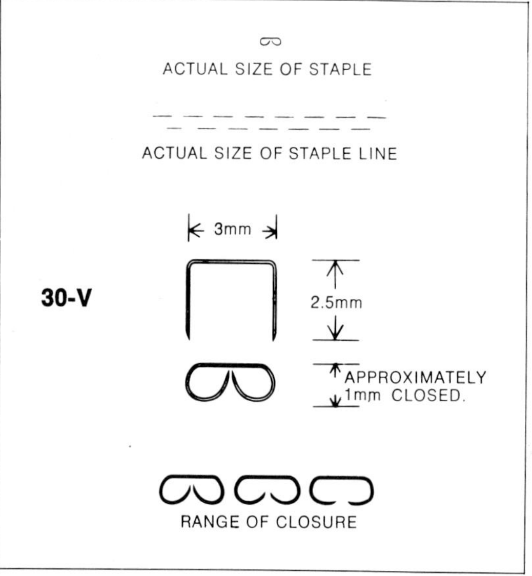

Fig II–3 (cont.).—C, staple dimensions and configurations for the TA 30[TM] instrument. The 3.5 and 4.8 mm staples are also used in the TA 55[TM] and TA 90[TM] instruments, but the suture lines are 55 and 90 mm long.

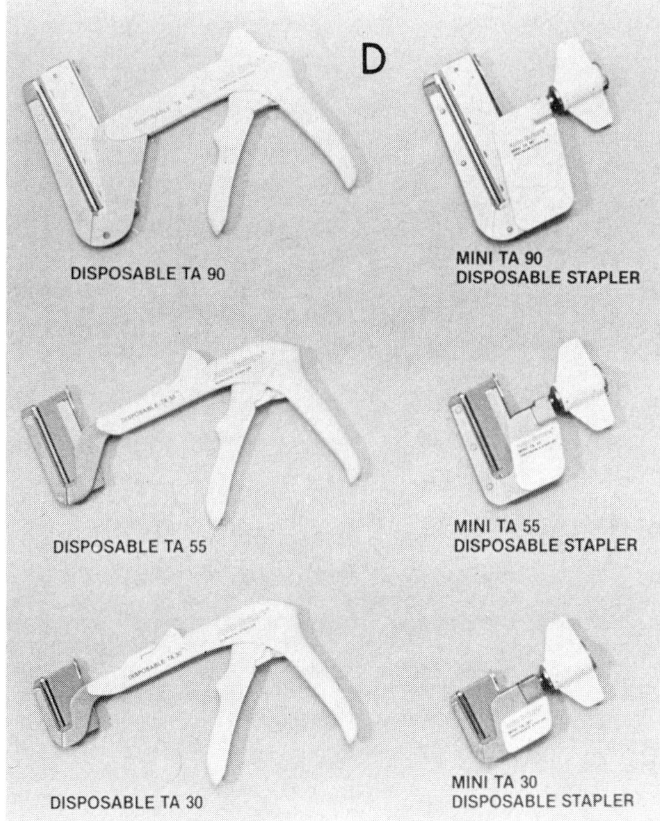

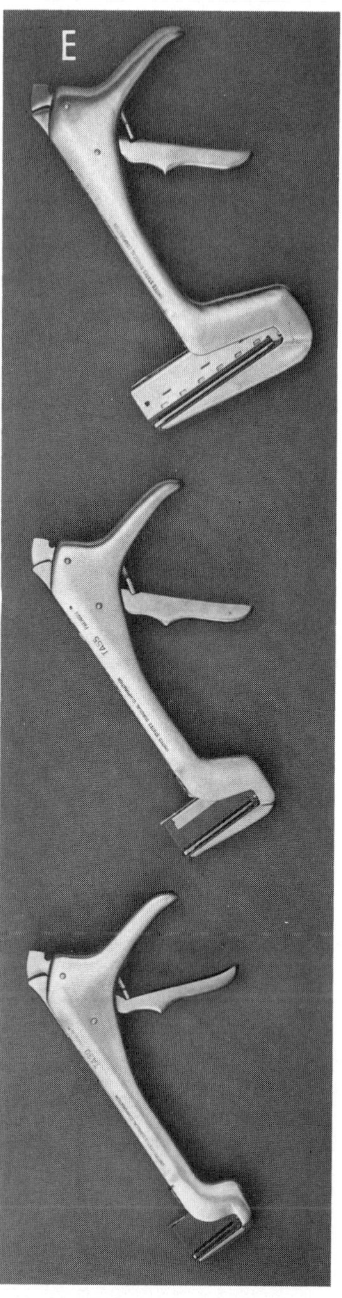

Fig II–3 (cont.).—D, the totally disposable TA™ instruments made available in 1980. These come in sterile packages, loaded with their integral cartridges and tissue-retaining pins. In the instruments in the left column, the jaws snap open by pressure on the projecting catch on the shaft and close by pressure on the lever just below the catch. In the truncated instruments in the right-hand column, the jaws are opened and closed by turning the wing nut. Pulling up on the ring, which is centered on the top of the wing nut, engages the wing nut in a second set of threads. Turning the wing nut now drives in the staples. Staples, configuration, and staple lines are identical to those shown in **A–C.**

E, the most recent (TA 90, 55, 30 Premium™) models of the steel instruments. Made available in 1981, these, like the conventionally shaped totally disposable TA™ instruments, have eliminated the need of a wing nut to close the jaws.   *(continued)*

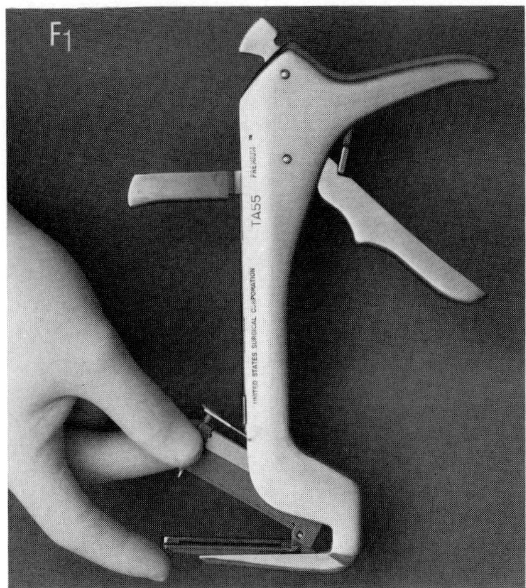

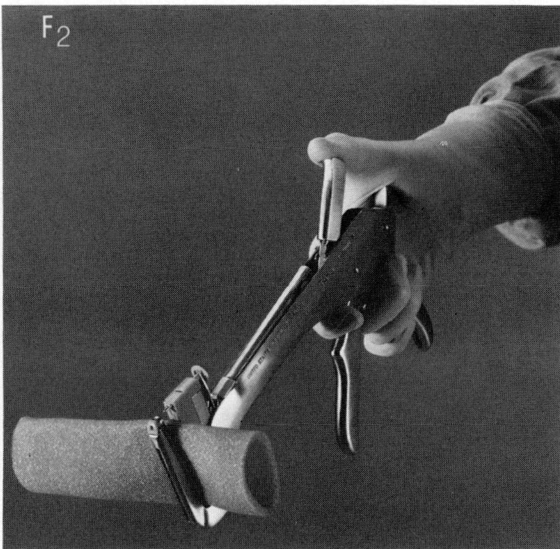

Fig II–3 (cont.).—F, the TA 55 Premium™ instruments. *(1)* The disposable staple cartridge and anvil are a hinged unit as in the totally disposable instruments, but now replaceable, and inserted into the open jaws in a single movement. *(2)* The jaw is opened by thumb pressure on the catch at top and closed by pressure on the lever below. The tissue-retaining pin, an integral part of the loading unit, presses into place as the jaw is closed. Staples, configuration, and staple lines are as shown in **(A–C)**. As the lever on the shaft, opposite the handle, is pressed down, the upper jaw of the staple cartridge-anvil assembly, hinged at the heel, closes on the tissue. The tendency for the tissue to slide forward requires attention on the part of the operator. To correct this, the fixed hinge is being replaced by a floating hinge, which will allow the jaws to come parallel as they start to close.

The TA 90^{TM} instrument (Fig II–4) finds greatest use in transection of the stomach and colon, in excision of pulmonary bullae and division of incomplete fissures, in stapling the undivided stomach, and in lateral closures of stomach and colon. The TA 55^{TM} instrument occasionally is large enough for gastric division or stapling, is the usual instrument for closing the transected duodenum, small or large bowel, and for excision and stapling of Zenker's diverticula, Meckel's diverticula, or mural lesions treated by a tangential resection, and for closing the opening left after a GIA^{TM} anastomosis. The pancreas is satisfactorily transected and stapled with the TA 55^{TM} instrument. The TA 55^{TM} instrument may be used for the main bronchus and for the pulmonary parenchyma as in biopsy wedge excision, "blebectomy," and division of incomplete fissure.

The TA 30^{TM} instrument often is large enough for the duodenum or small bowel and for most bronchi.

The TA 30^{TM} instrument, in addition to the cartridge containing the 3.5 mm and the 4.8 mm staples, has a third cartridge and corresponding anvil for fine, closely spaced staples for closure of pulmonary vessels, patent ductus, Potts' aortopulmonary shunt, portal vein, etc. The staple cartridge for this purpose is coded TA 30^{TM}-V and the cartridge delivers 15 staples of 0.21 mm sized wire, 3.0 mm across the bar, 1.5 mm apart, and in two rows separated by 1.5 mm, compressing tissue to approximately 1.0 mm. Figure II–4 shows the basic applications of the TA^{TM} instruments.

Disposable TA^{TM} instrument (see Fig II–3D). Entirely disposable TA^{TM} instruments with cartridge and stapler molded into a compact unit duplicate the specifications of staple size, shape, alignment, and length of suture lines of the standard instruments. However, they embody a hinge-like opening and closing mechanism for the upper staple cartridge jaw, as well as a tissue-retaining pin that moves into position automatically as the jaws are closed. The jaws are opened and closed by activating a lever in the vertical shaft of the instrument, obviating the need for turning a wing nut and eliminating the time required for that. The staples are driven in by the familiar compression of the handles. In an even simpler version of the TA^{TM} instruments (see Fig II–3D), likewise totally disposable and useful in deep cavities, the long shaft of the instrument is dispensed with, the jaws being opened and closed by a wing nut placed, for all intents and purposes, directly on the jaws so that there is no "handle" to the instrument. Once more, the tissue-retaining pin is integral to the instrument. The staples are discharged by pulling upward on a ring and then turning the wing nut again, which has been moved to a different set of threads by the pulling of the ring.

In using any of the TA^{TM} instruments, the jaws are opened, the lower jaw slipped under the tissue to be stapled, the retention pin introduced, the jaws approximated, and the staples fired. The instrument is brought down to the tissues, avoiding traction on them. The bronchus, vessel, or bowel is divided on the edge of the instrument before the instrument is removed. The bowel and bronchus closures are all mucosa-to-mucosa.

TA PROCEDURES

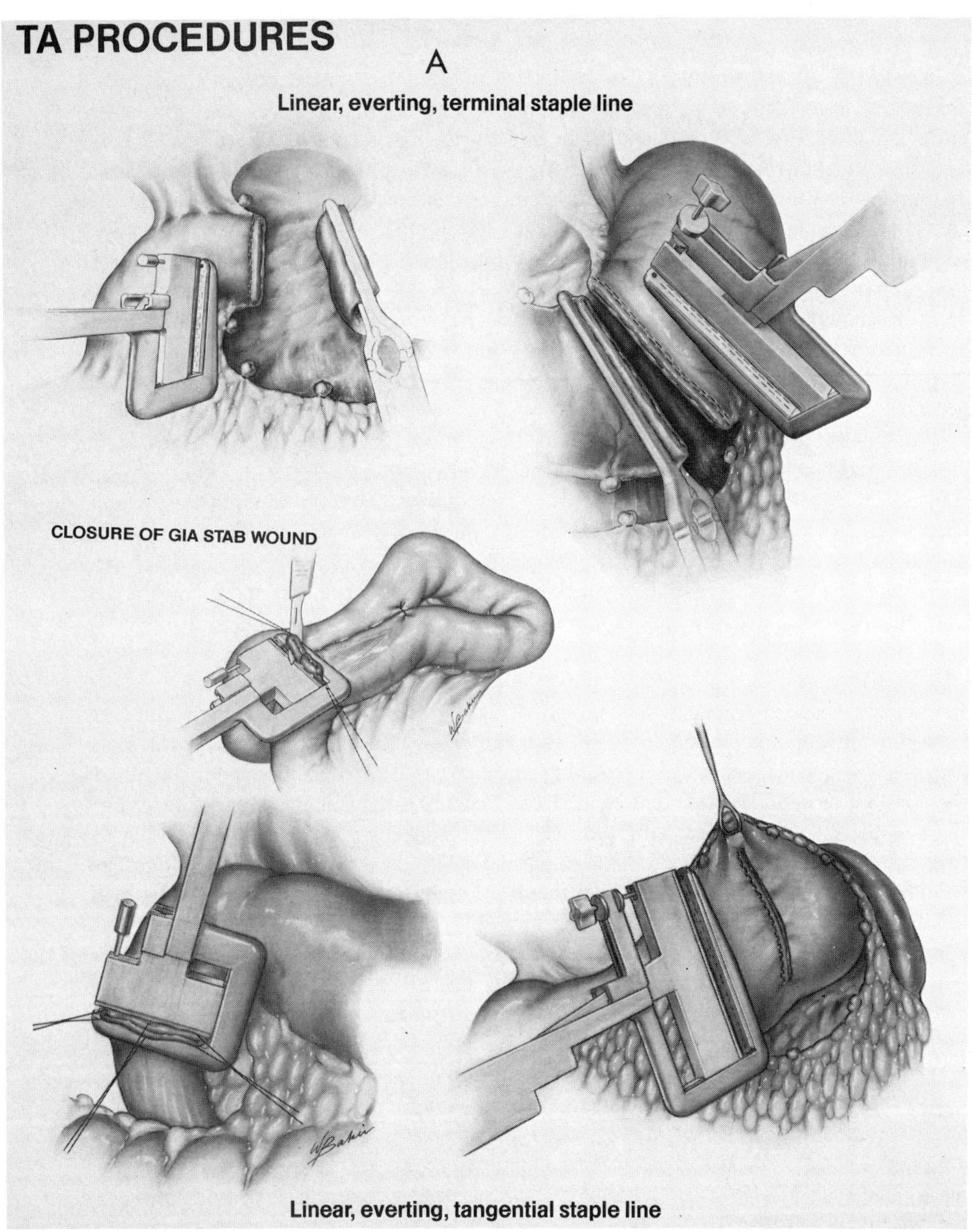

Fig II–4.—Basic uses of the TA™ instrument. In all its uses certain principles obtain: *(1)* One must bring the instrument down to the tissue to be stapled rather than pulling the organ up to the instrument. Stapling tissue on stretch invites the staple holes to tear. *(2)* The tissue-retaining pins always must be used, to keep the tissues from being squeezed beyond the staple line and to guarantee alignment of upper and lower jaw—i.e., of staples and anvil grooves. *(3)* The tissues should be cut, as shown in the drawings, on the edge of the stapler. This provides enough tissue for safety beyond the staple line, and no more. Cutting freehand after the stapler has been removed risks cutting into the staple line on the one hand or leaving an excessive stump of tissue on the other. *(4)* In the original steel TA™ instruments, one must close the jaws with the wing nut until the vernier markings are opposed. With the totally disposable instruments, and the steel Premium™ instruments, an automatic mechanism regulates jaw distance and tissue pressure when the lever is thrown, closing the jaws. *(5)* Do not include omentum or mesentery in the tissue to be stapled and divided. Bleeding will result. *(6)* In closing GIA™ stab wounds, be certain that

→

TA PROCEDURES

B

Linear, everting, terminal staple line

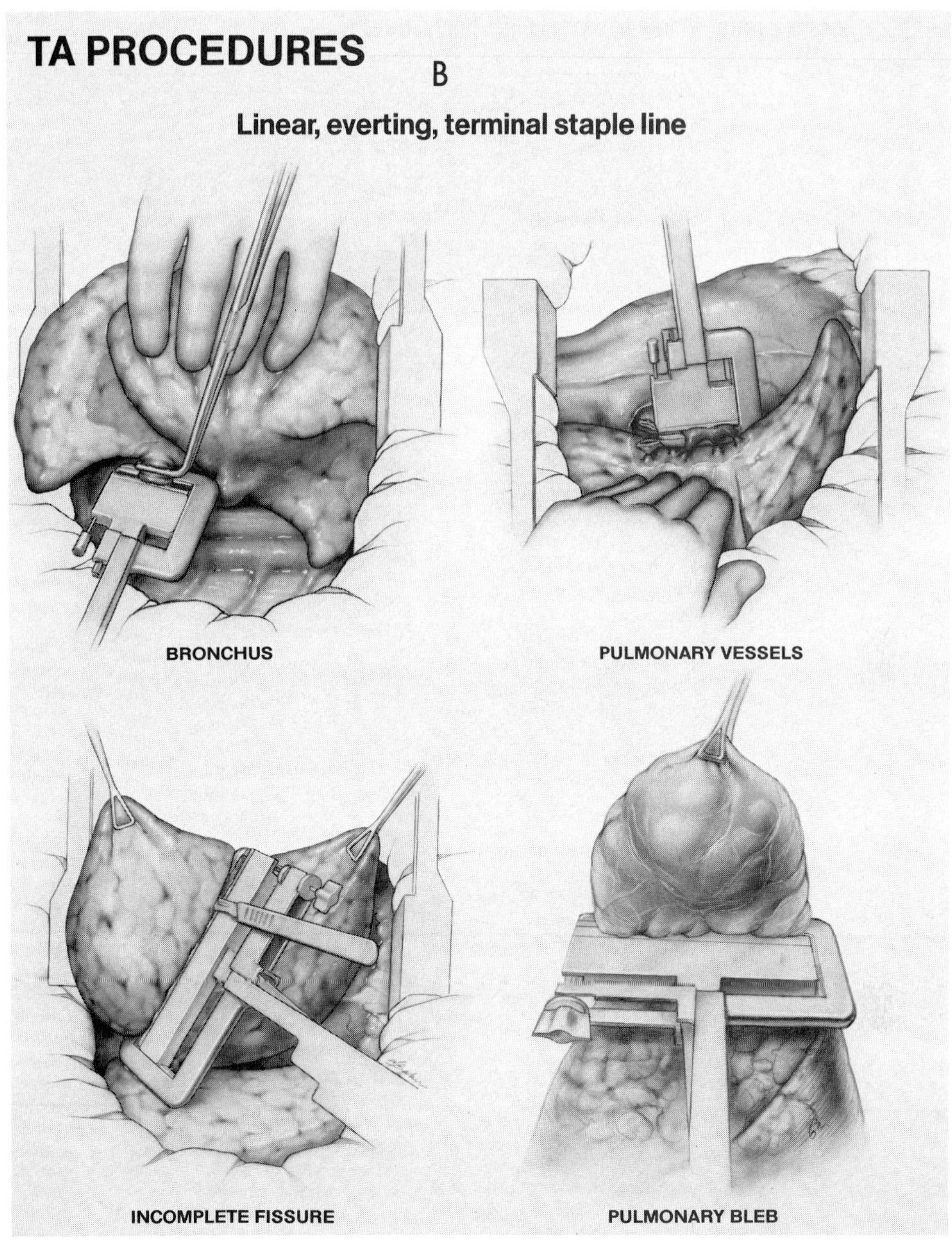

the TA™ jaws are on serosa the full 360 degrees of the opening. **A,** gastrointestinal tract. The instruments provide 30, 55, or 90 mm, double staggered staple lines for mucosa-to-mucosa closure of transected duodenum or stomach, as shown, or other portions of the gastrointestinal tract from the esophagus to the rectum. In the performance of anastomoses with the GIA™ instrument *(middle),* the single opening resulting generally is closed mucosa-to-mucosa with the TA™ instruments (see also Figs V–3 and V–4). Linear incisions in the bowel, as in duodenotomy for exposure of the ampulla of Vater *(bottom left),* are readily closed mucosa-to-mucosa with a TA™ instrument. Portions of bowel wall containing mural lesions are drawn through the jaws of the TA™ instrument, the bowel stapled and the specimen excised as in the lower right, showing the result after excision of a posterior wall gastric ulcer. **B,** basic uses of the TA™ instruments in pulmonary surgery. *Upper left:* mucosa-to-mucosa bronchial closure, TA 55™ or TA 30™ instrument. *Upper right:* stapling of the pulmonary vessels with the fine vascular cartridge in the TA 30™ stapler. *Lower left:* bloodless division and closure of an incomplete fissure, as between the upper and middle lobes in right upper lobectomy, TA 90™ or TA 55™ instrument. *Lower right:* amputation of a pulmonary bulla, TA 90™ or TA 55™ instrument.

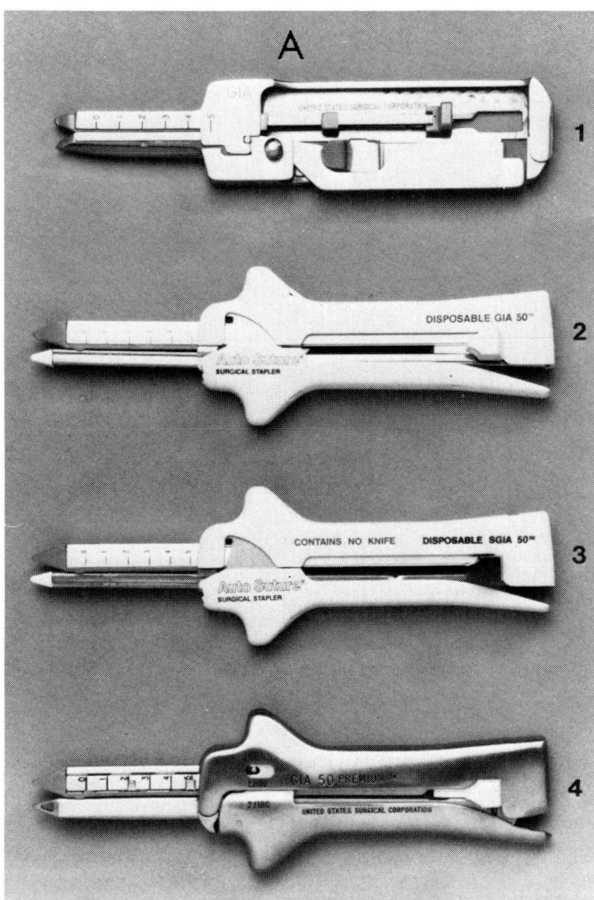

Fig II–5.—Instruments of the GIA™ series. **A,** GIA™ instruments: *(1)* steel, *(2)* totally disposable, *(3)* SGIA™, totally disposable and without knife blade, and *(4)* Premium GIA™. Each inserts two double staggered staple lines (i.e., four rows of staples) and all except the SGIA™ instrument have a knife that passes down the center between the two double rows. *(1), (2),* and *(4)* transect bowel, leaving both ends stapled, or perform side-to-side, end-to-side, end-to-end, or functional end-to-end anastomoses; *(3),* the SGIA™ instrument, applies four rows of staples without dividing the tissue.

The totally disposable SGIA™ instrument and the Premium™ instrument have more staples **(B),** closer together, and include a device to maintain compression of the jaws **(C).**   *(continued)*

B

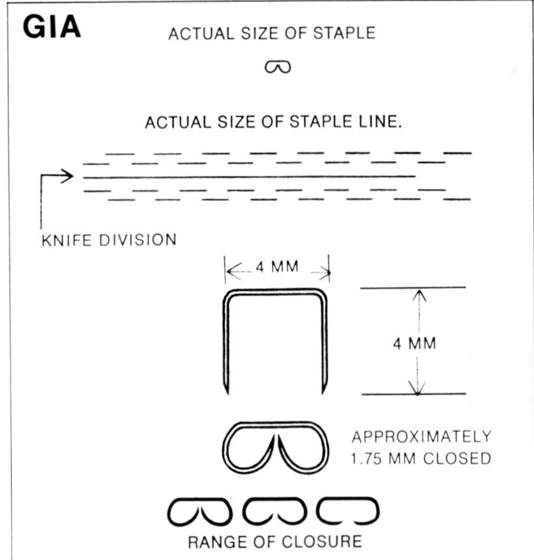

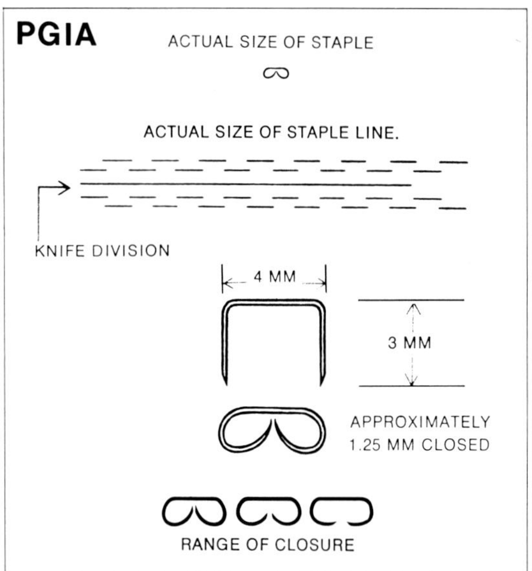

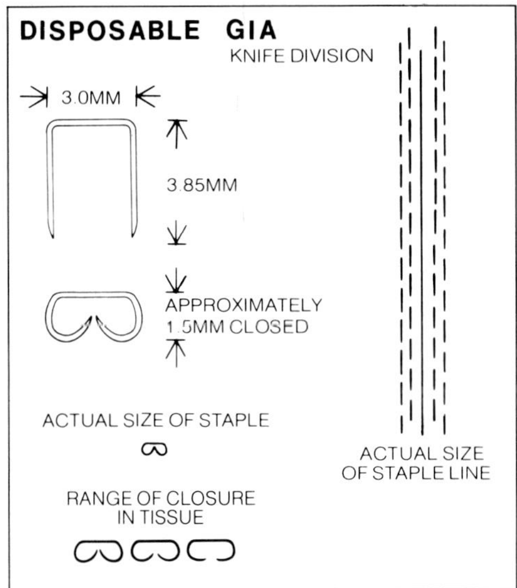

Fig II–5 (cont.).—B, staples, configuration, and staple lines of the GIA,[TM] P(Pediatric) GIA[TM], and disposable GIA[TM] instruments. Not shown is the S(Special) GIA[TM] cartridge for inserting four rows of staples without the knife, as used in control of gastric and esophageal varices and construction of the Kock pouch.   *(continued)*

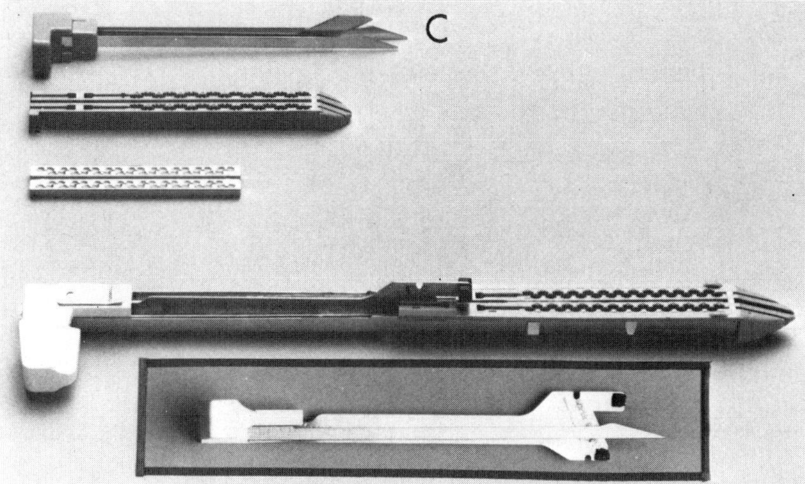

Fig II–5 (cont.).—C, the disposable loading units of the standard GIA™ instrument, in three parts, above, and of the Premium GIA™ instrument, below. The standard GIA™ disposable loading unit contains the metal anvil, the plastic staple-carrying cartridge, and the three-pronged assembly of two slightly staggered staple pusher elements and a knife between and a little behind them. In the Premium GIA™ instrument, the anvil recesses are carved in one limb of the instrument itself and the cartridge containing the staples—52 as against 32 (see **B**)—also contains the simplified pusher assembly. The insert shows the latter before it has been inserted during manufacture. The near staple pusher is visible, and behind it the knife blade to which are affixed, above and below, the small black shoes that fit into upper and lower jaws, above the midline slots. The effect, as the knife is pushed forward, is of a moving miniature I-beam that holds the jaws compressed to the same degree while the staples are driven in for the full length of the staple line.

II. The GIA™ instrument (Figs II–5 and II–6) consists of two interlocking halves that form a flat handle with two straight limbs. One limb accommodates the staple cartridge and the other accepts the anvil. Within the cartridge are two double staggered rows of staples, 16 staples in each double row, thus one double row on each side of a central groove through which the knife blade will advance. The staples are of 0.20 mm wire, have a bar of 4 mm, and a leg length of 4 mm. The two sets of staple lines are approximately 4 mm apart and each double row is 0.52 mm long. To divide bowel, the instrument is partially assembled, the loop of bowel to be divided slid between the two jaws and the instrument then locked and activated. The knife divides the bowel and both ends of bowel are closed mucosa-to-mucosa with a double staggered row of staples. In anastomosing two portions of the gastrointestinal tract, one limb is inserted into the lumen of each loop. As the instrument halves then are matched, mated, and locked, the double thickness of bowel wall is grasped between the limbs of the instrument. Operating the instrument now drives home the four rows of staples and, at the same time, divides the stapled tissue so as to leave a double row of staples on either side of the division, the knife stopping one and a half staples short of the end of the staple line. The assembly, which is driven home by the thumb, as in operating a piston-syringe, consists of three blades (see Fig II–5*C*), the two outer ones driving in the staples, the central one, the knife, dividing the tissues, each of the three blades sliding in a separate channel of the cartridge. The instrument is scored at 1-cm intervals up to 5 cm so that one can control the size of an anastomosis.

Anastomoses done with the GIA^{TM} instrument are serosa-to-serosa, but inconsequentially inverting. As the knife divides the stapled partition between the two loops, it converts the two stab wounds used for insertion of the instrument limbs into a single opening. This then is closed mucosa-to-mucosa with the TA^{TM} instrument. The GIA^{TM} stapler has been used by some surgeons for dividing the duodenum in gastrectomy, a practice that we have not adopted. It serves quite well for creating greater-curvature gastric tubes, or Janeway gastrostomies (see Fig V–9). If both walls of the stomach are transected with the GIA^{TM} instrument, because of the greater thickness of both gastric walls and the shorter GIA^{TM} staples, we reinforce the staple suture lines, the only time when reinforcing, manual sutures are routinely used by us. The GIA^{TM} instrument serves quite well for transection and stapling of pulmonary parenchyma, for whatever need (see Fig II–6).

The GIA^{TM} instrument is supplied with two sizes of staples. For adults (GIA^{TM}), 0.20 mm wire, 4 mm bar, 4 mm limbs, two sets of staple lines, the lines in each pair 1.2 mm apart and the two pairs 4 mm apart, and the PGIA^{TM} instrument for children, with staples of 0.20 mm wire, 4 mm bar, 3 mm limbs. Each 5.3-cm-long double row contains 16 staples. A special cartridge, SGIA^{TM} without the knife, inserts four rows of staples without any tissue division, as required in such special procedures as the stapling modification of the Tanner procedure for varices (see Fig VI–17) or the Kock ileal reservoir (see Fig VIII–12).

Disposable GIA^{TM} instrument. The GIA^{TM} instrument, too, now is provided in a totally disposable form, the basic instrument already being armed with staple-loaded cartridge and with anvil. The staples are shorter and closer together than in the standard GIA^{TM} instrument. There still are four rows of staples but these now are of 0.20 mm wire, 3 mm bar, 3.85 mm legs. The two sets of staple lines are approximately 3.5 mm apart. There are 26 staples in each double row, which is 5.3 cm long. The two jaws, instead of being held together only at their base by a lock, now are additionally held by a small shoe above and below the knife shaft. The shoes fit into slots in the cartridge and anvil and hold the two limbs constantly compressed to the same degree while the staples are progressively driven home the length of the instrument. It was thought that the original GIA^{TM} stapler had not been as regularly hemostatic as possible because of a tendency for the distal ends of the limbs to spread with repeated use. The mechanism described and the staple line changes are aimed at better hemostasis. The new approximating mechanism in the cartridge has altered the size and configuration of the instrument limbs. The disposable cartridge limb now has 1.34 sq. cm total cross-section as opposed to 0.99 sq. cm in the steel instrument. The anvil limb has been made smaller, 0.63 sq. cm as opposed to 0.93 sq. cm. The combined jaws now have a section of 1.97 cm^2 as opposed to the 1.92 cm^2 of the steel instrument. The newest steel instrument, GIA Premium^{TM}, incorporates all these features (see Fig II–5A).

GIA PROCEDURES
Transection between two staple lines

A

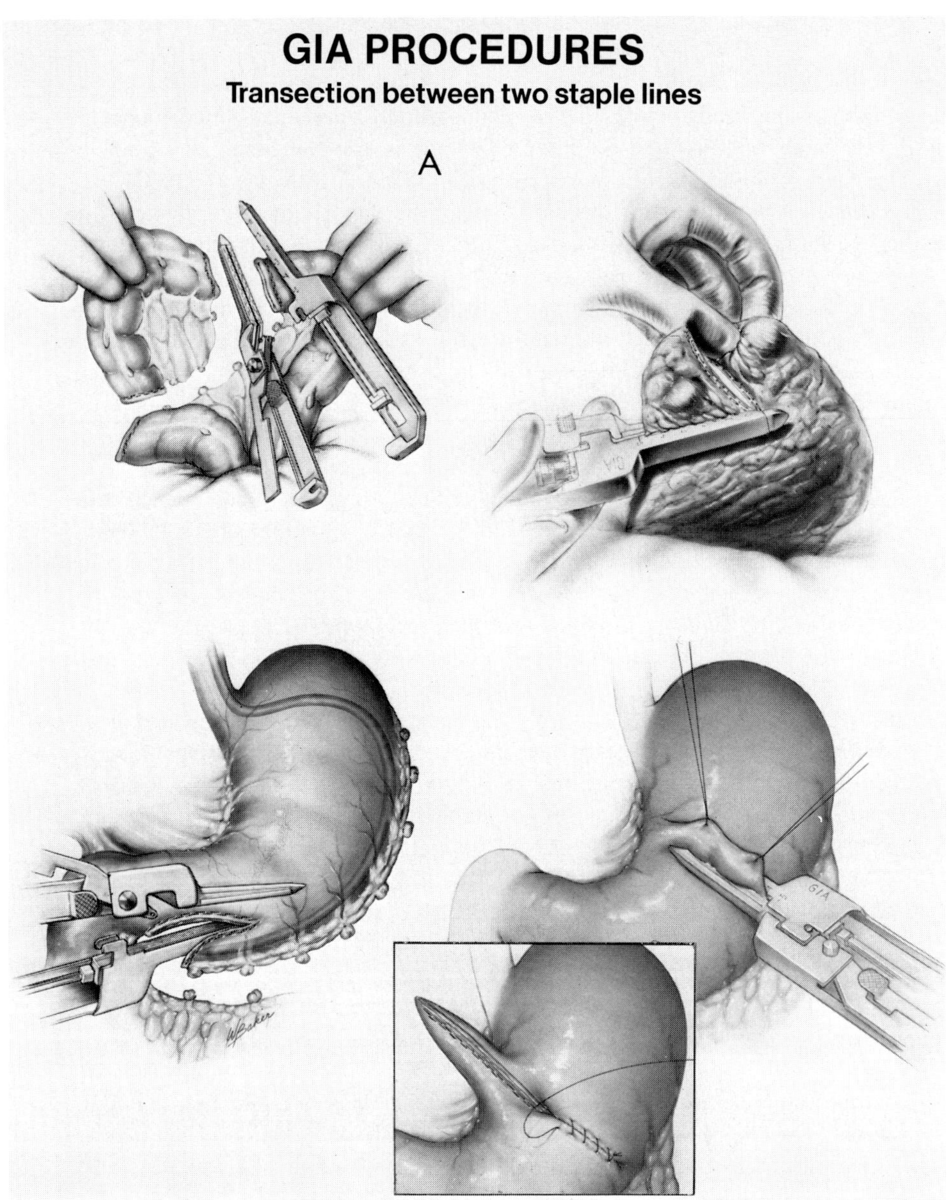

Fig II–6.—Basic uses of the GIA™ instrument. In all its uses, certain principles obtain: *(1)* The two limbs must be correctly mated and locked. This does not require force. If force is required to drive the staples home, the instrument limbs have been improperly assembled. *(2)* Be certain that the two staple drivers and the knife are each in their separate slots. *(3)* In dividing bowel or lung, be sure that the tissue to be divided is all within the graduations—i.e., in the staple-bearing portion of the jaws. *(4)* Do not attempt to include mesentery or omentum in the suture line. Bleeding will result. *(5)* Inspect anastomoses for bleeding. Reinforce with fine sutures if a bleeding point is seen. **A,** transec-tion and simultaneous stapling of lung and bowel. *Upper left:* shows the colon simultaneously transected and both ends stapled. Mesenteric vessels have been secured by the LDS™ instrument. *Upper right:* shows wedge resection of the lung. The staple lines cross. *Lower left:* shows the greater-curvature gastric tube produced by repeated applications of the GIA™ instrument, yielding a 5 cm increment in the length of the tube with each application of the instrument. *Lower right:* a Janeway mucosa-lined gastrostomy produced with a single operation of the GIA™ instrument. As shown, we usually oversew GIA™ suture lines when two layers of stomach are involved.

GIA PROCEDURES
Linear inverting anastomosis

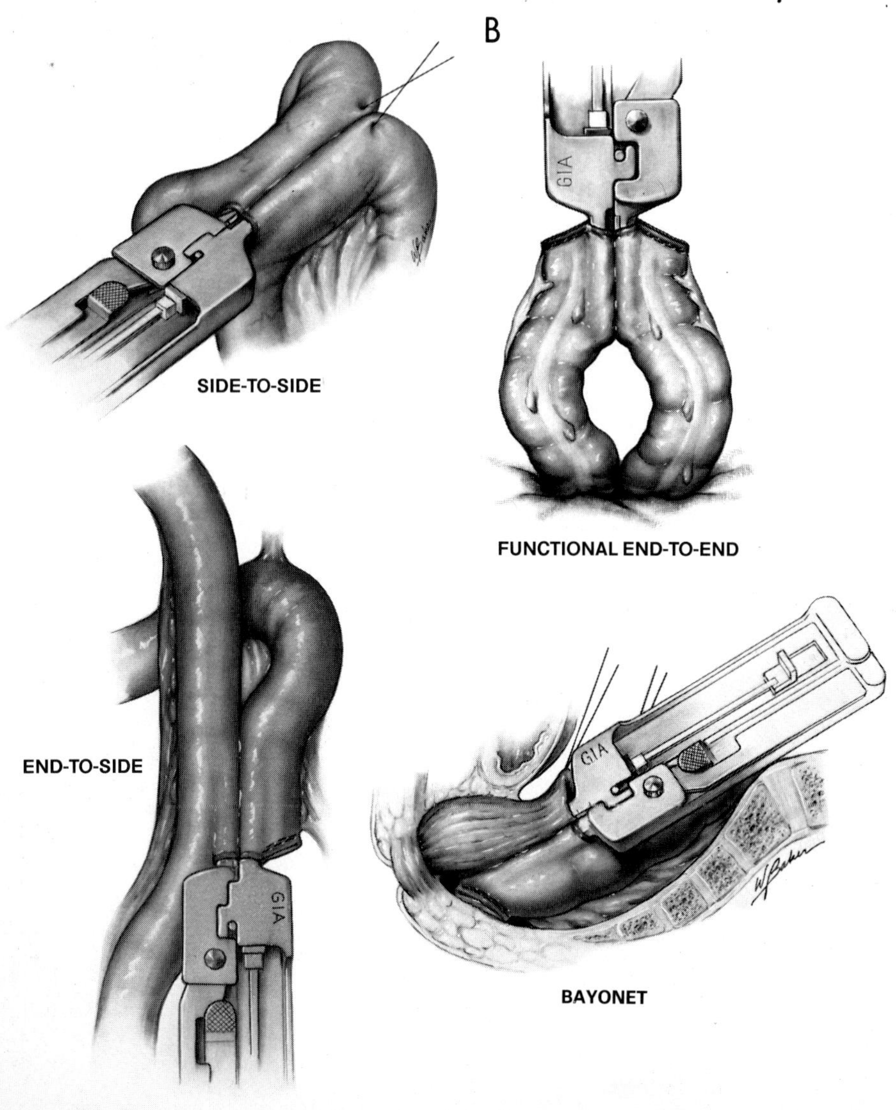

Fig II–6 (cont.).—B, Intestinal anastomoses. These are all serosa-to-serosa, minimally inverted and in each case the two openings, one for each prong of the GIA™ instrument, are converted into one when the two loops are stapled together and the stapled tissue divided by the knife in the instrument. The single opening that remains usually is closed mucosa-to-mucosa with the TA™ instrument, as shown in Figure II–4**A** (see also Figs V–3 and V–4). *Upper left:* side-to-side enteroenterostomy. *Upper right:* functional end-to-end colocolostomy. *Lower left:* end-to-side jejunojejunostomy as in the construction of a Roux-Y loop. *Lower right:* bayonet anastomosis as in low anterior resection.   *(continued)*

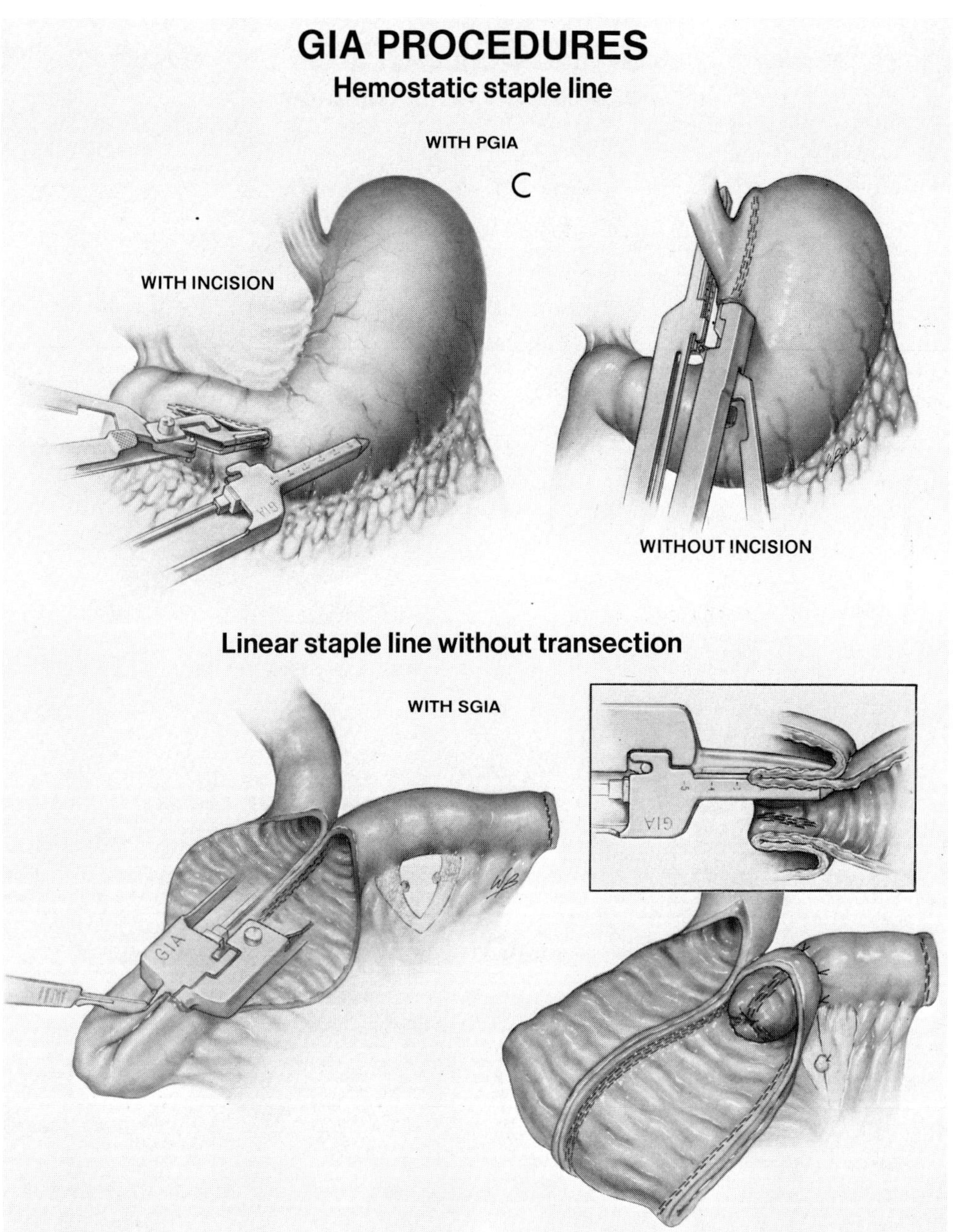

Fig II–6 (cont.).—C, special uses of the GIA™ instrument. *Upper left:* gastrotomy with the PGIA™ (P[ediatric] Cartridge) avoids troublesome bleeding from the gastrotomy during the intragastric manipulation. *Upper right:* application of the PGIA™ instrument *without the knife blade* to the anterior and posterior walls of the cardia for control of esophageal varices. *Lower left:* all four rows of staples, without the knife (SGIA™), anastomosing the two loops in a Kock pouch. *Inset and lower right:* the GIA™ instrument without the knife (SGIA™) is used to staple the inverted nipple to reduce the likelihood of loss of the nipple in a Kock pouch.

III. The EEA™ instrument (Figs II–7 and II–8) is a tubular instrument looking not unlike a sigmoidoscope. At what would be the obturator end of the sigmoidoscope, the tubular shaft of the EEA™ instrument can be loaded with a disposable cartridge that consists of a cylinder containing two circular rows of staggered staples, the pushers to drive the staples, and a circular knife just inside the inner ring of staples. A dome-shaped nose cone, carrying the anvils, screws onto the rod that passes through the center of the staple cartridge. Within the nose cone, just inside the inner row of anvil recesses, is a heavy plastic ring against which the circular knife cuts the bowel ends, purse-stringed around the central rod of the EEA™ instrument. The staples are of 0.28-mm wire, the bar 4 mm, the limbs 4.8 mm prior to closure. A wing nut in the handle separates or approximates the disposable staple and anvil portions of the instrument. The pursestringed bowel segments to be anastomosed are slipped over the dome-shaped anvil and the cylindrical cartridge, respectively, and the pursestrings tied tightly around the central shaft, the anvil and cartridge approximated, and the handles compressed, creating an instantaneous, minimally inverting, end-to-end or end-to-side anastomosis. The instrument can be positioned through a natural orifice, such as the anus in a low anterior resection of the rectum, the mouth in special circumstances for high esophago-gastric anastomoses, or through an opening made in the ordinary course of operation, as in the stomach for esophagogastrostomy, the small bowel for esophagojejunostomy, the terminal ileum for esophagocecostomy, or through a special gastrotomy, enteroto-my, or colotomy made only for the purpose of inserting the EEA™ instrument (see Fig II–8).

The EEA™ instrument is supplied with cartridges approximately 31, 28, and 25 mm in outside diameter, which produce anastomoses of 21, 18, and 15 mm internal diame-ter, respectively. The largest of these is designed for the adult rectum, although on occasion a smaller size is required. It is uncommon for the adult esophagus to accept the largest size. Ovoid sizers permit one to gauge the caliber of the bowel to assess which cartridge is to be used, to avoid making the anastomosis smaller than required, or alternatively to prevent injuring the bowel in the attempt to stretch it over too large a cartridge.

Disposable EEA™ instrument (see Fig II–7B,C). The Disposable EEA™ instrument comes fully assembled with any of the three cartridge sizes. The nose cone is removable for those procedures in which the instrument is passed into the lumen of a segment of the gastrointestinal tract, and the central rod, emerging through a puncture wound, then capped with the nose cone over which is slid the pursestringed segment of bowel to be anastomosed. The staple sizes and staple line specifications are unchanged. The instru-ment is opened and closed with a wing nut. The staples are easily fired, and the purse-stringed ends cut through, by compression of two handles, one on either side of the shaft. There has not yet been time to acquire experience with the new curved model of the totally Disposable EEA™ instrument. The instrument is a response to our long-term request for a curved shaft that would more easily be introduced from the anus or from the mouth and more comfortably placed deep in the chest or abdomen through thora-cotomy and laparotomy incisions. The demonstrated need for a smaller-diameter car-tridge in some applications, particularly the esophagus, has been met by the 20.9 mm diameter of the smallest cartridge and 11.4 mm knife diameter, made for the curved disposable EEA™ instrument, in addition to the same three sizes previously available for the steel instrument.

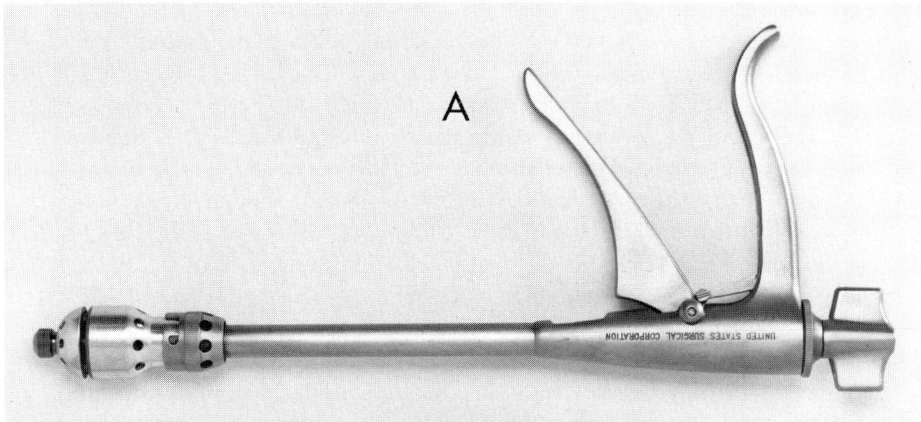

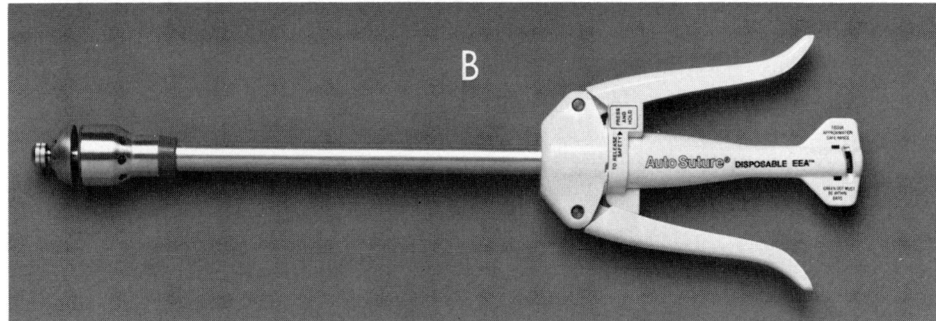

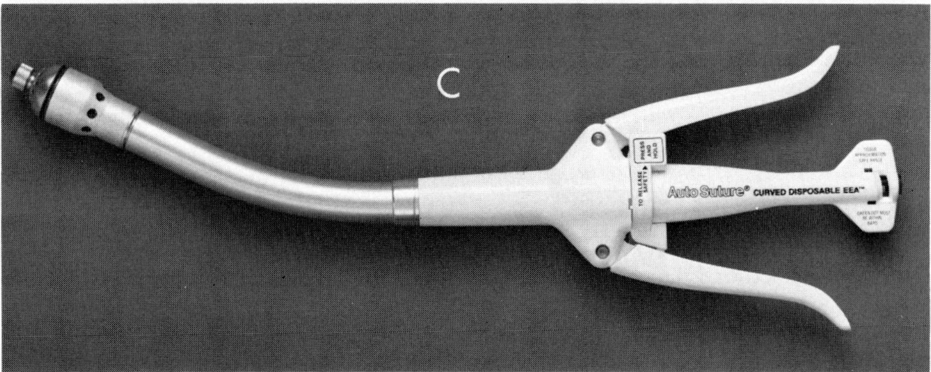

Fig II–7.—The EEA™ instruments. Utilized for end-to-end and end-to-side circular anastomoses, the EEA™ instruments find their chief use in esophageal and rectal anastomoses, although they have been used in every segment of the gastrointestinal tract. The instrument accepts cartridges of 25, 28, and 31 mm external diameter; the circular knives are of 15, 18, and 20.9 mm diameter. The totally disposable EEA™ instrument has an improvement in the closure mechanism, the two wing-like handles, which are readily compressed against the shaft. The curved EEA™ also has a smaller size cartridge, 20 mm outside diameter, and circular knife, 11.4 mm diameter. The EEA™ instrument produces a minimally inverting anastomosis with two staggered rows of staples. The disposable instruments are packaged sterile and loaded. **A,** the steel instrument with disposable cartridges. This accepts cartridges with outside diameters of 25, 28, and 31 mm. **B** and **C,** the disposable instruments. The straight instrument carries the same cartridges as the steel instrument and comes loaded. The curved instrument also carries a smaller 20.9 mm cartridge with an 11.4 mm diameter circular knife. *(continued)*

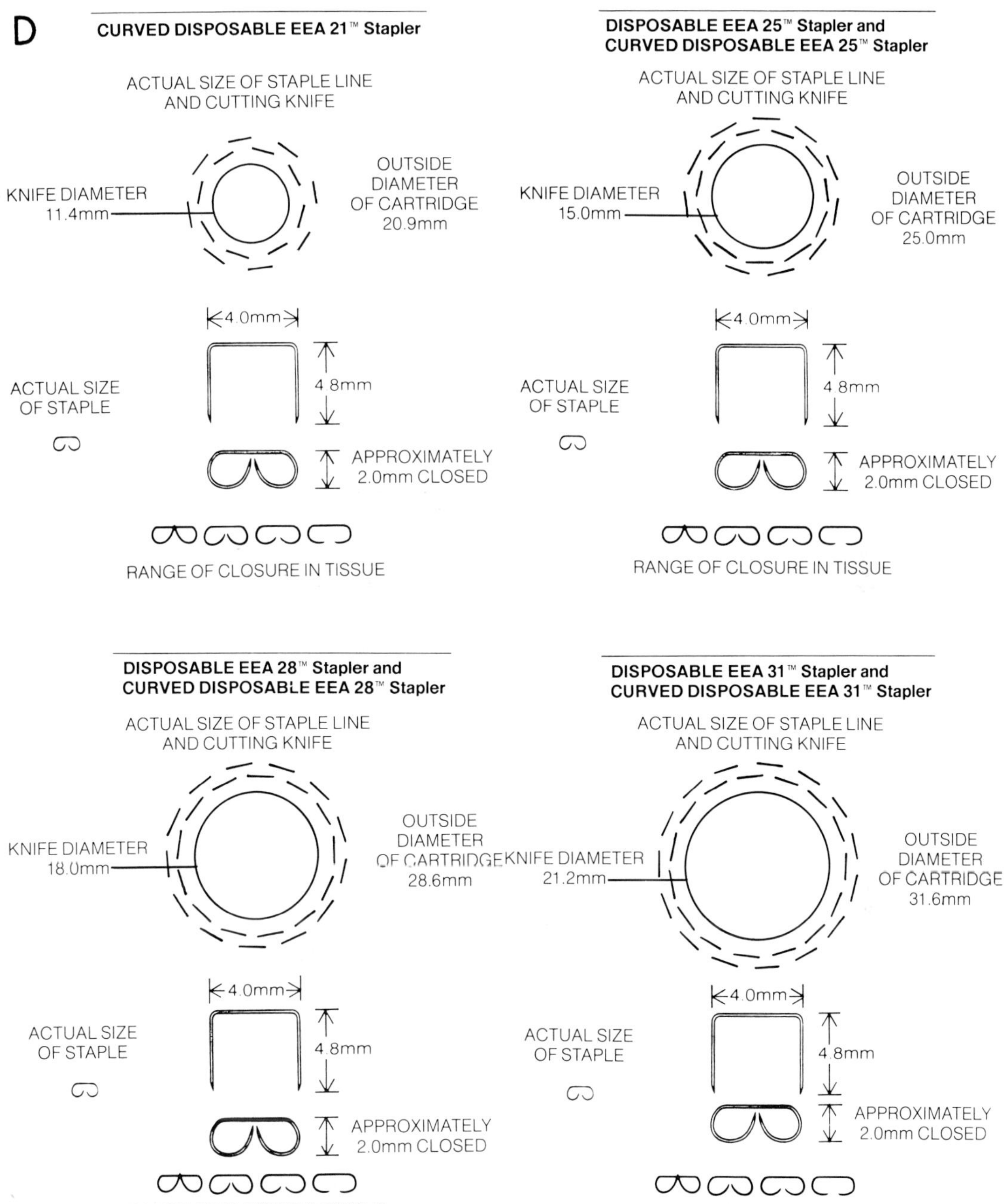

Fig II–7 (cont.).—D, staples, configuration, and staple lines of the EEA™ instruments only. Currently, the smallest size, 11.4 mm knife diameter, is supplied only with the curved, disposable instrument.

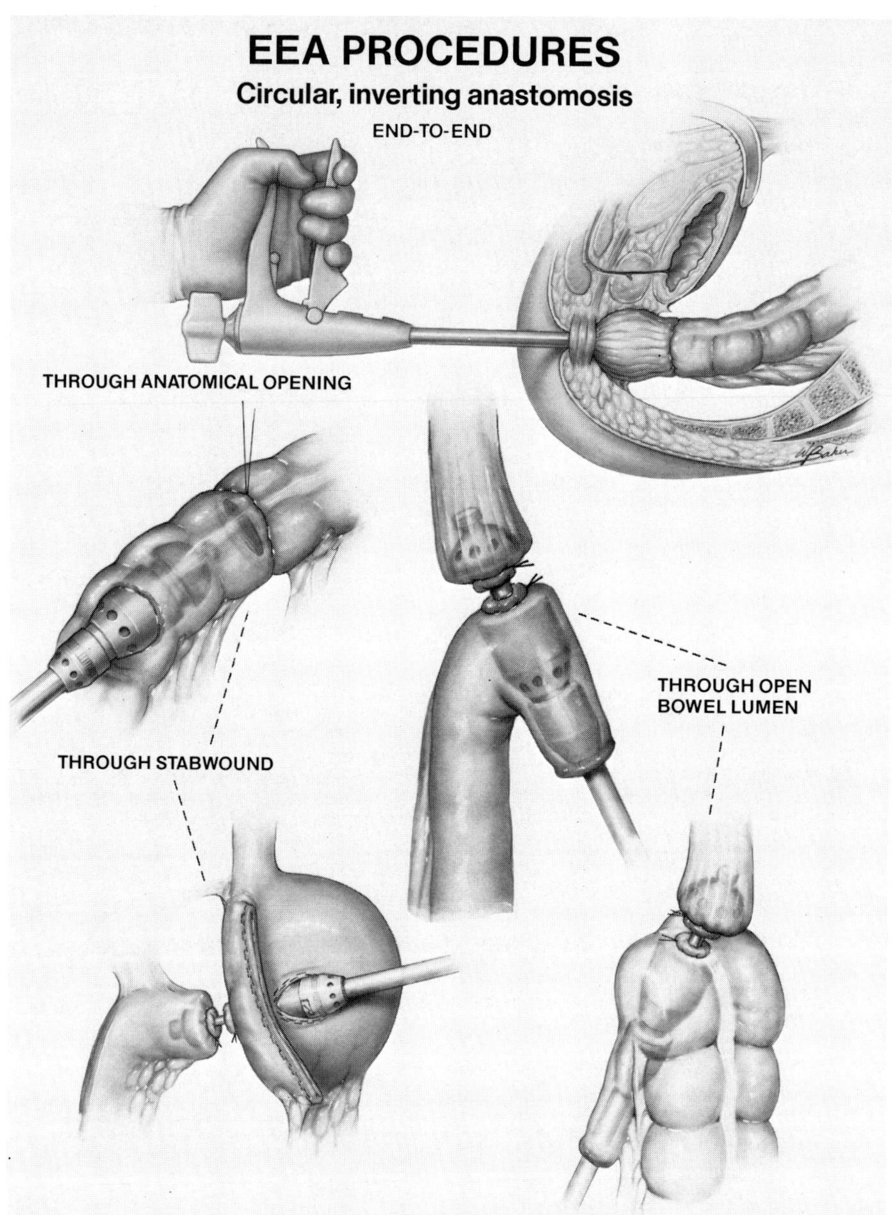

Fig II–8.—Basic uses of the EEA™ instrument. In all its uses, certain principles obtain: *(1)* Forcing the use of too large a cartridge risks tearing the bowel. *(2)* Secure closure of the pursestring about the central rod is essential to security. *(3)* Placing the pursestring back from the edge, or turning in a mass of fat, places more tissue in the capsule than can be held without tissue-destroying pressure. *(4)* The instrument must be opened before its gentle withdrawal. *(5)* The rings of tissue stamped out by the circular knife must be checked to see that they are unbroken.

The EEA™ instrument, for end-to-end and end-to-side anastomoses. As in the upper illustration, the instrument can be inserted through an anatomical opening—the anus in low rectal anastomoses, the mouth in esophageal reconstructions in the neck. The instrument can be inserted through a stab wound made for the purpose as in the end-to-end colocolostomy and the Billroth I operations pictured at the left. Finally, the instrument can be inserted through the open end of bowel divided in the normal course of the operation as in the end-to-side esophagojejunostomy or esophagocolostomy. The same technique can be used in passing the instrument back into the stomach through the open antral end, performing the EEA™ gastroduodenostomy or gastroenterostomy before the stapled amputation of the stomach (see Fig V–15). In the two right-hand operations, the stumps of the jejunum and of the terminal ileum will be stapled and amputated once the anastomosis has been completed.

102

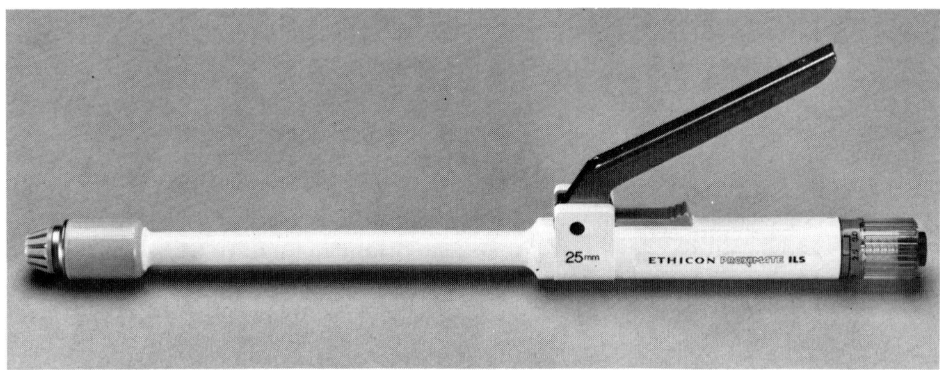

Fig II–9.—End-to-end and end-to-side disposable anastomotic instrument (Ethicon Corporation). The nose cone containing the anvils and the cutting ring is advanced or retracted by the knurled knob. The cartridge contains a double staggered row of staples. Closure of the handle drives in the staples and divides the two bowel ends. Currently, a single preloaded, presterilized, and totally disposable instrument is available, providing an anastomosis 25 mm in diameter. A disposable caliper is provided to measure tissue thickness and determine the degree to which the jaws are to be approximated by turning the knurled knob.

Another straight tubular, totally disposable instrument of quite similar design (Fig II–9) has appeared on the market.

IV. The LDS^{TM} instrument (Figs II–10 and II–11) places two metal clips of fine stainless steel on either side of the dividing blade, simultaneously suturing and dividing tissue contained within the recurved end of the instrument. The instrument itself consists of a squeeze handle and a short stem to accommodate the disposable cartridge. The cartridges contain 6 or 15 pairs of U-shaped staples of 5.8 mm width, 5.2 mm length, 5.3 mm closed width, and, for the wider staple, 8 mm width, 7.2 mm length, and 7.3 mm closed width. At the end of the cartridge there is a J-shaped jaw in which the structures—mesenteric or gastric vessels, cystic duct, etc.—to be ligated and divided

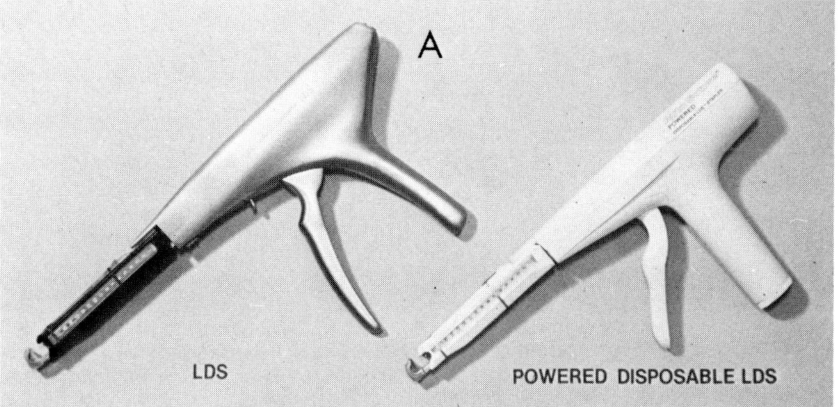

Fig II–10.—Ligating and dividing stapler (LDS^{TM}). **A,** the steel, reloadable and the powered, totally disposable instruments. *(continued)*

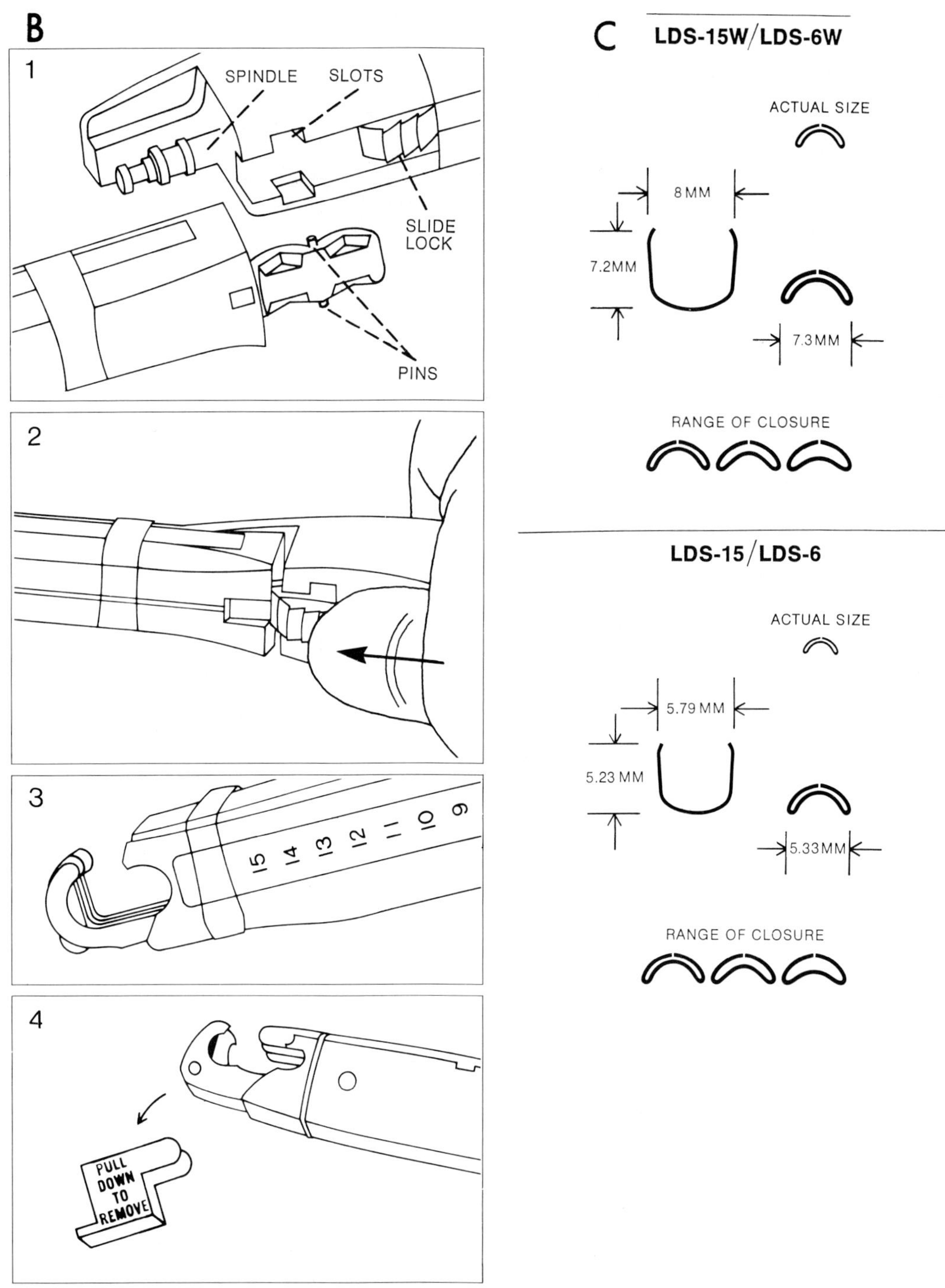

Fig II–10 (cont.).—B, detail of cartridge and mechanism for attachment to the steel handle. A squeeze of the handle encloses with two staples any tissue contained in the oval space in the jaw and simultaneously divides the tissue between the staples. In the case of the disposable instrument, the squeeze of the handle releases from a contained cartridge a puff of gas, which accomplishes the work of the instrument. The cartridges carry 15 pairs of staples and a knife. After the last staple has been discharged, the instrument locks so that an attempt at further use will not divide tissues that cannot be stapled. **C,** the initially U-shaped staples close in a double crescent within which the tissue is compressed.

LDS

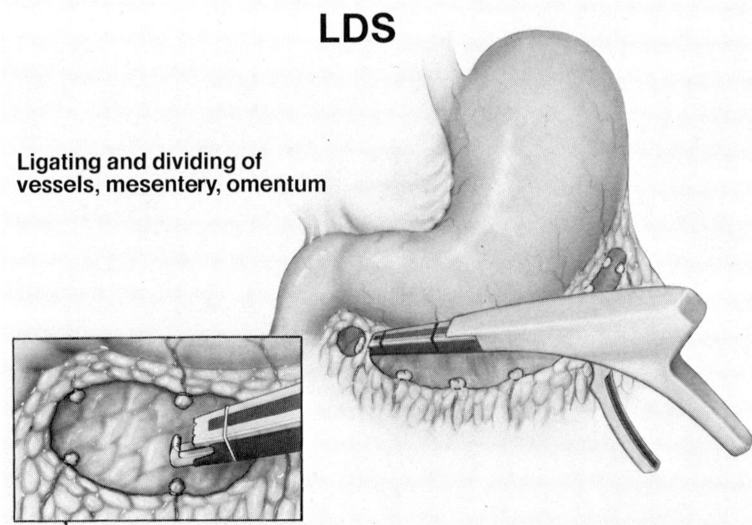

Fig II–11.—Use of LDS™ instrument in dividing vessels of omentum and mesentery. The instrument satisfactorily divides and clips splenic vessels, cystic duct, appendix, lateral rectal ligaments, esophageal vessels in resection of esophagus without thoracotomy, fallopian tube, and vas deferens. Like all the other instruments, it is held down to the tissue to be cut. One should resist the temptation to crowd an excess of tissue into the opening of the instrument. The staples compress the tissues, do not penetrate them, and, like other clips, can be dislodged if caught on laparotomy pads, etc.

are hooked and held. Each time the handle is squeezed, a U-shaped staple on each side is fired and closes in a crescent around the tissues, which are divided between the staples by the same squeeze of the handle. Designed for ligating and dividing mesenteric and omental blood vessels, the instrument has also been used to divide and secure the cystic duct, the fallopian tubes, appendix, and vas deferens. The staples are 6.35 mm apart so that there is a cuff of tissue 3.17 mm beyond each staple. The wide staples are 9.5 mm apart, leaving a cuff of tissue 4.75 mm beyond each staple.

The LDS™ instrument requires perhaps a little more skill in its use than do the other stapling instruments. The tissue placed into the confines of the jaw should not exceed the amount that can be fitted comfortably into the jaw. At least in the learning period, one should squeeze the handle with one hand, supporting the distal end of the instrument with the other. A firm squeeze and brisk release of the handles will insure the correct placement of the staples and the advancement of the knife. As with all of the staplers, one should avoid making traction on the tissues with the instrument. A slight down and back move of the hand after the instrument has been fired insures that the stapled tissue comes free from the instrument (see Fig II–11). When the cartridge is empty, the instrument locks automatically so that an attempt to use it will not cut tissue when there are no staples left to clip it.

The totally disposable LDS™ instrument. The instrument is substantially lighter than its metal precursor. The staple-feeding mechanism and activating mechanism have been modified, producing a smoother, recoil-free action, eliminating the principal disadvantage of the original instrument. A light pressure on a button releases with an audible

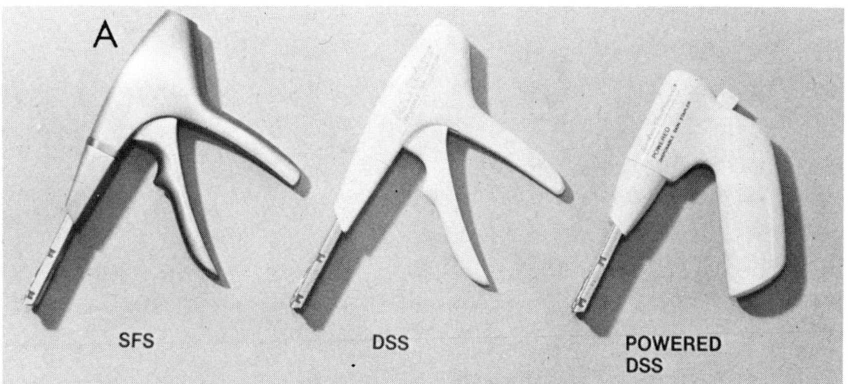

B

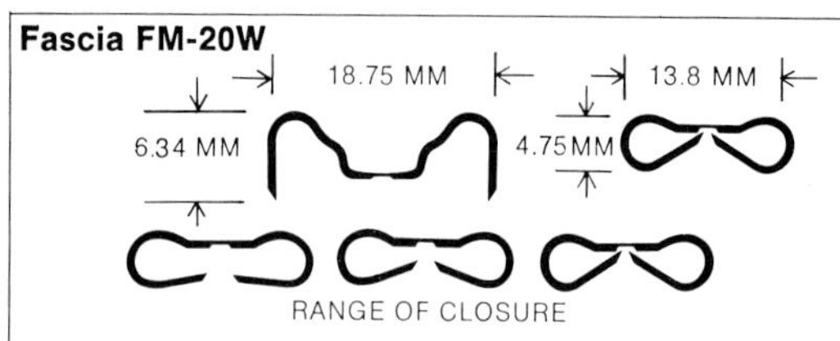

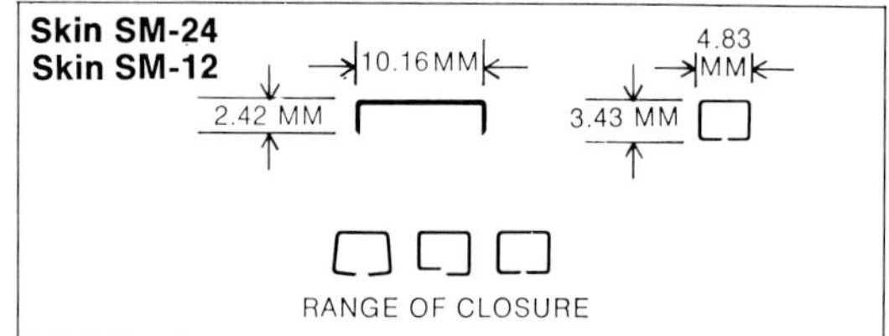

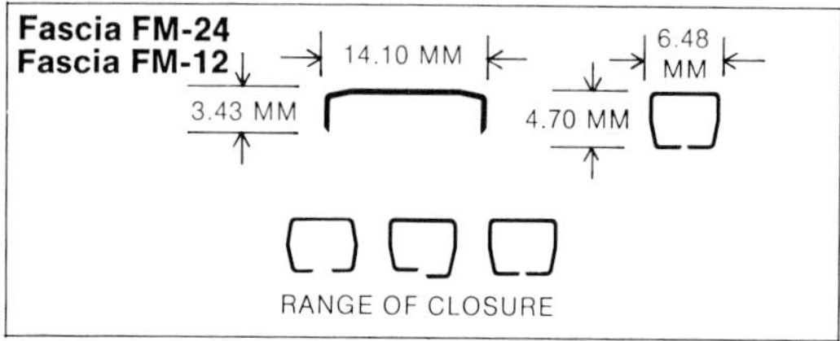

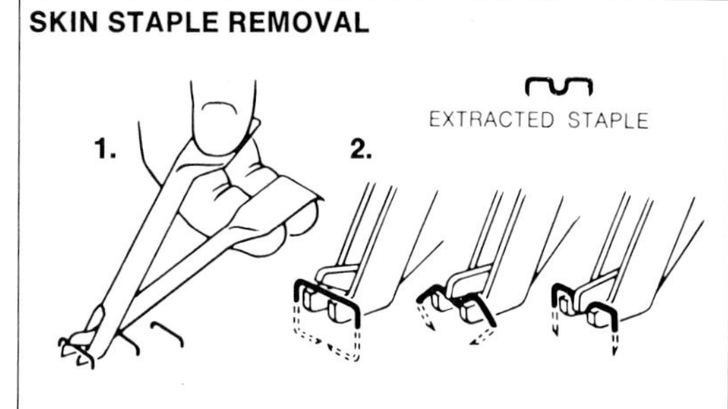

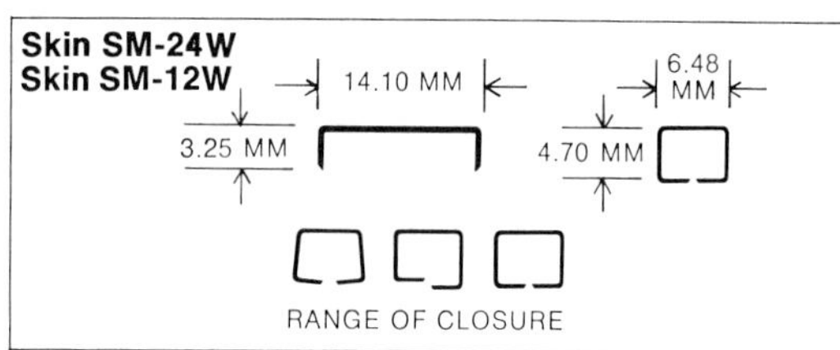

Fig II–12.—The skin and fascia staplers. **A,** from left to right—the steel cartridge-loaded instrument, the totally disposable instrument, and the totally disposable instrument powered by a contained gas cartridge. The disposable instruments come already loaded. In all three, the head can be swiveled, permitting stapling under direct vision, whatever the direction or position of the suture line. Only the SFS™ instrument accepts fascia staples. **B,** all three close skin staples in a rectangle ▭ and the SFS™ instrument closes fascia staples in a ∽ shape. Skin staples are removed by a disposable instrument that operates as shown. Fascia staples can be removed intraoperatively by placing the points of a hemostat into the oval-shaped loops of the staple and opening the clamp, thus spreading the staple arms apart.

SFS

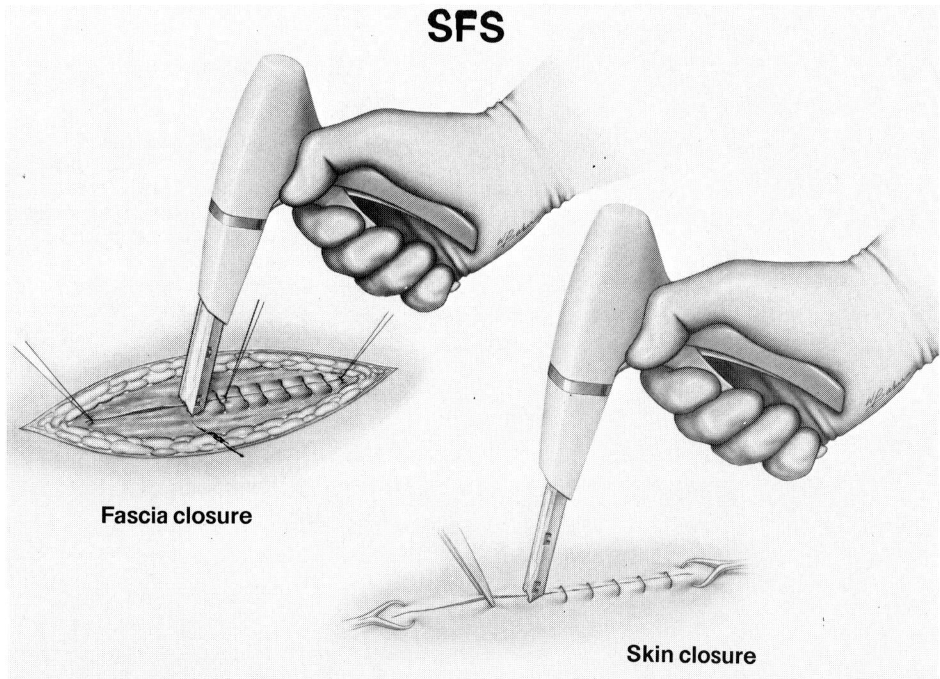

Fig II–13.—Use of skin and fascia staplers. The same stapler (SFS™) with different cartridge loads delivers heavy staples with a broad span, and a special principle of closure ᴄᴏ for fascia closure, or finer staples closed in a delicate rectangle ⊓ for skin closure. For fascia closure, the instrument is held firmly against the tissues; for skin closure, the instrument is held barely touching the skin so that the bar of the staples does not press on the skin.

puff a pulse of specially formulated, nontoxic gas from the integrally contained cartridge. The stapled and divided tissues seem literally to spring apart.

The LDS™ instrument is quite different in feeding mechanism, staple configuration, and closing mechanism from the Russian instruments, which at one time were advanced for the same clinical purposes (see Fig I–20*I*). The LDS™ instrument has a knife as well, which was not a part of any of the Russian models.

V. Skin and fascia stapler (Fig II–12). The skin and fascia stapler represents a radical departure in design and concept from the previously described staplers, and owes nothing to the Russian instruments. The same instrument accommodates either skin or fascia staple cartridges. The skin cartridges contain 12, 25, or 35 staples of 0.51 mm and 0.56 mm wire size, 3.4 mm and 4.7 mm closed leg length, bar 4.8 mm or 6.5 mm. The ingenious feature of the skin-stapling instrument is that the conventional ⊔ -shaped staples, when driven in by a stapler that rests lightly on the skin, close underneath the skin to form a complete rectangle, the outer bar of which is a millimeter or two above the skin. The instrument can be precocked before it is applied to the skin, so that a quite light touch is all that is required to drive the staple through. The instrument's nose, with cartridge attached, can be rotated, permitting one to place the staples at various angles while still maintaining direct visual control of insertion of each staple. The larger and stronger (0.7-mm-thickness wire) fascia staples culminate in a closed staple formed into a ᴄᴏ 13.8 mm long.

When the instrument is used for skin closure, the cartridge is placed in gentle contact

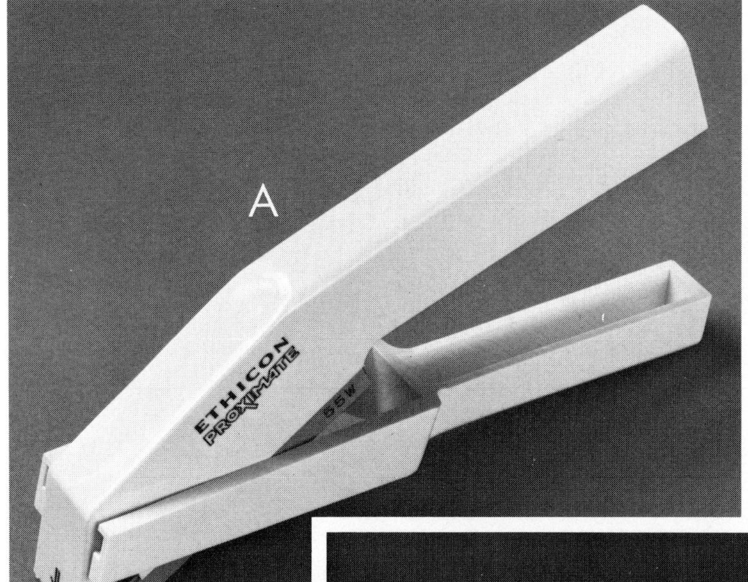

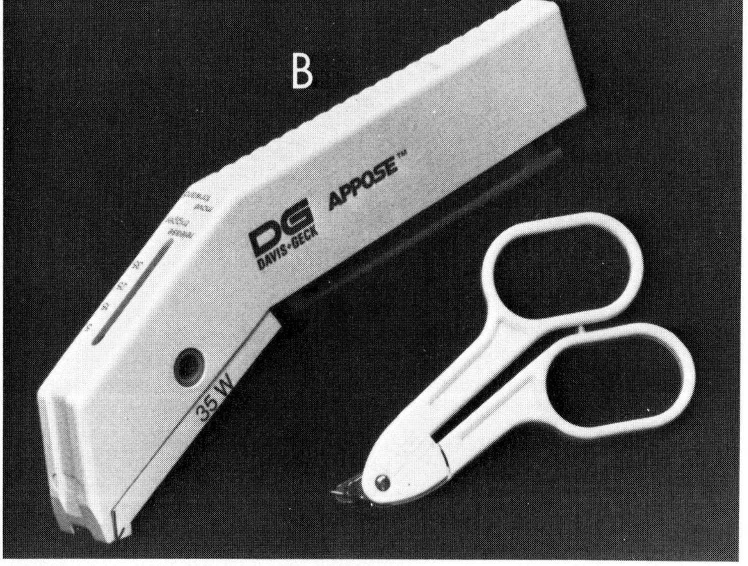

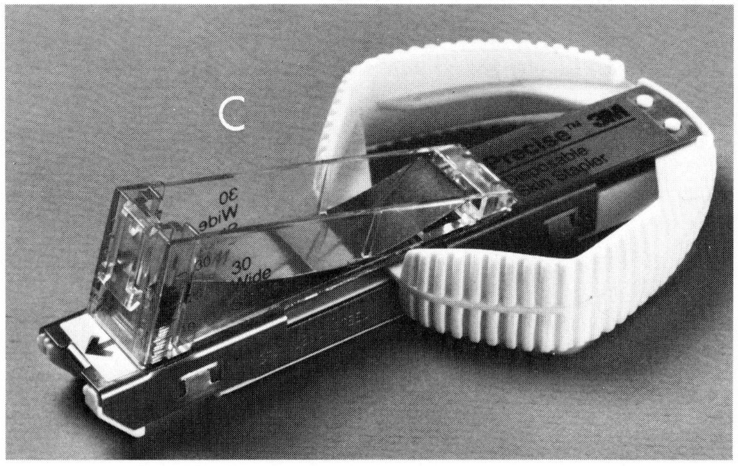

Fig II–14.—Varieties of skin staplers. **A,** Ethicon "Proximate". **B,** Davis & Geck "Appose". **C,** Minnesota Mining and Manufacturing "Precise". All three are magazine-loaded, totally disposable, and form their staples in a rectangle ▢ on the principle previously developed (Figs II–12 and II–13) and have disposable staple removers similar to those in use for the prior instrument (Fig II–12B).

with the skin, the skin edges held together slightly everted, and each skin staple placed by a gentle squeeze of the handle. The newest, totally disposable, skin stapler is powered by an integral gas capsule, which still further simplifies its use and speeds skin closures. The external bar of the staple "floats" above the skin, preventing cross-hatching even if the staple is left for many days. The skin stapler has also found wide use in the rapid suture of split-skin grafts in burn patients.

In stapling fascia, the end of the fascia stapler cartridge is applied firmly against the fascia to be sutured, which is held up by traction sutures placed at wide intervals. A narrow malleable retractor, or long knife handle, placed behind the fascia may be used to provide resistance to the pressure of the stapler against the linea alba. The cleaning off of the rectus sheath on both sides of the linea alba to facilitate stapling is best accomplished when the incision is being made, before entering the abdomen. The fascia staples can be removed readily, if need be, by spreading the points of a hemostat introduced into the oval loops of the staple. The removal of the skin staples is performed with a disposable extractor not unlike that used for Michel clips. For some time the skin stapler has been available as a totally disposable instrument. No disposable instrument is provided for stapling fascia, the weight of the instrument being considered an advantage in pressing down on the fascia during closure (Fig II–13).

Because of the saving in time and the results obtained, and probably the prior familiarity with Michel clips, the skin stapler has enjoyed wide use even among surgeons who have not utilized the other staplers for the various visceral uses.

The ready acceptance of staple closure of the skin has led to the introduction of skin staplers by a number of manufacturers (Fig II–14).

PRECAUTIONS AND SAFETY RECOMMENDATIONS

As with any mechanical device, there is the possibility of an inherent defect in an instrument or cartridge, or, in the case of the steel instruments, a defect due to faulty maintenance. In point of fact, such incidents have been relatively infrequent and such problems as we and others have had from time to time usually have been due to surgeon's error. It is perhaps not altogether surprising that the same surgeon who is accustomed to admit with candor, as occasion requires, that "I had an anastomotic leak," whatever the suture material he may have used, without seeking to blame the silk, catgut, or synthetic material, will say, when a similar mishap occurs in a stapled anastomosis, "the staples failed." Like anything else in the art of surgery, the use of the instruments, simple as they are, must be learned, preferably first in the animal laboratory and then in the operating room under appropriate supervision.

It is to be borne in mind that mechanical stapling instruments do not permit the surgeon to ignore the basic rules of clean atraumatic dissection, hemostasis, preservation of blood supply, avoidance of tension, and assurance that sutured tissues are free from disease. With the possible exception of the EEA^{TM} instrument in certain extremely low rectal anastomoses, and in esophageal anastomoses in the cupola of the thorax, the instruments will not enable the skillful surgeon to do what he could not do manually, although, in practically all situations, the stapled anastomoses are substantially simpler and easier than manual anastomoses. Particularly important is it, moreover, to understand that the instruments are not a quick road to surgery for the untrained and will not turn a neophyte into a virtuoso.

The tissue to be stapled should be easily compressed between the anvil and the staple cartridge of a given instrument. If the tissue is excessively thick or remarkably thin, one should resort to manual suture, as one should in any situation in which one has reservations about the applicability of the instruments. In every case, the instrument should be brought to the tissue, the surgeon resisting the temptation to elevate the tissue into the wound by mere force of traction on the instrument. Those instruments with handles are moderately heavy, they are long, and undue traction or leverage—not difficult to apply—may injure the blood supply or tear the tissues, since a relatively small movement of the handle can produce an unacceptably large movement of the cartridge end.

Obviously, one must take the elementary precautions required to be sure that all of the tissue to be anastomosed or closed is included in the staple line and that other tissues are not.

A paper (Wassner, Yohai, Heimlich, 1977), warning of problems with stapling, actually was a catalogue of instances, all but unbelievable, of misuse of the instruments. As for specific, less egregious errors in the use of the instruments, we give here the errors that we have experienced, heard of, or conceived of, and the precautions required to prevent them.

TA^{TM} INSTRUMENTS. (1) Failure to lock the safety so that the instrument is prematurely fired, resulting in an empty cartridge. (2) Loading the instrument with an anvil not corresponding to the staples to be used, viz., leaving a TA 30^{TM} anvil when changing the cartridge from the bronchial stapler to the TA 30^{TM}-V fine vascular stapler. This will result in malformed staples that will not be secure. (3) Failure to use an anvil, which will result in a staple closure that barely holds momentarily. (4) Failure to insert, at the end of the jaws, the pin that maintains the cartridge and anvil in alignment, insures that the staples are driven into the corresponding anvils forming the proper B shape, and prevents the tissue from slipping beyond the staple line in the jaw. In the case of the TA 90^{TM} metal instrument, the special pin is screwed into place with its little wing nut rather than merely dropped in, as in the TA 30^{TM} and TA 55^{TM} instruments, because the leverage exerted on the long jaw requires the support of the screwed tip to support it. (5) Forgetting to compress the handle and fire the staples, and then discovering as the stapler is removed that the divided bowel, bronchus, or pulmonary artery has not been stapled. (6) Transecting the viscus on the patient's side of the instrument. (7) Failure to incorporate a full thickness of bowel 360 degrees around the opening in closing the end of the bowel, or the opening after use of the GIA^{TM} instrument. (8) Removing the instrument before the tissue has been divided, then attempting to excise the excess tissue, or divide the bowel by cutting with knife or scissors, with the danger that one may cut too close to, or into, the staple line. The tissue always must be divided on the edge of the stapler before it is removed. (9) Failure to examine for and to control any bleeding that may occur when the instrument is removed. In transecting bowel or stomach, such bleeding practically always means that the mesentery and a mesenteric vessel have been included in the jaws of the instrument. The TA^{TM} instruments cannot be relied on for control of vessels in the mesentery or omentum. Oozing from the cut bowel end after use of the TA^{TM} stapler we consider reassuring, indicating, as it does, a blood supply that is good right to the edge of the divided bowel. Rarely in the bowel end is there a spurting vessel that may require suture or coagulation. One always checks the TA 30^{TM}-V fine vascular staple cartridge closure of the pulmonary artery, and occasionally a single fine silk suture may be necessary at some point in the suture line. (10) It is possible to crack a sclerotic pulmonary artery with the stapler just as it is with a vascular clamp. Occasionally, the partially calcified bronchus of an elderly male may crack with the stapler just as it may when seized with bronchial forceps. Excessively thick bowel squashed down in the stapler to the degree necessary to form the staples properly may be rendered avascular by the compression. We prefer not to use the instruments on excessively thick or excessively edematous bowel. (11) We suspect that a good many duodenal stump "blow-outs" were, in fact, leaks not from the stapled closure but from the ulcer itself left in place distal to the closure and unwittingly torn loose from the pancreas by rough use of the stapling instrument.

THE GIA[TM] INSTRUMENT. (1) Failure to use an anvil, failure to use a loaded cartridge, improper seating of the cartridge. (2) Improper mating of the instrument halves. If force is required to lock the instrument or to operate it, the halves probably are not appropriately mated. The steel instruments have serial numbers that must match for the two halves. (3) Failure to insure the entry of each of the three elements of the pusher and knife assembly into its appropriate slot. This should be controlled under direct vision, and the appropriate use of the integral spacer bar facilitates it. If two of the three elements of the assembly are fitted into a single slot, the knife will cut out one of the staple suture lines. Usually, if this is happening, it will be difficult to advance the knife and staple pushers. (4) In transecting the bowel, one should be sure that all of the bowel to be transected is within the area of graduation markings on the cartridge-carrying arm of the instrument. (5) Failure to examine for hemostasis as the GIA[TM] instrument is removed. Any bleeding that does not stop after brief gauze compression should be controlled with a fine catgut suture. (6) In anastomoses, excessive separation of the two halves as the instrument is removed. This invites tearing of the bowel. (7) In anastomoses, failure to separate and hold apart the GIA[TM] suture lines as the TA[TM] instrument is used to staple the bowel opening closed. Since the tissues are viable and nourished to the very edge of the cut beyond the staples, if the opening left after the use of the GIA[TM] instrument is closed so as to press the two edges of the stapled anastomosis incision together, it is theoretically possible and has, rarely, occurred that the apposed viable wound edges heal to each other (see Fig VIII–2).

Bleeding from bowel transected with the GIA[TM] stapler usually is minimal. When it is excessive, just as with the TA[TM] instrument, this generally is because mesentery and mesenteric vessels have been inappropriately included in the instrument jaws.

EEA[TM] INSTRUMENT. (1) Failure to draw either pursestring suture tightly enough around the shaft. The ring of staples and the circular knife thus fail to surround the entire proximal or distal opening. (2) Placement of the pursestring suture so that a portion of the circumference of the bowel escapes from it and is outside the suture line. (3) Placing the pursestring suture too far back from the cut end of the bowel. An unacceptably large mass of tissue then is compressed in the space within the closed cartridge, resulting in tissue damage. (4) Forcing too large a cartridge into esophagus or bowel, which may result in splitting or devascularization of the bowel. (5) Using too small a cartridge for a given organ, which may produce a relative stenosis. (6) Withdrawing the EEA[TM] instrument before it has been reopened, thus pulling on the completed anastomosis. (7) Failure to close the handle completely (which can be avoided by watching the appropriate vernier marks). Such a failure may drive in the staples without cutting out the two diaphragms with the circular knife, and obviously the instrument then cannot be disengaged. This is the only one of the instruments that requires a really firm squeeze of the handle. With the TA[TM] instrument, one can feel the staples as they yield. It is difficult to tell by the "feel" that the EEA[TM] instrument has been operated properly.

With the TA™, GIA™, and EEA™ instruments, it is obvious that the bowel to be stapled must have had its blood supply conserved, should be free from specific disease, such as cancer, tuberculosis, inflammatory bowel disease, etc., and should not be so excessively thick that the degree of compression required properly to form the staples will crush the bowel.

LDS™ INSTRUMENT. (1) Attempting to include too large a mass of tissue in the instrument. (2) Pulling up on the tissue to be stapled and cut, which may allow it to escape from the instrument as the staples are closing. (3) Catching a staple on a roughly withdrawn Mikulicz pad, which may tear it loose. (4) Reapplying the stapler so as to include a previous staple, blunting the knife.

REFERENCES

Amosov N.M., Berezovsky K.K., Zabroda G.S.: Experience of 100 resections of the lungs with UKL-60. *Eksp. Khirurg.* 6:3, 1958.

Amosov N.M., Berezovsky K.K.: Pulmonary resection with mechanical suture. *J. Thorac. Cardiovasc. Surg.* 41:325, 1961.

Ravitch M.M.: The use of stapling instruments in surgery of the gastrointestinal tract, with a note on a new instrument for end-to-end low rectal and oesophagojejunal anastomoses. *Aust. N.Z. J. Surg.* 48:444, 1978.

Ravitch M.M., Brown I.W., Daviglus G.F.: Experimental and clinical use of the Soviet bronchus stapling instrument. *Surgery* 46:97, 1959.

Ravitch M.M., Canalis F., Weinshelbaum A., McCormick J.: Studies in intestinal healing: III. Observations on everting intestinal anastomoses. *Ann. Surg.* 166:670, 1967.

Ravitch M.M., Hirsch L.C., Noiles D.: A new instrument for simultaneous ligation and division of vessels, with a note on hemostasis by a gelatin sponge-staple combination. *Surgery* 71:732, 1972.

Ravitch M.M., Lane R., Cornell W.P., Rivarola A., McEnany T.: Closure of duodenal, gastric and intestinal stumps with wire staples: Experimental and clinical studies. *Ann. Surg.* 163:573, 1966.

Ravitch M.M., Rivarola A.: Enteroanastomosis with an automatic instrument. *Surgery* 59:270, 1966.

Ravitch M.M., Rivarola A., VanGrov J.: Studies of intestinal healing. I. Preliminary studies of the mechanism of healing of the everting intestinal anastomosis. *Johns Hopkins Med. J.* 121:343, 1967.

Ravitch M.M., Steichen F.M.: Experiences with a second generation of stapling instruments in general and thoracic surgery. *Bull. Soc. Int. Chir.* 31:502, 1972.

Ravitch M.M., Steichen F.M., Fishbein R.H., Knowles P.W., Weil P.: Clinical experience with the Soviet mechanical bronchus stapler (UKB-25). *J. Thorac. Cardiovasc. Surg.* 47:446, 1964.

Steichen F.M.: The use of staplers in anatomical side-to-side and functional end-to-end enteroanastomoses. *Surgery* 64:948, 1968.

Steichen F.M.: Clinical experience with autosuture instruments. *Surgery* 69:609, 1971.

Steichen F.M., Ravitch M.M.: Mechanical sutures in surgery. *Br. J. Surg.* 60:191, 1973.

Steichen F.M., Ravitch M.M.: Mechanical sutures in esophageal surgery. *Ann. Surg.* 191:373, 1980.

Steichen F.M., Talbert J.L., Ravitch M.M.: Primary side-to-side colorectal anastomosis in the Duhamel operation for Hirschsprung's disease. *Surgery* 64:475, 1968.

Wassner J.D., Yohai E., Heimlich H.J.: Complications associated with the use of gastrointestinal stapling devices. *Surgery* 82:395, 1977.

CHAPTER III

The Healing of Wounds of the Intestines

BECAUSE so many of the techniques in which the instruments are used, particularly the TA™ instruments, involve a mucosa-to-mucosa closure of bowel, which appears to violate long-established surgical tenets, it seems appropriate at this point to consider the subject of the healing of intestinal wounds.

It was not until toward the end of the nineteenth century that surgeons undertook intestinal suture with any degree of frequency and secured healing with any degree of regularity. As late as the Civil War, penetrating wounds to the abdomen were considered to have a better prognosis without operation than with (Otis, 1876). Such attempts as had been made at intestinal suture were more remarkable for the ingenuity or symmetry of the sutures than for any successes achieved, and many operations were undertaken simply in the hope of attaching the wounded bowel to the external wound so as to create a fecal fistula. Heister (1743), in his section on "The Bubonocele Incarcerata," records what is generally accepted as the first successful intestinal resection and anastomosis—

". . .that the Parts will thus agglutinate or join together, is confirmed by a late Observation of Ramdohrius, present Surgeon of his serene Highness the Duke of Brunswick, who some Years ago cut off a large Part of a mortified Intestine in a Woman, that had an incarcerated Rupture, which broke of itself; and joining the two sound Parts of the Intestine together, he inserted one into the other, and tied them together loosely with a String and replacing them in the Abdomen, drawed them by the String to the Mouth of the Wound, by which means the divided Intestine inflamed, and surprizingly united; the Woman discharging her Feces afterwards, not through the Wound, but by the Anus as before. The woman afterwards lived in a State of Health, till in about a Year's Time she died of Pleurisy, and upon opening her, the divided Intestines appeared to be united with each other, of which he made a Present to me, together with part of the abdomen, to which they adhere, and I now keep them in Spirits, to convince such as are incredulous, and of a different Opinion."

It is worthy of note that Ramdohrius' intussuscepting technique continues to be rediscovered as a "new" method every decade or so (Lindenmuth and May, 1967). An occasional success with closure of a stab wound of the bowel had been reported from earlier times. However, Ramdohr probably was the first surgeon to have described a successful anastomosis of the divided bowel.

Travers (1812) pointed out that Astley Cooper had seized the edges of a small perforation with a clamp and tied off the nipple of bowel thus held, the patient recovering well from this crude mucosa-to-mucosa closure, and that Cooper in fact had been preceded in this by others. And, of course, the creation of an anastomosis between two limbs of bowel by slow, deliberate pressure necrosis of their apposed walls had been performed by Dupuytren (1828) in the treatment of fecal fistulas consequent upon the sloughing of a gangrenous, strangulated groin hernia. Dupuytren's spur crusher now is more generally given Mikulicz's name (Ravitch, 1979).

It is not altogether clear from this distance of time to what to attribute the infrequent success with simple closure of incised wounds of the bowel in those early days. Illustrations suggest that heavy needles and coarse suture materials were at fault. On the other hand, some drawings and the injunctions of the authors to use fine needles and fine threads would suggest that failure might not always have been attributable to the crudity of the suturing materials. In general, antisepsis, in dealing with patients with incised wounds of the intestine, can hardly have been the problem, and many authors advised cleaning out and sponging away feces, etc. Clearly, the absence of suction to minimize further contamination, and the straining of patients operated on without anesthesia or even with the poor anesthesia of the mid-nineteenth century, must have played some part in operative difficulty. The use of fine instruments to pick up the intestine appears not to have been common, and instructions usually specify how the fingers are to be placed in holding up the bowel for the suture.

Antoine Lembert (1826) proposed serosa-to-serosa apposition as the fundamental basis of successful intestinal suture, a doctrine that has been almost unchallenged until relatively recently. Nicholas Senn of Chicago (1893), in his Presidential Address on Intestinal Suture or "enterorrhaphy" before the Association of Military Surgeons of the National Guard of the United States in Chicago on August 8, 1893 said,

". . .To Lembert is conceded almost by universal consent the credit of having established the modern doctrine concerning the healing of intestinal wounds. . . .Lembert's work initiated the most important era in the history of the intestinal suture. . . .The great principle inculcated by Lembert to rely on the serous coat in procuring early internal adhesions will never be rejected."

It is utterly fascinating that while insisting on inverting, serosa-to-serosa closure of the bowel, and recognizing along the way that with end-to-end anastomoses, this might invite excessive inversion leading to obstruction, Lembert made reference to "les belles expériences" of Travers. Like Lembert, innumerable writers since have made a ritual obeisance to Travers' work without clearly drawing from it all the lessons that might be learned. Travers, certainly Astley Cooper's most distinguished pupil, described in a book devoted to the subject (Travers, 1812) his successful end-to-end anastomoses in dogs and made little of the difficulties of operative technique, stating

". . .I am not aware that any formal directions are required for the operation of sewing up a wound of the intestines. . . .The subject of gastrorrhaphy has occupied a space in most surgical works, greatly over proportioned to its claims. The triangular needles generally recommended for the suture of the intestines are certainly very ill-fitted for the occasion. Let a small round sewing needle, armed with a silk thread, be passed near to the lines formed at the bases of the *everted** lips. The thread is to be carried at short regular distances through the whole extent of the wound, the operator being mindful that an equal portion of the edges is included in each stitch. When the suture is finished, let the thread be securely fastened and cut close to the knot. The reduction of the prolapsed fold [loop] should then be conducted with the nicest caution; and when completed the wound of the teguments should be treated with a stitch, a plaster or a poultice, as circumstances dictate.

The practice embraces two points, 1st, The accurate closure of the intestinal wound, by which the case is reduced to one of simple prolapse [evisceration]. 2d. The careful reduction of the protruded part, and the union of the divided integuments. . .it remains only that I should point out the several stages of a process, which has not to my knowledge been described. It commences with the agglutination of the contiguous mucous surfaces, probably by the exudation of a fluid similar to that which glues together the sides of a recent flesh wound, when supported in contact. The adhesive inflammation supervenes and binds down the *reverted** edges of the peritoneal coat, from the whole circumference of which a layer of coagulable lymph is effused, so as to envelope

---

*Italics ours.

the wounded bowel. . .During this time, the lymph deposited becomes organized, by which further retraction is prevented, and the original cylinder, with the threads attached to it, are encompassed by the new tunic. . .but the opposed villous surfaces, so far as my observation goes, neither adhere nor become consolidated by granulation, so that the interstice linking the division internally is probably never obliterated. The union of a divided bowel requires the contact of the cut extremities in their entire circumference, effectively to resist the muscular action opposed to an artificial connection during the process of union. The species of suture employed is of secondary importance, if it secures this contact.''

So that Travers described, and his drawings illustrate, everting anastomoses. After observing that the transected dog intestine presented everted ends, with pouting mucosa, Travers said

''. . .the absolute contact of the *everted*∗ surfaces of a divided intestine in their entire circumference is requisite to secure the animal from the danger of abdominal effusion [of feces]. If the interrupted suture is employed it is therefore necessary to include such a portion of the *everting*∗ lips as will endure this contact. . .for the *eversion*∗ is permanent, and if the threads are passed as near as possible to the edges, with a view to overcome the eversion, effusion [of feces] is to be apprehended from laceration of the included substance of the gut.''

We have referred in Chapter I to Henroz' pin-and-hole articulated rings for producing end-to-end everting anastomoses in the dog. Senn seems not to have been aware that Travers produced everting anastomoses, and of Henroz' work blithely said that since the anastomoses were everting, they could not have healed.

Lembert himself, in fact, had indicated that Dupuytren was the first ''to conceive the idea of apposing the serosal surfaces to each other by looking for a method for a cure of the anus contre nature.'' It is of some interest that although it is generally stated that Lembert's suture does not penetrate into the lumen, his own account indicates that it was a matter of indifference to him whether the suture penetrated through into the lumen or passed between muscular coat and the mucosa. ''L'aiguille pénètre dans la cavité de l'intestin ou bien sa pointe glisse entre les tuniques musculeuse et muqueuse suivant que l'intestin est plus ou moins épais.'' The submucosa was not mentioned. The cardinal importance of the submucosa as the single strong layer in suturing the intestine was pointed out by Halsted (1887), who also strongly emphasized the importance of avoiding penetration into the lumen, in order to protect the suture tract from contamination. Writing in 1887, he said

''In looking through the literature of intestinal suture I cannot find that any one has called sufficient attention, from a surgical point of view, to the structure of the different coats of the intestine, particularly to their physical properties. . .my experiments have led me to attach great weight, in the successful performance of enterorrhaphy, to an accurate knowledge. . .of the submucous coat of the intestine and I am not aware that the importance of this coat in connection with this operation has hitherto been emphasized.''

He pointed almost scornfully to the descriptions of Madelung, Reichel, Maydl, and Kocher that (Madelung) ''The needle now penetrates in the usual manner the two ends of the intestine, passing between serosa and muscularis.'' They and others—Gussenbauer, von Winiwarter, Czerny, and Rydygier—ignored the importance of the submucosa. Halsted insisted that

''Each stitch should include a bit of the submucosa. A thread of this coat is much stronger than a shred of the entire thickness of the serosa and muscularis. It is not difficult to familiarize one's

---

∗Italics ours.

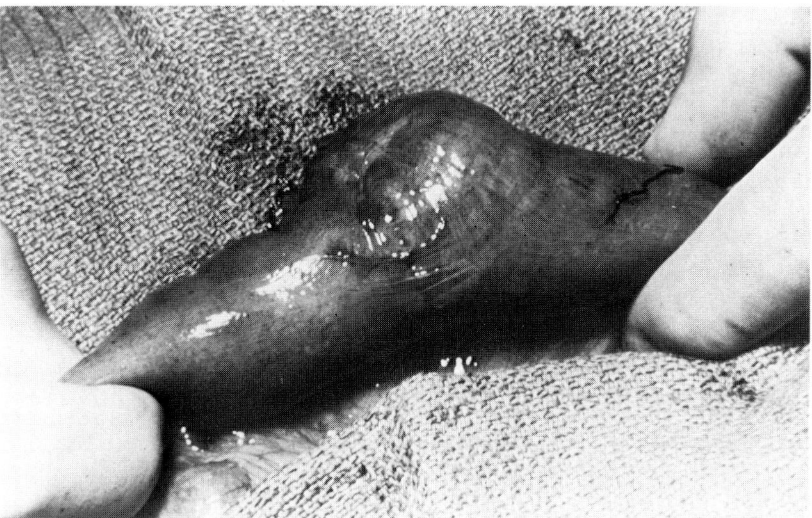

Fig III–1.—Healed functional end-to-end jejunojejunostomy—one year postoperatively (in a patient). At reoperation, for a different indication than the one that had led to this anastomosis, the area of bowel healing was clearly identifiable. There was one minor adhesion to the mesentery of the loop containing the anastomosis. The serosal surface is smooth and shiny. A little mesenteric fat is visible under the glistening serosa. The original functional end-to-end anastomosis has the appearance of an asymmetric end-to-end anastomosis.

self with the resistance furnished by the submucosa, and it is quite as easy to include a bit of this coat in each stitch as to suture the serosa and muscularis alone.''

In the course of the evaluation of the application of mechanical stapling devices to intestinal closure, we observed that healing regularly was achieved by the simple through-and-through, mucosa-to-mucosa closure of the flattened end of the stomach, duodenum, or large or small bowel, with two staggered rows of wire staples. Healing occurred without abscess formation, localized peritonitis, or excessive inflammation to suggest even a temporary leak (Fig III–1).

The success of such a simple mucosa-to-mucosa closure ran counter to what had been accepted surgical practice for 150 years, and it seemed worthwhile to examine the phenomenon more closely (Ravitch, Rivarola, and VanGrov, 1967). In the first place, it seemed possible that compression with the clamp alone could force the tissues to adhere in the way that a clamp on the distal loop of a colostomy will cause the bowel to remain sealed when the clamp is first removed, so that it seems as if the bowel had healed closed. When this possibility was tested by compressing the duodenum and the cut end of the stomach in a Billroth II gastric resection and reconstruction, with pressure for 15 minutes from the TA™ clamp, without the staples, the stomach invariably broke down subsequently, although the duodenum sometimes held. We next set out to see whether simple stapling across the undivided viscus would produce a permanent seal. In six animals in the mid-stomach, and in three animals in the duodenum just below the pylorus, two staggered rows of staples were driven home without dividing the viscus and a bypassing anastomosis was placed around the line of staples. The stapled duodenum in each animal remained sealed securely with mucosa-to-mucosa healing. Of the six animals whose stomachs had been stapled across, only one showed complete mucosa-to-mucosa healing. The other five showed a number of openings through the line of staples, most of them small, some perhaps a centimeter in diameter, obviously indicating that the staples had not all held and the two mucosal surfaces had not healed together. The thickness of the stomach wall and its strong muscular action presumably accounted for this difference from the results in the duodenum. Although this work on stapling the undivided stomach was published in 1967, a number of surgeons subsequently have attempted to compartment the stomach with a line of staples, without a transection, as in staged operations for babies with esophageal atresia without tracheoesophageal fistula. They confirmed clinically what we had reported to be true in dogs, that a staple suture line was not secure in the undivided stomach. More will be said of this below in the discussion of gastric stapling in antiobesity operations. We considered we had demonstrated that there was a difference in the healing of a stapled cut end of the transected stomach and the healing of a stapled line of closure of the intact stomach.

It seemed most reasonable to assume that with stapling of the undivided stomach the degree of compression trauma to the mucosa was not sufficient to produce a mucosal wound that would allow healing to occur, and that with the divided stomach, healing in fact occurred at the very cut end, perhaps on the basis of adhesions to the omentum or to the viscera, although in the course of our experiments we had not been aware of adhesions to an extent that would have supported that assumption.

We tested the necessity for adhesion to neighboring viscera in the prevention of leaks in the stapled, unreinforced, mucosa-to-mucosa closures (Canalis and Ravitch, 1968). In five dogs undergoing gastrectomy and Billroth II reconstruction, the stapled mucosa-to-mucosa closures of the duodenal and gastric stumps were loosely covered over with polyethylene sheeting. In three of them, the duodenal and gastric stumps failed to heal. We had never had a breakdown before. In six animals, the gastric and duodenal stumps, after a Billroth II resection, were inverted by interrupted silk sutures, and polyethylene film again sutured lightly over the cut ends. All of these animals healed uneventfully.

The thesis seemed to be supported that healing of an everting mucosa-to-mucosa closure in the gastrointestinal tract was dependent on external adhesions. Our interest in the clinical possibilities of mucosa-to-mucosa anastomoses had been aroused by the obvious advantages of everting end-to-end anastomoses, which are technically simpler than inverting anastomoses and which avoid inversion and the risk of some resultant intestinal obstruction. There had been prior studies of everting anastomoses by others (Galluzzi and Possenti, 1954; Healey, McBride, and Gallager, 1964; Getzen, 1966; Getzen, Roe, and Holloway, 1966), and more have appeared in the course of the years in which we have been working on the problem (Loeb, 1967; Guglielmi, Moschina, and Ricci, 1968; Brøyn and Helsingen, 1969; Getzen, 1969; Rusca, Bornside, and Cohn, 1969; Herzog, 1971; Kornfält, Okmian, and Jonsson, 1973).

We performed a variety of experiments in dogs to test everting anastomoses in the small bowel, with silk sutures or with staple closures, with and without resection of the omentum and with and without a loose protective wrapping of the anastomotic site with polyethylene film or glove rubber (Ravitch, Rivarola, and VanGrov, 1967). The stapled anastomoses were performed with a Russian vascular stapling instrument, which was designed for blood vessels, not for anything as heavy as bowel. This instrument inserted a single circular row of fine staples parallel to the cut edge of the everted bowel. In some animals, a single layer of staples was applied and in some the instrument was used twice, producing a double row. In the animals with silk anastomoses, an everted end-to-end anastomosis was performed with one layer of through-and-through silk mat-

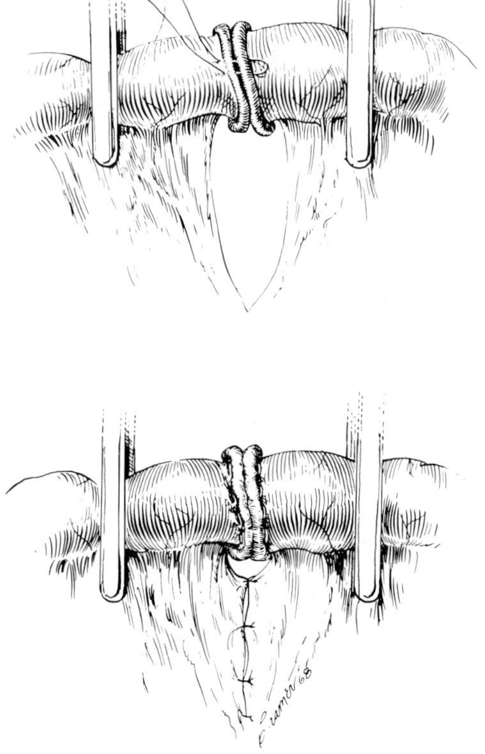

Fig III–2.—The everting anastomosis is made with a single layer of through-and-through everting mattress sutures of 4–0 silk, with the bar parallel to the cut edge of the bowel. The submucosa is necessarily penetrated with each stitch. This is a much more truly everting anastomosis than some utilized in studies of this problem. Infringement of the lumen is virtually impossible. The luminal surface is at once smooth and even, and the everted flange shows relatively little inflammation. Adhesions of the peritoneal surfaces are perhaps more extensive with everting anastomoses, and the final resolution of microscopic evidences of inflammation in the anastomosis is prolonged. (From M.M. Ravitch, *Surgical Clinics of North America,* 1969, used by permission.)

tress sutures, the bar placed parallel to the cut edge (Fig III–2). In both groups, half of the animals had omentum resected and half did not, and half of the animals had wrapping of the anastomosis with a thin sheet of polyethylene or glove rubber lightly held around the anastomosis with two or three sutures through an avascular section of the mesentery and half did not. All of the animals with polyethylene- or glove rubber-wrapped everting anastomoses suffered a breakdown of the anastomosis with abscess and peritonitis, 25 dogs in all. Of 31 dogs with one or another type of end-to-end everting anastomosis without such wrapping, only two had leaks. Our thesis seemed once more to be supported. But, almost as an afterthought, ordinary silk end-to-end inverting intestinal anastomoses were wrapped with polyethylene, and, to our astonishment, three of nine such animals developed leaks and abscess or peritonitis, an altogether unusual experience in our hands.

We thus had evidence that bowel closed mucosa-to-mucosa would heal, and that clinically the extent of adhesions formed did not seem to account for this healing, either to seal off the bowel or to bring new circulation to the end of the bowel. Healing must have been dependent on the intrinsic circulation of the bowel. The situation in this respect was quite comparable to that in the healing of the bronchial stump, which is, of course, sutured mucosa-to-mucosa. Rienhoff, Gannon, and Sherman (1942), in the bronchus, demonstrated a temporary sealing off by a fibrin plug at the end of the bronchus after suture (Fig III–3). In that situation also, the circulation on which the healing

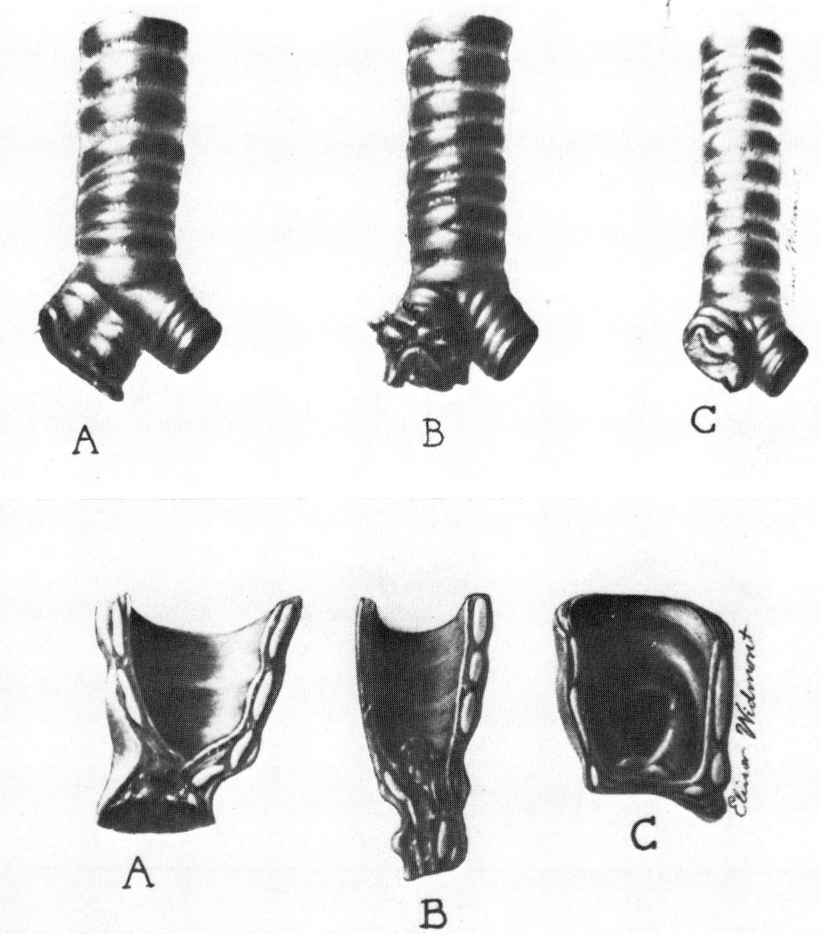

Fig III–3.—Apart from a few early clinical trials of inversion of the bronchial stump, thoracic surgeons have relied on mucosa-to-mucosa closure of the bronchus. The studies by Rienhoff and his collaborators demonstrated that for the most part the sutures served only as a temporary seal while healing was taking place at the cut end of the bronchus. (From W.F. Rienhoff Jr., J. Gannon Jr., and I. Sherman, *Transactions of the American Surgical Association,* 1942, used by permission.)

of the structure was dependent had to come from the end of the bronchus itself, the sutures serving as a temporary occluding mechanism.

When it was found that everting anastomoses of the small bowel regularly broke down when wrapped with a fine material and that a significant proportion of inverting anastomoses similarly wrapped also broke down, it became apparent that some factor was involved that was not unique to an everting anastomosis. The most reasonable explanation appeared to be that even with the ordinary inverting anastomosis, performed as an open anastomosis in an intestine not prepared with antibiotics, there was enough contamination of the peritoneal surfaces in the anastomotic area so that, if the anastomosis was isolated from the protective defenses of the peritoneum by interposed foreign material, infection around the suture line would result, progressing rapidly to necrosis, leak, and fatal peritonitis.

This thesis was tested by a series of systematic experiments with five groups of animals, 24 animals in each group (Ravitch, Canalis, Weinshelbaum, and McCormick, 1967): (1) everting open anastomosis, with one layer of interrupted through-and-through silk mattress sutures parallel to the cut edge; (2) everting open anastomosis, with a single row of staples parallel to the cut edge; (3) inverting open anastomosis, with a single layer of interrupted silk Lembert sutures; (4) inverting open anastomosis, with a two-layer closure, inner catgut, and outer silk; and (5) inverting closed anastomosis, with a one-layer silk closure. Twelve of the dogs in each of the five groups were prepared with orally administered antibiotics and 12 were not; six of the antibiotic-treated dogs and six of the dogs without antibiotics in each group had the anastomosis covered with a layer of silicone-rubber gauze membrane. Silicone rubber gauze sutured around intact intestine for several weeks elicited no discernible inflammatory response. Intestinal antisepsis was undertaken with a combination of neomycin sulfate and sulfathalidine. The silicone rubber membrane was placed lightly around the anastomosis and secured with two or three silk sutures passing through the mesentery, fastening both sides of the membrane together, above and below the anastomosis, without constricting the intestine or embarrassing its circulation. In short, if their anastomoses were not wrapped, virtually all of the animals in all five groups survived whether the anastomoses were inverting or everting with sutures or with staples, open or closed. Virtually all those died, with wrapped anastomoses, whether inverting or everting, open or closed, with silk or with staples. Among the few survivors were four dogs in whom the wrapping had been applied so loosely that it had become displaced. The use or withholding of antibiotics had no effect on survival, but there was a correlation in all surviving dogs between the use of antibiotics and the extent of adhesions, which tended to be less in dogs prepared with antibiotics.

To elucidate further the matter of bacterial infection after anastomoses (Kho and Ravitch, 1970), the everting and inverting anastomoses were cultured by the use of a precut strip of sterile velvet wrapped around the anastomosis for five seconds, pile surface down, and then imprinted on an agar plate. Few or no bacteria were cultured from the completed anastomoses of either type in the first two hours after operation. Increasingly thereafter, with exceptions in some animals with either type of anastomosis, more organisms appeared until, at six hours after operation, all anastomoses yielded more colonies than could be counted. By 12–24 hours, the number of organisms had decreased sharply. Rusca, Bornside, and Cohn (1969), in a follow-up of these studies, used a pigmented nonresident bacterium injected into the lumen of the bowel proximal to the anastomosis but after the anastomosis had been completed. The marked organism never was cultured from the surface, suggesting that the organisms recovered from the bowel surface at intervals following the anastomosis all had been implanted during the procedure and had not leaked out in the subsequent hours.

The malign effect of wrapping anastomoses with foreign material vitiated this approach to the study of the importance of adhesions in securing the healing of everting anastomoses. It was clear that loosely wrapping a fresh anastomosis with foreign material interfered with healing of the anastomosis, presumably because bacteria were protected against the normally effective peritoneal defenses. Manz, LaTendresse, and Sako, from the University of Minnesota (1970), and Crowson and Wilson (1973), from the University of Tennessee, carried the study one step further by investigating the effect of a drain fastened by a single suture near a colonic anastomotic suture line in dogs. Manz used a two-layer open anastomosis, inner catgut and outer silk, interrupted. The one-inch Penrose drain was brought out through the flank. There were no leaks, no abscesses, and few adhesions in the 15 control dogs. In the drained dogs there were massive adhesions, intestinal obstruction, and anastomotic dehiscence with abscess or peritonitis, even if the drain was left in place only two days. Crowson and Wilson brought the drain out into, but not through, the abdominal wall, and also used a two-layer open anastomosis. The drain—a stuffed Penrose, with either a 5-mm polyvinyl-chloride tube or a 5-mm Silastic tube—was fastened by a single suture 2 cm from the anastomosis. Although the stuffed Penrose drain produced the severest peritoneal reaction, all three drains were associated with a substantial incidence of abscesses and anastomotic disruption. The results correlated well with the presence or absence of bacteria in peritoneal washings after completion of the anastomosis.

We next undertook the use of promethazine and dexamethasone (Kho, Replogle, and Ravitch, 1969) to evaluate the effect of the resultant decrease in the extent of adhesion formation (Replogle, Johnson, and Gross, 1966). We utilized this regimen with inverting and everting end-to-end intestinal anastomoses to provide a test of the possible interference of these drugs with the healing of bowel anastomoses, as a stringent test of the ability of the regimen to prevent adhesions in a more clinically applicable situation than the brush-scrubbing serosal denudement of the original experiments, and, most of all, as a test of the role of adhesions in the successful outcome of everting anastomoses. The use of combined promethazine and dexamethasone did effectively reduce the incidence of intestinal adhesions in dogs with both types of anastomosis, less markedly in everting anastomoses than in inverting anastomoses. The drug regimen did not demonstrably hinder healing of anastomoses of either kind.

The need for inversion of mucosa-to-mucosa closures was further studied at Lincoln Hospital (Steichen 1964–69). In 38 distal gastrectomies and Billroth II reconstructions in dogs, the stapled duodenal closure was not inverted, in 12 others neither gastric nor duodenal stapled closures were inverted, and in 14 more the mucosa-to-mucosa stapled, gastric and duodenal ends and the GIA^{TM} openings closed by the TA^{TM} instrument were left uninverted. There were no leaks in any and in that period we began clinically not to invert stapled mucosa-to-mucosa closures. When the functional end-to-end anastomosis (Steichen, 1968) was developed, the mucosa-to-mucosa stapled closure was left uninverted in 24 dogs. There were no leaks and our clinical practice with this procedure, from the first, has been to leave the mucosa-to-mucosa stapled closure of the bowel ends without any inversion.

The comparative histology of everting and inverting anastomoses was studied (Ravitch, Canalis, Weinshelbaum, and McCormick, 1967) by performing manual inverting,

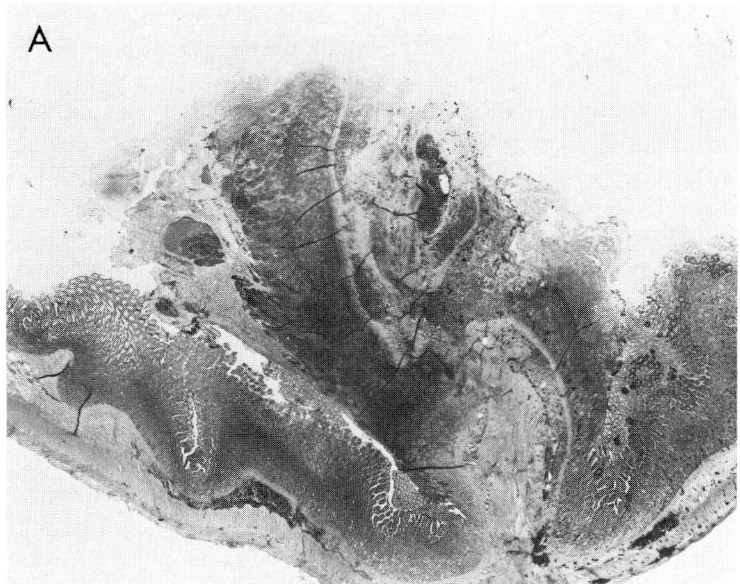

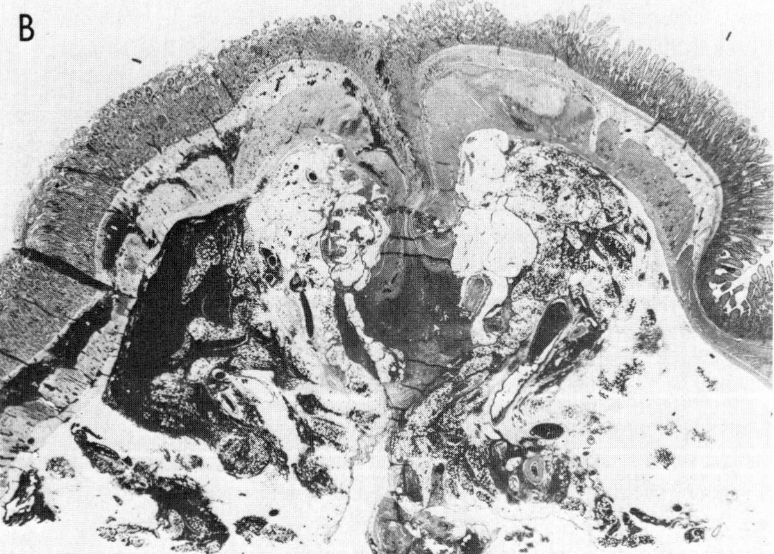

Fig III–4.—**A** and **B,** anastomoses at 12 hours. **A,** inverting anastomosis. The intraluminal protrusion of swollen hemorrhagic bowel wall covered by hemorrhagic coagulum is more prominent than at six hours. The inverted flange is firmly coapted at its base by the suture. **B,** everting anastomosis. The mucosal surface continues smooth and unbroken. There may be a little crossover of India ink and the everted mucosa is not recognizable. There is remarkably little inflammation anywhere along the line of union or in the everted coagulum. *(continued)*

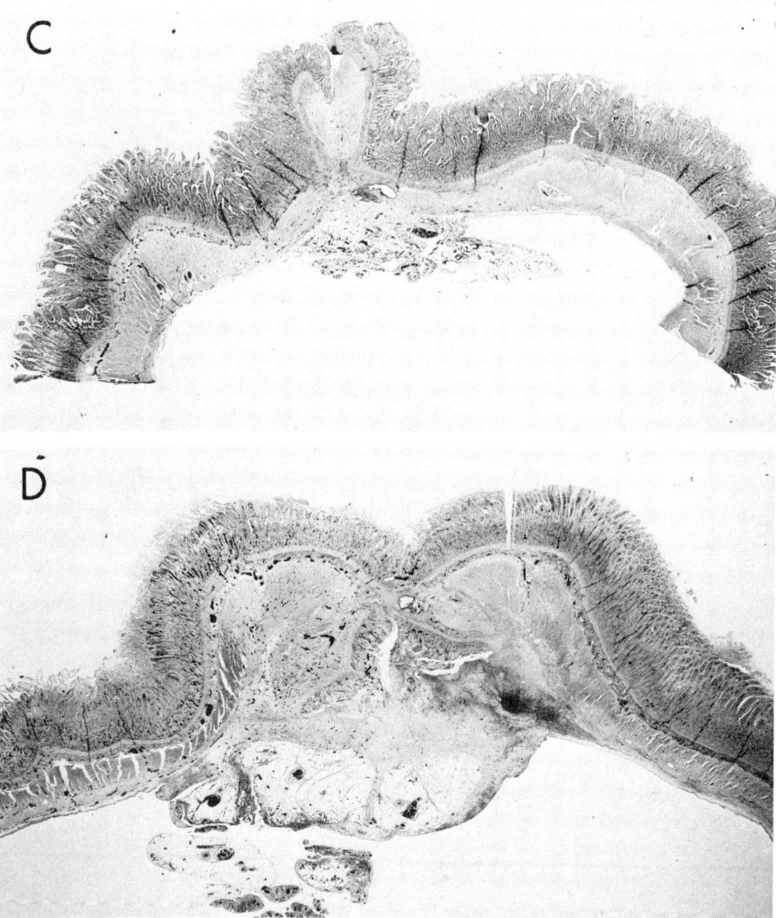

Fig III–4 (cont.).—C and **D**, anastomoses at seven days. **C**, inverting anastomosis. Intraluminal hemorrhagic plug has been resorbed. Submucosal layers of the two sides seem to have fused at the level at which sutures had been placed, but an intraluminal flange persists and its surface still is granulating and uncovered by mucosa. **D**, everting anastomosis. Mucosal surface healed and continuous, and one can see free crossover of the India ink. The serosal surface is quite smooth and most of the everted mucosa has been resorbed, although in this section one can see retained mucosa in a cleft at the line of eversion. It is happenstance whether the section is taken quite close to the sutures, in which case one will see a firm mucosal union, or between sutures, when one may see an open cleft going up into the everted flange. There is not now, nor has there ever been in the everting anastomosis, any inflammation on the mucosal side, although there still is, at seven days, more cellular reaction on the serosal side than is present in the inverting anastomosis. (From M.M. Ravitch, F. Canalis, A. Weinshelbaum, and J. McCormick, *Transactions of the American Surgical Association,* 1967, used by permission.)

and truly everting, anastomoses on dogs, harvesting the anastomoses at intervals of from six hours to six weeks and attempting at the time of harvesting to inject the arterial tree with India ink on one side of the anastomosis to demonstrate the extent of passage of the injected material across the anastomotic site. Mall (1896) had studied the histologic healing sequence in inverting anastomoses performed in his laboratory by William S. Halsted. It was these studies that led to Halsted's appreciation of the importance of the submucosa. At six hours in our everting anastomoses there was an almost unbroken mucosal lining. On the serosal surface, a wedge of coagulum filling in the cleft between the everted mucosal edges already was covered by a smooth monocellular layer of mesothelial cells without any significant inflammatory reaction. In the inverting anastomoses, at six hours, there was an astonishing degree of hemorrhage and edema of the inverted mucosa and submucosa. By 12 hours (Fig III–4*A,B*) in the everted flange, little mucosa was recognizable whereas in the inverted flange there was an intraluminal mass of hemorrhagic, necrotic, edematous mucosa and an intense polymorphonuclear response. In both types of anastomosis, the cleft in the inverted or everted flange was filled by a wedge-shaped plug of hemorrhagic coagulum. But in the everting anastomosis, this wedge had become laminated and smoothed out on the serosal side and the mucosal surface was smooth and neat. By 72 hours, the everting anastomosis showed apparent complete union of the mucosa on the luminal side, although there still was some recognizable mucosa either in the anastomotic cleft or superficial to it. India ink was injected into a mesenteric artery on one side of the anastomoses to be harvested. In general, there was an earlier crossover of the injected India ink in the everting anastomoses, beginning as early as 48 hours, although the differences may not have been significant. At the end of a week (Fig III–4*C,D*), the everting anastomoses showed a smooth mucosal continuity and usually a crossover injection of India ink, a modest external inflammation, and an organizing scar covering the serosal surface. Occasional islands of epithelium persisted in the scar between the united ends. The inverting anastomoses, at 72 hours, showed infrequent crossover of the injected India ink, a largely pyogenic plug on the mucosal side, and a sizable intraluminal projection of the inverted flange. It took about two weeks for the inverted anastomoses to develop continuous mucosa on the luminal side.

It was exciting to us to note that Travers (1812), describing the healing of the anastomoses that he performed with the bowel perforce everted, since he had not devised a technique for inverting the cut ends, said,

" . . . the opposed villous surfaces, so far as my observation goes, neither adhere nor become consolidated by granulation, so that the interstice marking the division internally is probably never obliterated . . . although the substance of the paries intestinalis is ever after deficient in the line of division, yet by inspection of the external surface, it would be difficult, if possible to say, where the division had taken place even at a recent period from the injury."

We have for many years been in the habit of treating or preventing paralytic ileus by pharmacologic stimulation of the paretic bowel with alternate doses of Prostigmin and Pitressin. In patients with ileus from peritonitis or from excessive manipulation of the bowel, as after the evisceration associated with resections of the abdominal aorta, this regimen has proved its value to our satisfaction. We have, however, religiously abstained from such stimulation of the bowel in patients with a recent anastomosis. Given our observation of the absence of edema and obstruction with stapled anastomoses (Ravitch and Rivarola, 1966), we thought it worthwhile to test the effect of pharmacologic stimulation on both sutured and stapled anastomoses, seeking at the same time to further our comparative evaluation of conventional and stapled anastomoses (Brolin and Ravitch, 1980). With Brolin, we performed enteroenterostomies, ileocolostomies, and colocolostomies, comparing the functional end-to-end stapled anastomosis, the one-layer silk everting "Navy" anastomosis of Getzen, our one-layer silk everting anastomosis and the conventional two-layer inverting anastomosis, 220 animals in all (Fig III–5A–D). Half the animals in each group received 1 ml of Prostigmin, 1:2,000, on each of the first three days after construction of the anastomoses and half of them received Prostigmin as well intravenously on the operating table and 30 ml of castor oil on each of the first two postoperative days. All 110 dogs so stimulated passed their first stool within the first three days whereas 33 of the 110 control animals passed their first stool on the fourth day or later. In the combined total of 60 pharmacologically stimulated, stapled or two-layer inverted anastomoses at these three levels of the gastrointestinal tract there were no leaks. Two leaks occurred in the 60 control animals who received no Prostigmin or castor oil. The "Navy" everting anastomosis in the colon proved less reliable than either the stapled or inverting techniques, which were equivalent, but induced peristalsis had no discernible effect on the incidence of leaks with the "Navy" technique. The end-to-end true everting one-layer silk colonic anastomosis, the silk placed as a mattress suture with its bar parallel to the cut end of the bowel, resulted in leaks in four of ten controls and nine of ten stimulated animals. Thus, in small and large bowel anastomoses with the stapled, two-layer inverted or one-layer everted "Navy" technique, pharmacologic stimulation had no deleterious effect on fresh anastomoses. As Poth (1950) and others have pointed out, the sutures in the simple interrupted "Navy" everting technique cut through the bowel edges sufficiently to produce, after a few hours, a true edge-to-edge, end-to-end anastomosis rather than an everting anastomosis. In this group of experiments, the one-layer silk everted anastomosis performed with horizontal mattress sutures in the large bowel of a dog was less secure than any of the other methods, and pharmacologically induced peristalsis accentuated the inadequacy of this technique. In our earlier studies, this single-layer true everting technique met with uniform success, but those earlier studies involved only the small bowel and obviously are not applicable to the colon in the dog. Goligher, Morris, McAdam, de Dombal, and Johnston (1970) have demonstrated that a single layer of such true everting sutures placed parallel to the cut end of the human colon is associated with an increased anastomotic failure rate.

Although from the start we have been reluctant to use the stapling instruments in patients with florid peritonitis, intestinal obstruction, etc., our house staff have not been so hesitant and have, in fact, obviously preferred to use the staples in these emergency conditions, just as Chassin (Chassin, Rifkind, Sussman, Kassel, Fingeret, Drager, and Chassin, 1978) found in his experience. And, like Chassin, we found no deleterious results. To put this to the test, we compared resection and stapled functional end-to-end anastomoses with resection and conventional inverting two-layer anastomoses, performed in dogs 48 hours after devascularizing a segment of ileum, 48 hours after producing obstruction by ligature of ileum or colon, and 24 hours after excision of a full-thickness button of wall of small or large bowel (Ravitch, Brolin, Kolter, and Yap, 1981). Ischemic bowel was produced by ligating the blood vessels of a segment of ileum 6–10 cm in length, obstructed bowel by ligating the ileum or colon with umbilical tape, perforated bowel by excising a 1-cm button of the ileum or colon. A control group of

TWO—LAYER INVERTED

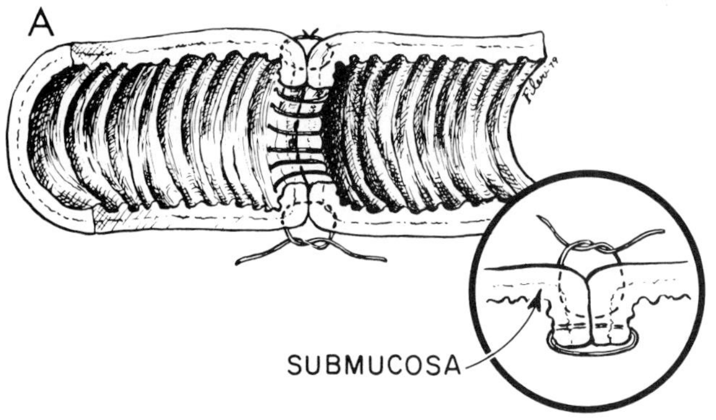

Fig III–5.—Suture techniques evaluated by pharmacologic stimulation of peristalsis. **A,** the two-layer inverted suture is the conventional anastomosis, done in this instance with the continuous inner row of 4–0 catgut and an interrupted outer row of 4–0 silk. **B,** the "Navy" stitch. One layer of interrupted sutures placed in the bowel to produce a minimal inversion. Within a few hours, the suture will have cut through sufficiently to produce a precise end-to-end anastomosis.

"NAVY"

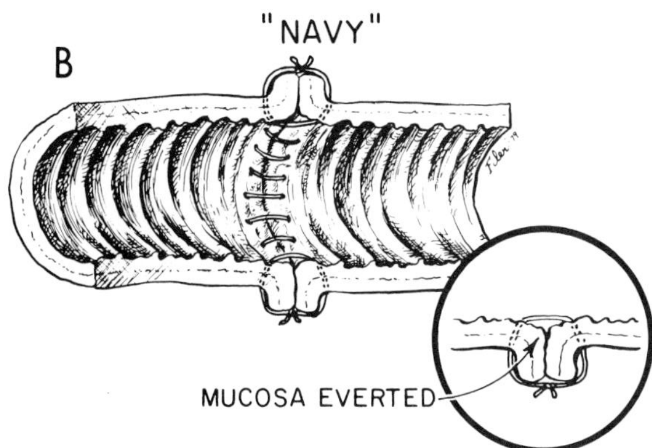

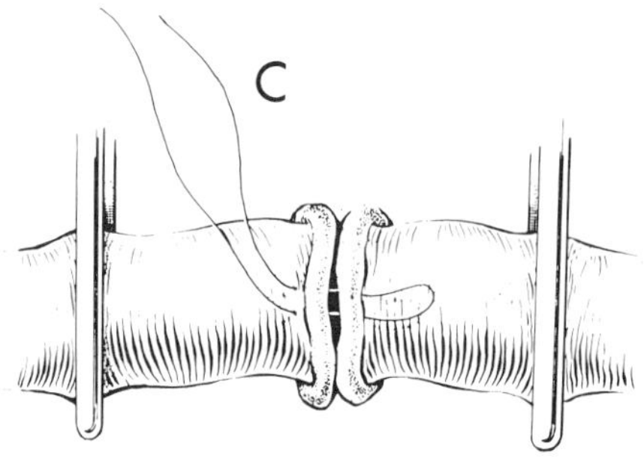

Fig III–5 (cont.).—**C,** the one-layer truly everting anastomosis performed with a single row of interrupted mattress sutures, the bar of the suture parallel to the cut edge of the bowel.

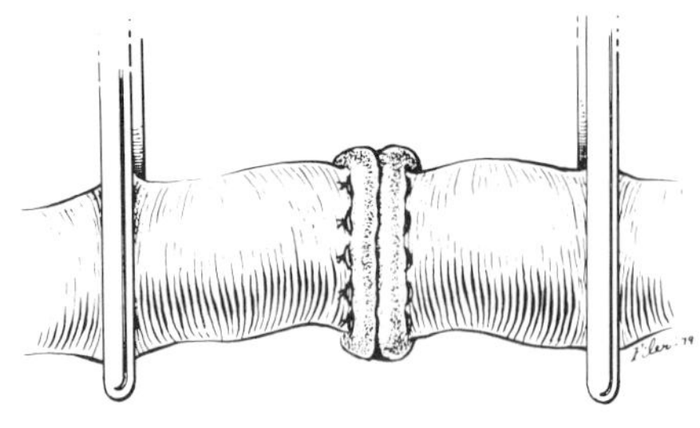

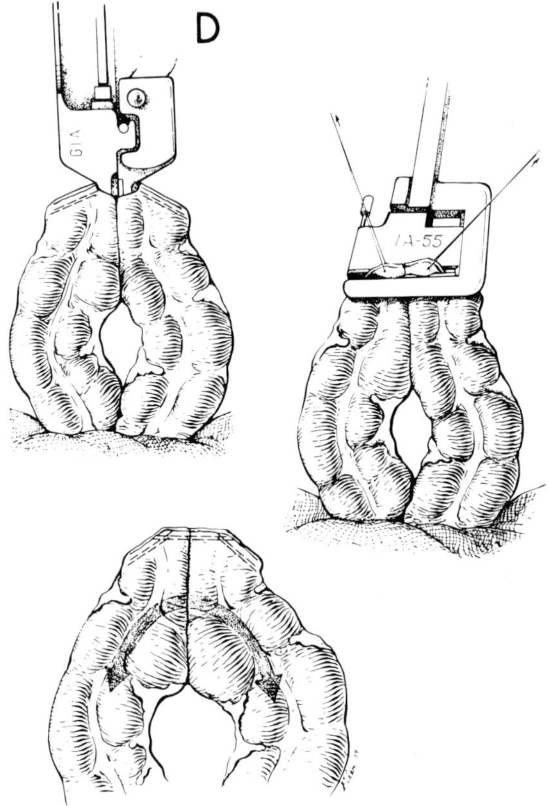

STAPLED FUNCTIONAL END-TO-END

Fig III–5 (cont.).—D, the stapled functional end-to-end anastomosis. The upper left of the figure shows the two loops of bowel stapled closed, mucosa-to-mucosa, and the septum between the two limbs being stapled and divided with the GIA™ instrument, which provides a serosa-to-serosa inverting suture for this portion of the anastomosis. The upper right-hand corner of the illustration shows the GIA™ instrument withdrawn, and the opening left by its withdrawal closed mucosa-to-mucosa. The lower drawing shows the anastomosis, which appears to have been made as a side-to-side anastomosis but in truth produces an end-to-end reconstruction of the intestine. (From M.M. Ravitch, R.E. Brolin, J.P. Kolter Jr., and S. Yap, *World Journal of Surgery,* 1981, used by permission.)

animals merely underwent ileal transection and reanastomosis, without any preliminary insulting procedure.

With each type of preparation, ten animals had a functional end-to-end stapled anastomosis after the resection and ten animals had a two-layer manual inverting anastomosis. At the time of resection, the ischemic bowel showed areas of gangrene or frank perforation; the bowel, at the levels of transection and anastomosis, was edematous, friable, and hyperemic. In the obstructed animals there was proximal distention and some edema, and a striking disparity in size between the proximal and distal bowel at the levels of transection. The animals with intestinal perforation had a severe exudative peritonitis with edematous, hyperemic, friable bowel both proximal and distal and no walling off of the perforation. In all animals of the three groups, peritoneal cultures yielded an array of pathogenic organisms, indicating that in both the obstructed and the ischemic preparations the bowel had been sufficiently injured to permit bacteria to pass through. The first five stapled functional end-to-end anastomoses in perforated or obstructed animals, performed by an operator new to the laboratory, all developed leaks where the GIA^{TM} staple line crossed the TA 55^{TM} staple line. In the next 30 dogs with the same operator, a single leak occurred, in a dog in the perforation group.

It was interesting that, in these experiments, the hand-sewn silk technique seemed to result in more postoperative adhesions, both around the anastomosis and throughout the abdomen. Adhesions with the stapled anastomoses usually were along the everted flange of the TA 55^{TM} closure of the functional end-to-end anastomosis.

Just as with bowel in which peristalsis was pharmacologically stimulated, so in bowel injured by experimentally created ischemia, obstruction, or perforation there was no significant difference between standard two-layer silk inverted end-to-end anastomoses and the functional end-to-end staple technique, which utilized both an inverting and an everting staple suture line (Ravitch, Brolin, Kolter, and Yap, 1981).

Greenstein, Rogers, and Moss (1978), in year-old beagle dogs, compared a continuous 4-0 end-to-end Dacron anastomosis with an EEA^{TM} anastomosis. After four days, the disruption pressures in the two preparations were compared. The average air pressure disruption in millimeters of mercury for the Dacron sutures was 23 mm Hg $\pm$ 25 and for the EEA^{TM} instrument was 138 mm Hg $\pm$ 46, an obviously significant difference despite the spread in individual pressures.

Bubrick (1981; Bubrick, Lundeen, and Hitchcock, 1981), from the Hennepin Medical Center, Minneapolis, compared two-layer, manual, inverting rectal anastomoses in dogs with EEA^{TM} stapled anastomoses, performing barium enemas at least four times in the first two weeks. In the 20 hand-sewn anastomoses there were 13 radiographic or clinical dehiscences—65%—and in the 20 dogs with stapled anastomoses there were four—20%. There were six deaths in the entire series, all due to anastomotic dehiscences, four in the hand-sewn group, two in the stapled group.

Polglase, Hughes, McDermott, and Burke (1981) compared the EEA^{TM} stapled anastomoses (12 dogs) with single-layer 0 polypropylene suture anastomoses, vertical mattress sutures posteriorly, and Gambee sutures anteriorly (12 dogs). In two of the sutured anastomoses there was radiologic evidence of leak, none in the stapled anastomoses. Fecal impaction occurred at one sutured anastomosis on the fourth day, ''The narrowing score was significantly higher for suture anastomoses compared with stapled anastomoses, p $<$ 0.001.'' The gross appearance of the anastomoses in the days following operation was all in favor of the stapled anastomoses on the second day, after which differences were less obvious, but there was a wider gap in the granulation tissue between the epithelial surfaces in the stapled group. Inversion was minimal after stapled, and significant after manual, anastomosis. There was no difference in the edema in the two groups. Both types of anastomoses were airtight and watertight to pressure testing from the time of their construction. ''The end-to-end staple anastomosis. . .may be considered mechanically sound and hermetic if the rings of tissue around the central rod are intact. This vital pointer to the integrity of the staple anastomosis may lead to increased confidence and to fewer unnecessary proximal stomas.'' There was a definite delay in mucosal healing of the stapled as opposed to the manual anastomoses.

Harrison, at the University of British Columbia (Harrison and Oka, 1982; Oka, Harrison, and Burhenne, 1982), as part of a continuing series of experiments on the healing of intestinal anastomoses in dogs, evaluated the possible usefulness of a fibrin glue

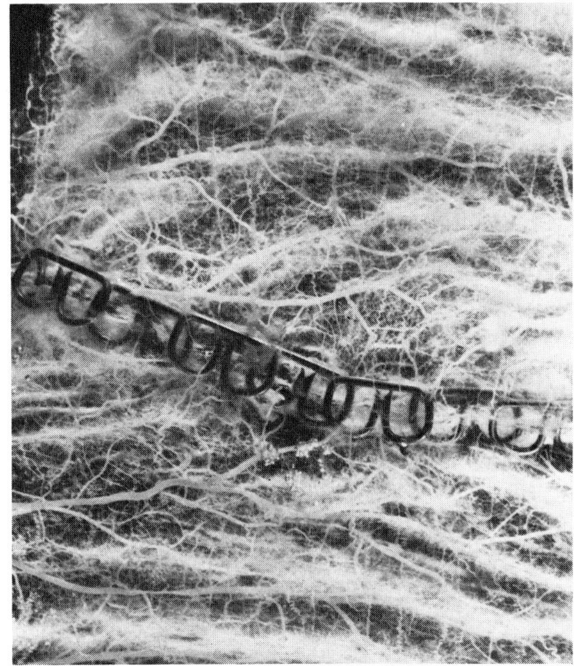

Fig III–6.—Microangiogram of staple sutured rectum in the dog. One can clearly see vessels going through the loops of the staple Bs. (Courtesy of R.C. Harrison, Vancouver, British Columbia.)

inserted just before the two ends of bowel were compressed by the stapler. The animals were deliberately jeopardized by ligating mesenteric vessels, in order to provide a severe test. Before the seventh day there were four fatal leaks in the 17 animals without the glue and one in the 17 animals with the glue. Radiologic studies of leaks on the seventh day and studies at autopsy afterward showed a total of 11 leaks out of the 17 animals without glue and six out of the 17 animals with glue, not a statistically significant difference. Harrison makes the interesting suggestion that the stapler would make it quite simple, if an appropriate glue were available, to perform anastomoses without any suture material whatsoever, which might be ideal, since all suture techniques cause some interference with the circulation in the sutured tissue. For studies as yet unpublished, Harrison (1982) has obtained brilliant microangiograms (Fig III–6) showing remarkably little disturbance of the vascularity of stapled bowel.

Although we have stressed throughout that the adequacy of a technique of anastomosis is determined by its clinical success and not by bursting strength or tensile strength of the anastomosis or by injection studies with vital dyes or radiocontrast material, Harrison's studies have, for instance, demonstrated the striking decrease in vascularity with a continuous suture anastomosis as opposed to an interrupted suture anastomosis, and such studies do add considerable information to our understanding of the healing of intestinal wounds.

In clinical practice, we have come to rely on stapling instruments in performing every type of operation on the gastrointestinal tract, and regularly rely on stapled, mucosa-to-mucosa closure of esophagus, stomach, duodenum, and small and large bowel, without inverting or covering over the stapled ends. Although the time saved by the appropriate use of the staples is not inconsiderable, we stress the advantages of the stapling instruments in terms of precision, neatness, reduction of trauma, decrease of the likelihood

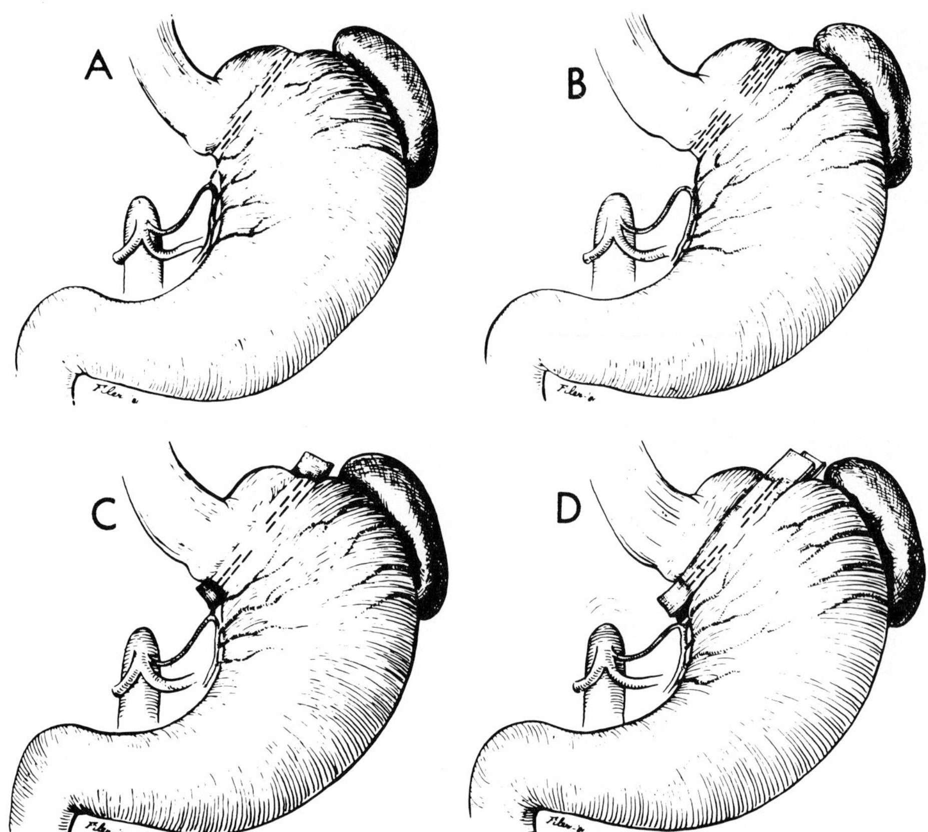

Fig III–7.—The cause of disruption of in-continuity gastric stapling. We had shown in 1967 (Ravitch, Rivarola, and VanGrov) that dogs' stomachs, stapled in continuity and provided with a bypassing gastroenterostomy, did not remain securely partitioned. We had presumed then that the uninjured gastric mucosa would, of course, not heal, and that the staples pulled out in response to the gastric effort to force food by. **(A)** The original technique for gastric partitioning as described by Pace and associates (Pace, Martin, Tetirick, Fabri, and Carey 1979) using one application of the TA 55™ stapler with three central staples removed from the cartridge. **(B)** Modification of the original technique described by Ellison and colleagues (Ellison, Martin, Laschinger, Mojzisik, Hughes, and Carey 1980) using two applications of the TA 55™ stapler, placing four rows of staples side-by-side with three staples removed from each cartridge. **(C)** One application of the TA 55™ stapler, as in **(A),** but reinforced with a strip of Marlex mesh or Teflon. The strip is attached to the lower jaw of the instrument and secured on the posterior aspect of the stomach, the crimped side of the staples. **(D)** One application of the TA 55™ stapler, again as in **(A),** but reinforced with strips of Marlex mesh placed anteriorly and posteriorly, creating a sandwich of the stapled stomach between the strips of Marlex mesh. (From R.E. Brolin and M.M. Ravitch, *SG&O,* 1981, used by permission.)

of soiling, and the elimination of the problem resulting from disproportion in size between bowel ends to be anastomosed.

Mechanical suture techniques do not release the surgeon or the patient from the basic rules of surgery or the penalties for their violation. Bowel deprived of its blood supply, or diseased or abused bowel, may no more be relied on to heal when stapled than when sutured with silk. The instruments, with the possible exception of the EEA^{TM} instrument in extremely low rectal anastomoses, and in some esophageal anastomoses, will not permit a surgeon to do what he could not otherwise do manually. They will not permit the safe performance of operative maneuvers by untrained or unskilled personnel, nor do they eliminate the necessity for rigorous surgical training, due regard for tissues, and of course training in the various manual techniques of resection and anastomosis.

The paper by Pace and Carey (Pace, Martin, Tetirick, Fabri, and Carey, 1979) on staple partitioning of the stomach in the treatment of morbid obesity, which aroused so much initial enthusiasm, ran counter to our experimental observations in stapling of the undivided stomach, in which presently the stapling line opened up (Ravitch, Rivarola, and VanGrov, 1967). Our brief experience with this operation in patients showed a disquieting frequency of ''disruption'' of the staple line. Alden (1977), who had modified the gastric bypass of Mason (Mason, Printen, Hartford, and Boyd, 1975) by a double row of staples across the undivided stomach just distal to the high gastroenterostomy, confirmed to us (Alden, August, 1977) that in fact, on subsequent barium swallow, at least in some patients, the stapled gastric closure no longer was complete. In studying this anew in dogs (Brolin and Ravitch, 1981) (Fig III–7), we found that within five weeks the double staple line across the stomach no longer was complete and that staples had ''pulled out.'' On the assumption that vigorous peristalsis had allowed the staples to be literally torn out of the posterior gastric wall, we attempted to study the effect of putting a strip of prosthetic material such as Marlex, Dacron, or Teflon on one or both gastric surfaces to provide a secure purchase for the staples so that they would not ''pull out.'' The results were somewhat surprising. In a number of dogs, fatal leaks occurred from necrosis in such reinforced staple lines. The staples ''pulled out'' presently in many of the animals who survived. It was particularly interesting to observe in x-rays of the autopsy specimens of those animals who survived (Fig III–8) that the staples had not torn through the stomach but had gradually opened up, sometimes widely, and slipped out. It appears to us that the progressive muscular action of the stomach, repeatedly stressing the fine wire staples, gradually opened them. There have been reports of staples in the vaginal cuff, after hysterectomy, coming open and being discharged, so the gynecologists have resorted to speculum examination at postoperative visits and withdrawal of any open staples seen. The presumption that such staple opening is due to repeated physical stress is being evaluated by serial postoperative roentgen study of women who are sexually active compared to those who are not (Beresford, 1982). The insecurity of the staple lines in the undivided stomach obviously has been a problem to many of those working in the field of operations on the stomach to combat morbid obesity, and variations remarkable in number have been introduced, one following another (Mason, Printen, Hartford, and Boyd, 1975; Mason, Printen, Barron, Lewis, Kealey, and Blommers, 1979; Ellison, Martin, Laschinger, Mojzisik, Hughes, Carey, and Pace, 1980; Gomez, 1980; Eskind, Massie, Born, O'Leary, and Scott, 1981; Mason, 1982). The basic fact, however, is that the stapling instruments do not produce necrosis of the mucosa and, therefore, the stapled, intact stomach cannot be relied on to heal. Compression sufficient to necrose the bowel, or the use of multiple applications

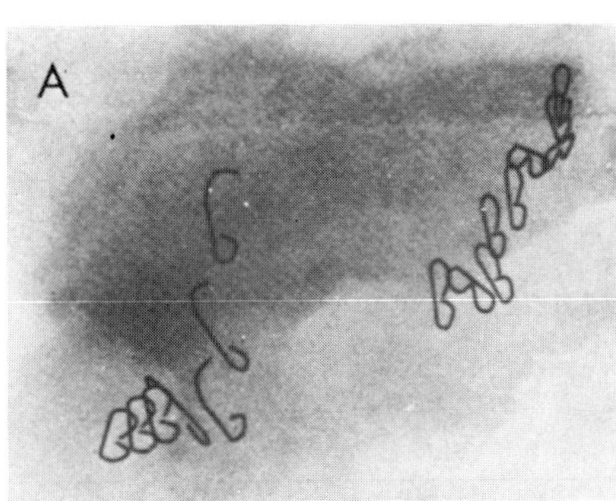

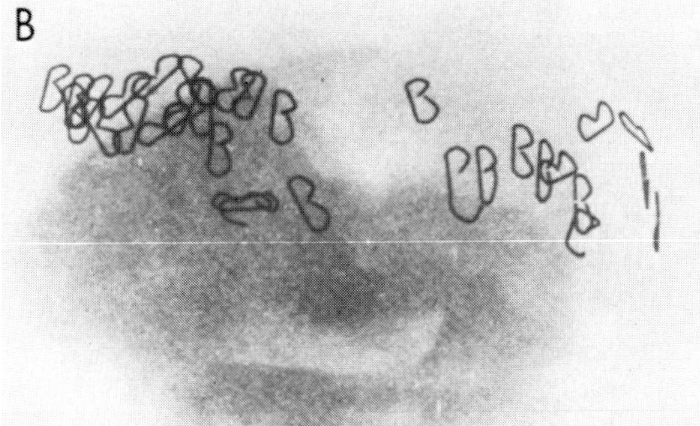

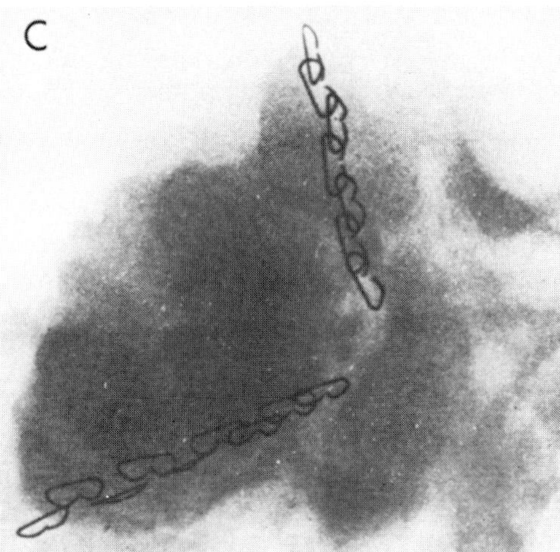

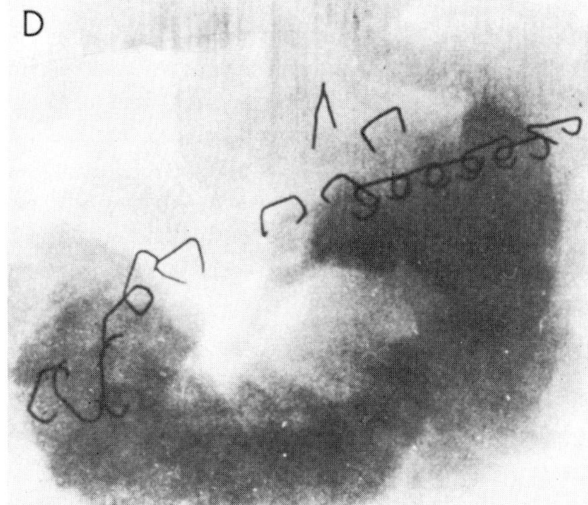

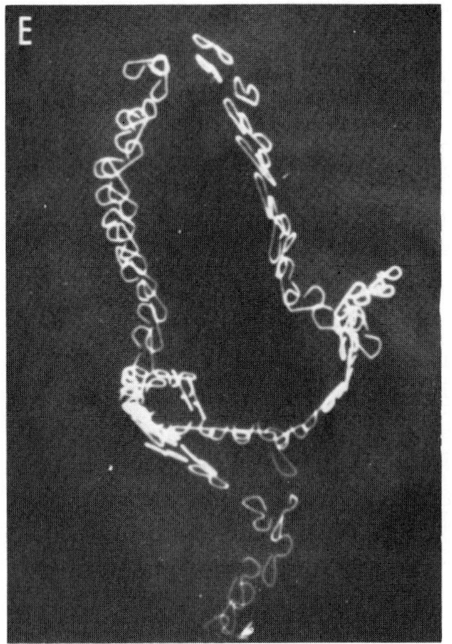

Fig III–8.—Fate of staples in undivided stomach (Brolin and Ravitch 1981). In dogs in which the undivided stomach was partitioned with staples, immediate radiologic study always showed all staples perfectly formed. **A,** partition made with one application of the TA 55™ stapler, five weeks after operation. Original stoma 0.9 cm. Stoma diameter now 2.7 cm. The staples have opened up on one side of the stoma. **B,** partition made with two side-by-side applications of the TA 55™ stapler five weeks after operation. Stoma diameter now 2.9 cm. Some staples have begun to open whereas others have remained closed but pulled through the anterior wall of the stomach. One staple is missing. **C,** partition made with one application of the TA 55™ stapler reinforced posteriorly with Marlex mesh. Five weeks after operation, stoma diameter is 0.9 cm, which is the original size of the opening. None of the staples have opened or pulled through. Such a result occurred only irregularly. **D,** partition at five weeks made with one application of the TA 55™ stapler reinforced anteriorly and posteriorly with Marlex mesh strips. At five weeks, stoma diameter is 2.0 cm. Staples have completely opened on one side of the stoma but have remained embedded in the Marlex. **E,** functional end-to-end anastomosis in jejunoileal shunt five years after construction. Note the perfect B shape of all staples forming the circular anastomosis. (From R.E. Brolin and M.M. Ravitch, *SG&O,* 1981, used by permission.)

of the stapler, or reinforcing through-and-through sutures threaten the circulation and the viability of the stomach. At this writing, we do not believe that stapling the undivided bowel has solved the problem of providing an operation for morbid obesity that is at the same time safe and reliably effective.

THE USE OF METAL SUTURES

Wire sutures of bronze, silver, steel, aluminum, tantalum—monofilament, twisted, or braided—in every size and range of ductility and tensile strength have been used by several generations of surgeons. Currently, most of these have been abandoned except for stainless steel, which still is used by many for intestinal (Cowley, 1969; Kratzer and Onsanit, 1974), bronchial, vascular, and soft tissue suture. Except for the suture manufacturers, we are long past the day of heated debate over the relative virtues of sutures of animal, vegetable, mineral, or petrochemical origin, recognizing the various virtues and deficiencies of each. The steel used in modern staples is relatively reactionless in the tissues, does not corrode, and possesses the appropriate physical properties. In the various uses described in these pages, the staples are not deformed by mechanical forces of peristalsis or distention, except as noted in stapling the undivided stomach, nor weakened by the process of closure, and do not change in shape or break with the passage of time. The fine stainless steel staples have presented essentially no foreign body problem. The bronchus provides a particularly good opportunity to evaluate this problem. Silk or synthetic sutures, not rarely, present in the bronchial lumen, causing chronic cough and requiring bronchoscopic removal. Staples, however, either are not seen at all through the bronchoscope or are visible through a thin layer of epithelium without any granulation tissue or evidence of inflammation. We have neither seen nor heard of a staple in the bronchus requiring removal for chronic cough or persistent granulating infection. If it does occur, it must be exceedingly rare.

If one applies a suture line longer than the tissue being closed or anastomosed, the excess staples beyond the tissue generally remain on the cartridge. We pick out any that may fall into the wound if they are obvious, but over the years we must have left a good many individual staples loose within the abdomen or chest and have yet to see a problem result from this.

The bowel is not devitalized by the instruments, heavy as they seem, and the B form of the staples allows vessels to pass through the openings in the staples and between the staples, so that the transected and stapled duodenal or bronchial stump or gastric or colonic cut end is viable beyond the line of staples, out to its very edge. Goldman (1964) demonstrated in the lung, by injection, open vessels passing through the stapled suture line (Fig III–9). Schwarzbart and Lubin (1978) studied the fate of stainless steel staples applied in the gastrointestinal tract and found that those staples used in an inverting suture line ultimately were evacuated into the GI tract whereas those placed in a mucosa-to-mucosa closure usually remained in their original position. Neither technique seemed to influence healing, solidity of suture line, or presence or absence of inflammation. The cut and stapled end of lung or bowel can be seen to ooze a little fresh blood, which is taken as a pleasant sign that the tissue is viable to the very edge. An occasional frank arterial bleeder is sutured or coagulated.

Healing of the transected bowel end, stapled mucosa-to-mucosa with a double row of staggered staples, occurs securely without the necessity for inversion or covering with adjacent tissues and without any remarkable formation of adhesions. Nutrition of the

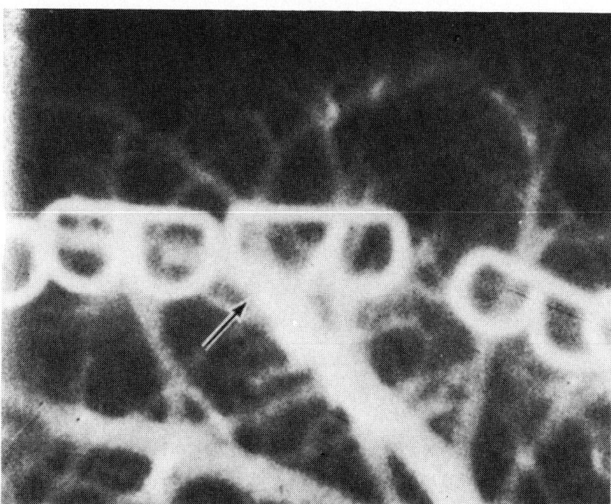

Fig III–9.—Dog lung magnified 10X at suture line. Note vessels approximately 1 mm in size passing through the openings in the "B" of the staples. (From A. Goldman, *Diseases of the Chest,* 1964, used by permission.)

ends of the stapled bowel, and healing, are dependent on the intrinsic circulation of the bowel wall, and not derived from adhesions to adjacent tissues. We have been informed of the remarkable strength of a terminal mucosa-to-mucosa closure of the sigmoid colon in a patient who had what was planned as a Hartmann procedure after sigmoid resection. No gas or stool emerged from the "terminal colostomy" for five days. At this point, it was realized that it was the proximal stapled end of the colon that had been dropped into the abdomen and the distal rectosigmoid that had been brought out the abdominal wall. At operation after five days, although the colon was enormously dilated, the staple line was intact and the colon was viable to the very stapled edge. There was no evidence of leakage or infection.

COMPARATIVE STUDIES OF MANUAL AND MECHANICAL SUTURE TECHNIQUES

Substantially less trauma is inflicted on the bowel by introducing 12 or 32 sutures with a single application of an instrument than by picking up the bowel, inserting the needle, and passing the suture material through the tissues as many times. Gross and microscopic comparison of stapled and manually sewn suture lines shows, in the stapled tissues, extraordinarily little edema, hemorrhage, or necrosis in the first week or ten days, at a time when manual inverting closures and anastomoses show edema, ecchymosis, ragged tags of mucosa and muscularis, and loosened sutures hanging into the lumen. Healing of stapled anastomoses has been as reliable, in controlled experiments in dogs, as conventional inverted two-layer anastomoses of small bowel-to-small bowel, small bowel-to-large bowel, and large bowel-to-large bowel.

There have been a number of experimental studies of the strength of stapled and of sutured anastomoses tested by bursting pressure, or resistance to tension. The results have been equivocal. In any case, it seems to us that the test of an anastomotic technique is healing under natural conditions, and stresses produced by mechanical inflation of the bowel or distraction of the two ends would appear to have little meaning.

Dunn and associates, from the University of Minnesota (Dunn, Robbins, Decanini, Goldberg, and Delaney, 1978), reported triangulated everted-inverted stapled true end-to-end and inverted hand-sewn end-to-end anastomoses in dogs, 12 in each group, performing two anastomoses in each colon, one with each technique alternating the location of the stapled and of the manually sutured anastomoses as to whether they were proximal or distal (an experiment flawed by the performance of both types of anastomosis in the same animal). The anastomoses were inspected at autopsy or at 14 days after operation. Bursting pressure was determined. The stapling technique was by our original end-to-end triangular method. Six of the 12 stapled anastomoses were found to leak but none of the 12 inverted sutured ones. The everted staple anastomosis was also compared with everted suture anastomosis, single row through-and-through. Two of the ten stapled anastomoses leaked and nine of the ten sutured ones. In all the experiments, the anastomoses were stressed by our technique (Ravitch, Canalis, Weinshelbaum, and McCormick, 1967) of loosely wrapping the anastomosis with polyethylene. They considered that they had demonstrated that the inverted one-layer anastomosis "provides a more secure approximation of the colon under adverse circumstances, i.e., wrapping, than the everted stapled anastomosis. . .the mucosal eversion and not the staples, *per se*, was responsible for the high dehiscence rate."

Many surgeons report their impression that anastomoses "open" faster when stapled than when sutured by hand. This certainly is our own impression, strikingly reinforced by the behavior of patients with a primary jejunoileal Scott-type shunt or in their subsequent reconnection, with its two anastomoses and an additional closure. For that matter, in our series of jejunoileal shunts there were no leaks in either the primary or the secondary operations, a total of 465 anastomoses and closures, all with staples (Ravitch and Brolin, 1979). The function of the bowel after anastomosis and resection depends as well on the condition of the bowel before operation, the amount of handling of the bowel, the medication given after operation, whether a long tube or a short tube is used and how long suction is maintained, so that a controlled comparative study of the time an anastomosis "opens up" presents difficulties. In any case, our conviction of the superiority of the stapled procedures prevents us from undertaking a clinical trial. Our own experience in comparing small bowel-to-small bowel, small-to large, large-to-large bowel anastomoses operated on electively in a non–randomized fashion in the same hospital, over the same period of time, by resident surgeons, has led us to the conclusion that stapling is at least as reliable as manual suturing.

Clinical comparative studies are discussed in Part II, Chapter IV, Introduction.

REFERENCES

Alden J.F.: Gastric and jejunoileal bypass. A comparison in the treatment of morbid obesity. *Arch. Surg.* 112:799, 1977.
Alden J.F.: Personal communication, August 9, 1977.
Beresford J.M.: Personal communication, February 26, 1982.
Brolin R.E., Ravitch M.M.: Studies in intestinal healing. VI. Effect of pharmacologically induced peristalsis on fresh intestinal anastomoses in dogs. *Arch. Surg.* 115:339, 1980.
Brolin R.E., Ravitch M.M.: Experimental evaluation of techniques of gastric partitioning for morbid obesity. *Surg. Gynecol. Obstet.* 153:877, 1981.
Brøyn T., Helsingen N. Jr.: Tumour implantation in colon surgery. The effect of everted versus inverted type of anastomosis. An experimental study in rats. *Acta Chir. Scand.* 135:635, 1969.

Bubrick M.P.: Effect of technique on anastomotic dehiscence. *Dis. Colon Rectum* 24:232, 1981.

Bubrick M.P., Lundeen J.W., Hitchcock C.R.: A comparative radiographic study of low anterior colon anastomoses in dogs. *Surgery* 89:454, 1981.

Canalis F., Ravitch M.M.: Study of healing of inverting and everting intestinal anastomoses. *Surg. Gynecol. Obstet.* 126:109, 1968.

Chassin J.L., Rifkind K.M., Sussman B., Kassel B., Fingeret A., Drager S., Chassin P.S.: The stapled gastrointestinal tract anastomosis: Incidence of postoperative complications compared with the sutured anastomosis. *Ann. Surg.* 188:689, 1978.

Cowley L.L.: One layer end-on intestinal anastomoses using fine monofilament steel sutures. *Am. J. Surg.* 118:177, 1969.

Crowson W.N., Wilson C.S.: An experimental study of the effects of drains on colon anastomoses. *Am. Surg.* 39:597, 1973.

Dunn D.H., Robbins P., Decanini C., Goldberg S., Delaney J.P.: A comparison of stapled and hand-sewn colonic anastomoses. *Dis. Colon Rectum* 21:636, 1978.

Dupuytren G.: Mémoire sur une méthode nouvelle pour traiter les anus accidentels. *Mém. Acad. Roy. Méd.*, Paris, 1 Sec. de Méd., pp. 259–316, 1828.

Ellison E.C., Martin E.W. Jr., Laschinger J., Mojzisik C., Hughes K., Carey L.C., Pace W.C.: Prevention of early failure of stapled gastric partitions in treatment of morbid obesity. *Arch. Surg.* 115:528, 1980.

Eskind S.J., Massie J.D., Born M.L., O'Leary J.P., Scott H.W. Jr.: Experimental study of double staple lines in gastric partitions. *Surg. Gynecol. Obstet.* 152:751, 1981.

Galluzzi W., Possenti B.: La sutura evertente applicata all'anastomosi termino-terminale del tenue. Studio experimentale. *Minerva Chir.* 9:1008, 1954.

Getzen L.C.: Clinical use of everted intestinal anastomoses. *Surg. Gynecol. Obstet.* 123:1027, 1966.

Getzen L.C.: Intestinal suturing. Part II: Inverting and everting intestinal sutures. *Current Problems in Surgery*, September, 1969.

Getzen L.C., Roe R.D., Holloway C.K.: Comparative study of intestinal anastomotic healing in inverted and everted closures. *Surg. Gynecol. Obstet.* 123:1219, 1966.

Goldman A.: An evaluation of automatic suture with UKL-60 and UKL-40 devices by pulmonary resection. *Dis. Chest* 46:29, 1964.

Goligher J.C., Morris C., McAdam W.A.F., de Dombal F.T., Johnston D.: A controlled trial of inverting versus everting intestinal suture in clinical large-bowel surgery. *Br. J. Surg.* 57:817, 1970.

Gomez C.A.: Gastroplasty in the surgical treatment of morbid obesity. *Am. J. Clin. Nutr.* 33(supp.):406, 1980.

Greenstein A., Rogers P., Moss G.: Doubled fourth-day colorectal anastomotic strength with complete retention of intestinal mature wound collagen and accelerated deposition following immediate full enteral nutrition. *Surg. Forum* 29:78, 1978.

Guglielmi M., Moschini A., Ricci G.: Le anastomosi intestinali evertenti (Studio sperimentale). *Acta Chir Ital.* 24(supp.):397, 1968.

Halsted W.S.: Circular suture of the intestine—An experimental study. *Am. J. Med. Sci.* XCIV:436, 1887.

Harrison R.C.: Personal communication, July 22, 1982.

Harrison R.C., Oka H.: Rectal anastomosis: Sutures vs staples and glue. *Contemp. Surg.* 21:17–19, 22–26, 1982.

Healey J.E. Jr., McBride C.M., Gallager H.S.: Is serosa-to-serosa approximation necessary in intestinal anastomosis? *Surg. Forum* 15:297, 1964.

Heister L.: *A General System of Surgery.* London, W. Innys, etc., 1743.

Herzog B.: Mikroangiographische Studien am Rattendarm zur Prüfung verschiedener Anastomosenarten. *Helv. Chir. Acta* 38:179, 1971.

Kho E., Ravitch M.M.: Studies in intestinal healing. V. Bacterial population in intestinal anastomoses. *Am. J. Surg.* 120:32, 1970.

Kho E., Replogle R., Ravitch M.M.: Studies of intestinal healing. IV. Prevention of adhesions following inverting and everting bowel anastomoses with promethazine and dexamethasone. *Arch. Surg.* 98:764, 1969.

Kornfält S.Å., Okmian L., Jonsson N.: Everted and end-on esophageal anastomosis in the piglet. *Z. Kinderchir.* 12:304, 1973.

Kratzer G.L. Onsanit T.: Single layer steel wire anastomosis of the intestine. *Surg. Gynecol. Obstet.* 139:93, 1974.

Lembert A.: Mémoire sur l'entéroraphie. *Rep. Gen. d'Anat. et de Physiol. Pathol.* II:101, 1826.

Lindenmuth W.W., May C.J.: Anastomoses in the alimentary tract using a sero-muscular tubular cuff technic. *Ann. Surg.* 165:590, 1967.

Loeb M.J.: Comparative strength of inverted, everted, and end-on intestinal anastomoses. *Surg. Gynecol. Obstet.* 125:301, 1967.

Mall R.: Healing of intestinal suture. *Johns Hopkins Hosp. Rep.* 1:76, 1896.

Manz C.W., LaTendresse C., Sako Y.: The detrimental effects of drains on colonic anastomoses: An experimental study. *Dis. Colon Rectum* 13:17, 1970.

Mason E.E.: Vertical banded gastroplasty for obesity. *Arch. Surg.* 117:701, 1982.

Mason E.E., Printen K.J., Barron P., Lewis J.W., Kealey G.P., Blommers T.J.: Risk reduction in gastric operations for obesity. *Ann. Surg.* 190:158, 1979.

Mason E.E., Printen K.J., Hartford C.E., Boyd W.C.: Optimizing results of gastric bypass. *Ann. Surg.* 182:405, 1975.

Oka H., Harrison R.C., Burhenne H.J.: Effect of a biologic glue on the leakage rate of experimental rectal anastomoses. *Am. J. Surg.* 143:561, 1982.

Otis G.A.: Surgical history, in Vol. II, *The Medical and Surgical History of the War of the Rebellion.* Washington, D.C., Government Printing Office, 1876.

Pace W.G., Martin E.W. Jr., Tetirick T., Fabri P.J., Carey L.C.: Gastric partitioning for morbid obesity. *Ann. Surg.* 190:392, 1979.

Polglase A.L., Hughes E.S.R., McDermott F.T., Burke F.R.: A comparison of end-to-end staple and suture colorectal anastomosis in the dog. *Surg. Gynecol. Obstet.* 152:792, 1981.

Poth E.J.: A technique for suturing bowel. *Surg. Gynecol. Obstet.* 91:656, 1950.

Ravitch M.M.: Some considerations on the healing of intestinal anastomoses. *Surg. Clin. North Am.* 49:627, 1969.

Ravitch M.M.: Dupuytren's invention of the Mikulicz enterotome with a note on eponyms. *Perspect. Biol. Med.* 22:170, 1979.

Ravitch M.M., Brolin R.E.: The price of weight loss by jejunoileal shunt. *Ann. Surg.* 190:382, 1979.

Ravitch M.M., Brolin R.E., Kolter J.P. Jr., Yap S.: Studies in the healing of intestinal anastomoses. *World J. Surg.* 5:627, 1981.

Ravitch M.M., Canalis F., Weinshelbaum A., McCormick J.: Studies in intestinal healing: III. Observations on everting intestinal anastomoses. *Trans. Am. Surg. Assoc.* 85:368, 1967.

Ravitch M.M., Rivarola A.: Enteroanastomosis with an automatic instrument. *Surgery* 59:270, 1966.

Ravitch M.M., Rivarola A., VanGrov J.: Studies of intestinal healing. I. Preliminary studies of the mechanism of healing of the everting intestinal anastomosis. *Johns Hopkins Med. J.* 121:343, 1967.

Replogle R.L., Johnson R., Gross R.E.: Prevention of postoperative intestinal adhesions with combined promethazine and dexamethasone therapy: Experimental and clinical studies. *Ann. Surg.* 163:580, 1966.

Rienhoff W.F. Jr., Gannon J. Jr., Sherman I.: Closure of the bronchus following total pneumonectomy. Experimental and clinical observations. *Trans. Am. Surg. Assoc.* 60:481, 1942.

Rusca J.A., Bornside G.H., Cohn I. Jr.: Everting versus inverting gastrointestinal anastomoses: Bacterial leakage and anastomotic disruption. *Ann. Surg.* 169:727, 1969.

Schwarzbart G., Lubin J.: Experience with Auto Suture® surgical stapling instruments. Fate of enterically applied staples. *Int. Surg.,* 63:146, 1978.

Senn N.: Enterorrhapy: Its history, technique and present status. *J.A.M.A.* 21:217, 1893.

Steichen F.M.: Unpublished data, 1964–69.

Steichen F.M.: The use of staplers in anatomical side-to-side and functional end-to-end enteroanastomoses. *Surgery* 64:948, 1968.

Travers B.: *An Inquiry Into the Process of Nature in Repairing Injuries of the Intestines.* London, Longman, etc., 1812.

PART II

Staplers in the Operations of Surgery

CHAPTER IV

Introduction

WE HAVE COMMENTED BEFORE that we have not felt properly justified in performing a prospective randomized comparison of stapling and manual suture techniques and that few such studies have been performed. In fact, in the past, the initial adoption by surgeons of one or another suture technique, whether with silk or with catgut or with synthetic absorbable sutures or with wire, in one layer or in two layers, of whatever specific type of suture, usually has depended merely on the appearance of one or several convincing series of what appeared to the general surgical public to be good results. We have clearly already arrived at the point where the use of staples is widespread and safely established. We accept for ourselves the conclusion that although the instruments and the details of staple suture line, staple closure, and staple material may change, the principle has been established by such widespread use that one can reasonably assume that mechanical visceral suturing is here to stay. It is difficult to ascertain how many visceral procedures are done annually with the stapling instruments—probably in the hundreds of thousands.

There has been a large number of publications on stapling over the years from the Soviet Union and from other Eastern European countries. There have been a few publications in the past 20 years from Western Europe also dealing with the Russian stapling instruments and an increasing number in recent years dealing with the American Auto Suture® instruments.

Surgeons the world over, despite long familiarity with the von Petz stapler, showed understandable reluctance to embark on stapling and to rely on staples alone for closures and anastomoses. We are artisans, after all, proud of our skill and it was discomforting to believe that mechanical methods could achieve results equal or superior to those we could achieve with the artistry of our nimble fingers. Most difficult of all to accept was the recommendation for mucosa-to-mucosa closure.

Reichel of Hannover (1975) pointed out the problems for all surgeons trained in standard techniques who undertake stapling: "For a surgeon who has learned as the overriding principle of anastomosis in gastrointestinal surgery, the apposition of the serosa as a condition sine qua non for a watertight and bacteria-safe closure of an anastomosis, it is not easy at first to observe that everting suture with a stapling apparatus results in complication-free healing." His animal studies of gastroenterostomies and end-to-end triangulation sutures showed good healing and without ulceration or defects.

It will be seen, too, that many surgeons began by using the TA™ instruments for

---

NOTE: Where the term "American instruments" or "U.S. instruments" is used, this refers specifically to the Auto Suture® stapling instruments of the United States Surgical Corporation pictured in the various operative drawings in Part II, unless instruments of another origin are specifically identified.

closures, then the GIA™ instrument for transections and closures, and finally risked anastomoses. When the EEA™ instrument arrived, with the reassuringly inverted anastomosis, its acceptance finally swept along many who had viewed the other instruments with suspicion and now were prepared to accept them all.

Gritsman (1966), who has been long associated with the Scientific Research Institute for Experimental Surgical Apparatus and Instruments in Moscow, analyzed the advantages of the stapling instruments as used in Russia. Proceeding from the observation that in his country the leading complication of gastric or intestinal surgery had to do with suture line leaks, he argued that the mechanical suture line, when compared to a manual one, does not depend to the same degree on the skill of the surgeon. He made the point that precision and accuracy in the hands of the occasional bowel surgeon were enhanced. He considered this particularly important in their country, where, for urgent abdominal surgery, distances and weather made it difficult to transport patients from the periphery to a sophisticated hospital center. He reported essentially uncontrolled statistics, comparing a large number of gastrectomies performed manually by one group of 62 surgeons to a smaller number of gastrectomies performed with the stapling instruments by a somewhat smaller group of different surgeons. In 42,528 gastrectomies done manually for ulcer, the mortality was 3.2% and in the 958 gastrectomies performed with the staplers the mortality was 1%. In the 10,358 gastric resections done manually for cancer, the mortality was 10.4% and in the 668 performed with the stapler the mortality was 3.6%. Although the differences, of course, are statistically significant, nothing is said about the relative skill of the surgeons in the two groups, the nature of the patients, the hospitals, etc. It was the observation of one of us, at that time, that in the Soviet Union, by and large, the staplers were being used by adventurous innovators in major hospitals and one might have expected, in fact, that the same surgeons and the same hospitals would have had lower mortalities than the other group, even if the staple users had performed their operations manually.

OVERVIEW OF EXPERIENCE WITH MECHANICAL SUTURES

After some nine years of experience with the Russian instruments (Ravitch, Brown, and Daviglus, 1959; Ravitch, Steichen, Fishbein, Knowles, and Weil, 1964; Ravitch,

TABLE IV–1.—STAPLE-RELATED MORBIDITY
AND MORTALITY
(June 6, 1967–June 30, 1976)

OPERATIONS	NUMBER	MORBIDITY		DEATHS	
		No.	%	No.	%
Gastric	278	13	4.6	2	0.7
Biliary	7	—	—	—	—
Pancreatic	48	1	2.0	1	2.0
Intestinal	157	5	3.1	3	1.9
Colon	264	12	4.5	1	0.4
Gynecologic	19	—	—	—	—
Genitourinary	20	—	—	—	—
Vascular	31	—	—	—	—
Pulmonary	188	9	4.7	2	1.0
Esophageal	33	3	9.0	2	6.0
Miscellaneous	1	—	—	—	—
TOTALS	1,046	43	4.1	11	1.0

Lane, Cornell, Rivarola, and McEnany, 1966; Ravitch and Rivarola, 1966; Ravitch, Rivarola, and VanGrov, 1966; Ravitch, Snodgrass, and Rivarola, 1966), on June 6, 1967, we performed the first operation—a gastrectomy with Billroth II reconstruction—with the TA 55™, TA 90™, and GIA™ instruments, which then had become available essentially in their present form. By June 30, 1976, a total of 1,046 operations had been performed with the American instruments either by us or under our guidance (Table IV–1). At that point, we discontinued the systematic tabulation of all patients treated with the instruments, since we were satisfied that the techniques had been largely standardized and our experience (Steichen, Talbert, and Ravitch, 1968; Ravitch, Hirsch, and Noiles, 1972; Ravitch and Steichen, 1972; Ravitch and Steichen, 1972; Steichen and Ravitch, 1973; Ravitch, Ong, and Gazzola, 1974; Talbert, Seashore, and Ravitch, 1974; Webster, Carey, and Ravitch, 1975) and an increasing number of reports from others (Weber, 1972; Vankemmel, 1974, 1976; Lawson, Hutchison, Longland, and Haque, 1977; Fortin, Poulin, and Leclerc, 1979; Risch, Weydert, Mandres, and Bleser, 1980; Turbelin, Arnaud, Welter, and Adloff, 1980) indicated that results were at least as good as with the previously standard techniques of manual suture.

EXPERIENCE WITH STAPLING INSTRUMENTS IN GASTRIC SURGERY

During our own period of evaluation of the stapling instruments from June 6, 1967, to June 30, 1976, 278 gastric operations were performed for the indications listed in Table IV-2. For gastric ulcers and gastric cancer, we performed either the Billroth I or Billroth II operation and an occasional total gastrectomy. For duodenal ulcers, during the time of this evaluation, we performed truncal vagotomy with antrectomy or with a drainage procedure, the latter most commonly a Heineke-Mikulicz pyloroplasty. Gastroenterostomies, and Roux-en-Y gastroenterostomies, performed alone, generally were for bypass of malignant obstructions with or without stapled transection of the stomach. The Janeway gastrostomies almost always were performed in patients with neurologic lesions who were expected to require tube feeding indefinitely and to survive for a significant period of time.

A total of 13 complications (Table IV-3) attributable to the staples was encountered in these 278 gastric procedures. In seven patients there was postoperative bleeding, confirmed in six of them by aspiration through the nasogastric tube. An unexplained postoperative drop in the hematocrit, without blood recoverable from the stomach and without any physical sign of intraperitoneal irritation, occurred in a single patient with an antral wedge resection for a nodule of ectopic pancreas. It is presumed that he bled into the peritoneal cavity from the everted TA 55™ closure of the gastric wall, the only episode of this kind in our records and, of course, it is possible also that he bled from an omental vessel unconnected with the TA 55™ closure. In one of the six patients, gastroscopy showed gastritis and it was difficult to determine whether bleeding was from the area of the gastritis or from the gastroenterostomy performed with the GIA™ stapler. Two patients required blood transfusion, but spontaneously stopped bleeding. Three patients required operation for bleeding, in each case from the gastroenterostomy suture line. In one patient, the single bleeding point required suture ligation, and in the other two patients, the entire GIA™ suture line oozed and required to be oversewn with a running suture of catgut. One of these two patients, reoperated on too late, died of multisystem failure after a protracted course.

As in the series of others, most instances of postoperative bleeding occurred in our

TABLE IV-2.—OPERATIONS ON THE STOMACH
(June 6, 1967–June 30, 1976)

INDICATIONS

Ulcer—Gastric	56
Duodenal	117
Hemorrhagic gastritis	12
Mallory-Weiss	1
Adenocarcinoma	54
Secondary carcinoma with involvement of stomach	1
Leiomyosarcoma	2
Lymphoma	1
Leiomyoblastoma	1
Polyps	3
Ectopic pancreas	1
T-E fistula	1
Marginal ulcer	4
Retained antrum	1
Gastroenterostomy malfunction	4
Bile gastritis	4
Gastric volvulus	1
Afferent loop syndrome	2
Brain tumor	3
Chronic brain syndrome	5

OPERATIONS—278

Billroth I	20
Billroth II	90
Antrectomy and vagotomy	104
Vagotomy and drainage procedure	6
Total gastrectomy	2
Total gastrectomy with a jejunal reservoir	8
Esophagogastrectomy	4
Esophagogastrectomy with jejunal interposition	1
Gastroenterostomy	20
Gastric wedge resection	5
Roux-Y gastrojejunostomy	3
Braun jejunojejunostomy	1
Janeway gastrostomy	9
Gastrotomy	5

early experience and we have long since made it a matter of course to inspect the anastomotic staple line from within the stomach after the GIA™ instrument has been removed.

In four of the 278 patients, suture line leaks were recognized, three of the duodenal stump, one of both duodenal and gastric stumps. In the patient with both leaks, the leak was only known to be localized to the region of the duodenal stump, possibly from behind the suture line where the penetrating ulcer, left in place, might have been elevated from the pancreas, and had as well a perforation of the greater curvature angle of the gastric closure by a stiff nasogastric tube. We were not successful in determining just how the operation was performed. That patient died. After returning home on gen-

TABLE IV-3.—278 OPERATIONS ON THE
STOMACH
(June 6, 1967–June 30, 1976)

COMPLICATIONS - 13/4.6%	DEATHS - 2/0.7%	
Postoperative bleeding: 7	Reoperation: 3	Death: 1
Suture leak: 4	Reoperation: 1	Death: 1
Anastomotic stenosis: 2	Reoperation: 1	Death: 0

eral diet, two patients drained a small amount of bile through the old duodenal stump drainage site. We do not, ourselves, ever drain the duodenal stump, and at least wonder whether drainage does not invite a suture line failure. In a third patient, who had had two previous gastric operations, a duodenal leak became manifest in the postoperative period, and with drainage and hyperalimentation closed spontaneously. It had been noted that the duodenum was thick and scarred. In this connection, it is worthwhile recounting a leak we have had in the period after this series. In that patient, a fistula became manifest during the period of convalescence from a gastrectomy for ulcer. One of us was invited to perform the reoperation. The fistula was found to come from a small opening in the stapled gastrojejunostomy, and could readily be stapled off without compromising the size of the anastomosis. Again a fistula developed some days after operation, but this time closed spontaneously. It was commented on that at reoperation the stomach wall was extremely thick and we then were told that that had been the case at the time of the original operation. A preternaturally thick or hypertrophied portion of the gastrointestinal tract should not be stapled, since the degree of compression obligatory to insure proper formation of the staples may be more than is tolerable by the thick tissues and may result in a degree of compression that produces ischemia (see also Chapter V).

Two patients were readmitted to the hospital with delayed gastric emptying through the gastroenterostomy, requiring nasogastric suction and intravenous feeding. In one of these, the problem resolved spontaneously. In the second, the anastomosis had to be taken down and reconstructed.

There were two deaths (see Table IV–3) attributable to the stapling procedure in the series of 278 gastric operations. One was the patient who bled, mentioned above, in whom reoperation was long delayed, death occurring subsequently from multiple organ failure, although there was no further bleeding. The gastrectomy had been undertaken for uncontrollable bleeding due to heavy ingestion of salicylates for severe osteoarthritis. The other death was in the patient mentioned above with leakage of both the gastric closure and the duodenum. He developed overwhelming sepsis and respiratory insufficiency and could not be salvaged.

EXPERIENCE WITH STAPLING INSTRUMENTS IN ESOPHAGEAL SURGERY

In our initial study period (Table IV-4), 33 operations with stapling instruments were performed on the esophagus for a variety of conditions, mostly malignant tumors of the cervical and thoracic esophagus. All of these procedures were before the EEA™ instrument became available, and in fact quite satisfactory esophagogastric resections and anastomoses can be made with the TA™ instruments and the GIA™ instruments. Figures VI–10, 12, and 13 show the techniques developed at that time, many of which we still will use from time to time, despite the availability of the EEA™ instruments.

That earlier experience included one use of the GIA™ instrument for the management of bleeding varices (see Fig VI–17). Our experience with that technique now is just under 20 patients, all of whom have had satisfactory cessation of their bleeding with the use of the GIA™ hemostatic procedure.

STAPLE COMPLICATIONS.—There were three postoperative complications due to the staple suture lines: (1) A salivary fistula, which developed in the neck after esophagocolostomy performed by the GIA™–TA™ technique, closed spontaneously. (2) A month after operation, in a patient with carcinoma of the esophagus in whom a reverse gastric tube was brought up retrosternally, it was found that there was a mediastinal

TABLE IV-4.—OPERATIONS ON THE ESOPHAGUS
(June 6, 1967–June 30, 1976)

INDICATIONS	
Cervical squamous cell carcinoma	4
Thoracic squamous cell carcinoma	17
Thoracic adenocarcinoma	3
Caustic stricture	2
Reflux stricture	3
Bleeding varices	1
Esophageal atresia	1
Epiphrenic diverticulum	2
TOTAL	33

OPERATIONS—33	
Esophagectomy, reverse gastric tube I	7
Laryngoesophagectomy, reverse gastric tube II	2
Esophagectomy, coloplasty	8
Esophagogastrectomy, colon interposition	2
Esophagogastrectomy and esophagogastrostomy	3
Colon bypass	3
Reverse gastric tube I, bypass	5
Epiphrenic diverticulectomy	2
Ligation of bleeding varices	1

COMPLICATIONS (3)—9%	
Salivary fistula, neck	1—closed spont.
Late leak mid-reverse gastric tube I	1—reoperation, died
Bleeding cologastrostomy	1—reoperation, died
MORTALITY (2)—6%	

abscess. It was drained from above through the cervical incision and from below through a subxiphoid incision. At the time of this re-exploration, the gastric tube appeared innocent at both ends, and the site of the fistula was not visualized. The patient ultimately went on to die with metastatic disease in both lungs. Autopsy was not granted. (3) An elderly patient, who had undergone total esophagectomy with colon replacement, required reoperation for gastric bleeding. This proved to be from the manually closed GIA^{TM} introduction site. The patient, who had a background of chronic obstructive pulmonary disease and a progressively worsening general condition, died of postoperative respiratory failure.

EXPERIENCE WITH BILIARY SURGERY

Seven operations were performed for conditions involving or relating to the biliary tree (Table IV-5). In most of these operations a manual biliodigestive anastomosis was created and the stapling instruments then were used in the construction of a Roux-en-Y loop or an Omega loop with a Braun anastomosis at the foot of such a loop.

For benign conditions, such as cholangitis, choledochal and pancreatic cysts, and echinococcal cysts, these operations were performed for a permanent cure. In all the patients with carcinoma obstructing the biliary tree, the biliodigestive bypasses were palliative.

There were no complications related to the use of staplers in these operations.

Subsequent to the original series, we have performed direct stapled anastomosis of intestine—usually Roux loops—to enlarged common ducts, gallbladder, and choledochal cysts.

TABLE IV-5.—BILIARY SURGERY
(June 6, 1967–June 30, 1976)

INDICATIONS	
Ascending cholangitis	1
Choledochal cyst	1
Pancreatic cyst, C.D. obstruction	1
Echinococcal cyst, C.D. obstruction	1
Carcinoma gallbladder	1
Carcinoma common duct	1
Metastatic carcinoma, C.D. obstruction	1
OPERATIONS—7	
Cholecysto-Roux Y jejunostomy	1
Choledocho-Roux Y jejunostomy	3
Choledochal cyst–Roux Y jejunostomy	1
Braun jejunojejunostomy	1
Gastrojejunostomy	1
COMPLICATIONS	NONE
MORTALITY	NONE

EXPERIENCE WITH PANCREATIC SURGERY

Forty-eight operations (Table IV-6) were performed for pancreatic disease. These operations can be subdivided into two principal groups: those performed for palliation, in the bypass of biliary and duodenal obstruction from malignancy, most often a carcinoma of the head of the pancreas, and those in which pancreaticoduodenectomy was performed in the treatment of operable lesions of the head of the pancreas and the ampulla of Vater. Although in the bypass operations the instruments were used in the

TABLE IV-6.—PANCREATIC SURGERY
(June 6, 1967–June 30, 1976)

INDICATIONS	
Carcinoma pancreas	30
Carcinoma ampulla Vater	4
Leiomyosarcoma duodenum	1
Islet cell carcinoma	1
Islet cell adenoma	1
Chronic pancreatitis	8
Pseudocyst	3
OPERATIONS—48	
Choledocho-Roux Y gastroenterostomy	14
Cholecystojejunostomy, ± gastrocntcrostomy	9
Braun jejunojejunostomy	2
Gastroenterostomy	1
Pancreatic cyst-jejunostomy	3
Duval procedure	1
Puestow procedure	1
Whipple procedure	15
Total pancreatectomy	2
COMPLICATIONS	
Leak Roux Y closure	1—died
Reoperation	0
MORBIDITY and MORTALITY	
2%	

creation of the Roux-en-Y or Omega loops, in patients with pancreatic and duodenal resection, the instruments were used in the gastrointestinal closures and anastomoses, after gastroduodenal resection. Roux-en-Y loops were also used in the operations for pancreatic pseudocyst and the various operations for chronic pancreatitis.

One patient, whose jejunum had been divided with the stapler and the Roux-en-Y jejunojejunostomy performed with the stapler, had her choledochojejunostomy performed manually. A leak developed and was demonstrated by contrast study through the fistula to be located at the staple closure line of the bowel, near the hand-sewn choledochojejunostomy, which appeared to be intact. This patient died after a protracted course in which the drained staple line leak was only one of many factors.

EXPERIENCE WITH SMALL BOWEL SURGERY

A total of 157 operations (Table IV-7) was performed for a wide variety of indications concerned with various pathologic conditions of the small bowel. The vast majority of these operations consisted in the resection of a variable amount of small bowel with the GIA™ and LDS™ instruments, using the functional end-to-end or the modified functional end-to-end anastomosis for reconstruction. Of interest is a second group of pa-

TABLE IV-7.—Operations on the Small Bowel
(June 6, 1967–June 30, 1976)

INDICATIONS	
Jejunal atresia	1
Meckel's diverticulum	7
Penetrating trauma	11
Postoperative fistula	9
Aorta-jejunal fistula	1
Ileo-vesical fistula	1
Ischemic gangrene	19
Strangulation gangrene	23
SMA syndrome	1
Radiation fibrosis	1
Intussusception	1
Foreign body perforation	1
Gallstone ileus	2
Bezoar	1
Anastomotic ulcer	3
Stricture	1
Morbid obesity	49
Takedown of JI shunt	1
Crohn's ileitis	4
Ulcerative colitis	2
Carcinoma duodenum	1
Carcinoid	1
Carcinoma invasion (from adjacent organ)	8
Metastatic cancer	6
Sarcoma	1
Lymphoma	1
OPERATIONS—157	
Resection and anastomosis	91
Tangential diverticulectomy	6
Enterotomy and closure	7
Duodenojejunostomy	2
Jejunoileal shunt	49
Continent ileal reservoir	2

tients in whom a jejunoileal shunt was performed for morbid obesity, using the functional end-to-end anastomosis for the reconstruction of jejunoileal continuity and the end-to-side anastomosis for the anastomosis of the excluded small bowel to the ascending or transverse colon (see pg. 135). We have since abandoned this operation because of the many metabolic difficulties patients with jejunoileal shunt suffer postoperatively (Ravitch and Brolin 1979).

COMPLICATIONS. In the 157 operations there were four suture line leaks, three in patients who had been operated on for superior mesenteric artery thrombosis and one in a patient operated on for bypass of a locally invasive, posteriorly fixed metastatic carcinoma.

One patient, operated on for a questionable superior mesenteric artery syndrome, developed a "stricture" of the duodenojejunostomy performed with the GIA^{TM} instrument. Reoperation showed a widely patent anastomosis. Although the original upper gastrointestinal series had shown an impression on the duodenum by the superior mesenteric artery and the postoperative barium swallow showed free passage from the duodenum into the jejunum through the bypassing duodenojejunostomy, a new anastomosis was constructed manually and the patient continued to vomit.

MORTALITY. The three patients with anastomotic leaks after resection and anastomosis for gangrene of the small bowel died. All three patients were quite elderly, all had diabetes and past histories of involvement of the brain, the heart, or the kidneys with atherosclerosis. In two of the patients, the resection of small bowel was a quite extensive one, making ultimate survival with nutrition through the remaining intestinal tract questionable. In one of the patients, a large segment of small bowel was removed and two separate fistulas developed, possibly from progressive necrosis. No autopsies were obtained in any of the three patients and hence it is difficult to decide what lesion led to leakage from the small bowel.

EXPERIENCE WITH STAPLING INSTRUMENTS IN LARGE BOWEL SURGERY

A total of 264 operations was performed for various conditions related to the large bowel (Table IV-8). Most of these procedures were resections of various lengths of large bowel and immediate reanastomosis. In some patients, a two-stage operation was selected, with resection, proximal colostomy, and distal closure of the bowel (Hartmann's procedure).

The functional end-to-end anastomosis (see Figs VIII–2–5) or the bayonet overlapping anastomosis (see Fig IX–2) were both used for low rectal anastomoses by us, as well as the modified functional end-to-end (see Fig VIII–5), but much less commonly by other members of our staffs. With the availability now of the EEA^{TM} instrument, this has become the preferred instrument and technique for anastomosis after truly low anterior resections. Some 50 cases operated on in this fashion are not part of the original series here commented on.

COMPLICATIONS. A total of nine postoperative leaks occurred, four after ileocolectomy, three after left colectomy, one after anterior resection, and one after subtotal colectomy.

Of the four leaks after ileocolectomy, one occurred in a ten-day-old baby who had had an emergency operation for in utero perforation of the cecum. At operation, a functional ileotransverse colostomy was performed, in fact proximal to what turned out to be Hirschsprung's disease, which declared itself on the nineteenth day after birth.

TABLE IV-8.—OPERATIONS ON THE LARGE BOWEL
(June 6, 1967–June 30, 1976)

INDICATIONS

Adenocarcinoma	160	Villous adenoma	4
Carcinoma invasion (from adjacent organ)	1	Metastatic carcinoma	1
Polyps	14	Abscess	1
Diverticulitis	23	Diverticulosis	5
Crohn's colitis	9	Ulcerative colitis	2
Radiation colitis	1	Ischemic colitis	3
Volvulus	8	Strangulation gangrene	5
SMA aneurysm	1	Penetrating trauma	7
Anastomotic stricture	3	Colovesical fistula	2
Hirschsprung's disease	13	Total aganglionosis	1

OPERATIONS—264

Ileocolectomy	98	Transverse colectomy	25
Left colectomy	64	Anterior resection	6
Hartmann procedure	17	Subtotal colectomy	6
Duhamel procedure	11	Martin procedure	1
Closure colostomy	22	Colotomy	8
Bypass ileocolostomy	5	Colocolostomy	1

COMPLICATIONS (12)—4.5%

Leak ileocolectomy	4	2—Closed spontaneously 2—Reoperation
Leak left colectomy	3	1—Closed spontaneously 2—Reoperation
Leak anterior resection	1	Reoperation, died
Leak subtotal colectomy	1	Reoperation
Stricture ileocolectomy	1	Reoperation
Stricture left colectomy	1	Reoperation
Late bleeding ileocolectomy	1	Reoperation

MORTALITY (1)—0.4%

This patient evacuated a small amount of feces on one occasion through the upper end of his extended McBurney incision. The leak healed spontaneously without reoperation. At the age of eight months, the patient underwent a successful Duhamel procedure with the GIA^{TM} instrument (see Fig IX–14) without having ever required a proximal colostomy.

One patient operated on by a right colotomy for pedunculated villous adenoma, followed during the same hospitalization by ileocolectomy for histologically proved carcinoma in the stalk, developed a leak and a fistula, which, although prolonged, closed without reoperation.

In two patients, both operated on for carcinoma of the right colon, anastomotic leaks occurred and required drainage. In one patient, the carcinoma had invaded the abdominal wall, and a large abdominal wall resection was performed en bloc with the carcinoma. In the other patient, persistent fever led to reoperation, at which time a phlegmon was found near the ileocolostomy and drained. No leakage was observed at the stapled functional end-to-end anastomosis. The condition of the patient did not improve; a second exploration was performed and a small abscess was drained. After the second operation, the patient developed a fistula that ultimately had to be closed operatively.

In the group with left colectomy, one patient developed a leak of 24 hours' duration after operation for extensive diverticulitis and anastomosis of the transverse colon to the upper rectum. This patient did not require a proximal colostomy and was discharged on the tenth postoperative day with a minimally granulating upper end of the incision and perfectly normal transit through the bowel.

In a second patient, with a descending colostomy performed some eight years previously for radiation colitis in the treatment of uterine carcinoma, closure of the colostomy was attempted. On the fourth day after operation, the patient developed local tenderness, a leak was found, and the colostomy restored.

In a third patient, a young man with acute volvulus of the sigmoid, resection of the gangrenous loop and reanastomosis in healthy tissue with the GIA[TM] instrument, reoperation became mandatory some 24 hours postoperatively because of tenderness, guarding, and fever. In this patient, a leak was found at the level of the hand-closed GIA[TM] introduction site. The TA[TM] instrument had not been used for the closure of the GIA[TM] introduction site, a technique that we began to use routinely only sometime later.

In two other patients, one with an anterior resection for carcinoma and the other with a subtotal colectomy for bleeding diverticulosis, reoperation was undertaken for signs of pelvic sepsis. In the patient with ileorectostomy for bleeding diverticulosis, a small leak in the anterior aspect of the functional end-to-end anastomosis was closed manually and a double-barreled ileostomy created. The patient with anterior resection for carcinoma had a transrectal drainage of a pelvic abscess on the twelfth postoperative day. She had coronary artery disease, aortic stenosis, and postoperative pulmonary embolism and died 22 days after operation.

Stricture formation was observed on two occasions, one after ileocolectomy and one after left colectomy. The circumstances of the stricture after left colectomy led to the belief that in this instance the instrument was used on distended bowel, which, after regaining its normal tone, simply led to a small-sized anastomosis. At reoperation, in the one, relief was achieved by manual reanastomosis of the ileocolostomy and, in the other, by a stapled reanastomosis of the left colocolostomy.

In one patient, a dramatic, late episode of bleeding occurred at the time she was eating and ready to go home. The patient had undergone an ileocolectomy and developed sudden and substantial rectal bleeding on the ninth postoperative day. Arteriography showed the bleeding to come from the anastomosis. At immediate reoperation, an active bleeding point was found at the posterior lip of the GIA[TM] functional anastomosis. This point was oversewn and the colotomy was closed. We have had no other such experience, nor heard of a similar complication.

MORTALITY. The patient with a leak after anterior resection, and drainage of a pelvic abscess some time later, died 22 days after operation of a combination of pre-existing conditions and postoperative complications, the only staple-related death.

COMPLICATIONS IN STAPLED GASTROINTESTINAL ANASTOMOSES AND CLOSURES

The analyses in each chapter, of the published work of others, with stapling operations is almost entirely from the literature dealing with the use of the American instruments described in Part I and illustrated in the various operative drawings in Part II. There is, of course, an extremely large literature from the Soviet Union and countries in Eastern Europe concerning the use of the stapling instruments developed at the Scientific Research Institute for Experimental Surgical Apparatus and Instruments in Moscow. There also is a moderate Western European literature dealing with the use of these instruments. In an earlier day, when the mere validity of surgical suturing with stapling instruments was in question, we did quote the Russian and Eastern European literature, and our own earliest experience, of course, was with the Russian stapling instruments. At this point, the major experience in the world, outside the Soviet Union and the countries of Eastern Europe, is with the American instruments here described and is likely to be for the foreseeable future. For this reason, most of the reports cited are those from North America and Western Europe.

The lessons learned in our experience are described at various points in this text. In general, it may be said that the learning curve on the way to skilled use of the instruments is fairly steep, and that inevitably, as with any other procedure, there will remain a small but finite incidence of morbidity and mortality. The mechanical suturing instruments are not proof against operations performed for inappropriate indications, tissues inappropriately chosen for anastomosis or closure, errors in use of the instruments, rough technique, or, for that matter, mechanical failure. A significant portion of the complication rate in most series has been due to early inexperience and poor surgical judgment, which may occur in the use of any suture technique and without relation to the instruments utilized. Since even at autopsy it may not be possible to determine what went wrong, much less why, in evaluating our own experience we have listed all of the complications and deaths in patients who suffered from leaks, hemorrhage, or stenosis as due to the use of stapling instruments.

In esophageal, gastric, and intestinal closures and anastomoses, essentially the only complications have been anastomotic leaks or bleeding into the lumen from the anastomoses. We have had only one, suspected, instance of bleeding into the peritoneal cavity. Stapled anastomoses, in our experience and in the generally reported experience, appear to open much more rapidly than those made by manual techniques. This is just what experimental evaluation of the amount of edema and hemorrhage in manually anastomosed tissues (see Chapter III) would lead one to expect.

BLEEDING

We had one patient with an ileotransverse colostomy who passed tarry stools and gradually lowered his hemoglobin until he required a transfusion and another, who nine days after operation, bled massively and suddenly as she was getting dressed to leave the hospital. Immediate exploration showed a pumping vessel in a tiny ulcer at the suture line in which a staple was visible.

In our initial experience using the Russian staplers for anastomosis (Ravitch, Lane, Cornell, Rivarola, and McEnany, 1966), in the interest of minimizing the possibility of contamination, we placed a Connell suture around the anastomosing instrument and pulled it tight as we withdrew the instrument, never inspecting the anastomosis, and had no patient who bled. Reports from around the country and our own observations, however, have convinced us of the wisdom of inspecting the anastomosis as the GIA™ instrument is withdrawn. Our usual practice is to place a small curved hemostat at the upper end of each GIA™ suture line (in tissue that will be excised) before withdrawing the GIA™ instrument (see Figs V–10*H* and VIII–2–5). As the anastomosis is held apart, if there appears to be any bleeding from within, a dry gauze sponge is packed into the stomach or bowel and removed in two minutes. If there is no further bleeding, the two clamps are held widely apart and the opening closed with the TA™ instrument. If there appears to be any continued bleeding, one starts a suture of 4–0 catgut and continues whipping over the anastomosis from within the lumen until it is clear that the bleeding point is reached, seeing no need to continue all the way around the anastomotic suture line. One of us places the sutures in the cut edge, outside the staple line; one of us includes the staple line in the whipstitch. Many surgeons do not hesitate to apply the electrocautery to a bleeding spot either on an anastomosis or at the mucosal edge of a mucosa-to-mucosa bowel closure. We have preferred not to do this. Fortin and associates (Fortin, Poulin, and Leclerc, 1979) had similar experience with occasional bleeding during the earlier phase of their use of stapling instruments and, like us, most of their instances of bleeding were with procedures on the stomach. One presumes that this is due to the thickness of the gastric wall, its muscular activity, and its rich vascular supply. Fischer (1976) had three episodes of bleeding in elderly patients, two with gastroenterostomy and one with colocolostomy, coming after a satisfactory two-year experience. He ascribed these to defective closing of the GIA^{TM} instrument, attributed to repeated use and either metal fatigue or poor maintenance. Indeed, there is a need for periodic checking of heavily used stapling instruments, just as, for that matter, with other instruments. Obviously, one of the advantages of totally disposable instruments is the elimination of this need. There has not yet been sufficient experience with the totally disposable GIA^{TM} instruments and the newest, Premium^{TM} GIA instruments (see Fig II–5), and their more closely spaced staples, to determine whether, as expected, the small incidence of annoying bleeding will be entirely eliminated or not. The mechanism of action of these instruments is somewhat different from that of the previous GIA^{TM} instrument, holding the blades as firmly together at the very tip of the instrument as at the base, so that one would expect that, in fact, bleeding will be eliminated.

ANASTOMOTIC LEAKS

The problem of anastomotic leaks occurring at the different levels of the gastrointestinal tract is discussed more extensively in the sections dealing with individual operations. In addition to using a properly maintained instrument, it remains necessary to preserve the blood supply of the bowel, avoid contamination by bowel contents, avoid stapling of diseased bowel, and avoid any undue traction on the anastomosis. Lawson and associates (Lawson, Hutchison, Longland, and Haque, 1977) choose to add a few supporting sutures in order to protect against any undue traction, just as one of us routinely adds a suture in the crotch of the functional end-to-end GIA^{TM} anastomosis. Similarly, we frequently anchor the stomach to the duodenum below a Jaboulay gastroenterostomy. We essentially never, but for division of both walls of the stomach with the GIA^{TM} instrument, as in the Janeway gastrostomy (see Fig V–9) or reverse gastric tube (see Fig VI–7), put in a supporting row of sutures, or invert our mucosa-to-mucosa closures, but have no objection to a reinforcing suture if any member of the operating team is concerned that the staple closure may have come too close to the edge of the bowel or that a spot seems ischemic or discolored.

Our own experience and the published experience of others do not suggest any difference in anastomotic leak rates between stapled and manual anastomoses except in the case of EEA^{TM} anastomoses to esophagus or rectum. In these situations, most of the evidence suggests that there are substantially fewer leaks when the staplers are used for these anastomoses in the portions of the gastrointestinal tract offering the greatest technical problems in reconstruction.

We illustrate, largely for historical reasons, the true end-to-end anastomosis made with three successive applications of the TA^{TM} instrument on the triangulated ends of the bowel, developed in the laboratory by Turi Josefsen and Gershon Efron (1969) (see Fig VIII–1). We described (Ravitch and Steichen, 1972) the application of the TA^{TM} instrument to the posterior third of the anastomosis to produce a serosa-to-serosa inverting suture line while the two sides of the triangle were stapled mucosa-to-mucosa, each staple line overlapping the other two at its ends. McGinty (1970) reported a technique with eversion of all three sides and has more recently updated his experience (McGinty, Kasten, Kinder, and Hunt, 1979). Others have also used a true end-to-end anastomosis by the triangulating technique (Rinecker and Danek, 1975; Reichel, 1975; Turbelin, Arnaud, Welter, and Adloff, 1980). It seems to us laborious and invites contamination. Neither in its creation nor in its function is it as simple and trouble-free as the functional end-to-end anastomosis (see Figs VIII–2–5) or the bayonet anastomosis (see Fig IX–2), the techniques we generally use for end-to-end reconstruction, unless we are using the EEA^{TM} instrument.

ANASTOMOTIC STENOSES

Strictured anastomoses, or "delayed opening" of anastomoses, probably occur with less frequency with the staplers. One of us has twice had a stricture at the site of a GIA^{TM} functional end-to-end anastomosis for primary resection of volvulus of the sigmoid. Elliott (Elliott, Albertazzi, and Danto, 1977) from Davis, California, reported two cases of anastomotic stenosis after the use of the GIA^{TM} stapler, one after functional end-to-end anastomosis of the colon for sigmoid volvulus, and one after a Billroth II gastrectomy. The gastroenterostomy seemed indeed to have healed across the lumen. For the sigmoid, our presumption is that the greatly thickened and hypertrophied bowel may have been unduly compressed by the instrument, producing enough ischemia to result in stricture. However, we have seen two specimens of GIA^{TM} anastomoses that required resection for postoperative obstruction. It was clear that the TA^{TM} closure of the GIA^{TM} stab wounds, as probably in Elliott's gastroenterostomy, was such as to appose the GIA^{TM} suture lines, so that the cut bowel edges, alive beyond the staple line, adhered and fused, almost completely closing off the lumen. This mechanism has several times been reported to cause obstruction after a Duhamel operation for Hirschsprung's disease (see Fig IX–14). In that circumstance, digital rectal examinations in the postoperative period are prophylactic. In the case of functional end-to-end and other GIA^{TM} anastomoses, the precautions shown in Figures VIII–2–5 should be followed to keep the GIA^{TM}-cut bowel edges apart.

EXPERIENCE WITH THE STAPLING INSTRUMENTS IN CLOSURE OF MAJOR VESSELS

The vascular procedures performed with the instruments described in this volume are solely the terminal closure of large vessels—the pulmonary artery, the pulmonary veins, the proximal end of the portal vein, and the compartmentation of the inferior vena cava in the prevention of pulmonary embolism (Ravitch, Snodgrass, and Rivarola, 1966). (That technique for trapping pulmonary emboli in the vena cava, like a variety of others, has essentially been rendered obsolete by the development of the intracaval filters insertable by instrument passage from the groin or neck. The special TA 30^{TM} cartridge devised for compartmentation of the inferior vena cava, therefore, no longer is provided.) We have had no clinical experience with the Russian stapling instruments used

TABLE IV–9.—VASCULAR SURGERY
(June 6, 1967–June 30, 1976)

INDICATIONS	
Pulmonary embolus	14
Inferior vena cava gunshot	1
Portal hypertension	14
Aortic aneurysm	2
OPERATIONS—31	
IVC compartmentation	14
IVC staple closure	1
Portacaval shunt	13
Mesocaval shunt	1
Closure distal aorta	2
COMPLICATIONS:	NONE
DEATHS:	NONE

to perform end-to-end and end-to-side vascular anastomoses and to close tangential vascular incisions.

In the 1967–76 period, 31 operations were performed for various conditions relating to vascular structures (Table IV–9). In these operations, the TA 30^{TM} instrument was used with two different cartridges. One (no longer available) contained special staples placed at a right angle to the long axis of the cartridge. These staples allowed for the compartmentation of the inferior vena cava in patients with recurrent pulmonary emboli.

The second cartridge is the vascular, white cartridge (30V) containing fine, closely spaced staples for the closure of vessels in pulmonary surgery and of vessels in the abdomen, such as inferior vena cava ligation in trauma patients, closure of the hepatic end of the portal vein in shunt operations for portal hypertension, and closure of the aortic bifurcation in special circumstances. No complications were observed in any of the vascular operations.

Keshishian, Vasarhelyi, Smyth, Garcia, and Mispireta (1978), in treating an aorto-enteric fistula, successfully stapled the aorta above and below the fistulous segment, which was excised and an axillo-femoral bypass constructed, making two applications of the stapler (i.e., four rows) at each end. Keshishian further wrote (1978), ''we have used it in quite a few instances.''

The uses of stapling instruments in vascular surgery as such will not be discussed in this volume.

EXPERIENCE WITH STAPLING INSTRUMENTS IN PULMONARY SURGERY

It was our opportunity to observe pulmonary resections by Amosov, in Kiev, that involved us with the use of stapling instruments in surgery. There was then and continues to be a huge literature in the Soviet Union and countries of Eastern Europe with the use of the Russian staplers in the various fields of surgery. In our initial experimental and clinical studies (Ravitch, Brown, and Daviglus, 1959; Ravitch, Steichen, Fishbein, Knowles, and Weil, 1964), we had only the Russian UKB, the bar of whose staples is across the cartridge, thus in the long axis of the bronchus, the only structure it was used for. We reported 139 pulmonary resections, 25 pneumonectomies, 80 lobectomies and bilobectomies, 21 segmentectomies, and 13 lobectomies with segmentectomy. There were three bronchial fistulas and one empyema without bronchial fistula and two of the fistulas occurred in diabetics, both tuberculars, one of whom was sputum positive.

TABLE IV–10.—PULMONARY SURGERY
(June 6, 1967–June 30, 1976)

BLEBECTOMY—12	
Complications: None	
WEDGE RESECTION—43	
Complications: Postoperative bleeding	2 (4.6%)
Air leak	1 (2.3%)
Reoperation	None
SEGMENTECTOMY—11	
Complications: Postoperative bleeding	1 (9%)
Air leak	1 (9%)
Reoperation	None
LOBECTOMY—88	
BILOBECTOMY— 3	
Complications: Bronchopleural fistula	3 (3.3%)
Air leak	1 (1.1%)
Reoperation	1
Deaths (BPF)	2 (2.2%)
PNEUMONECTOMY—31	
Complications: None	
BRONCHIAL CLOSURES	— 122
BRONCHOPLEURAL FISTULAS	— 3 (2.4%)

We shortly after obtained a fuller range of Russian instruments and became satisfied that the double staggered staple line, bars parallel to the axis of the cartridge of the UKL series (as in the later Auto Suture® TA™ series), was equally satisfactory for the bronchi, and of course could also be used for the vessels and parenchyma.

During the period June 6, 1967 to June 30, 1976 of our tabulated evaluation of our stapling experience, we performed the procedures shown in Table IV–10.

Resection of pulmonary blebs and bullae was performed in 12 patients. There were no complications related to the use of stapling instruments for this condition.

Forty-three wedge resections were performed for both therapeutic and diagnostic reasons. Except for the treatment of bleeding penetrating wounds, excised at the same time open thoracotomy was performed for penetrating wounds of the heart, most of the wedge resections were done for diagnostic reasons. All the various techniques, such as tangential wedge resection, pie-shaped resection, and resections into the body of a lobe, were used. In two patients there was postoperative bleeding and in one patient there was an air leak. In one of the patients with bleeding there also was decortication of the lung and section of adhesions between the parietal and visceral pleura. Both the bleeding and air leaks were of short duration and of no real consequence in the postoperative course of these patients. They are mentioned because we have come to expect total hemostatic and airtight closure when the staplers are used on pulmonary parenchyma.

A modified segmentectomy was performed on 11 patients using the TA 90™ stapler and removing all the involved segment, together with minimal adjoining areas from other segments, after the artery to the involved segment and, at times, the veins from that segment were interrupted. In some diseases such as tuberculosis and localized bronchiectasis, as well as unresolved inflammation, the operation was performed for both diagnosis and treatment. In the patients with necrotic carcinoma where intraoperative findings precluded a more extensive operation, the segmentectomy was performed for palliation. Postoperative bleeding occurred in one patient who had undergone a decortication and then segmentectomy for apical tuberculosis. In this patient, the bleeding was moderate and did not persist beyond 24 hours. In a second patient there was a moderate air leak that ceased spontaneously within 24 hours. Neither of these patients required reoperation.

Pulmonary lobectomy was performed in 88 patients, *bilobectomy* in three patients, and *pneumonectomy* in 31 patients. Lobectomies and pneumonectomies are discussed here together, since the complications related essentially to closure of the bronchus. In all cases, we used the TA 30™ V cartridge for closure of the pulmonary vessels. We have had no immediate or delayed mishaps with this utilization of the TA 30™ instrument. In a total of 122 bronchial closures, 91 after lobectomy and 31 after pneumonectomy, there were three bronchopleural fistulas, all after lobectomy. In one woman, suffering with severe and advanced Wegener's granuloma, a right lower lobectomy was performed for a lobe entirely destroyed by sepsis. In this patient, the bronchial closure failed almost immediately and she ultimately died both of her far-advanced underlying disease and from an ill-advised last-stand procedure resulting in a serious complication.

The second patient, an elderly man, had a right lower lobectomy for an excavated lesion thought to be a carcinoma. Postoperatively, this lesion was found to be an excavated and infected pulmonary infarction, secondary to a silent pulmonary embolus suffered by the patient while he was normally active. During an open thoracotomy performed under local anesthesia for drainage of the empyema resulting from bronchial suture failure, the patient aspirated infected material into the left lung and, after a complicated course, died of progressive respiratory failure.

In a third patient there was a continuous air leak for more than ten days, when the leak arrested spontaneously. The patient suffered no further ill effects.

Another air leak occurred in a patient after lobectomy and lasted for more than 48 hours. Again, since we have come to expect almost complete airtight sutures with the use of staplers, any leak that lasts for more than 48 hours is considered to be abnormal, even though it may be only parenchymal in nature.

The reported experience of others with use of the American staplers is given in Chapter XI.

REPORTED GENERAL EXPERIENCE WITH STAPLING IN THE GASTROINTESTINAL TRACT

Papers describing initial experience with the Auto Suture® instruments in gastrointestinal surgery frequently allude to a broad range of operations. The presentations of these experiences, given below, provide a panorama of the results that might be expected and the concerns and comments of the users of the instruments. In most cases, the reports are of initial experiences, and, as the authors frequently remark, the complications tended to be in their earliest cases.

Weber (1972), from Rudler's Clinic in Geneva, reported his Auto Suture® experience with 100 patients, 208 suture lines—120 closures, 88 anastomoses—mostly for gastric procedures. One patient bled after subtotal gastrectomy, required reoperation, and recovered. One patient who had an obstructing antral cancer was not relieved by the gastroenterostomy. One esophagogastric anastomosis leaked briefly. The staples tended to be used in bad-risk cases, but there were no deaths due to staple closures or anastomoses.

The report by Painter, Park, and Hochberg (1974), from the Kimball Hospital, in Putnam, Connecticut, covers their experience from November 1, 1971 through October 31, 1972. They reported a wide variety of operations, 84 in all—20 pulmonary, 26 gastric, seven small bowel, 28 large bowel, four esophageal, two "miscellaneous"—by six surgeons, although two surgeons performed 74 of the 84 procedures. In some cases, all suture lines were with the staplers, in some cases not. In some cases, the staple line was". . .buttressed with additional sutures." In the entire group of patients, seven died, all had autopsies, ". . .none showed complications related to the use of the stapler," and all staple lines were intact. The surviving patients did have three staple-related complications—one bleeding from the GIA^{TM} gastrojejunostomy, requiring reoperation; one with a fistula from a side-to-side ileocolostomy, repaired by re-resection and a second stapled anastomosis; and the third, a ten-day-long air leak in a patient who had a stapled resection of an apical pulmonary bulla, in which "the leak was caused by an improperly assembled stapler and incompletely closed staples."

Latimer, Doane, McKittrick, and Shepherd (1975) reported the two-and-a-half-year experience of three surgeons with 104 patients having operations on the gastrointestinal tract—167 closures of esophagus, stomach, or bowel and 80 anastomoses, plus nine other procedures, such as polypectomy or excision of ulcer. Four complications thought to be staple related resolved without operation, respectively, an "infected intramural hematoma" after sigmoid colotomy, two instances of stomal dysfunction after gastric procedures, and one efferent loop dysfunction. One patient who developed a fecal fistula in irradiated bowel after lysis of adhesions and enterotomy required reoperation and resection of a segment of bowel, and recovered. One patient, unautopsied after total gastrectomy, died of gram-negative septicemia with a radiologically intact esophagojejunal anastomosis. It was presumed that some other anastomosis or closure had broken down. A jaundiced patient with carcinoma of the ampulla of Vater, who bled seriously after a GIA^{TM} cholecystojejunostomy, required reoperation, developed progressive hepatorenal failure, and died.

Rinecker and Danek (1975) of Munich, early converts to the use of mechanical sutures, reported on 140 gastrointestinal procedures involving duodenal closure, of which 25 were subtotal gastrectomies. Prior to that series of 140, they had done 14 Billroth I resections with triangulating gastroduodenostomy and 11 Billroth II resections. They had no instance of postoperative bleeding and no leakage from the closed ends of stomach or duodenum. They tested all Billroth I anastomoses for security with injection of indigo carmine solution, apparently without finding leaks, and do not even mention gastric outlet obstruction. In their Billroth II reconstructions, they commented that they had no necroses in the strip of stomach between the gastroenterostomy and the gastric staple line. They had no leaks, no intraluminal or intraperitoneal bleeding, and no intra-abdominal abscesses. In a single case, a Billroth I anastomosis proved stenotic but improved spontaneously and required no operation. This was their single complication. Radiologic studies suggested remarkably early function of the anastomosis. They now reported 13 duodenal stump closures; 23 duodenotomy closures; 14 triangulating, partially inverting, partially everting gastroduodenostomies—Billroth I; 17 Heineke-Mikulicz pyloroplasties; and 32 Finney or modified Finney pyloroplasties. They used reinforcing sutures in nine operations, one gastroduodenostomy, and eight pyloroplasties. They recognized two temporary stenoses not requiring operation. A single patient with intraperitoneal bleeding following a modified Finney pyloroplasty was treated nonoperatively.

Subsequently, Rinecker (1977) described his experience with 300 varied gastrointestinal operations with six deaths from anastomotic leaks—one after Billroth I resection, one after Billroth II resection, one after a small bowel resection, and three after left colon resections. He had postoperative bleeding in a patient with GIA^{TM} stapling of esophageal varices and in a patient with a pyloroplasty, in both of whom the bleeding might have come from the staple lines. Four patients, two with pyloroplasty, one with a Billroth I, and one with a Billroth II, had "temporary stenoses." In addition to the six patients with fatal leaks there were seven patients who either had temporary leaks or were diagnosed as probably having leaks.

Rignault, Pailler, Berthet, and Tardat (1976), from France, reported operations on 105 patients for a variety of lesions of the gastrointestinal tract, of which 35 were gastroenterostomies, 18 were Whipple procedures, 12 were total gastrectomies for carcinoma, and eight were esophagogastrectomies for carcinoma. In the 105 patients, they had one esophageal fistula, one duodenal fistula, and two pancreatic leaks, but in each case they demonstrated that the leak came from a manual suture line and not the stapled one. (One of the advantages of a stapled anastomosis is that its sufficiency can be accurately determined by contrast radiologic studies, since one can see the ring of staples.) Two of the 20 duodenal stump closures leaked bile through the drainage tract for the first 48 hours after operation. Their conclusion was that they had not had a single fistula attributable to the staples. There were no late fistulas. In five patients, after gastric procedures, there was significant bleeding, requiring only transfusion in two cases and reoperation in three. One of the bleeders was a cirrhotic and two of the others had a long-standing jaundice.

de Ruiter (1977), from The Netherlands, described his early experience with the Auto Suture® stapling instruments, using the GIA^{TM}, TA^{TM}, and LDS^{TM} instruments in gastrointestinal surgery. Like many surgeons, he began using the GIA^{TM} instrument cautiously, only for transection and closure of the bowel, gradually moving on to its use for anastomoses. In his moderate total experience in gastric, biliary (three cholecystojejunostomies), and colonic surgery of 68 cases, in which there were 15 bowel transections and 43 anastomoses, there was one episode of bleeding, no leaks, no stenoses. He agreed that ". . .The tissues can be handled with less manipulation. . . . Soiling with bacteria and tumor cells can be reduced. . . . The saving of time is substantial. . . ." and made the observation, that we and others had made, that the original LDS^{TM} instrument was a somewhat more difficult instrument to use and less secure than the GIA^{TM} and TA^{TM} instruments. de Ruiter was particularly pleased with his eight colorectal anastomoses with the GIA^{TM} instrument without complication, pointing out his previous experience of a 46% anastomotic dehiscence rate with manual anastomoses.

Lawson and associates (Lawson, Hutchison, Longland, and Haque, 1977) from the Royal Infirmary, Glasgow, reported 113 abdominal stapling procedures, gastric and colonic, with one duodenal stump leak and one fatal colocolostomy leak. Like many surgeons reporting the use of the staples, they point out that the complication rate should be calculated on the number of staple applications rather than the number of patients, and in this group of 113 patients there were 188 staple suturing procedures. They had two "intraoperative failures." In one, the duodenal stump was clamped, but the surgeon failed to fire the staples. The duodenum then was sutured and the patient did well. In the other "failure," a colocolonic anastomosis performed on loops approximated under tension pulled apart at once. That patient ultimately died. One patient had a minor duodenal leak and one a minor leak from an ileocolostomy. They concluded that "The staple-suturing methods described are safe and straightforward, and it is believed that they represent a significant advance in the techniques of thoracic and abdominal surgery, which can usefully be applied in many situations."

We had some initial uncertainty about the use of staples in emergency conditions. Our experimental studies and Chassin's clinical series (Chassin, Rifkind, Sussman, Kassel, Fingeret, Drager, and Chassin, 1978), and our own progressive experience, have reassured us about the safety of staples in moderately edematous bowel or bowel exposed to peritonitis.

The papers by Wheeless and Dorsey (1981) and Photopulos and associates (1979) now provide a suggestion that after abdominal irradiation, stapling may be more reliable than suture anastomosis, and this has been our own recent experience in a moderate number of such patients (Barber and Steichen 1982).

Photopulos, Delgado, Fowler, and Walton (1979), from the University of North Carolina at Chapel Hill and from Georgetown University Hospital, reported the use of Auto Suture® stapling instruments in 17 patients previously irradiated for malignant disease who required intestinal operations. "No patient suffered a complication as a direct result of the intestinal anastomosis. . . . There were no anastomotic leaks and no obstruction at the anastomotic site." They thought that the reduction in operating time and the reduction of the possibility of intra-abdominal soiling was significant in achieving this result. In general, results in malnourished patients who had undergone heavy irradiation for pelvic malignancies were thought to be unusually encouraging.

Wheeless and Dorsey (1981) report from Baltimore on 283 stapling operations on small or large bowel for 1,162 patients with gynecologic malignancy. Of these patients, 53 had received prior abdominal irradiation. There was one disruption of a small bowel anastomosis in heavily altered, irradiated bowel, "temporary stricture" in three anastomoses of colon to rectum, and one low rectal leak and pelvic abscess. There were no operative deaths. "The low complication rate in gastrointestinal anastomoses performed with the automatic surgical staplers supports the conclusion that this is a technically superior method which provides better utilization of operating time on radical pelvic procedures."

Like many other surgeons, Risch, Weydert, Mandres, and Bleser (1980) from Luxembourg convinced themselves in pulmonary surgery of the advantages of mechanical suture with the Auto Suture® instruments, and then embarked on a program of gastrointestinal surgery with them. In a total of 410 gastrointestinal procedures, they listed two cases of bleeding, 14 fistulas, and four deaths—one from an esophagogastric leak, one from a leak after a total gastrectomy, one after a side-to-side anastomosis for Crohn's disease, and one after a colocolic side-to-side anastomosis for cancer. Of the 14 gastrointestinal fistulas four were temporary duodenal fistulas after Billroth II gastrectomies, the two esophagogastric leaks, already mentioned as resulting fatally, and eight after colonic procedures, all of which closed after being drained. In a number of cases, endoscopic examination showed granuloma at the level of the gastroenterostomy, but this always was where, for the GIA^{TM} opening, they had used a manual closure with nonabsorbable sutures. Both cases of bleeding from the stomach required reoperation. In 277 pulmonary operations, they had five deaths, one after reoperation for bronchial fistula, one from hemoptysis, and three from cardiorespiratory insufficiency because of late bronchial fistula.

Turbelin, in his extensive and well-documented Doctoral Thesis at the University Louis Pasteur School of Medicine in Strasbourg (1980), reviews in detail the history of mechanical sutures in the gastrointestinal tract, as well as the various operative techniques and results obtained by authors in Europe and the United States with the use of the American-made instruments. In a series of 373 patients, operated on in Strasbourg with the American instruments, Turbelin reports six deaths (1.6%) related to the use of staplers. Mortality related to the total number of anastomoses was 1.97%, in triangulating anastomoses 1.17%, in functional end-to-end anastomoses 1.86%, and in end-to-end EEA™ anastomoses 3.44%. He makes the point that mortality and morbidity rates should be related to the number of anastomoses, since in his experience anastomotic suture lines and not linear closures represent the real risk.

There were additionally 11 complications (2.9%) in patients who survived. If all complications, even those questionably related to the use of the instruments were counted, the morbidity rose to 5.6%. In relation to the type of instrument, the morbidity was as follows: GIA™ stapler—1.34%, TA™ stapler—0%, EEA™ stapler—1.60%

Anastomotic leakage occurred six times (2.94%). Five patients died. The total incidence of suture failure was highest with the EEA™ instrument (6.89%), followed by the GIA™ instrument (2.48%) and the TA™ instrument (1.17%). It is reasonably certain that the EEA™ instrument was used exclusively in esophageal and low rectal anastomoses.

Suture line hemorrhage developed in one patient in whom the GIA™ instrument was used. In another eight patients with postoperative bleeding, the responsibility of the staplers could not be established. Turbelin notes that in the collected European and American series (2,095 patients), suture line bleeding rarely led to death (0.09%); in 14 patients (36.8% of bleeders), reoperation was required and the bleeding was stopped each time. In another 22 patients of the collected series (57.8% of bleeders), bleeding ceased spontaneously.

Anastomotic strictures were noted on four occasions by Turbelin, all with the EEA™ instrument. In reviewing the experience of others, Turbelin noted that strictures were more frequent in circular stapled anastomoses than in anastomoses made with the linear instruments. In three of the four strictures observed by him personally, the smallest of the three EEA™ cartridges had been used.

In reviewing their results, analyzed by site of staple closure and/or anastomosis in gastric procedures, Turbelin reported 37 duodenal closures, 45 gastric closures, three triangulation and eight EEA™ gastroduodenotomies, and 38 GIA™ gastrojejunostomies. There were no deaths. Morbidity was 4.39%: one duodenal fistula, one hemorrhage, and two strictures. Counting complications questionably related to the staplers, the morbidity rose to 10.9%: four patients with hemorrhage, two stenotic dysfunctions.

Operations performed on the small bowel did not lead to any deaths or complications, and Turbelin noted that the small bowel, whether sutured manually or mechanically, "has a good reputation."

In 201 patients operated on for colonic or rectal disease there were 159 anastomoses and 60 bowel closures. The mortality related to the staplers was 2.5% (five patients) and the morbidity 6.5% (eight patients). Four patients suffered fistulas, two had suture line bleeding, one stricture developed and one anastomosis leaked.

Fahrenkrug and Clemmesen (1981), reporting from Frederiksborg, Denmark, reported their experience in 100 operations, performing 104 anastomoses with the EEA™ instrument, six esophagojejunostomies, two esophagogastrostomies, four cholecystojejunostomies, two ileoileostomies, ten ileotransversostomies, 41 colocolostomies, and 35 low anterior resections. The EEA™ instrument, for the low rectal anastomoses, was placed either through the anus or from above through a colotomy and, in all other anastomoses, was inserted through a colotomy or an enterotomy, which was closed manually. They report one clinical leak with an esophagogastrostomy, two clinical leaks with ileo- or colocolostomies and two clinical leaks with low anterior resections, but four other radiologically demonstrated "leaks." The esophagogastrostomy leak resulted fatally. The leaking ileotransverse colostomy was in a patient with a perforated recurrent carcinoma of the colon and, like the colocolostomy leak, was not fatal. The two deaths, in the low anterior resections, were associated with anastomotic leaks.

REPORTED COMPLICATIONS WITH STAPLING INSTRUMENTS

Only a few communications are addressed specifically to complications. The paper by Wassner, Yohai, and Heimlich (1977) from the Jewish Hospital of Cincinnati is notable in this regard.

Reviewing 55 operations involving the colon and 77 the proximal gastrointestinal tract, they had the following to say about complications. Four anastomoses bleeding at the time of the operation required additional sutures. Two patients had significant postoperative bleeding after gastroenterostomy but required no reoperation. There was bleeding from two colocolostomies, requiring reoperation in one. In many cases, a variety of difficulties was experienced by the surgeons. For instance, with two duodenal stumps and one gastric stump it was found that the stapler had not been placed across the full length of the cut end of the viscus and had to be reapplied. In three other patients, duodenal stump leak occurred, all of whom recovered; one colonic anastomosis disrupted. In a total gastrectomy there was an "inadvertent stapling of the common duct." They concluded that ". . .complications can result from the use of these instruments" and wished to "alert surgeons to specific complications. . . ." The comments of the discussers at the meeting of the Central Surgical Association were not kind.

Griffen of Lexington, Kentucky (1977) indicated that the use of staples had to be learned, bleeding was no more certainly controlled with staples than with thread, and suggested that the problem might have been not with the staplers but with the surgeons. Furste (1977), in the same discussion, said ". . .all of us who have used the staplers have been impressed with (1) the decrease in anesthesia time and tissue exposure time, which use of the stapler makes possible; (2) the decrease in the tissue handling; and (3) the decrease in tissue trauma which is the result of tissue manipulation and handling." Furste went on to say, similarly emphasizing the responsibility of the surgeon in any technical maneuver, "May I emphasize that we look upon the surgical blade and gastrointestinal stapling devices in a similar light. . .both the surgical blade *and* gastrointestinal devices may be responsible for complications and *should be used only when indicated, and correctly."*

In general, stapled suture lines have been remarkably free from any complications due to the presence of the staples. This is most notable in the bronchi, where chronic cough, requiring removal of staples, simply does not occur whereas, with a variety of nonabsorbable sutures, it is not at all rare, at some time after operation, to have to remove bronchoscopically one or several sutures exposed in a tuft of granulation tissue.

As is noted in the section on construction of urinary diversion ileal loops, if a loop does not drain well, concretions may attach themselves to the staples in the mucosa-to-mucosa stapled loop. This is, of course, the reason that the current stapling instruments are not used for closure of the urinary bladder. Dickinson (1971) reports a polypoid granuloma causing substantial bleeding from the recent suture line of the Duhamel operation for Hirschsprung's disease: "Polypoid lesions, up to 1.5 cm in diameter, were noted along the anastomotic lines. . .were excised with cautery and snare and proved to be granulomatous polyps about the staples." This seems to be an exceedingly rare occurrence. One of us recently has seen a woman with a single small granuloma in the suture line a year after a functional end-to-end, very low anterior anastomosis of the rectum.

COMPARATIVE STUDIES OF ANASTOMOTIC TECHNIQUES

We have stated, as have other surgeons, that we are sufficiently convinced of the superiority of staple techniques that we cannot ourselves ethically undertake a controlled trial of stapled versus manual suture techniques. Most of the published evaluations are not properly controlled prospective comparative studies, but we provide below such information as can be gleaned.

Maillard, Goyer, and Lortat-Jacob (1971), from Paris, compared Russian stapled (PKS 25) esophagogastric anastomoses and sutured anastomoses by the same surgeons in the same time interval. Anastomotic leaks were more frequent with hand-made anastomoses. There were 30 fistulas in 72 manual anastomoses and eight fistulas in 39 machine-made anastomoses. They placed a protective layer of sutures over the one-layer stapled anastomosis of the Russian instrument.

Kabanov (1973) reported from Russia what appears to be one of the few prospective, controlled comparisons of stapled and manual closure and anastomosis after gastric surgery, using the Russian instruments comparable to the TA^{TM} series, to the GIA^{TM} series, and to the EEA^{TM} series, the principal staple line differences being that the Russian equivalents of the GIA^{TM} instrument and the EEA^{TM} instrument place only a single row of sutures, which usually is reinforced by a manual suture. Details are not given as to whether the suture lines were oversewn or not, although our observation has been that most Russian surgeons oversew the mucosa-to-mucosa closures, as of the duodenal stump or the cut end of the stomach, and all oversew the single staple line of the GIA^{TM} and EEA^{TM} analogues. In their total of 826 patients, 415 had procedures performed manually and 411 of the procedures were performed with the stapling instruments. Indications for operation were almost identical in the two groups. Bleeding occurred in 2.9% of the stapled patients, 1.9% of the manual operations; duodenal stump failure was 0.6% in the stapled cases and 2.2% in the manual closures. No leaks occurred in stapled gastroenterostomies, seven leaks (1.6%) in manual gastroenterostomies. Gastric outlet obstructions occurred in 0.07% of the stapled anastomoses and 0.09% of the manual anastomoses. Subdiaphragmatic abscesses occurred in 0.07% of the mechanical cases and 1.9% of the manual cases; wound infection occurred in 0.7% of the stapled cases and 1.9% of the manually closed cases. Definition of wound infection, for these extremely low percentages, was not given.

Kabanov's conclusion was that "(1) The suture instruments insure the certainty of a leak free anastomosis, permit a less traumatic resection of the stomach, shorten operative time and lead to better healing of anastomoses.

"(2) The number of postoperative complications and fatalities after gastrectomy is significantly lower with the use of the suturing instrument than with manual techniques.''

One of the more interesting papers comparing the results of anastomoses performed with the staplers with those performed manually is that by Chassin and colleagues (Chassin, Rifkind, Sussman, Kassel, Fingeret, Drager, and Chassin, 1978) from the New York University School of Medicine and Booth Memorial Medical Center in Flushing, New York. They reviewed 812 operative procedures in the gastrointestinal tract performed in one hospital over a four-year period by the same group of surgeons on entirely similar indications, the choice of manual or staple suturing having been at the pleasure of the operator. All stapling operations were with the TA^{TM} and the GIA^{TM} instruments. The principal difference between the two groups of patients was that traumatic perforation or suppuration, gangrene of the bowel, intestinal obstruction, Crohn's disease, or carcinoma were all more frequent in the patients who were stapled than in the patients who were sutured, i.e., the surgeons tended preferentially to use stapling in critically ill patients with systemic or local disease that might a priori have been considered to predispose to suture line complications. Nevertheless, the complication rates were almost identical—2.8% in 472 stapled anastomoses and 3.0% in 296 sutured anastomoses.

In a retrospective study of ileal bladder urinary diversions performed by resident surgeons at the University of Pittsburgh Health Center (Karamcheti, O'Donnell, Hakala, Schwentker, and Steichen, 1978), the operators were a changing group of residents, but the attending urologists, first assistants, were constant over the same period. The patients were matched for age, associated disease, and severity of primary disease. The decision to perform a stapled anastomosis and loop closure or a manual one was not randomized but depended on the preference of the attending surgeon. Some always chose to use the staplers, others always preferred the manual anastomosis. No attending surgeon ever used a stapled anastomosis at one time and a manual anastomosis at another. All of the operations were performed by residents in Urology, regardless of the type of anastomosis, e.g., mechanical or manual. There were significant differences in the duration of the operation, postoperative ileus, and hospital stay, as well as postoperative fever and wound infection, all favoring the use of staplers. There were no suture line leaks in either group. It should be stressed that all of these anastomoses were performed by surgeons who only occasionally performed intestinal operations.

Three years ago, we reviewed 129 patients who had undergone elective colon resection with anastomosis from January, 1971 through August, 1978 at the Oakland VA Medical Center in Pittsburgh (Thompson, Stremple, Loubeau, and Steichen, 1980). All operations were performed by the surgical house staff; all but 12 of the hand-sewn anastomoses were by the conventional two-layer technique. The 12 were with a single layer. All but two of the stapled anastomoses were functional end-to-end, the two most recent having been done with the EEA^{TM} instrument. The case material was similar and the surgeons were identical, but the study was entirely retrospective. In the 44 right colectomies with ileocolic anastomosis, 21 hand-sewn and 23 stapled, the operating time was shorter with staples, but not to a statistically significant degree, nor was the time of resumption of oral intake significantly different. There were two anastomotic leaks in each group. One, in the hand-sewn anastomosis, resulted fatally. Of the 85 colocolic anastomoses, 64 were hand-sewn and 21 were stapled. Mean operative time was significantly shorter for the stapled group, $P = 0.07$. There were five documented leaks and one obstructed anastomosis requiring reoperation in the hand-sewn cases, a complication rate of 9.4%. A single patient in the stapled group developed postoperative fever and left lower quadrant pain, which resolved with antibiotics and without operation, a complication rate of 4.8%. Wound infection rates were nearly identical—9.4% hand-sewn, 9.5% stapled.

Reiling and colleagues (Reiling, Reiling, Bernie, Huffer, Perkins, and Elliott, 1980), from Dayton, Ohio, undertook a prospective controlled study of gastrointestinal anastomoses between March, 1976 and May, 1977, the operations being performed by five general surgeons. The anastomosis was the true end-to-end triangulation technique, which we did describe in 1972 (Ravitch and Steichen, 1972) but have not used clinically because it is somewhat more difficult than the functional end-to-end and invites more contamination. They had 50 patients in each group and the procedures up and down the gastrointestinal tract were equally divided between the two groups. They found no difference in operating time, no difference in hospital stay. Patients with sutured anastomoses tended to be a day longer on gastric suction and two days longer on intravenous fluids. There were no fistulas in either group and paralytic ileus occurred in two patients in the suture group and three in the stapled group. There were six abscesses in the sutured group and three in the stapled group. There was no bleeding in either group. They admitted that time was lost in loading the staples, etc., because of inexperience of the nursing staff and technicians. Nevertheless, their published paper states, ''The study was stopped prematurely at 100 cases because all of the authors felt that the staples were more time efficient. No one wanted to have to suture the bowel for the sake of controls when the staplers were available and desired.'' In the discussion, Hinchey of Montreal, Canada (1980) said, ''I have had a complication applying the TA-30 to the duodenum in the presence of a chronic penetrating duodenal ulcer. The suture line remained intact, but the ulcer cracked away from the pancreas. This was not recognized until later on in the procedure, when a bile leak was noted by a medical student. . . .'' Price of Salt Lake City (1980) pointed out that the failure to find a significant time differential probably was a function of inexperience of the surgeons and thought that it required a substantial experience before one was adept in the use of these instruments. In his analysis of the operation sheets of three busy and experienced surgeons, he compared ''. . . 150 gastric resections before the advent of stapling and the first 150 done after stapling. . .'' and similarly 100 stapled colon anastomoses. He found that stapling yielded an average saving of 56 minutes in a Billroth I or II procedure, 42 minutes for a vagotomy and pyloroplasty and 21 minutes for colon resection.

The excitement over the possibilities of the EEA^{TM} stapler, and often its use by surgeons who had had no experience with the previous stapling instruments, led to a number of papers comparing results in manual and stapled end-to-end rectal and colonic anastomoses.

Cady, Godfroy, Sibaud, and Mercadier (1980) extensively studied and compared a series of 64 patients (1975–1977) with a second series of 85 patients (1977–1979) in whom colic and colorectal resections and anastomoses were performed by the same surgeon, helped by the same team, over this five-year period. In the 64 earlier patients, the anastomosis was manual, one-layer inverting, with interrupted sutures of linen or vicryl. In 52 of the patients, the anastomosis was primary, in 12 patients there was a two-stage operation; ''protective'' colostomy for 35 left-sided resections was used in 16 instances (46%).

In the second series of 85 patients, primary staple anastomosis was used in 81 patients. This anastomosis was a functional end-to-end in 62 patients, an end-to-end triangulating anastomosis in two patients, and an end-to-end anastomosis with the EEA™ instrument placed through the anus in 21 patients. "Protective" colostomy was performed in 23 patients of 63 who had a left colectomy (37%).

There were more elderly patients in the stapled group (24% versus 14%). Factors such as general condition, age, and type of lesion appeared to have no influence on the end results in either series, although a greater number of septic complications, especially wound infection, was noted in patients with unprepared bowel. In both groups, the patients were evenly matched for diagnosis (the stapled anastomosis group contained more patients with liver metastases in patients with cancer, 17% versus 7%), extent of colon resected, and emergency or elective character of the operation.

RESULTS. In 56 patients with colon resection and manual colocolic anastomosis there were 16 (28.5%) leaks, seven (12.5%) reoperations, and eight (14%) deaths. In 61 patients with functional end-to-end stapled anastomoses there were five (8%) leaks, three (5%) reoperations, and four (6.5%) deaths.

Mercadier and his colleagues concluded from this that stapling suture techniques are superior to manual techniques for intraperitoneal colon anastomoses, but expressed reservations about the use of mechanical sutures in low anterior resections—a conclusion strikingly at variance with that of others. They recognized the increased technical difficulties inherent in the use of a new instrument and new technique in a difficult anatomical location. To this one must add that, as with all new approaches, there is a learning curve, results improving as more experience is gained. The principle of mechanical sutures and healing is a priori no different in colocolic than in colorectal anastomosis, and the conclusion of most surgeons is that the EEA™ instrument introduces a technical facilitating factor that becomes of particular importance in low anastomoses.

Adloff, Arnaud, and Beeharry (1980), from Strasbourg, but writing in the *Archives of Surgery,* compared 26 stapled colorectal anastomoses and 25 manually sutured anastomoses, all performed between 1975 and 1979. The manual suture was a single-layer inverting technique with interrupted 4–0 Dacron sutures, and in all patients the pelvis was drained suprapubically. The patients were not randomized, and it would appear that the lower tumors were preferentially selected for the stapling operations. There was no difference in the mean operating time. Two of the stapled anastomoses had wound infections, as did four of the sutured anastomoses. Two of each had external fistulas. No stapled anastomosis resulted in leakage or peritonitis, but two of the sutured anastomoses did, and one resulted fatally. There was one long-term stenosis in each group.

Buchmann, Uhlschmid, and Hollinger, from Senning's Clinic in Zurich (1980), compared 13 hand-sutured and 22 EEA™-stapled low anterior anastomoses, the stapled anastomosis series following consecutively on the hand-sutured anastomoses. There were three clinical anastomotic leaks in the manually sutured group and none in the stapled group. There were two radiologically demonstrable leaks in the stapled group and one in the manually sutured group.

Bolton and Britton, from St. Martin's Hospital in Bath, England (1980) compared ten conventional two-layer low rectal anastomoses and ten EEA™ low rectal stapled anastomoses, all 20 protected by tube cecostomy, and ten additional stapled anastomoses without fecal diversion. There was one anastomotic leak in the ten hand-sutured patients and one in the 20 stapled patients. There were two strictures in the hand-sutured cases and none in the stapled cases, two wound infections in the ten hand-sutured cases and four in the 20 stapled cases. The stapled anastomoses were somewhat lower, and the patients left the hospital on the average of four or five days earlier. Bolton and Britton were impressed that "the ability of the stapler to produce a low extraperitoneal anastomosis in the pelvis is unique" and that "this technique has almost certainly reduced the incidence of permanent colostomies over the past year. . . ."

We have commented before that, particularly with the GIA™ anastomoses, the tissues being alive beyond the line of staples to the cut edge of the bowel, it has occurred that the two sides fall together in apposition and heal together. From Ann Arbor, Michigan, Brain, Lorber, and Fiddian-Green (1981) report something similar with an EEA™ anastomosis performed 3 cm from the anal verge. The patient had been doing well, when seven weeks after operation she presented with abdominal distention and incontinence of feces and decreased caliber of her stool. Gastrografin® enema showed narrowing of the lumen of the bowel at the anastomosis but no contraction of the ring of staples. There proved to be a pinhole opening at the level of the anastomosis ". . .with a membrane stretching across the lumen of the bowel. This was broken with ease. . . . The full diameter of the bowel was restored." She did well thereafter. It is difficult to see how this could have formed in a woman who was having regular bowel movements, but the evidence is unequivocal.

Probst, Becker, and Ungeheuer of Frankfurt (1981) compared 52 EEA™ anterior resections and anastomoses with 52 manual anastomoses performed between September, 1979 and August, 1980, using three rows of sutures for the manual anastomoses. Their abstract provides only a partial analysis. The staples saved 30 minutes per operation. There was no mortality in the stapled cases and there were three anastomotic insufficiencies with the stapler versus four for the manually sutured cases. There was no bleeding with the staples. The wound infection rate was 9% in both groups, and the length of hospitalization was similar in both groups. They considered placement of the distal pursestring suture difficult and thought that the stapler should be used only by experienced rectal surgeons.

Beart (1981) conducted a prospective randomized trial at the Mayo Clinic, evaluating the EEA™ stapler in performing the anterior anastomosis. He compared the use of the stapler with the traditional two-layer hand-sewn anastomosis by randomization, when the surgeon thought that either technique could be used. "If, however, it was decided that one method, for any one of a number of conceptual reasons, offered an advantage to the patient then that procedure was utilized and the patient was excluded and followed in a separate group. . . ." There were 70 patients in the randomized groups, 35 in each. All ten of the excluded patients were patients in whom ". . . it was felt, at the time of surgery, that a standard two-layered anastomosis could not be done whereas a stapled anastomosis could be created." The average level of the anastomosis in the nonrandomized, stapled group was 3 cm from the dentate line (2–6 cm) and it was 9 cm in the randomized group.

In the total group of 80 patients there was one death, a 3.75% dehiscence rate, and a 3.75% rate of pelvic infection. No analysis is given comparing the two groups of 35, except that, "It does appear that the stapler is faster. . . . Lower anastomoses can be created than with a traditional two-layer handsewn anastomosis. . . ."

At the proctologic clinic in Recklinghausen, Athanasiadis, Barry, and Girona (1981) performed a comparative study of the EEA™ and Soviet SPTU staplers for colorectal anastomoses in 260 patients. However, their experience was much greater with the EEA™ instrument, 225 cases, than with the SPTU, 35 cases. There was an 11% anastomotic leakage rate with the EEA™ instrument and a 17% leakage with the SPTU. There were three stenoses in the 225 EEA™ anastomoses and one stenosis out of 35

SPTU anastomoses. They did point out that their first trials in this experience were with the Russian instruments.

Weil and Scherz (1981), from the Albert Einstein College of Medicine retrospectively analyzed 545 Billroth II gastrectomies. In 385, the duodenal stump was sutured conventionally with 18 leaks (4.7%) whereas in the 160 with stapled duodenal stump closure there were four leaks (2.5%). In the 474 hand-sutured anastomoses there were 12 complications—leaks, hemorrhage, or obstruction—and none in the 71 stapled anastomoses. The technique used was based solely on the choice of the individual surgeon. They expressed a strong preference for the stapling techniques, stating also that ". . . there is no doubt that the use of the staplers cuts down on the length of the operation."

Scher, Scott-Connor, and Ong (1982) analyzed 112 consecutive patients undergoing gastric operations in Huntington, West Virginia, by a number of surgeons using whichever technique they preferred. Forty-four gastric operations were reported with conventional suture techniques and a Billroth II reconstruction and 36 gastrectomies and reconstructions were reported using the staple techniques and a Billroth II reconstruction. Forty-two patients underwent gastrojejunostomy alone, 24 with the staples and 18 manually sutured. The patients in the sutured and stapled series turned out to be alike in terms of age, underlying disease, hemoglobin and serum albumin levels, and other risk indicators. In the 36 stapled gastrectomies there was a single duodenal stump leak, in a patient with carcinoma of the stomach, resulting in death. There were no leaks in the sutured gastrectomies. Bleeding from the gastrojejunal anastomosis occurred in two of the 36 stapled gastrectomies and two of the 44 sutured gastrectomies, requiring reoperation in all four patients. Gastric outlet obstruction occurred in a single gastrectomy patient in the sutured series and in none in the stapled series. There were four superficial wound infections in the 36 stapled gastrectomies, only one in the 44 sutured gastrectomies. In the gastrojejunostomies there were two anastomotic leaks, one fatal in the 24 stapled procedures and one in the 18 sutured procedures. Two deaths occurred in the sutured group, one attributable to anastomotic failure. Bleeding after gastroenterostomy requiring reoperation occurred in one of the stapled patients and none of the manually sutured patients. There was temporary outlet obstruction in two of the 24 stapled procedures and none after the manual procedures. Superficial wound infection occurred in four of 24 stapled patients and two of 18 sutured patients. The duration of the operations, although not significant statistically, actually was a little greater for the stapled procedures, as can be the case in initial procedures. Patients in the sutured gastrectomy group regained intestinal function more rapidly than when the staples were used. After gastrojejunostomy alone there was no significant difference in the duration of operation. Oral feeding resumed later for the stapled group and postoperative hospital stays were identical.

The conclusion was that stapling devices were safe and that complication rates of stapled and sutured procedures were similar and operative time was not reduced nor intestinal function restored more rapidly. As in other uncontrolled studies, it is not possible to compare the general expertise of the surgeons using staples with that of those using manual techniques. It is not possible to say whether feeding was resumed later in the stapled cases because of persistence of profuse nasogastric tube drainage or because the surgeons distrusted the staples, and the significance of the leaking anastomoses is thrown into doubt because of the high rate of leakage from the standard manual procedures. The figure regarding the time consumed in the stapling procedure and the statement that "The reloading of the disposable cartridges consumes substantial amounts of time'' suggest unfamiliarity with the instruments on the part of surgeons or nurses.

Pimenta's ingenious stapling device (see Fig I–3) applies modern stapling instrument technology to Henroz' 1826 (see Fig I–2) articulated half rings with alternating pins and holes, for everting end-to-end anastomoses. His most recent account (Pimenta, Cardoso, and Rodrigues 1982) reports 28 anastomoses in 25 patients—six esophagogastrostomies, ten esophagojejunostomies, three jejunojejunostomies, seven colocolostomies, one ileocolostomy, and one colorectal anastomosis—with no deaths, one fistula, and one (esophagojejunal) stricture. Whatever the merits of the instrument in terms of convenience and ease of use, the results obtained clearly further substantiate the validity of the use of everting stapled anastomoses at the several levels of the gastrointestinal tract.

As in all the other reviews of the literature that follow, those above are given chronologically. All the earlier reports represent initial experience with the staplers in the earlier days of use of the Auto Suture® instruments. In addition, the reports almost invariably include a surgeon's entire experience with the staplers, including his first ventures. As will be seen, particularly in the more demanding and more dangerous anastomoses, those of the esophagus and rectum, a number of the surgeons now reporting state that complications that were experienced initially now are seen rarely or not at all.

REFERENCES

Adloff M., Arnaud J-P., Beeharry S.: Stapled vs. sutured colorectal anastomosis. *Arch. Surg.* 115:1436, 1980.

Athanasiadis S., Barry B.A., Girona J.: Vergleich der Behandlungsergebnisse bei Dickdarmanastomosen mit den Klammernahtgeräten EEA und SPTU in einem Kollektiv von 260 Patienten. *Langenbecks Arch. Chir.* 354:111, 1981.

Barber H.K., Steichen F.M.: Unpublished data, 1982.

Beart R.W.: A clinical comparison of handsewn vs. stapled anastomoses. *Dis. Colon Rectum* 24:234, 1981.

Bolton R.A., Britton D.C.: Restorative surgery of the rectum with a circumferential stapler. *Lancet* 1:850, 1980.

Brain J., Lorber M., Fiddian-Green R.G.: Rectal membrane: An unusual complication following use of the circular stapling instrument for colorectal anastomosis. *Surgery* 89:271, 1981.

Buchmann P., Uhlschmid G., Hollinger A.: Erfahrungen mit dem EEA-Stapler bei Kolonanastomosen. *Helv. Chir. Acta* 47:645, 1980.

Cady J., Godfroy J., Sibaud O., Mercadier M.: La désunion anastomotique en chirurgie colique et rectale. Étude comparative des procédés de suture manuelle et mécanique à propos d'une série de 149 resections. *Ann. Chir.* 34:350, 1980.

Chassin J.L., Rifkind K.M., Sussman B., Kassel B., Fingeret A., Drager S., Chassin P.S.: The stapled gastrointestinal tract anastomosis: Incidence of postoperative complications compared with the sutured anastomosis. *Ann. Surg.* 188:689, 1978.

Dickinson J.: Foreign body granuloma following anastomosis with the anastomotic stapler. *J. Pediatr. Surg.* 6:489, 1971.

Elliott T.E., Albertazzi V.J., Danto L.A.: Stenosis after stapler anastomosis. *Am. J. Surg.* 133:750, 1977.

Fahrenkrug L., and Clemmesen T.: Anvendelse af et autosuturinstrument i gastroenterologisk kirurgi. *Ugeskr. Laeger* 143:263, 1981.

Fischer M.G.: Bleeding from stapler anastomosis. *Am. J. Surg.* 131:745, 1976.

Fortin C.L., Poulin E.C., Leclerc Y.: Evaluation de l'utilisation des appareils d'autosuture en chirurgie digestive. *Can. J. Surg.* 22:580, 1979.

Furste W.: In discussion of Wassner J.D., Yohai E., Heimlich H.J. *Surgery* 82:395, 1977.

Griffen W.O.: In discussion of Wassner J.D., Yohai E., Heimlich H.J. *Surgery* 82:395, 1977.

Gritsman J.J.: Mechanical suture by Soviet apparatus in gastric resection: Use in 4,000 operations. *Surgery* 59:663, 1966.

Hinchey E.J.: In discussion of Reiling R.B., Reiling W.A. Jr., Bernie W.A., Huffer A.B., Perkins N.C., Elliott D.W. *Am. J. Surg.* 139:147, 1980.

Josefsen T., Efron G.: Personal communication, 1969.

Kabanov N.Ya: Comparative evaluation of complications after gastric resection made by mechanical and hand sutures in ulcer disease. *Khirurgiia* (Mosk) 49:16, 1973.

Karamcheti A., O'Donnell W.F., Hakala T.R., Schwentker F.N., Steichen F.M.: Autosuture ileal conduit construction: Experience in 110 cases. *J. Urol.* 120:545, 1978.

Keshishian J.M.: Personal communication, February 13, 1978.

Keshishian J.M., Vasarhelyi L., Smyth N.P.D., Garcia J.M., Mispireta L.: Aorto-enteric fistula following renal artery bypass graft. *Contemp. Surg.* 12:17, 1978.

Latimer R.G., Doane W.A., McKittrick J.E., Shepherd A.: Automatic staple suturing for gastrointestinal surgery. *Am. J. Surg.* 130:766, 1975.

Lawson W.R., Hutchison J., Longland C.J., Haque M.A.: Mechanical suture methods in thoracic and abdominal surgery. *Br. J. Surg.* 64:115, 1977.

McGinty C.P.: A new method of bowel anastomosis. *Cape County J.* (Missouri), November, 1970.

McGinty C.P., Kasten M.C., Kinder J.L., Hunt R.S.: Update on stapled bowel anastomosis. *Mo. Med.* 76:145, 1979.

Maillard J-N., Goyer B., Lortat-Jacob J-L.: Comparaison chez l'homme des anastomoses oesophagogastriques. A la pince PKS 25 et à la suture. *Ann. Chir.* 25:569, 1971.

Painter R.L., Park S., Hochberg D.T.: One year's experience with the auto-suture stapling device at the Day Kimball Hospital. *Conn. Med.* 38:59, 1974.

Photopulos G.J., Delgado G., Fowler W.C. Jr., Walton L.A.: Intestinal anastomoses after radiation therapy by surgical stapling instruments. *Obstet. Gynecol.* 54:515, 1979.

Pimenta A.P.A., Cardoso V.M.B., Rodrigues J.S.: A mechanical suturing method for the gastrointestinal tract: Clinical experience with a new stapling instrument. *World J. Surg.* 6:786, 1982.

Price R.R.: In discussion of Reiling R.B., Reiling W.A. Jr., Bernie W.A., Huffer A.B., Perkins N.C., Elliott D.W. *Am. J. Surg.* 139:147, 1980.

Probst M., Becker H., Ungeheuer E.: Vergleich der Ergebnisse von konservativer Nahttechnik und maschinelle Anastomosierung bei anteriorer Rektumresektion (abstract). 98th Kongress Deutsche Gesellschaft für Chirurgie, Munich, April 22–25, 1981.

Ravitch M.M., Brolin R.E.: The price of weight loss by jejunoileal shunt. *Ann. Surg.* 190:382, 1979.

Ravitch M.M., Brown I.W., Daviglus G.F.: Experimental and clinical use of the Soviet bronchus stapling instrument. *Surgery* 46:97, 1959.

Ravitch M.M., Hirsch L.C., Noiles D.: A new instrument for simultaneous ligation and division of vessels, with a note on hemostasis by a gelatin sponge-staple combination. *Surgery* 71:732, 1972.

Ravitch M.M., Lane R., Cornell W.P., Rivarola A., McEnany T.: Closure of duodenal, gastric and intestinal stumps with wire staples: Experimental and clinical studies. *Ann. Surg.* 163:573, 1966.

Ravitch M.M., Ong T.H., Gazzola L.: A new, precise, and rapid technique of intestinal resection and anastomosis with staples. *Surg. Gynecol. Obstet.* 139:6, 1974.

Ravitch M.M., Rivarola A.: Enteroanastomosis with an automatic instrument. *Surgery* 59:270, 1966.

Ravitch M.M., Rivarola A., VanGrov J.: Rapid creation of gastric pouches with the use of an automatic stapling instrument. *J. Surg. Res.* 6:64, 1966.

Ravitch M.M., Snodgrass E., Rivarola A.: Compartmentation of the vena cava with the mechanical stapler. *Surg. Gynecol. Obstet.* 122:561, 1966.

Ravitch M.M., Steichen F.M.: Technics of staple suturing in the gastrointestinal tract. *Ann. Surg.* 175:815, 1972.

Ravitch M.M., Steichen F.M.: Experiences with a second generation of stapling instruments in general and thoracic surgery. *Bull. Soc. Int. Chir.* 31:502, 1972.

Ravitch M.M., Steichen F.M., Fishbein R.H., Knowles P.W., Weil P.: Clinical experiencs with the Soviet mechanical bronchus stapler (UKB-25). *J. Thorac. Cardiovasc. Surg.* 47:446, 1964.

Reichel K.: Nahtgeräte in der Bauchchirurgie. 16. *Jahrestagung der Österreichischen Gesellschaft für Chirurgie,* 5.-7. June, 1975.

Reiling R.B., Reiling W.A. Jr., Bernie W.A., Huffer A.B., Perkins N.C., Elliott D.W.: Prospective controlled study of gastrointestinal stapled anastomoses. *Am. J. Surg.* 139:147, 1980.

Rignault D., Pailler J-L., Berthet A., Tardat M.: Les sutures mécaniques automatiques en chirurgie digestive. Appréciation de la méthode après 3 ans d'utilisation de l'appareillage americain. *Chirurgie* 102:945, 1976.

Rinecker H.: Indikationsbereiche maschineller Nahtmethoden am Gastrointestinaltrakt. Operationsergebnisse bei 300 Fallen. *Chirurg* 48:241, 1977.

Rinecker H., Danek N.: Maschinelle naht—und skeletiermethoden am Gastro-intestinaltrakt: 2/3-magenresektionen nach B I und B II. *Langenbecks Arch. Chir.* 340:1, 1975.

Risch F., Weydert N., Mandres G., Bleser F.: Les sutures mécaniques en chirurgie. Bilan de 11 ans d'utilisation. *Bull. Soc. Sci. Méd. Grand-Duché Luxemb.* 117:13, 1980.

de Ruiter P.: Automatic stapling devices in gastrointestinal surgery. *Arch. Chir. Neerl.* 29:187, 1977.

Scher K.S., Scott-Conner C., Ong W.T.: A comparison of stapled and sutured anastomoses in gastric operations. *Surg. Gynecol. Obstet.* 154:548, 1982.

Steichen F.M., Ravitch M.M.: Mechanical sutures in surgery. *Br. J. Surg.* 60:191 1973.

Steichen F.M., Talbert J.L., Ravitch M.M.: Primary side-to-side colorectal anastomosis in the Duhamel operation for Hirschsprung's disease. *Surgery* 64:475, 1968.

Talbert J.L., Seashore J.H., Ravitch M.M.: Evaluation of a modified Duhamel operation for correction of Hirschsprung's disease. *Ann. Surg.* 179:671, 1974.

Thompson B., Stremple J., Loubeau J-M., Steichen F.M.: Unpublished data, 1980.

Turbelin J.M.: Les sutures mécaniques en chirurgie digestive. Thèse de Docteur en Médecine, Faculté de Médecine de Strasbourg, Université Louis Pasteur, 1980.

Turbelin J.M., Arnaud J.P., Welter R., Adloff M.: Etude comparative des surfaces anastomotiques obtenues par utilisation des sutures mécaniques en chirurgie digestive. *J. Chir.* 117:541, 1980.

Vankemmel M.: La ''viscéro-synthèse'' par agrafes métalliques après résection digestive segmentaire. Modalités et résultats. *Lyon Chir.* 70:339, 1974.

Vankemmel M.: La résection-anastomose de l'oesophage suscardial a l'appareil PKS 25 ou SPTU 26 pour rupture de varices oesophagiennes. *Ann. Chir.* 30:187, 1976.

Wassner J.D., Yohai E., Heimlich H.J.: Complications associated with the use of gastrointestinal stapling devices. *Surgery* 82:395, 1977.

Weber M.: Utilisation de l'autosuture par agrafes en chirurgie digestive. Technique et résultats. *Helv. Chir. Acta* 39:263, 1972.

Webster M.W. Jr., Carey L.C., Ravitch M.M.: The permanent gastrostomy: Use of the gastrointestinal anastomotic stapler. *Arch. Surg.* 110:658, 1975.

Weil P.H., Scherz H.: Comparison of stapled and hand-sutured gastrectomies. *Arch. Surg.* 116:14, 1981.

Wheeless C.R. Jr., Dorsey J.H.: Use of the automatic surgical stapler for intestinal anastomosis associated with gynecologic malignancy: Review of 283 procedures. *Gynecol. Oncol.* 11:1, 1981.

CHAPTER V

Operations on the Stomach

A NUMBER OF general principles are found to apply to the various gastric operations. As in all portions of the gastrointestinal tract, stapling and transection of the stomach and duodenum are carried out at the selected level, along the very edge of the viable portion of the remaining viscus. This closure and transection should be within the immediate proximity (literally millimeters) of the intact vascular supply and should not staple the vessels outside the stomach. The cut ends of the stomach and duodenum stapled mucosa-to-mucosa by the TA^{TM} instruments are essentially never reinforced. A little bleeding from the cut edge coming through the staples is a reassuring sign of good blood supply up to the very cut edge. An occasional spurting vessel requires a single suture. Very rarely is there enough bleeding to suggest the need for reinforcing the suture line and, after closure of the abdomen, only on one occasion have we suspected bleeding from the cut surface of a tangential gastric excision. There was a significant drop in hemoglobin, no abdominal or systemic signs, and no intervention was required. If there is significant bleeding when the TA^{TM} instrument has been removed from the duodenum or stomach, it almost invariably will be disclosed that the extragastric, omental vessels to the residual stomach or duodenum have been included in the clamp. The TA^{TM} instruments do not provide secure hemostasis of such vessels. Until the advent of the EEA^{TM} instrument performing circular, minimally inverting anastomoses, we made all Billroth II anastomoses with the GIA^{TM} instrument, one limb inserted into the stomach and one into the jejunum, the opening left after withdrawal of the GIA^{TM} instrument being closed mucosa-to-mucosa with the TA^{TM} instrument. It is possible to perform a Billroth II with the EEA^{TM} instrument, either inserting it into the open and unstapled end of the stomach and thence through the gastric wall into the jejunum, in the manner analogous to the use of the EEA^{TM} instrument for Billroth I anastomosis, shown in Figure V–15, or inserting the EEA^{TM} instrument through a gastrotomy in the already amputated and stapled stomach by analogy with the Billroth I technique shown in Figures V–14 and V–16. We have been so satisfied with the GIA^{TM} anastomosis that we have not ourselves used this technique, although we gather that it is becoming popular (Nance, 1979). Prior to the use of the EEA^{TM} instrument, the anastomosis in the Billroth I operation was performed manually. Walker Reynolds of Alabama (1972, 1982), in performing a Billroth I, created a distal gastric tube by two applications of the GIA^{TM} stapling instrument at right angles to each other and then performed, by hand, an end-to-end Billroth I gastroduodenostomy (see Fig V–17). We have not used this technique ourselves. The EEA^{TM} instrument lends itself admirably to the performance of the Billroth I reconstruction by either of the two techniques pictured. It will be noted that in several of the operative descriptions we have pointed out a hazard of dealing with the duodenal stump. If the duodenum is transected and stapled proximal to the ulcer, it is possible that with the leverage of the long instruments, one may unwittingly separate the ulcer borders away from the pancreas, inviting a duodenal leak, which in the postoperative period will be diagnosed as a "duodenal stump blowout" (Hinchey, 1980). Similarly, it is conceivable that if the staple line is made through the indurated tissue of the ulcer that has been mobilized, this thick and brittle tissue will be crushed through and will leak. In a single instance in one of our affiliated hospitals there was a leak from a stapled Billroth II anastomosis. The stomach had been noted to be extremely thick and edematous and the explanation appears to be that under these circumstances the degree of tissue compression required to permit the staples to form correctly resulted in injury to the tissues, causing the leak and the resultant fistula.

It is occasionally useful to transect the stomach, or form tubes, with the GIA[TM] instrument, as in a Janeway gastrostomy or the greater-curvature Beck-Jianu-Gavriliu tube. We have insisted on reinforcing such suture lines, involving both walls of the stomach, with a continuous inverting suture or an over-and-over whipstitch placed behind the staples, because of the shorter length of the staples in the GIA[TM] instrument.

The use of the staples on the stomach and the duodenum, avoiding the necessity for clamps of various kinds dangling from the organs, permits one to perform the gastrojejunostomy immediately on the transection of the stomach, providing a steady flow in the operative procedure—gastric transection, gastrojejunostomy, duodenal transection.

A number of surgeons have used the LDS[TM] instrument in the serial division of the branches of the vagus nerve in parietal cell vagotomy. Engelke, Kamphausen, and vom Rath (1977) of Krefeld, Germany, in the performance of parietal cell vagotomy in 216 cases, found the LDS[TM] instrument useful for the serial division of the vessels and vagal branches on the lesser curvature.

Waugh (1971), from the Army Hospital in Fort Benning, Georgia, reported the use of the GIA[TM] instrument for providing a bloodless gastrotomy, using the shorter PGIA[TM] staple as we recommended.

In this instance, as in many others, procedures that we had devised, and were using, were first published by others, sometimes with attribution, as in this case, sometimes without.

Jascalevich (1972) described the same technique.

Awe and Loehden (1973) of Portland, Oregon reported satisfaction with stapled gastrotomy in six cases.

Harrison, Anderson, Rosen, Ross, and Hendricks (1982) applied the same GIA[TM] technique to experimental hysterotomy in monkeys to achieve a dry uterine incision, subsequently closing the hysterotomy with the TA 90[TM] instrument.

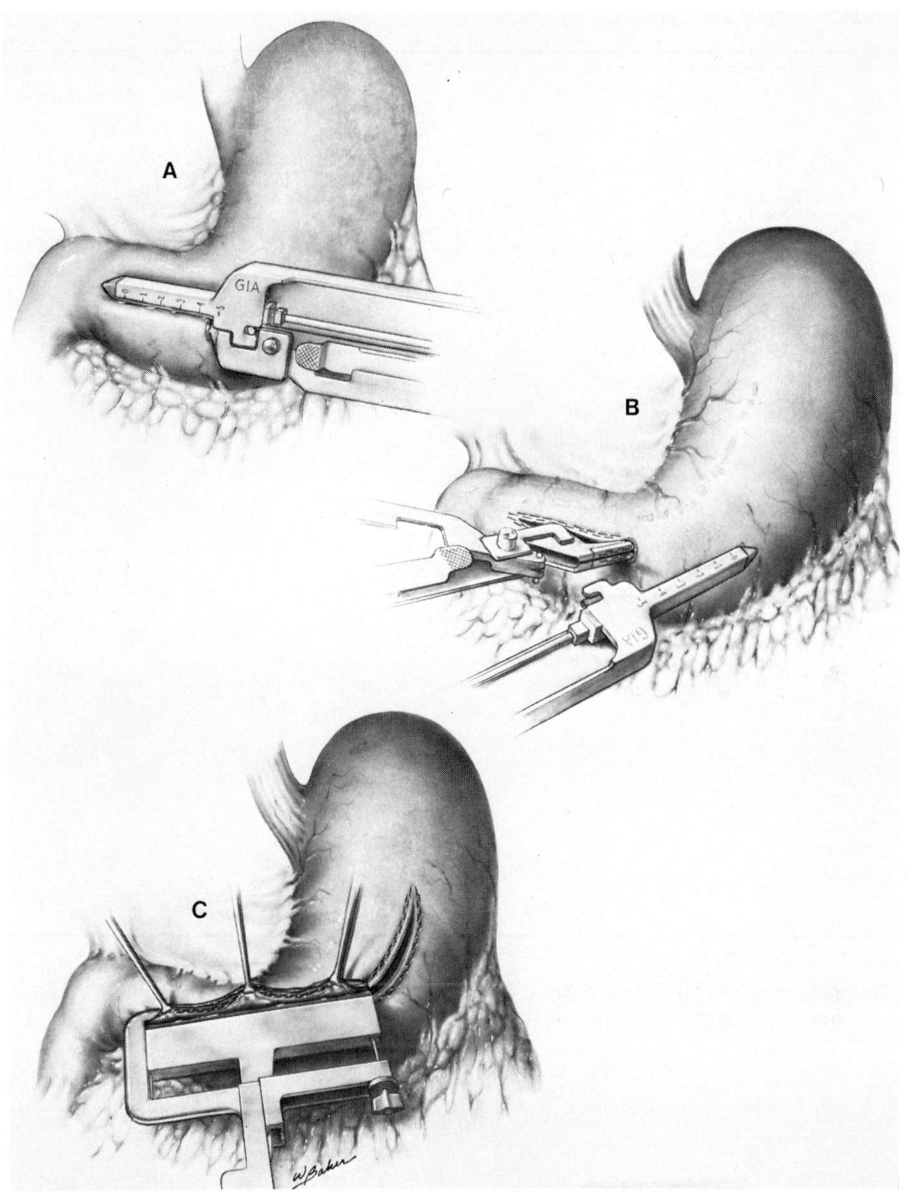

Fig V–1.—Gastrotomy. In a variety of situations, the bleeding from an ordinary gastrotomy can be annoying. With the use of the P(pediatric)GIA™ cartridge, whose staple legs are 3 mm long as opposed to 4 mm of the standard GIA™ instrument and compress to 1.25 mm as compared to 1.75 mm for the standard GIA™ instrument, so as to be hemostatic when stapling only a single thickness of stomach, a 5-cm gastrotomy is performed, which is hemostatically sutured by the staples. **A,** a small cautery opening has been made in the stomach, the assembled but not locked GIA™ instrument is placed on the anterior gastric wall, the anvil limb inside the stomach and the cartridge limb outside. The instrument is closed, the slide pushed, and the gastrotomy formed. **B,** if a longer gastrotomy is desired, the staple cartridge is replaced and the instrument reapplied proximally. **C,** at the completion of the procedure, if it is desired to close the stomach, this is done mucosa-to-mucosa, holding the lips of the incision up through the TA 90™ instrument, which, in this case, would be applied twice. The excess tissue beyond the jaws is excised each time before the jaws are removed. No reinforcing sutures are required. (**B** and **C** from M.M. Ravitch and F.M. Steichen, *Annals of Surgery,* 1972, used by permission.)

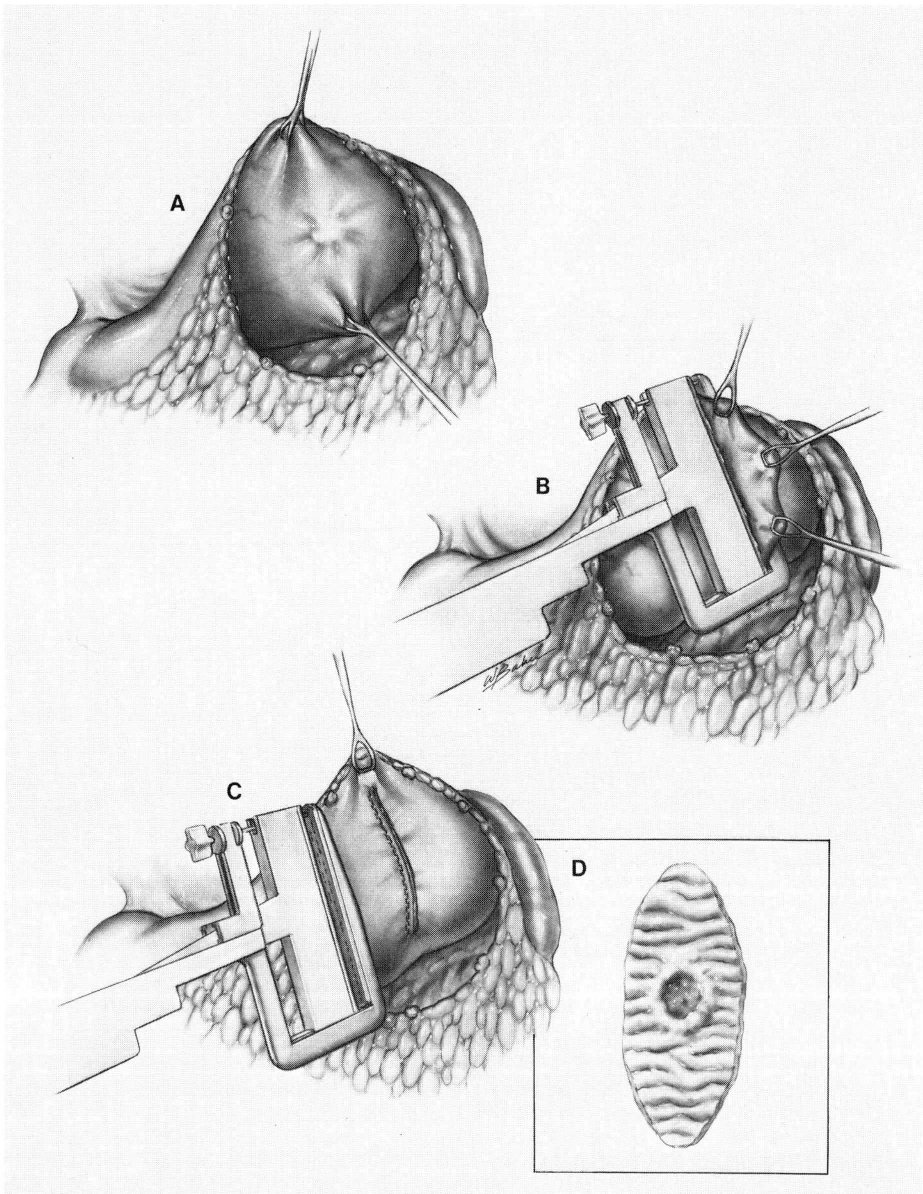

Fig V–2.—Tangential excision of a mural lesion. Shown is the excision of a posterior gastric ulcer, the nature of which was not certain. **A,** the stomach is freed as required and seized near the greater and lesser curvature with Babcock clamps, so that **B,** the palpable lesion in the posterior wall of the stomach can be held up and the TA™ instrument, here the TA 90™ instrument, can be placed down on the stomach, well beyond the lesion to be excised. The instrument is placed to produce a transverse staple line, which does not deform or narrow the stomach. **C,** the staples having been delivered and the specimen cut away, the TA™ instrument is removed. The opportunity for contamination or bleeding is minimal. **D,** the oval specimen containing the lesion, in this case, a benign ulcer.

The same technique is admirably suited to the excision of leiomyomas, mural polyps, nodules of ectopic pancreatic tissue, benign intestinal tumors, etc. If the nature of the specimen indicates an operation of greater magnitude, the viscus already is closed and sealed and the operation can be proceeded with without concern for contamination, bleeding, etc.

Engelberg and Lifschitz, from Tel Aviv (1980), report the amputation of a pedunculated villous adenoma, presenting rectally, by drawing it out the anus and amputating it with the TA 90[TM] instrument.

Freed, Christodoulides, and Szuchmacher (1978) describe the use of the GIA[TM] stapling instrument in the excision of gastric polyps. They approach such polyps through an anterior gastrotomy and, if the lesion is not located near the cardia or near the pylorus, it is grasped by a Babcock instrument, elevated, and the GIA[TM] instrument is applied to the base of the polyp. In this fashion, an inverting gastric wall wedge resection is performed. Although this approach is useful in patients who may have several lesions and the TA[TM] instruments can also be used for it, it invites contamination, requires a second suture line to close the gastrotomy, and does not appear to possess advantages over the tangential resection pictured, for the usual solitary, intramural lesion of the stomach.

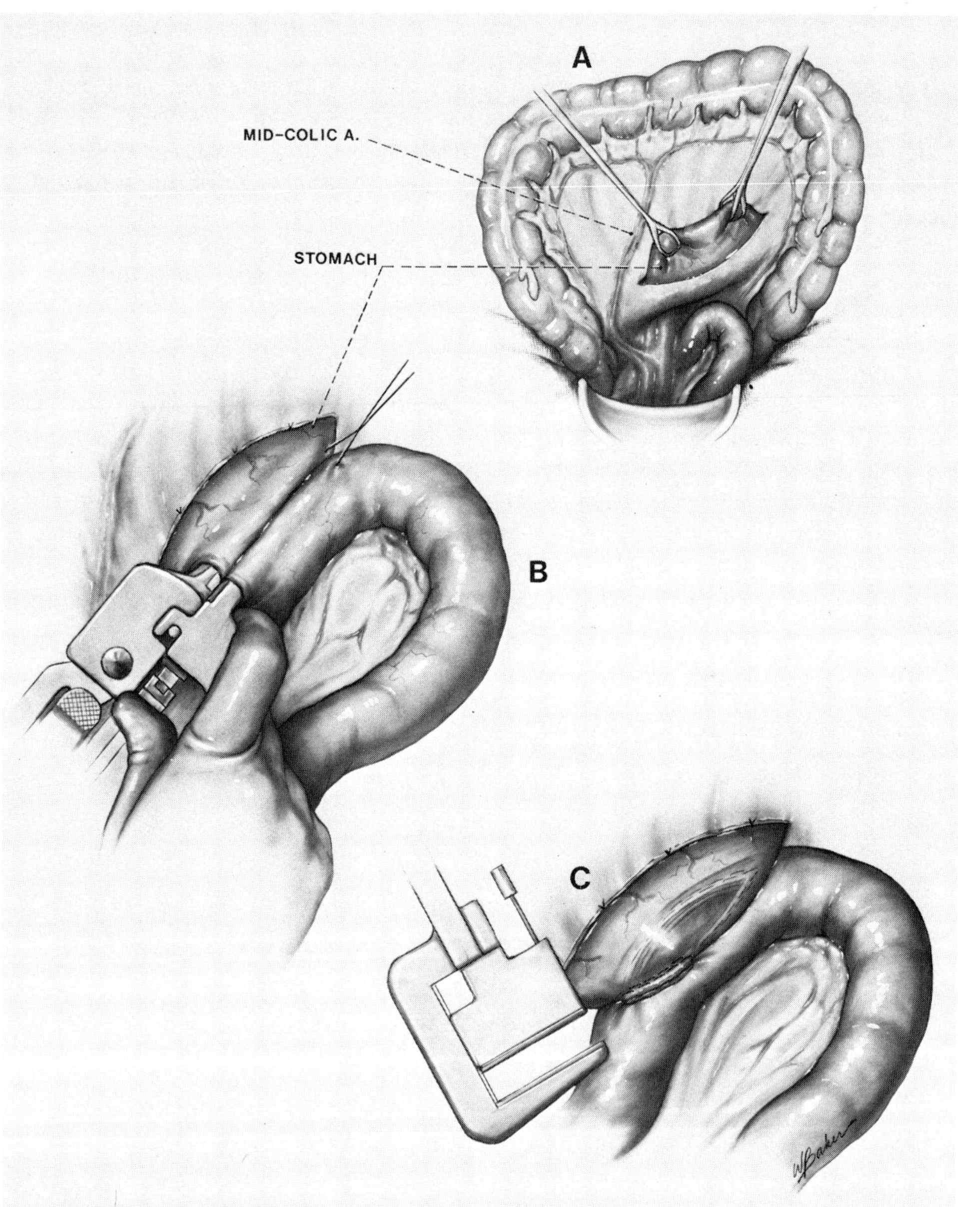

Fig V–3.—Gastroenterostomy. **A,** the posterior wall of the stomach is drawn through an avascular rent in the mesocolon. **B,** the edges of the rent in the mesocolon have been sutured to the stomach. The stomach and the appropriate loop of jejunum are held together, either with traction sutures, as shown, or with Babcock clamps. Matched cautery openings are made in the stomach and jejunum and the limbs of the assembled GIA™ instrument slipped into the two lumina, matched and locked. Driving forward the three-pronged assembly of staple pusher bars and central blade, the jejunum and stomach are united with four rows of staples. The central blade divides the stapled union of the two viscera between the two middle rows of staples, the knife cut ending one and a half staples from the end of the staple line. **C,** the lips of the single opening, made as the blade divides the partition between the two puncture wounds, are held up by clamps. One must insure that full thickness of viscus wall is sutured on both sides. The clamps holding the GIA™ staple lines are held widely apart, the lips of the opening usually held in the middle with a Babcock clamp and the TA 30™ or TA 55™ instrument applied just below the three clamps, thus insuring a through-and-through stapled closure of full thickness wall completely around the opening. One must not take so much tissue with the TA™ clamp as to risk narrowing the anastomosis. The drawing shows the TA™ instrument being withdrawn and, in transparency, the anastomotic opening. (See Fig V–4) (From M.M. Ravitch and F.M. Steichen, *Annals of Surgery,* 1972, with permission.)

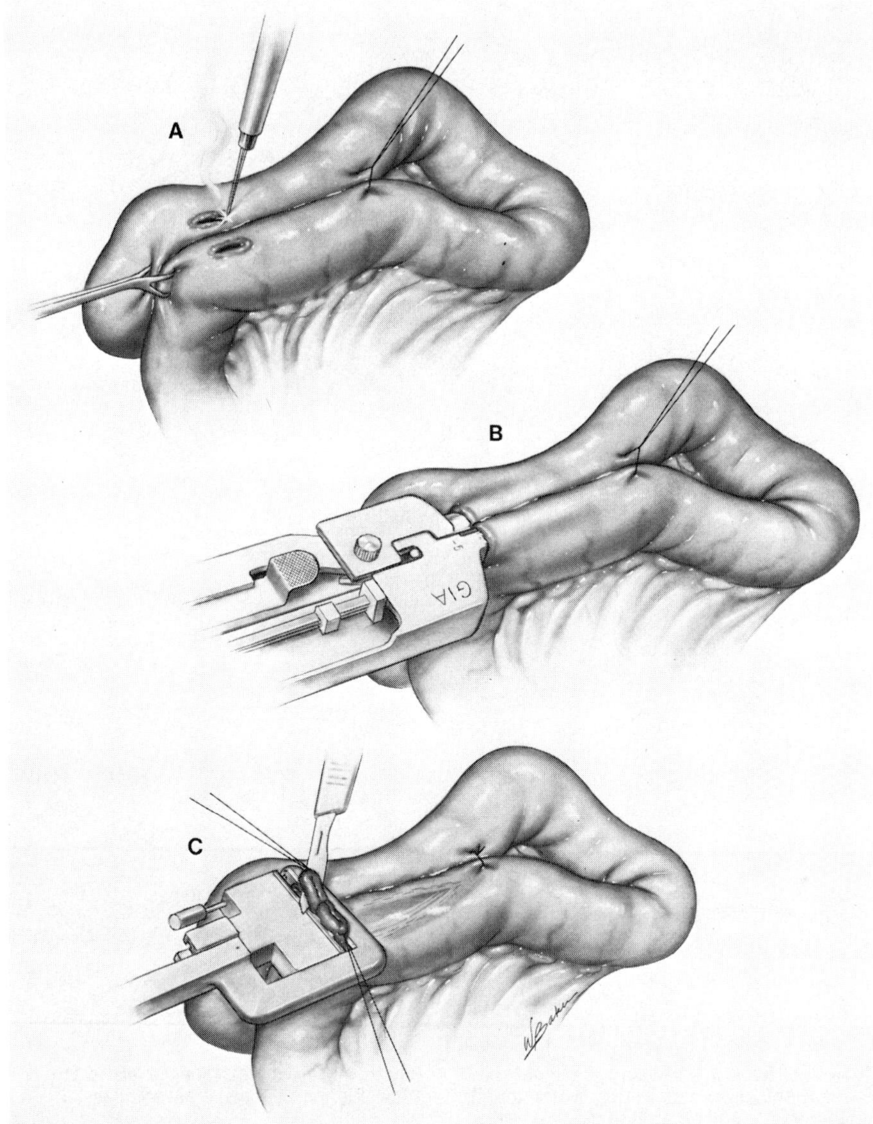

Fig V–4.—Enteroenterostomy in continuity for omega loop. **A,** the two loops of bowel being held in position with a Babcock clamp or stay sutures, the appropriate stab wounds are made with a fine needle-tipped electric cautery. **B,** the blades of the GIA™ instrument inserted well away from the mesentery, the anastomosis is created. **C,** the opening left by the action of the GIA™ instrument is closed mucosa-to-mucosa, taking the precautions mentioned in Figure V–3. With antecolic gastroenterostomy and an undivided stomach, the obligatory Braun's loop is created in this way. Although for esophagojejunal and choledochojejunal anastomoses we prefer to use a Roux-Y loop, the omega loop shown here can be used there as well.

This technique of lateral anastomosis is used, with variations, in almost every portion of the gastrointestinal tract. The anastomosis itself is serosa-to-serosa, but the staple closure of the openings made for insertion of the GIA™ instrument is mucosa-to-mucosa and is not reinforced. At times, but quite infrequently, the situation of the GIA™ opening in the two viscera is such that one cannot conveniently apply the TA™ instrument. We then close this opening with manual sutures.

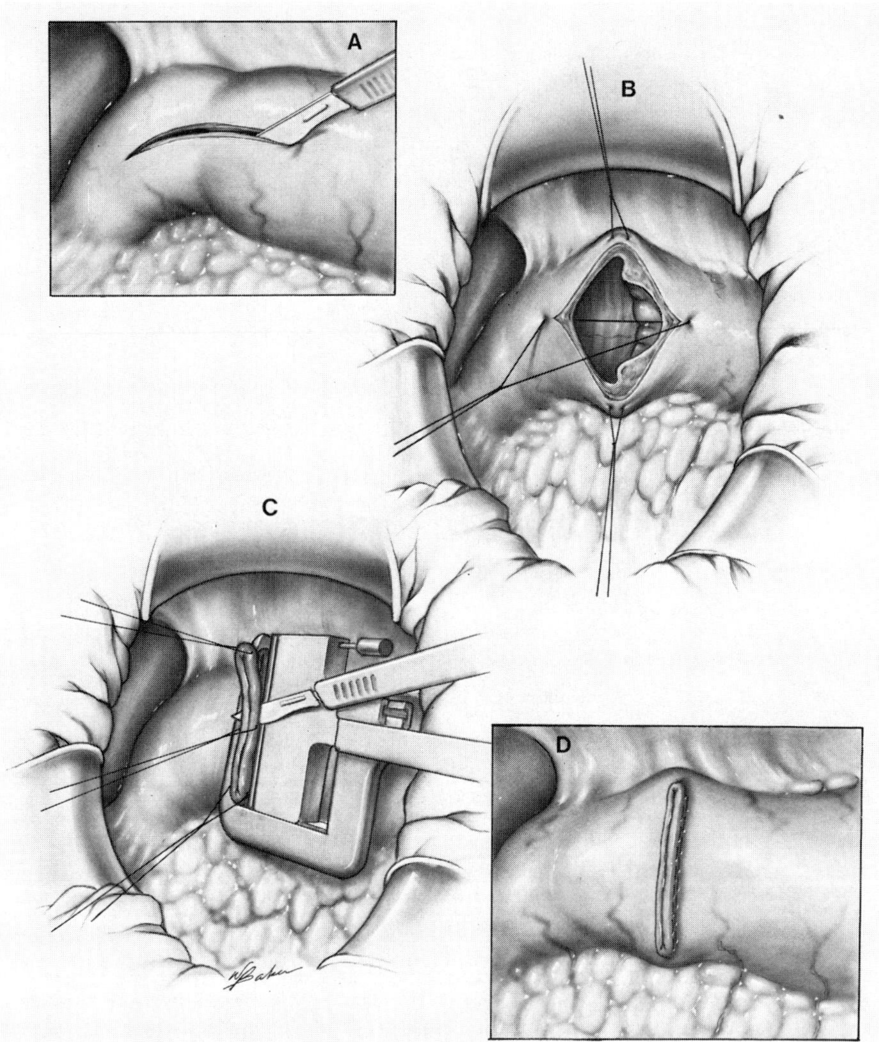

Fig V–5.—Heineke-Mikulicz pyloroplasty. **A,** the usual longitudinal incision is made across the pylorus. **B,** traction sutures transform the longitudinal incision into a transverse opening. **C,** the TA 55™ instrument is placed around the lips of the opening. As in all such mucosa-to-mucosa closures, operator and first assistant must agree that serosa and mucosa are seen completely around the circumference of the closure, so as to be certain that there is a stapling of full thickness of the viscus. The staples having been fired, the tissue excess beyond the instrument is cut away before the instrument is opened. **D,** the completed pyloroplasty. No additional sutures are required.

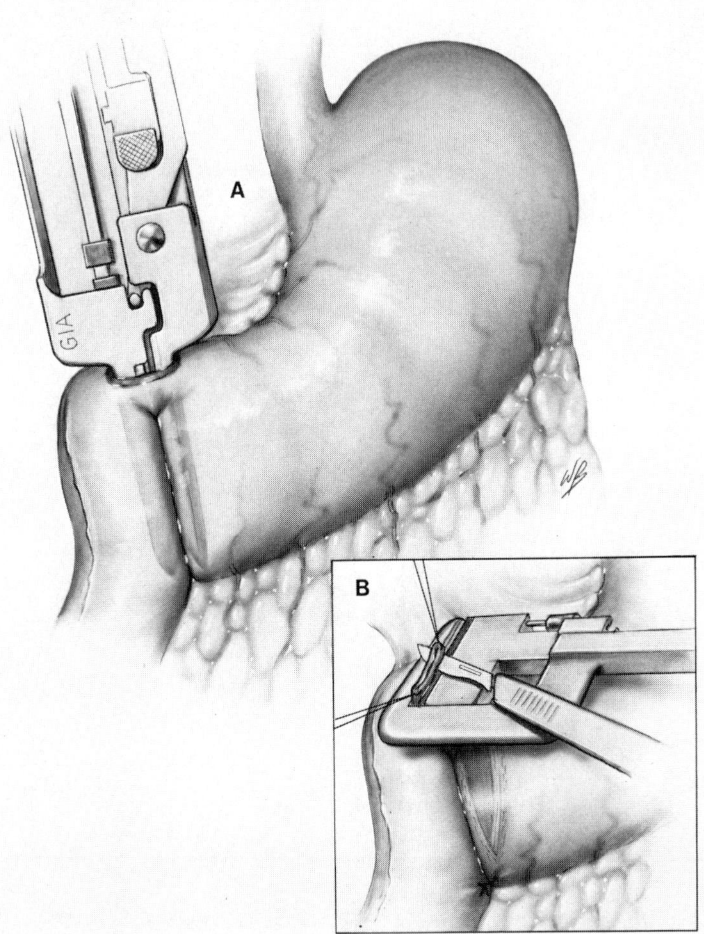

Fig V–6.—Finney pyloroplasty. **A,** the blades of the GIA™ instrument have been inserted through an opening in the pylorus, one blade into the duodenum and one into the stomach. The fatty tissue between duodenum and stomach has been depressed with a Kelly clamp while the instrument is being locked, insuring serosa-to-serosa apposition of the two viscera without any interposition of fat or vessels. **B,** the GIA™ instrument having been fired, a long pyloroplasty, or gastroduodenostomy, has been fashioned with a double staggered row of staples on each side of the opening. The lips of the stab wound made for the GIA™ instrument are held up with sutures or clamps, the TA™ instrument applied far enough down to insure a full-thickness stapling of the bowel, and the excess tissue beyond the instrument cut away. A single suture is placed to unite stomach and duodenum, below the anastomosis, as shown, in order to provide support against possible pull by a dilated stomach.

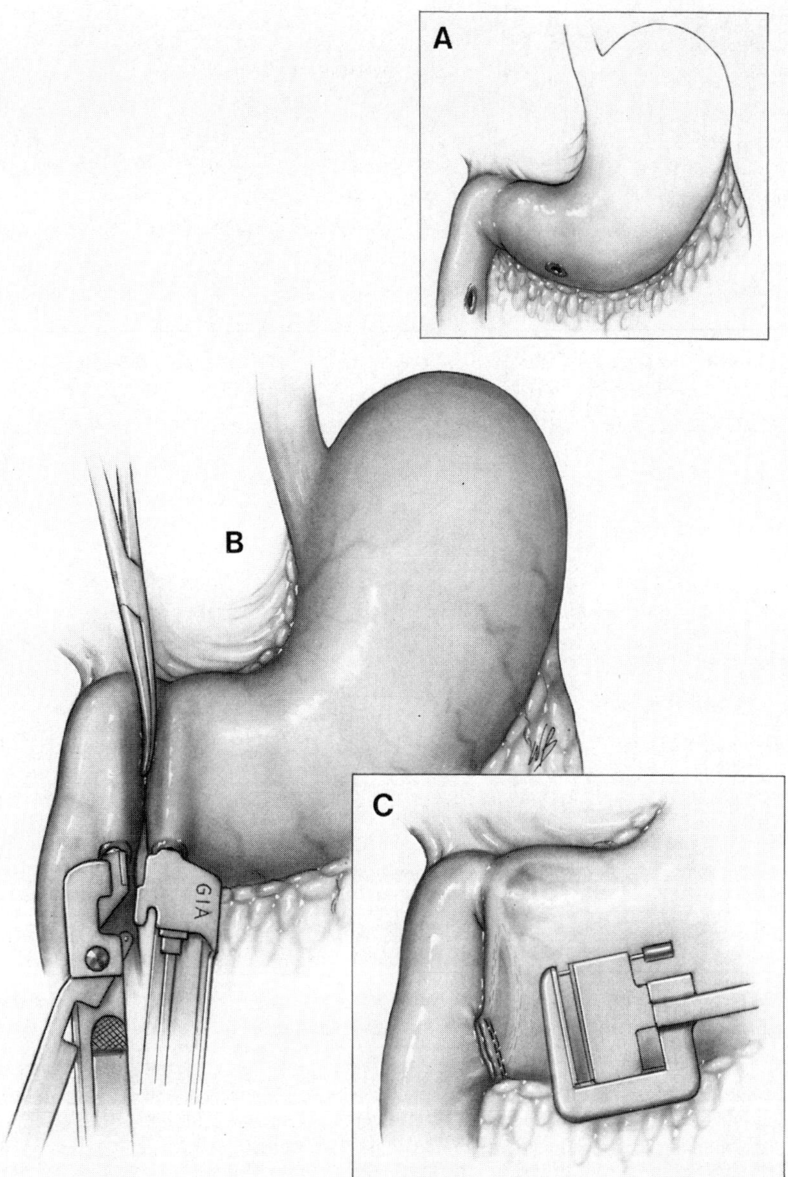

Fig V–7.—Jaboulay pyloroplasty. **A,** appropriate cautery openings are made in the duodenum and stomach. **B,** the GIA™ instrument is placed and the duodenum and stomach are approximated. A Kelly clamp is used to depress the fat and vessels out of the way while the blades of the GIA™ instrument are locked. **C,** the single opening, left by the action of the GIA™ instrument, is closed mucosa-to-mucosa with the TA 55™ instrument, securely anchoring the lower corner of the gastroduodenostomy. It is not material whether the upper end of the anastomosis fuses with the pyloric lumen or terminates a little below it.

The choice of technique of pyloroplasty depends on preference and on the nature of local disease. The Finney and Jaboulay techniques are readily used even in the face of the sort of duodenal ulcer disease that might make the Heineke-Mikulicz pyloroplasty difficult.

The use of Auto Suture® instruments for the various varieties of pyloroplasty was reported by Rinecker in 1975 (Heineke-Mikulicz, Finney, and Aust-Willenegger [transverse oval excision and transverse closure]), Fortin, Poulin, and Leclerc, in 1979 (Finney), and others.

Nance of New Orleans, in 1978, presented before the Southern Surgical Association (Nance, 1979) an EEA™ technique for gastroduodenostomy inserting the instrument through a gastrotomy.

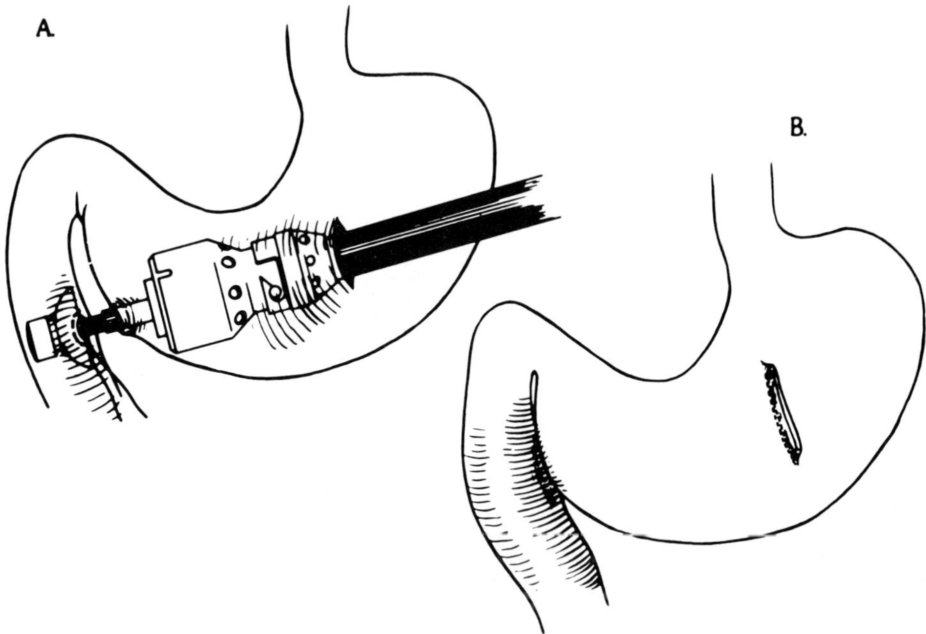

Fig V–8.—Nance's EEA™ Jaboulay gastroduodenostomy technique (1979). **A,** the EEA™ instrument is inserted through a gastrotomy, the threaded rod passing out through the greater curvature of the prepyloric antrum. The anvil-carrying nose cone is screwed on and slipped into the duodenum inside a pursestring, the pursestring tied, and the anastomosis created with the EEA™ instrument. The gastrotomy is closed with a TA 55™ instrument. **B,** completed anastomosis and closed gastrotomy. (From F.C. Nance, *Annals of Surgery,* 1979, used by permission.)

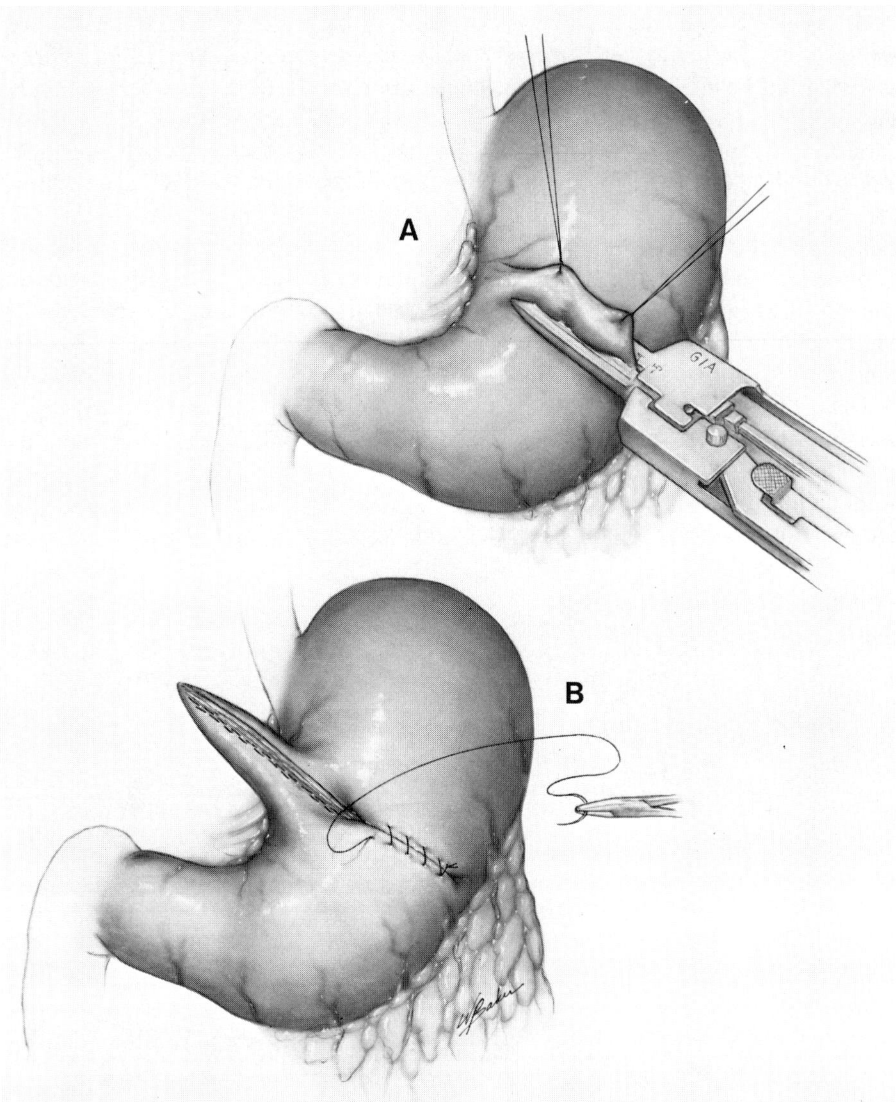

Fig V–9.—Janeway gastrostomy **A,** the portion of the stomach to be used for the construction of the mucosa-lined gastrostomy is held up with sutures or Babcock clamps and the GIA™ instrument used to divide the tube from the stomach, simultaneously stapling both the tube and anterior gastric wall as seen in **B. B,** we normally reinforce at least the gastric portion of the suture lines, fearing to trust the shorter staples of the GIA™ instrument on a double thickness of stomach wall. As frequently as not, the staple line on the tube has not been inverted. However, we recommend a reinforcing suture placed as a running over-and-over whipstitch behind the staple line. The tube then is brought through the abdominal incision or a stab wound, its tip amputated, and the mucosa sutured to the skin edges. The circulation of the stomach is such that one can make the base of the tube at either the greater or lesser curvature, or direct the tube longitudinally, making the base either proximal or distal.

This type of gastrostomy is preferred for neurologic patients and others who will need permanent gastrostomies. The mucosa-lined tube will not close off if the catheter has been withdrawn and not replaced whereas conventional gastrostomies begin to close off their sinus tracts within hours.

The Janeway gastrostomy had been used clinically by us for some time when Gerald Moss of Troy, New York, at the Rensselaer Polytechnic Institute, described his successful use in 50 dogs (Moss, 1972). Our first animal experiments of this kind, not reported, date back to the 1960s, when we did report the creation of Heidenhain pouches for experimental work in gastric secretion (Ravitch, Rivarola, and VanGrov, 1966).

In 1974 (Webster, Carey, and Ravitch, 1975), we presented our clinical experience with 29 tube gastrostomies, mostly in elderly patients requiring permanent gastrostomy for neurologic disorders. There were no deaths attributed to the gastrostomy, no suture line leaks, and no peritonitis. There were two partial wound dehiscences requiring secondary closure, no bleeding, and no discharge of feedings on the abdominal wall.

A more recent study of our experience (Cobb, 1981) evaluated the 25 tube gastrostomies performed in 1980. Once more, all operations were under local anesthesia. There were no intra-abdominal leaks or infections, no wound infections, and no deaths attributable to the gastrostomy, but three patients had postoperative upper gastrointestinal bleeding, one requiring transfusion. The source of bleeding was not sought and in these patients might well have been from stress ulceration.

→

Fig V–10.—Gastrectomy and Billroth II reconstruction. **A,** the omental vessels are being stapled and divided with the LDS™ instrument, each operation of which fires two staples and divides the tissue between them. **B,** the TA 30™ or TA 55™ instrument has been slipped under the duodenum, the duodenum stapled and divided with a knife on the edge of the instrument. The mucosa-to-mucosa closure is safe without further reinforcement. The greatest hazard probably lies in the possibility that one is transecting the duodenum just proximal to an ulcer eroding into the pancreas, and that manipulation with the instrument unwittingly cracks open the ulcer posteriorly, without discovery. We understand that many surgeons use the GIA™ instrument for transecting and stapling the duodenum. We prefer the TA™ instrument. **C,** the stomach has been stapled proximally and is being transected with the scalpel on the edge of the TA 90™ instrument. Unless the stomach is unusually thick, one of us prefers to use the blue cartridge with the 3.5-mm staples, which are better for hemostasis. In this and in all other situations using the TA™ instruments on the gastrointestinal tract, bleeding from the stapled visceral edges rarely is more than momentary. Occasionally, a single spurter will require a silk suture and extremely rarely will a portion of the closure have to be sutured over or inverted. Vigorous bleeding from the cut edge of the stomach or bowel almost always turns out to be due to the fact that mesentery was drawn up into the clamp and a vessel transected. The TA™ instruments will not secure omental or mesenteric vessels with any degree of safety. *(continued)*

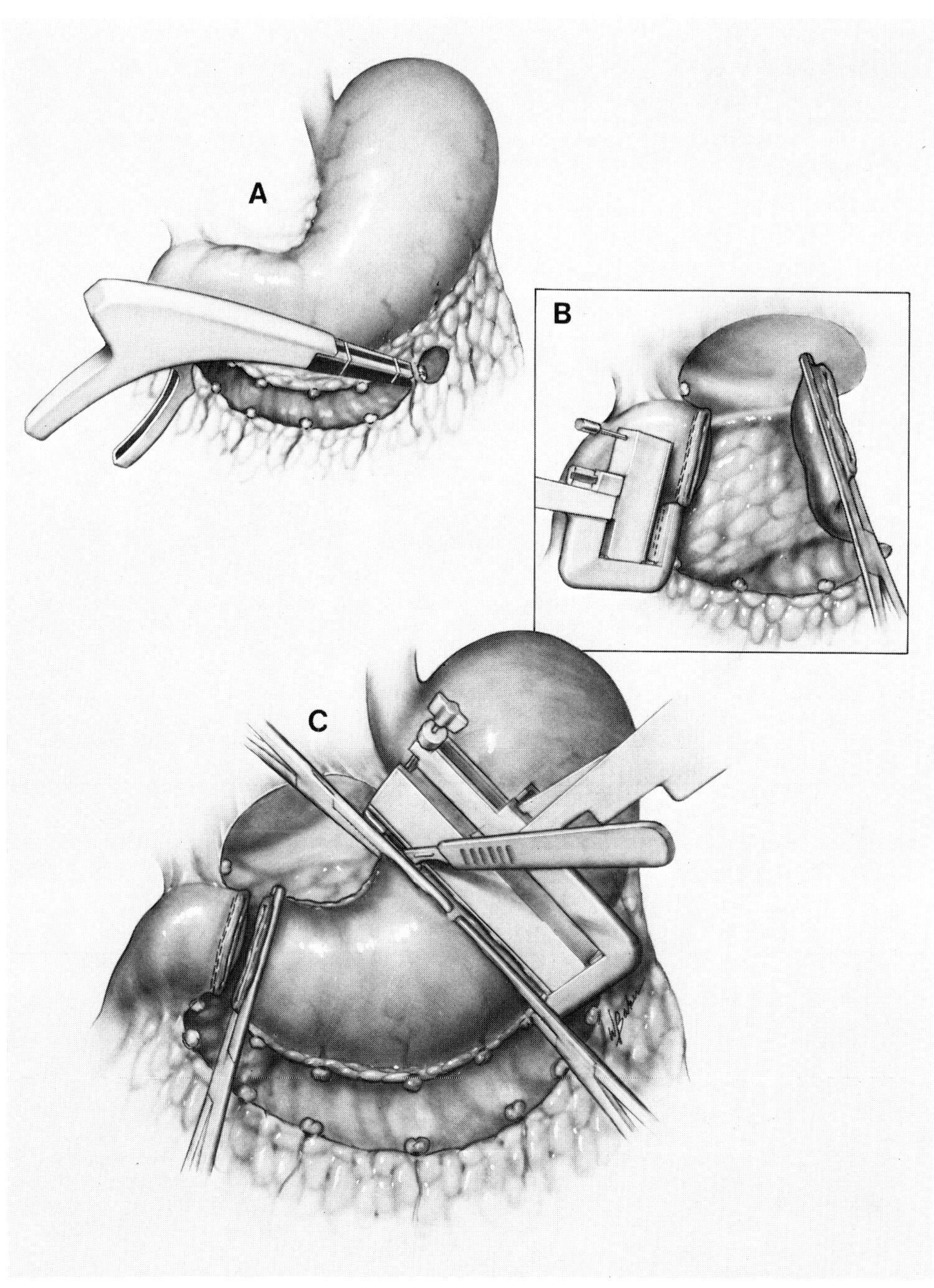

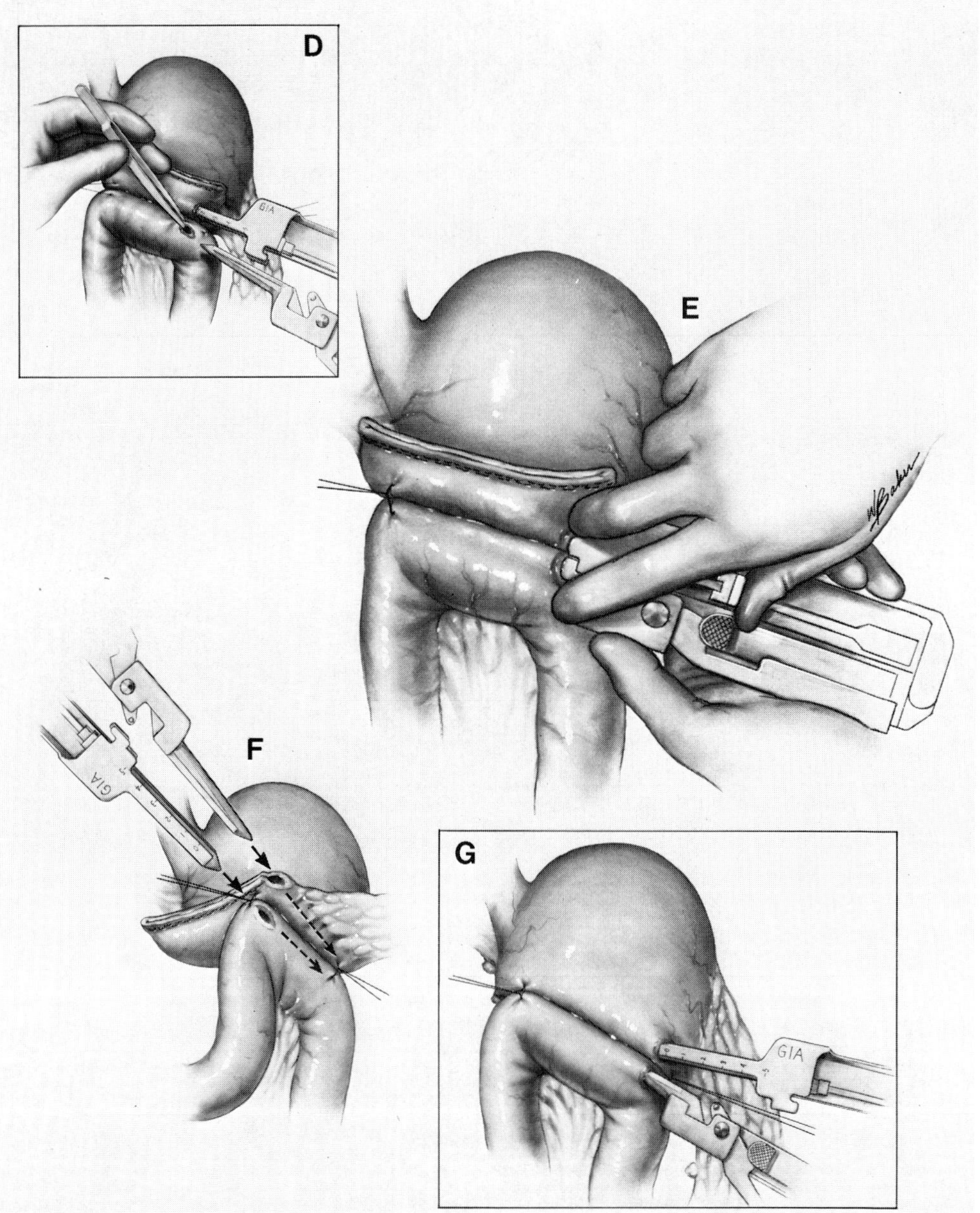

Fig V–10 (cont.).—D and **E,** gastroenterostomy on the posterior gastric wall, parallel to the gastric transection. The jejunum and the stomach are apposed with stay sutures or Babcock clamps and the GIA™ blades inserted through cautery-made stab wounds. The length of the anastomosis can be determined by the depth to which the calibrated limbs are inserted. **F,** alternatively, the axis of the gastroenterostomy can run longitudinally in the stomach, and we often insert the gastric limb of the GIA™ instrument through the cutaway greater-curvature end of the gastric staple line. **G,** if one prefers, the gastroenterostomy can be performed on the anterior wall of the stomach. *(continued)*

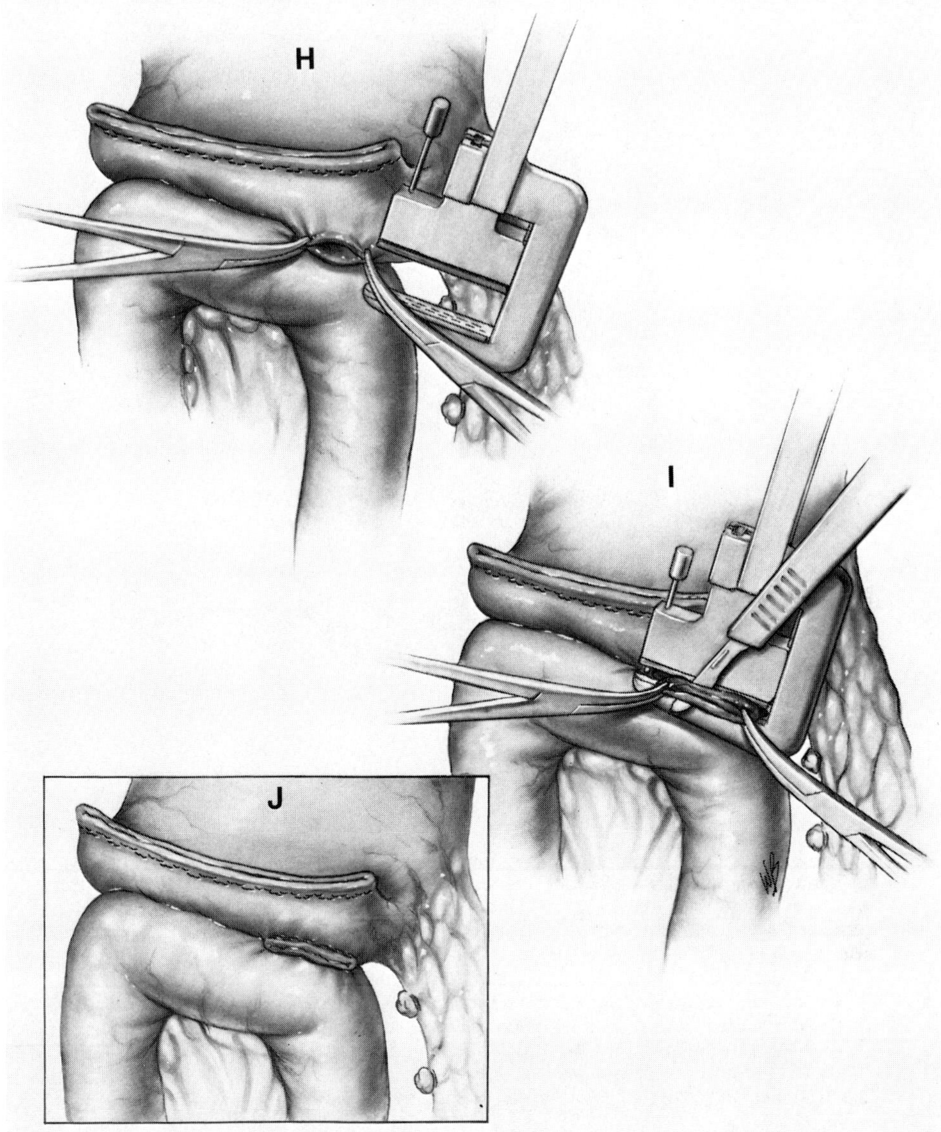

Fig V–10 (cont.).—H, as the GIA™ instrument is withdrawn, in this case from the gastroenterostomy being performed as in **D** and **E,** the suture line is inspected to be sure that there is no bleeding. In the uncommon event that there is significant bleeding that does not stop in a moment or two, the anastomotic edges within are whipped over with 4–0 catgut. The two GIA™ staple lines are held apart with fine clamps and the TA™ instrument passed behind them to be certain to staple a full thickness of stomach above and jejunum below. **I,** the lips of the gastrojejunal opening beyond the staple line are cut away from the stapler. **J,** the completed gastroenterostomy. Not infrequently, the stomach is anchored to the jejunum on the lesser curvature side with a single suture to take any possible strain off the stapled anastomosis and closure. Although questions often are raised about the distance that the GIA™ staple line must be from the gastric transection staple line, as in **E** and **G,** in point of fact, we never have seen a leak or necrosis arising from lack of blood supply to the distal end of the stomach from this cause, and generally consider 2 cm a safe distance. We have had a communication from Dr. T.K. Hunt (1981) of the University of California, San Francisco describing perforation in the strip of stomach between cut end and gastroenterostomy.   *(continued)*

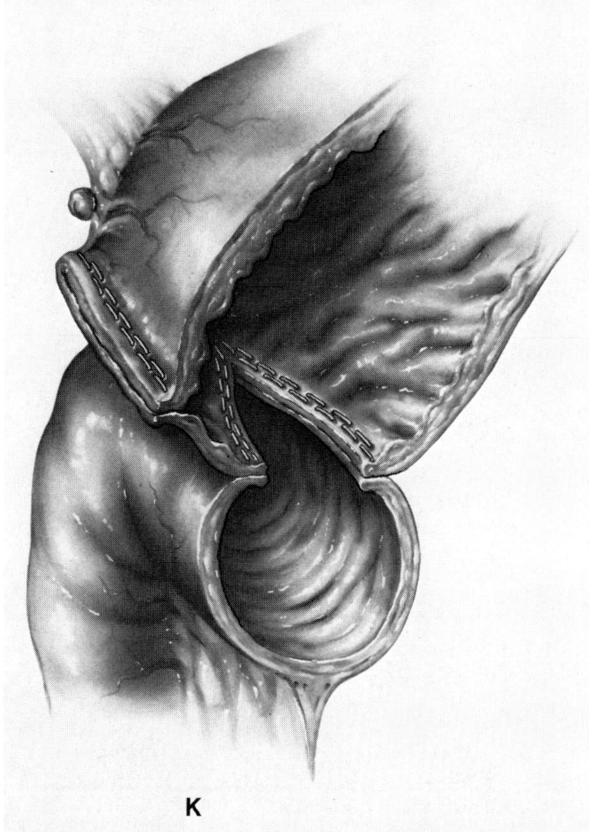

K

Fig V–10 (cont.).—K, cutaway view of the GIA™ stapled gastroenterostomy made parallel to the stapled gastric closure after Billroth II resection. The gastric and jejunal edges are viable beyond the staple lines. The TA™ closure of the GIA™ opening should be across the end of the GIA™ anastomosis widely separating the GIA™ staple lines at the base, as shown. On the other hand, if the TA™ closure of the GIA™ opening is made so that the TA™ line of staples is at right angles to the GIA™ staple lines, the GIA™ wound edges will be held approximated and there is some danger that these edges will heal together. This has been recorded by Elliott (Elliott, Albertazzi, and Danto 1977) and we know directly of two such occurrences in ileocolic anastomoses, resulting in severe stenosis. (**A–J** from M.M. Ravitch and F.M. Steichen, *Abdominal Operations,* 7th ed. New York, Appleton-Century-Crofts, 1979, Rodney Maingot [ed.], used by permission. **K** from T.E. Elliott, V.J. Albertazzi, and L.A. Danto, *American Journal of Surgery,* 1977, used by permission.)

The general discussion of the reported clinical experience with stapling in gastric surgery appears after Figure V–18.

Roux, of course, first described his Y-anastomosis for the gastroenterostomy in a Billroth II and the operation seems to be in the process of a revival in both primary and secondary reconstructions, whether with the linear or circular anastomosis instruments.

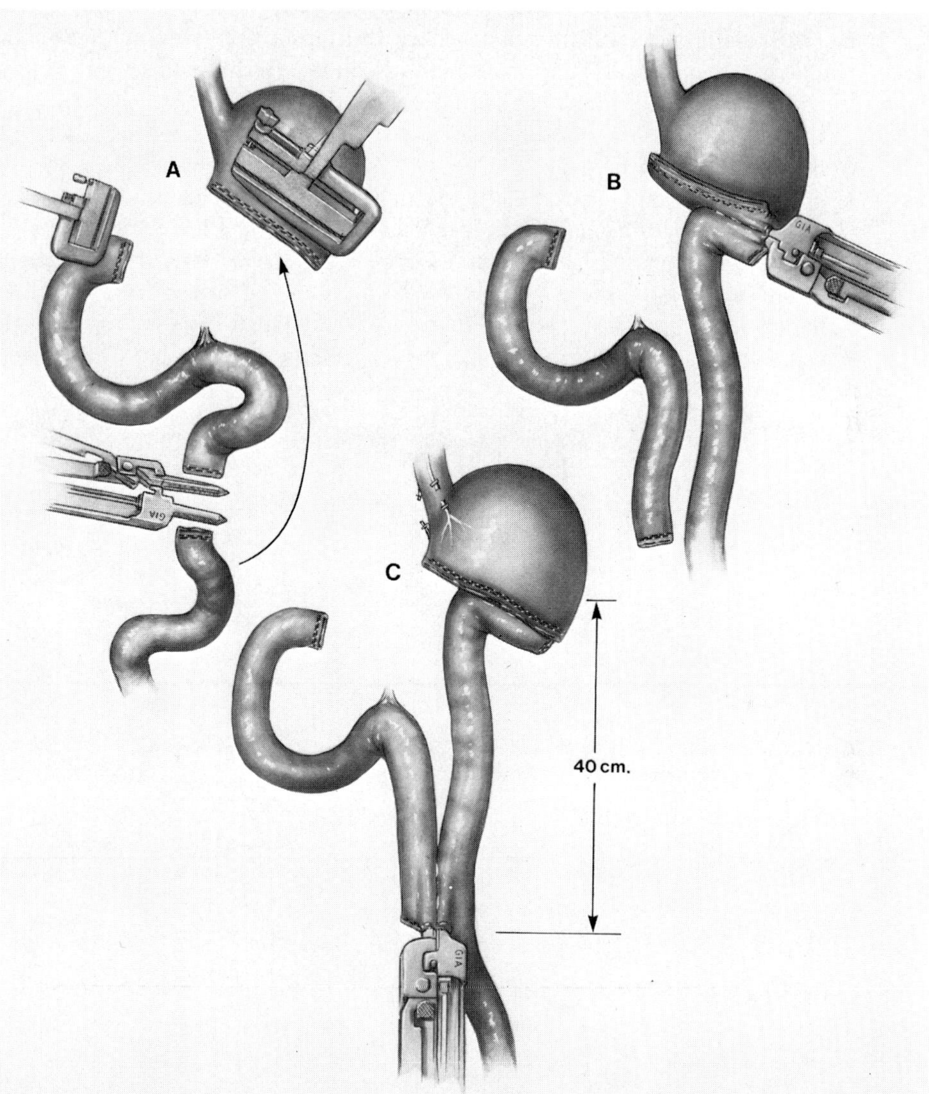

Fig V–11.—Gastrectomy—primary—Billroth II with Roux-Y. **A,** Stomach and duodenum are stapled and transected as in Figure V–10, and the jejunum divided with the GIA™ instrument. **B,** the proximal end of the distal jejunal loop is anastomosed to a convenient point on the stomach with the familiar GIA™ and TA™ technique (see Fig V–10**D,E,H,I,J**). **C,** the distal end of the proximal jejunum now is anastomosed to the distal jejunal limb by the end-to-side Roux-en-Y technique (see Fig VII–1**E**).

Welter, Turbelin, and Charlier (1981) of Luxembourg have described a technique developed by Welter, in which the gastrojejunostomy is performed before removing the gastric specimen. After the duodenum has been stapled and transected, the gastric specimen is used to exert gentle traction and to gain easy exposure of the posterior aspect of the stomach for the gastrojejunostomy. A single application of the TA 90™ instrument excludes the GIA™ stab wound and closes off the gastric remnant.

We have utilized this principle (stapling and resecting the specimen *after* completing the anastomosis) for some time in esophageal reconstruction (see Fig VI–10) and in the modified functional end-to-end anastomosis (see Fig VIII–5), but had not envisioned the useful application to gastrectomy here described.

Alain Charlier (1981), in his doctoral thesis, reviewed 50 patients operated on by Welter, using this technique, from January 4, 1973 to December 31, 1980. Of these, 33 patients had benign ulcers (11 gastric, five pyloric, 16 duodenal, and one marginal) and 17 patients had malignancies (15 adenocarcinoma, one leiomyoblastoma, and one malignant lymphoma). Eight operations were done as emergencies. Two patients had stapler-related complications—one duodenal leak, closed successfully with one suture on the day after operation, and one stenosis of the efferent loop due to faulty construction of the original anastomosis, requiring reoperation on the twenty-fifth postoperative day.

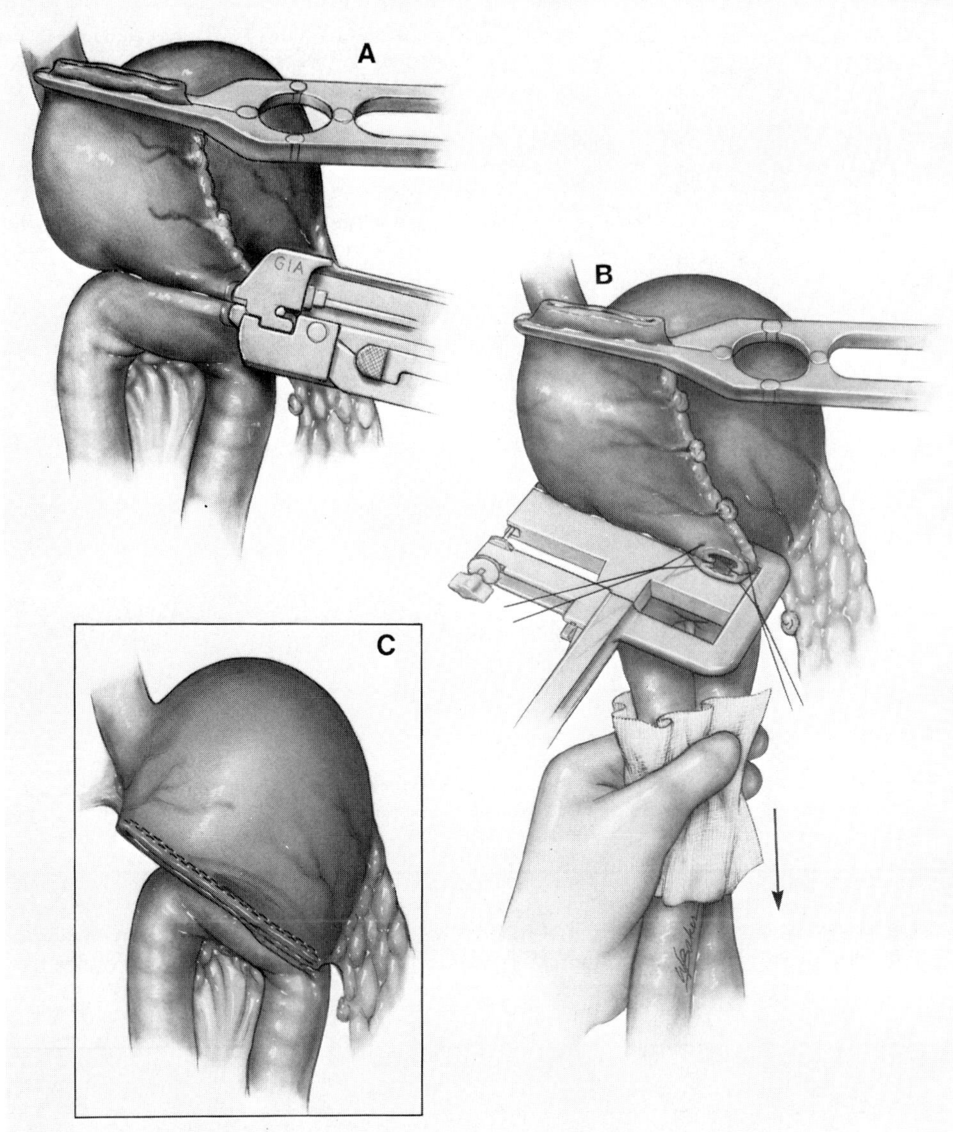

Fig V–12.—Billroth II with Welter gastrojejunostomy. **A,** The gastrojejunostomy is performed at the elected level on the posterior surface of the stomach near the greater curvature. The duodenum already has been stapled. **B,** after removal of the GIA™ instrument, and assurance of hemostasis in the gastroenterostomy, the TA 90™ stapler is placed so as to surround the now common GIA™ stab wound consisting anteriorly of the anterior gastric wall and posteriorly of the posterior jejunal lip, near the greater curvature. The TA 90™ instrument includes also both walls of the gastric remnant beyond, to the lesser curvature. As the TA 90™ instrument is closed, care is taken to include the two lips of the now common GIA™ stab wound, so as to have 2 mm of tissue protrude beyond the jaws of the TA 90™ stapler. At the level of the future gastric stump, great care is taken not to include other structures, pads, etc. in the TA 90™ closure. Including an excessive amount of the lips of the anastomotic opening would result in a stenosis; therefore, at the time of the TA 90™ application and closure, gentle traction is exerted on the afferent and efferent jejunal loops so as to make them conform to the legs of a pair of pants. Following closure with the TA 90™ instrument, the excess tissue—e.g., the posterior lip of the jejunal stab wound and the anterior lip of the gastric stab wound along the greater curvature, as well as the distal stomach—is excised, using the TA 90™ jaw as a guide, thus delivering the specimen. **C,** after completion of the TA 90™ suture line and excision of the gastric specimen, the closure is composed of anterior gastric wall to jejunal loop wall toward the greater curvature and anterior to posterior gastric wall toward the lesser curvature.

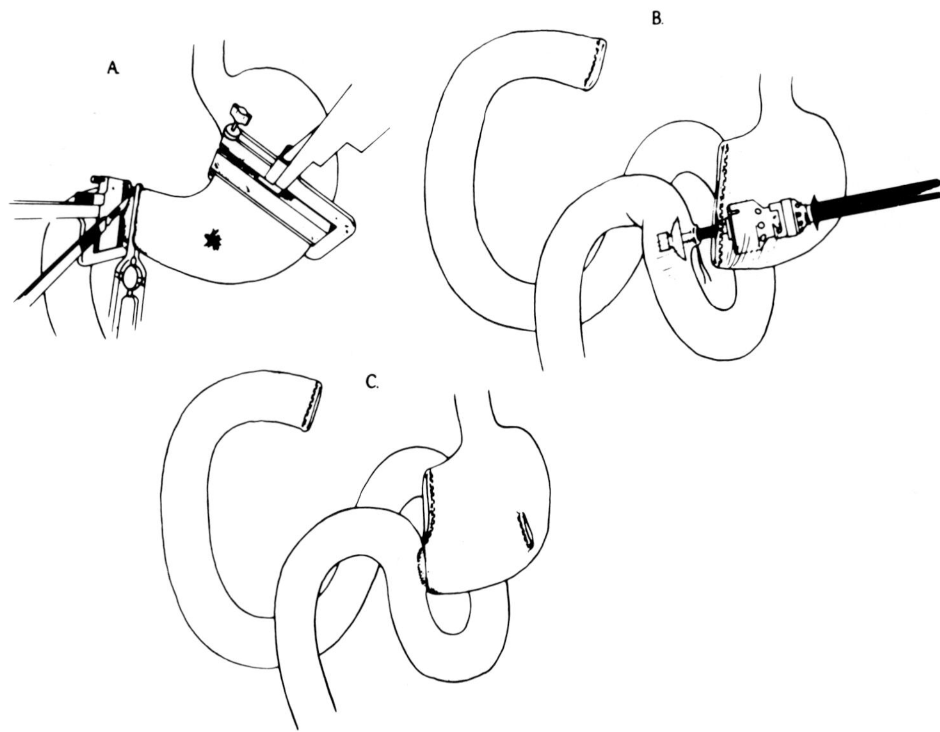

Fig V–13.—Nance's EEA™ Billroth II reconstruction (1979). Billroth II gastrectomy. **A,** the duodenal stump is closed with a TA 55™ staple line. The proximal stomach is closed with the TA 90™ stapler. **B,** the EEA™ instrument has been inserted through a proximal gastrotomy, the central spindle passed through the posterior gastric wall, and the nose cone screwed on and slipped into the jejunum through a pursestring. **C,** completed anastomosis. The gastrotomy has been closed with a TA 55™ staple line. The EEA™ instrument could have been inserted through the pyloric end of the stomach, the anastomosis performed, and the specimen then amputated, avoiding the need for a gastrotomy. In any case, we are not quite ready to accept the intersecting EEA™ and TA™ suture lines, fearing disruption by the EEA™ knife, although our experiments in progress thus far support the safety of that technique. (From F.G. Nance, *Annals of Surgery,* 1979, used by permission.)

Nance, in 1978 before the Southern Surgical Association (Nance, 1979) presented, in a wide variety of uses of the EEA^{TM} stapler, a gastroenterostomy performed with it in the Billroth II reconstruction. The instrument is inserted through a gastrotomy and out close to the TA 90^{TM} staple line, a technique about which we still have some reservations, despite its successful use by Nance and by Knight and Griffen (1980) and others, the problem being the possible disruption of the TA^{TM} staple line by the knife of the EEA^{TM} instrument. Given Knight's continued success with this technique in anterior rectal anastomoses (see Fig IX–13), it may be safer than we thought. We are studying the problem in the laboratory and thus far the safety of the technique seems to be supported.

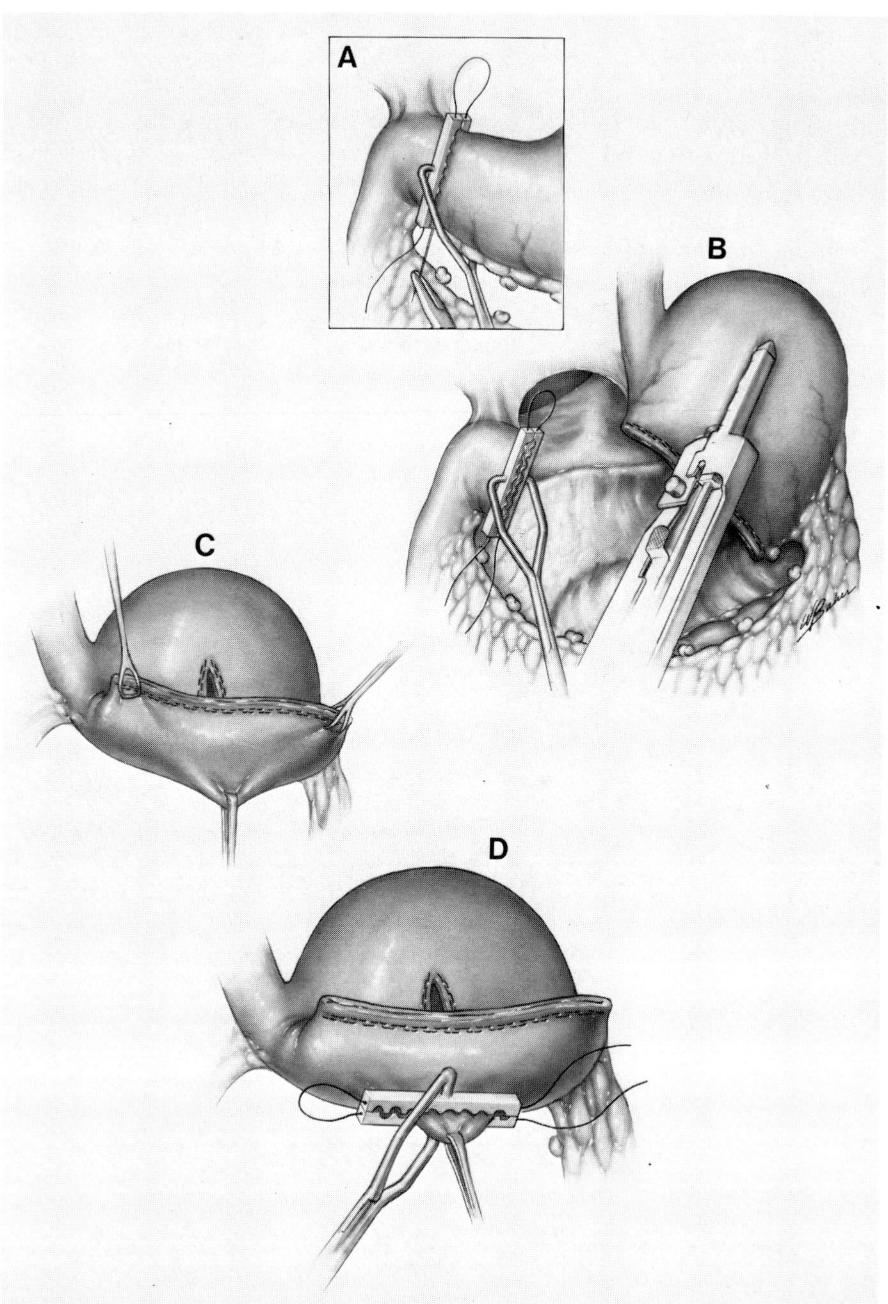

Fig V–14.—Gastrectomy and Billroth I reconstruction—alternative techniques. I—with EEA™ instrument inserted through gastrotomy. **A,** the duodenum is transected and either a heavy monofilament prolene suture whipped over the edge for a pursestring or the special modified Furniss pursestring clamp applied. The jaws of that clamp (shown in **B**) are such that a straight needle passed down the appropriate passage on one blade of the clamp and back the other seizes only one wall of the enclosed portion of the gastrointestinal tract on each side, so that as the clamp is withdrawn, a purse-string suture has been properly placed close to the level of division of the bowel, which is made on the edge of the clamp. **B,** the stomach in this case has been resected and stapled shut and a PGIA™ gastrotomy is being made in the proximal gastric pouch. **C,** the posterior wall of the stomach, through which the threaded rod of the EEA™ instrument will be passed, is pulled out. **D,** the tit of stomach is seized in the pursestring clamp, a pursestring inserted, and the tit cut away on the edge of the clamp.

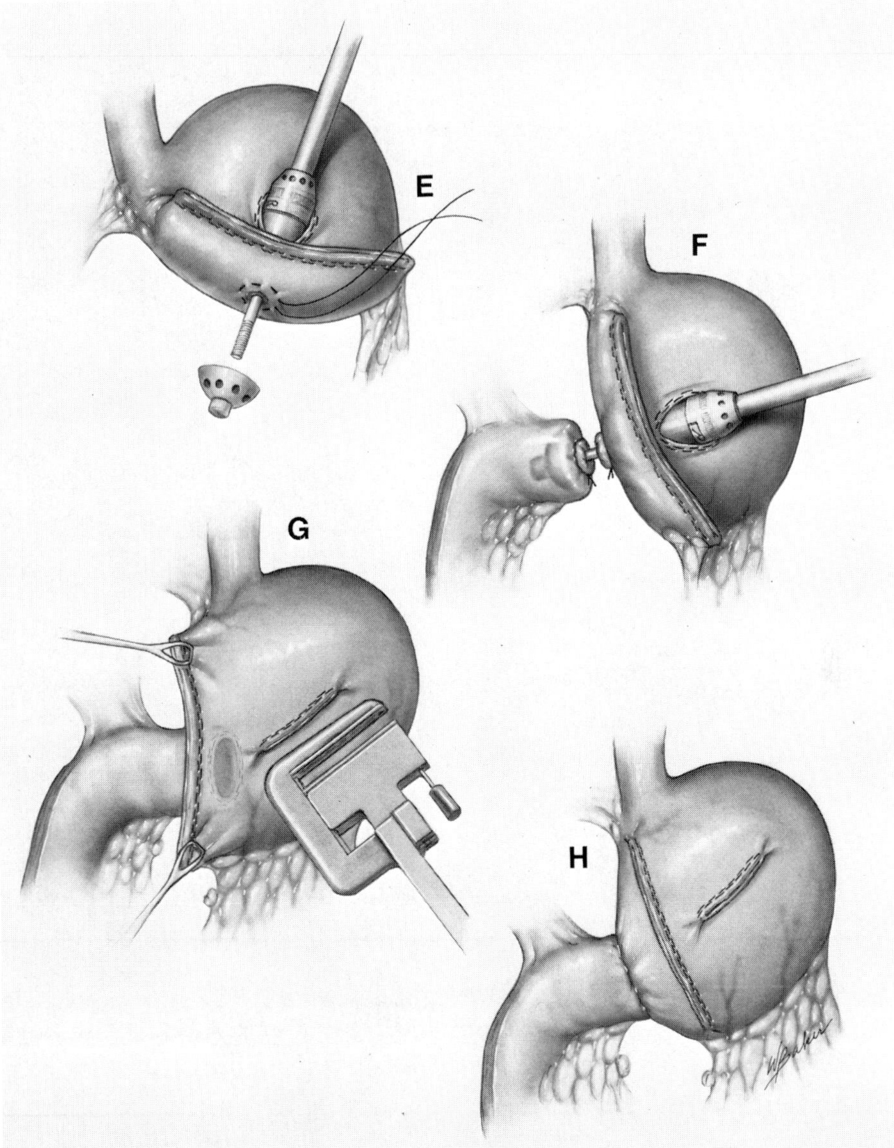

Fig V–14 (cont.).—E, the EEA™ instrument with the cartridge mounted on the center rod, but without the nose cone, is passed into the stomach through the anterior gastrotomy and the center rod passed out through the pursestring suture around the posterior gastrotomy. In point of fact, one can merely make a small stab wound in the posterior gastric wall on the center rod as it is pushed forward, without or with a manual pursestring suture, although the suture provides extra assurance. The nose cone containing the anvil for shaping the staples now is screwed onto the tip of the center rod. **F,** the nose cone has been passed into the duodenum and duodenal and gastric pursestrings tightly tied. Turning the wing nut on the EEA™ handle to the right approximates stomach and duodenum to the required degree, and squeezing the handles of the instrument then puts in a double, staggered, circular row of staples. The circular knife just inside the staples simultaneously cuts out the double diaphragm, with the two pursestrings, completing the anastomosis. As in all uses of the EEA™ instrument, one must examine the two rings of tissue to be sure that they are complete and unbroken. Care is taken to note the orientation of the instrument and that of any deficiency found in the ring or doughnut, so that the portion of the anastomosis in question may be specifically checked. **G,** the anastomosis is shown in translucency. The lips of the gastrotomy have been closed mucosa-to-mucosa with the TA™ instrument. **H,** interestingly enough, as the stomach readjusts, the final result is as shown, the gastroduodenostomy being at the most distal portion of the gastric remnant. (From M.M. Ravitch and F.M. Steichen, *Surgery of the Alimentary Tract,* 2d ed. Philadelphia, W.B. Saunders Co., 1981, R.T. Shackelford and G.D. Zuidema, [eds.], used by permission.)

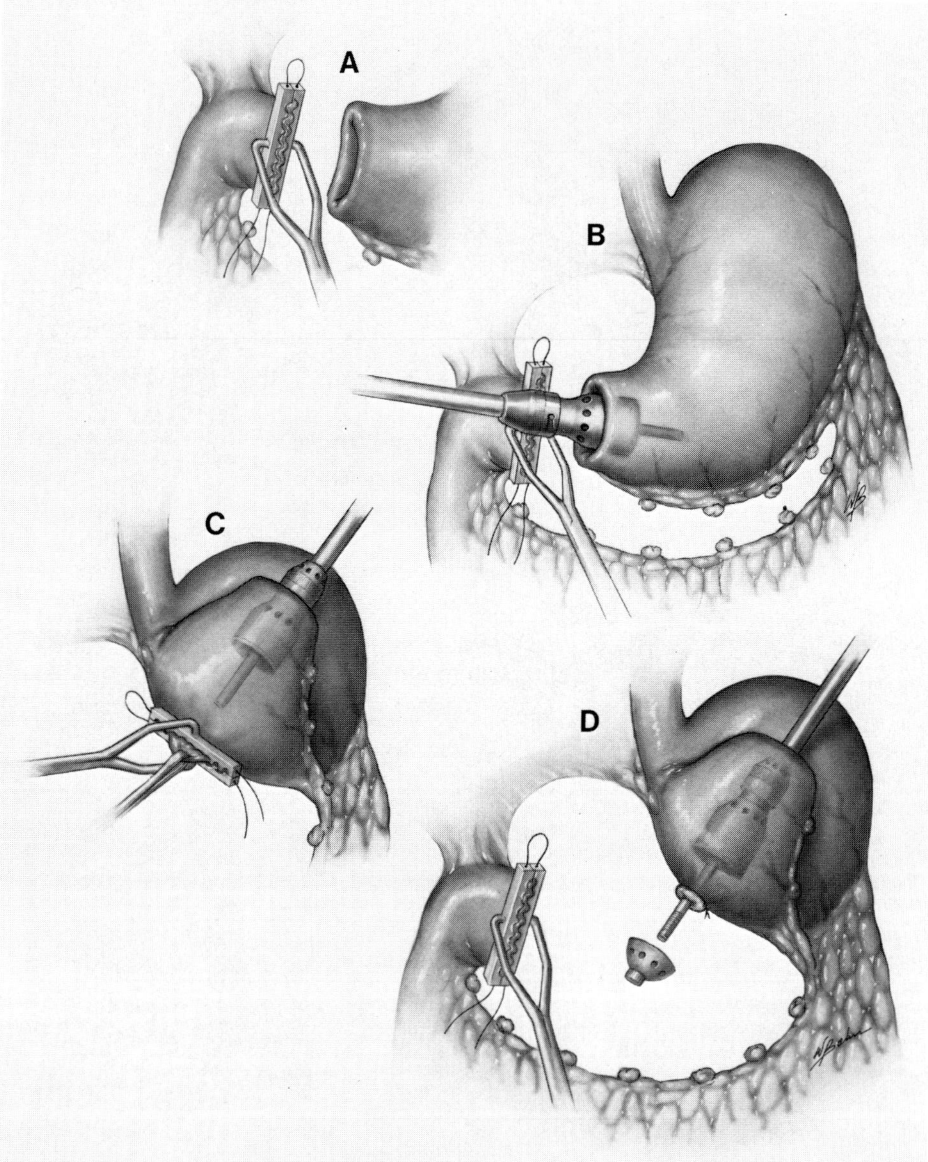

Fig V–15.—Gastrectomy and Billroth I reconstruction—alternative techniques. II—with EEA™ instrument inserted through open end of stomach. Technique of L.B. Pemberton, presented before the American College of Surgeons Clinical Congress in 1979. **A,** the duodenum is divided on the pursestring clamp and the end of the stomach is left open. **B,** the EEA™ instrument armed with the staple cartridge, but without the anvil-nose cone, is inserted into the stomach through the open pyloric end, the stomach having been freed from its vascular supply for the distance required for the gastrectomy. **C** and **D,** the center rod of the EEA™ instrument is passed through the posterior wall of the stomach, the pursestring (as in Fig V–14**D** and **E**) made with the pursestring instrument, or manually, around the stab wound, or on the center rod simply pushed through a tight-fitting perforation of the posterior gastric wall. The nose cone is threaded onto the center rod.

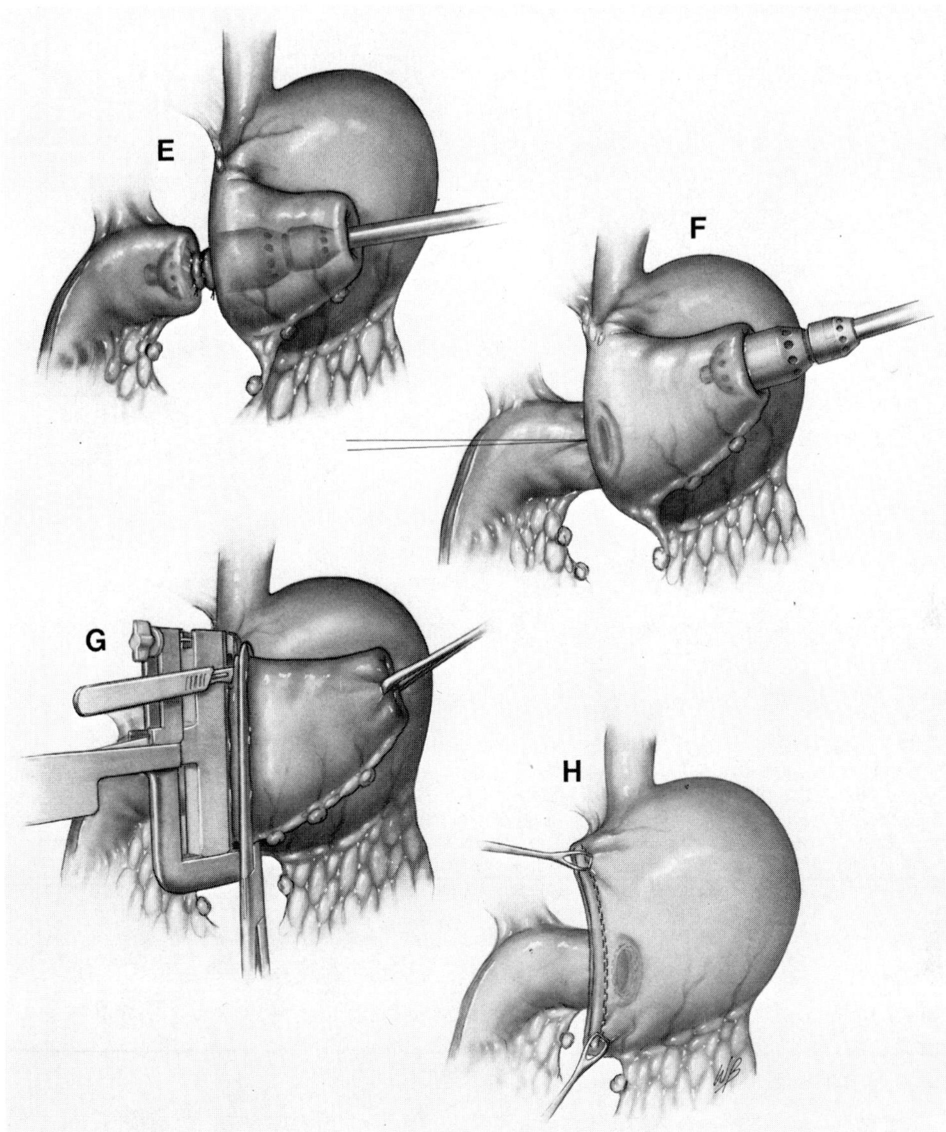

Fig V–15 (cont.).—E, the nose cone is placed in the duodenum and the pursestring suture tied. The anvil and nose cone are approximated and the instrument fired, producing **F,** the completed anastomosis. The EEA™ instrument is withdrawn. **G,** the TA 90™ instrument is applied to staple and transect the devascularized distal portion of the stomach, delivering the specimen and leaving **H,** the completed reconstruction. In general, in using the EEA™ instrument, we prefer to use techniques that will not, as in Fig V–14, require for introduction of the instrument an additional gastrotomy or enterotomy, which subsequently will have to be closed, creating an additional suture line that must heal. The pursestring instrument is ingenious and extremely quick. The over-and-over whipstitch (Fig IX–3B) is a little slower but more secure, although care must be taken to see that each bite secures a full thickness of the bowel and that the bites are not too far separated.

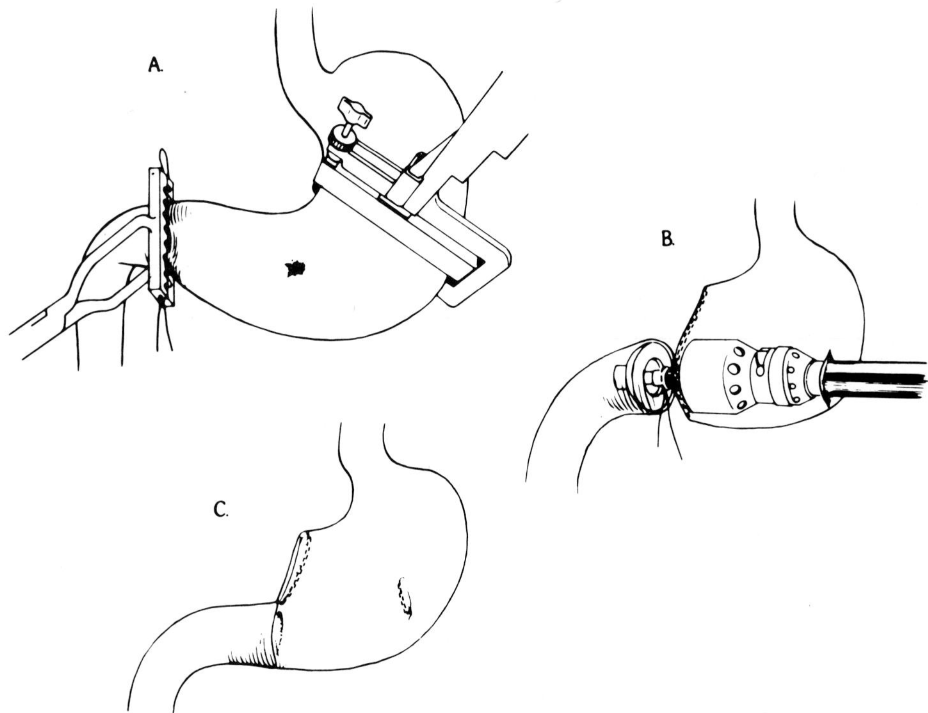

Fig V–16.—Nance's EEA™ Billroth I reconstruction (1979). Billroth I gastrectomy. **A,** the proximal stomach is stapled with a TA 90™ stapler. The pursestring instrument is used to put a pursestring suture line in the proximal duodenum, which then is divided on the edge of the instrument. **B,** the EEA™ instrument has been inserted through a proximal gastrotomy, the spindle emerging through the posterior gastric wall, the nose cone attached, inserted into the duodenum, and the duodenal pursestring tied. The instrument now will be closed and fired. **C,** completed anastomosis. The EEA™ staple line may intersect the TA 90™ staple line. (From F.G. Nance, *Annals of Surgery*, 1979, used by permission.)

Other surgeons (Knight and Griffen, 1980) also use EEA™ techniques that involve overlapping a TA™ staple line, but we still have some concern about possible tearing of the TA™ staple line by the EEA™ knife. Our ongoing laboratory studies are beginning to reassure us.

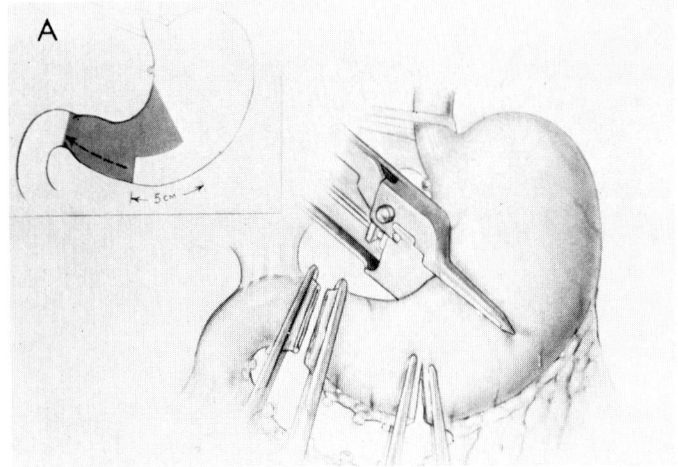

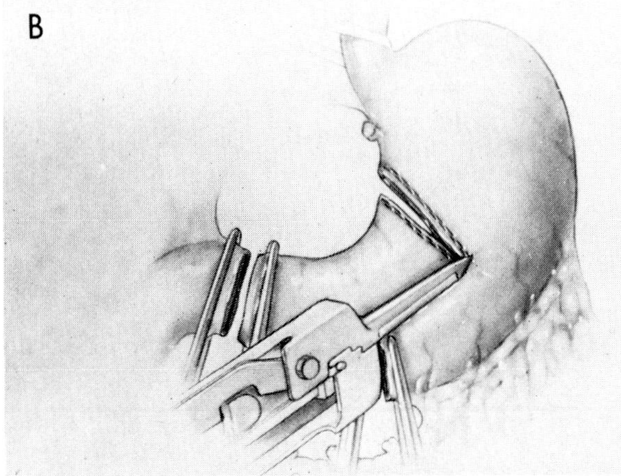

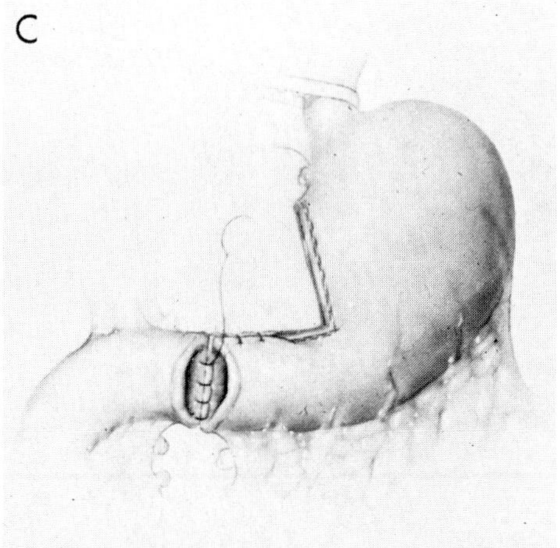

Fig V–17.—Distal greater-curvature tube—method of Dr. Walker Reynolds of Anniston, Alabama (1972, 1982). **A,** the duodenum is transected between clamps and, at the selected level of gastric resection, the greater curvature is incised perpendicular to the long axis of the stomach, for a distance equivalent to the diameter of the duodenum. The GIA™ instrument is applied from the lesser curvature, perpendicular to the long axis of the stomach, at a point some 5 cm proximal to the greater-curvature incision. **B,** the GIA™ instrument is used to construct a greater-curvature tube between the distal gastric incision and the proximal GIA™ partial gastric transection. **C,** the gastric tube is anastomosed manually to the duodenum and the GIA™ gastric suture lines will be completely reinforced, as is our policy as well when the GIA™ instrument is used on two thicknesses of stomach. (From W. Reynolds, used by permission.)

Dr. Reynolds (1982) has employed this procedure 20 times, in three of the cases connecting the gastric tube to the jejunum, a Billroth II procedure. In one of the Billroth I cases, the gastroduodenal anastomosis was with the EEA™ instrument; in all the others, by hand. Reynolds had one leak, salvaged by conversion to a Billroth II. The only death was of a patient readmitted for suspected pulmonary embolism and dying of heparin-caused hemorrhage.

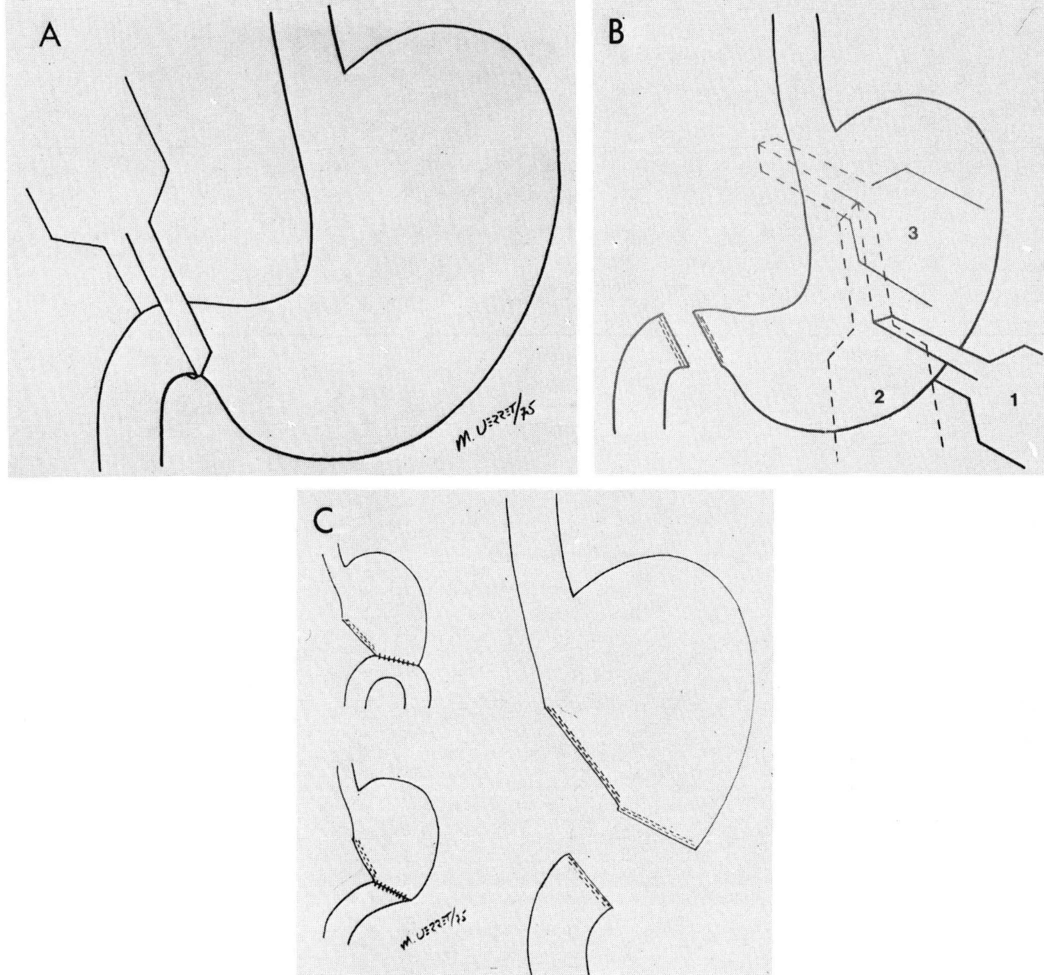

Fig V–18.—Gastrectomy and Billroth I and II reconstruction. Techniques of Dr. Wu Lu of Montreal, Quebec (unpublished illustrations) (1981). **A,** duodenal transection with the GIA™ instrument. **B,** gastrectomy effected by three, serial, applications of the GIA™ instrument, resecting the antrum and almost all of the lesser curvature. **C,** Billroth II and Billroth I reconstructions, effected manually. Doctor Lu states that he has used these techniques—and those shown in Figures V–26 and VI–4—for many years with entire satisfaction. No details are available. (From Dr. Wu Lu, used by permission.)

Korshunov (1968, 1969) reported the experience with the Soviet stapling instruments in a number of regional hospitals from 1963 to 1966. In the course of 225 gastrectomies performed with the stapling instruments, he discovered the following problems: (1) On performing the gastrojejunostomy in a Billroth II reconstruction, closure by pursestring suture of the opening left after withdrawal of the anastomotic instrument resulted in a stenotic deformation of the anastomosis. (See Ravitch and Rivarola [1966] for a technique of preventing this.) (2) In high subtotal gastrectomies, particularly for bleeding, the staples placed across the stomach could include a portion of the esophagus on the lesser curvature side, constricting the esophagogastric junction. (3) In a distal duodenal ulcer invading the pancreas, tunneling under the duodenum distal to the ulcer and stapling it resulted in stapling of the duodenum distal to the papilla of Vater. (4) He also warned against the possibility that a branch of the anastomosing instrument forming a gastroenterostomy could be inserted not into the lumen but submucosally. In 16 cases, the duodenum could not be closed with a stapler and had to be closed with manual sutures. Korshunov also mentioned the fact that occasionally with the Russian anastomosing instrument, the knife having been worn down by repeated sharpening would be too short and would not cut through the stapled gastrojejunal walls. There were five deaths in this series (2.2%) from causes unassociated with the stapler. In a previous series of 40 manual gastrectomies, three patients died of anastomotic leaks. The one suture line death in the present series was from a duodenal stump blowout. Another patient, who did not die, developed a temporary duodenal stump fistula. There was no mention of bleeding or of any other complications.

Dickman (1971) of Minneapolis, in one of the earliest American papers by others showing the use of the stapling instruments, reported 19 consecutive gastrectomies with the American instruments. Dissatisfied with one of the techniques we had reported, placing the GIA^{TM} anastomotic suture line parallel to the stapled cut end of the stomach, he inserted the gastric arm of the GIA^{TM} apparatus through the cutaway corner of the greater curvature (one of our other recommended techniques) and also whipped over the entire anastomotic suture line from within. He also reinforced the GIA^{TM} suture line from the outside. The duodenal stumps were inverted manually. In a total of 19 patients there were no deaths and no leaks. One patient required two transfusions after operation.

Korshunov (1973), reporting from a regional hospital, reported 161 gastric resections for bleeding gastroduodenal ulcer with the use of the Russian instruments. In 113, the instruments were used for all closures and anastomoses. In 48 patients, some part of the operation was done with manual suturing. There were six duodenal stump leaks, four stapled and two stapled with suture reinforcement, resulting in one death. Eight patients bled after operation, of whom one died. There was one obstructed gastroenterostomy that resulted fatally, one fatal leak from the lesser curvature in which the staples had been reinforced with sutures, one fatal peritonitis without obvious anastomotic leakage, and two subdiaphragmatic abscesses. There were two pancreatic fistulas and two instances of injury to the common duct.

The paper by Piksin, Surin, Bobkov, and Yarlikov (1974) provides a further insight into the use of the Soviet stapling instruments for gastric surgery in the Soviet Union in hospitals remote from Moscow. From 1965 through 1972, they performed 78 operations on the stomach, 58 for ulcer disease, eight for malignant disease, five for postresection syndrome, and seven for a variety of lesions. After a single duodenal fistula in a stapled duodenum in their first six cases, they resorted entirely to manual closure of the duodenum and had two deaths from leakage from such manually sutured stumps. The opening for the anastomotic instrument, made in the stomach and jejunum, was closed manually. The anastomotic suture line (only a single layer of staples in the Russian instrument) and the stapled cut end of the stomach were manually oversewn. There was one more death, from gastric outlet obstruction. Several patients had intraluminal bleeding.

At the 1975 meeting of the Austrian Gesellschaft für Chirurgie, K. Reichel (1975) from Hannover discussed only the use of the TA[TM] instruments, having, like many surgeons, first tested the water with these. In 165 Billroth I resections, 262 Billroth II resections, 41 cardia resections, and 13 antrectomy and vagotomy procedures, the anastomoses also apparently were made by the triangulation technique with the TA[TM] instruments. Additional sutures were taken only infrequently. The duodenal stump frequently was closed over manually. They had no gastric or duodenal stump or anastomotic leaks. The stapled duodenal stump was specifically stated to be inverted by four interrupted sutures. No mention of sutures is made in respect to the gastric closures. Use of the TA[TM] series for small bowel and large bowel closures was discussed favorably, without statistics.

Rinecker (1975) used the American TA[TM] instruments in 100 cases—13 duodenal stump closures, 23 duodenotomy closures, 14 Billroth I reconstructions, 17 Heineke-Mikulicz pyloroplasties, one Finney pyloroplasty, and 32 Aust-Willenegger pyloroplasties. (The Aust-Willenegger pyloroplasty involves a transverse oval excision.) A Billroth I reconstruction was performed by the triangulation method described in our 1972 report (Ravitch and Steichen 1972), the posterior row inverting and the two lateral rows everting, the staple suture lines overlapping. Additional manual sutures were used in nine cases, five of which were Heineke-Mikulicz pyloroplasties. In three of the earliest cases, the duodenal stump was closed manually. The only complications were one stenosis of a Billroth I gastroduodenostomy and one stenosis of a pyloroplasty in a patient in whom there also was suspected intraperitoneal bleeding. Rinecker specifically stated that the overlapping staple lines in the Billroth I TA[TM] anastomosis caused no problem. They controlled bleeding from the everted bowel edges with the cautery ". . . in spite of the cautions of Ravitch and Steichen."

An early report from France by Rignault, Pailler, Berthet, and Tardat (1976) covered their three-year experience from January, 1973 with the TA[TM], GIA[TM], and LDS[TM] instruments in 105 patients. There were ten esophageal operations, 74 gastric procedures, 18 Whipple operations, five colectomies, three Duhamel procedures, three ileal loops, and a variety of others. None of their six deaths was anastomosis related. They had four fistulas in a total of 158 anastomoses and closures, but all from suture lines made manually and not with staples. They had five significant hemorrhages after gastroenterostomy with the GIA[TM] instrument, two patients requiring transfusion and four patients requiring reoperation. They were impressed by the saving in time and the reduction in infections (no reoperation for abscesses).

From the Scott and White Clinic in Temple, Texas, Hardin (1977) reported 60 gastric resections for a variety of causes, including total gastrectomy. Like so many surgeons, Hardin was convinced that stapled anastomoses opened up more rapidly than manually sutured anastomoses. No patients needed transfusion or reoperation for bleeding. The 1.7% incidence of wound infection was considered to be remarkably low. One patient had a leak, which was found at operation to be from the manually closed stab wound made for the GIA[TM] instrument and one patient had gastric outlet obstruction, which resolved in three weeks.

Lawson and associates (Lawson, Hutchison, Longland, and Haque, 1977) from the Royal Infirmary, Glasgow, reporting their initial stapling experience with the TA^{TM}, GIA^{TM}, and LDS^{TM} instruments, included in their account 65 gastroenterostomies with no complications and 19 gastrectomies with one "minor biliary leakage" from the duodenal stump from the fourth to the eighth postoperative day.

Fortin, Poulin, and Leclerc from Quebec (1979) reported an experience with 148 gastric stapling procedures, of which 113 were gastrectomies. There were ten complications—four duodenal fistulas, one of which required reoperation, two gastrojejunal fistulas, and one instance of bleeding from the gastrojejunostomy requiring reoperation. Three patients had efferent loop problems, two of them requiring reoperation. There were four deaths in 148 patients (2.7%), none of them related to the technique of suture, the deaths being from pulmonary embolism, cardiac arrest, coagulopathy in a cirrhotic, and the fourth from metastases. They tended to reinforce the suture lines with occasional sutures for hemostasis. They pointed out that their single patient requiring reintervention for bleeding represented an incidence of 0.6%, and that Pearce, Jordan, and DeBakey (1957), describing 406 patients operated on by conventional techniques, had a 1% incidence of bleeding requiring reoperation.

Reuter's doctoral thesis (1982) from the Université Louis Pasteur, Faculté de Médecine in Strasbourg reports 806 stapling procedures at the St. Thérèse Clinic in Luxembourg. In 275 gastric procedures, 239 of them gastrectomies, three deaths were attributed to the stapling technique. Three patients with duodenal stump leaks closed their fistulas spontaneously and a fourth had a successful reoperation. Three patients required reoperation for bleeding, which was successfully controlled. One patient required reoperation and a Braun's loop for outlet obstruction. Gastroscopy never showed granuloma of the staple lines, but several times showed granulomas of the manual suture closures of the GIA^{TM} introduction site.

Hollender, Meyer, Blanchot, and Castellanos (1980, 1981) from Strasbourg, in a general discussion of their experience with the American staplers, reported their experience with 53 partial and 23 total gastrectomies. There were no deaths, and a single occult leak of an esophagojejunal anastomosis demonstrated radiologically and healing spontaneously. In 26 duodenal closures, they had one leak from a Heineke-Mikulicz procedure. There were two patients with gastric outlet obstruction for ten and 15 days, respectively. They reported some postoperative bleeding in two of 46 gastroenterostomies, neither requiring reoperation.

Jacobs and Ulrich from the City Hospital in Hildesheim, Germany (1981) reported their use of the American stapling instruments in gastric and small bowel surgery at the 98th Congress of the Deutsche Gesellschaft für Chirurgie. In a large clinical experience, they found postoperative bleeding from the use of the LDS^{TM} instrument requiring operation in 0.7% of cases, anastomotic leaks in GIA^{TM} anastomoses in 1.1% of the patients, and bleeding from the anastomoses in 0.8% of the patients. They observed no bleeding from the TA^{TM} closures, which had a 0.8% leak rate overall, but 2.7% for closure of the duodenum. Their conclusion was that greater operative speed and diminished leak and infection rates outweighed the cost of the staples.

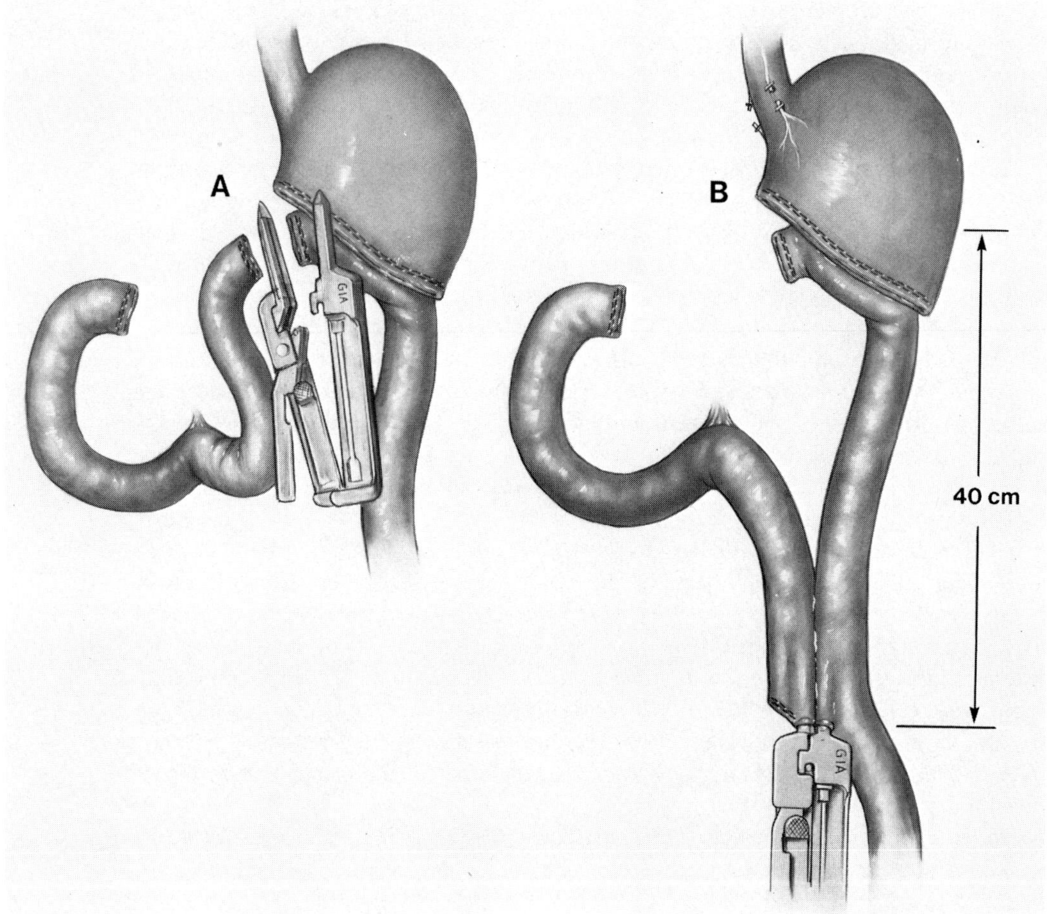

Fig V–19.—Application of the instruments to special problems in gastric surgery—Roux-Y conversion of Billroth II. In a patient with bile gastritis, or with afferent loop obstruction after gastrectomy and Billroth II reconstruction, it is remarkably simple with the stapling instruments to make the conversion to a Roux-Y. **A,** the proximal loop is divided close to the stomach with the GIA™ instrument. **B,** the stapled distal end of the proximal loop is brought down as shown for a GIA™ end-to-side Roux-en-Y anastomosis, the TA™ clamp then closing the GIA™ opening.

In converting standard Billroth II reconstructions for postgastrectomy syndromes, Albert Barrocas of New Orleans (1979) demonstrated the division of the proximal jejunal limb of the Billroth II with the GIA™ instrument and construction of a Roux-Y loop. Alternatively, he simply stapled the proximal limb with the TA™ instrument, then formed an enteroenterostomy between proximal and distal loops with the GIA™ instrument. In other cases, after a Billroth II, he anastomosed the proximal and distal jejunal loops together with two applications of the GIA™ instrument, providing a reservoir. He reported ". . . uniformly good results in approximately 25 cases" over five years.

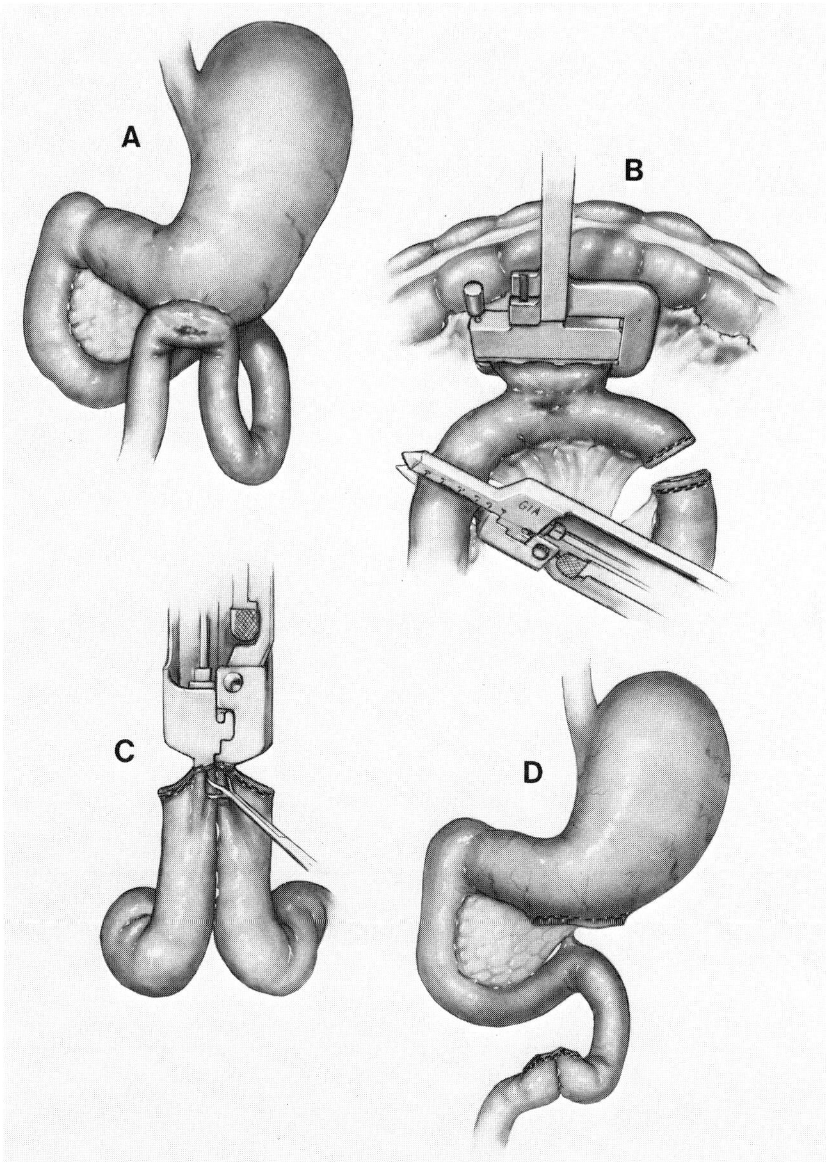

Fig V–20.—Application of the instruments to special problems in gastric surgery—Simple takedown of a retrocolic gastroenterostomy. **A** and **B,** with the index finger slipped under the gastroenterostomy, one need only dissect enough to be sure that one can place the lower jaw of the TA 55™ instrument through the same channel and then pass the instrument up on the stomach just above the anastomosis. The jejunum, in most cases, will be divided with the GIA™ instrument on either side of the gastroenterostomy, although at times if the gastroenterostomy is small enough and the jejunum innocent enough, the jejunum can be simply closed transversely with a TA™ instrument on the jejunal side of the old anastomosis, the attached cuff of stomach being cut away before the TA 55™ instrument is removed. **C,** the stomach having been stapled and cut away on the instrument and the jejunum having been divided, the two jejunal limbs are apposed in gun-barrel fashion. The two antimesenteric corners of the jejunal closures are cut away, one blade of the GIA™ instrument slipped into each side and the instrument operated, making the anastomosis (see Fig VIII–2). **D,** a TA™ instrument—not shown—then is applied across the GIA™ introduction site so as to transform the side-to-side anastomosis into what is in effect a U-shaped, functional end-to-end anastomosis.

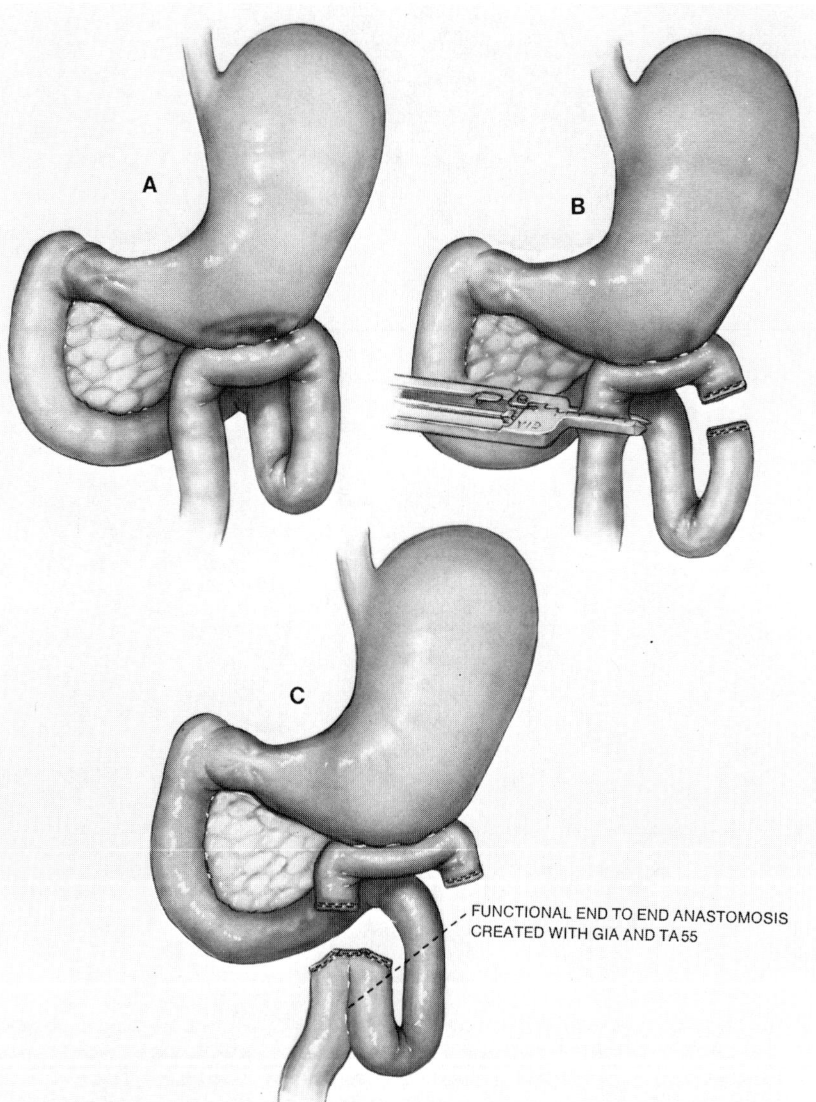

Fig V–21.—Application of the instruments to special problems in gastric surgery—Takedown of gastroenterostomy, with gastrectomy and Billroth II anastomosis in patient with duodenal ulcer persisting after gastroenterostomy. **A,** the gastroenterostomy is sufficiently far distal so that it cannot be retained for the gastric reconstruction. **B,** the afferent and efferent jejunal loops are divided with the GIA™ instrument, which seals them both. **C,** the usual functional end-to-end anastomosis, with the GIA™ instrument inserted through the excised antimesenteric corners of the stapled closures of the two jejunal ends, and the TA 55™ instrument to close the GIA™ opening, restores intestinal continuity (see Fig VIII–2).

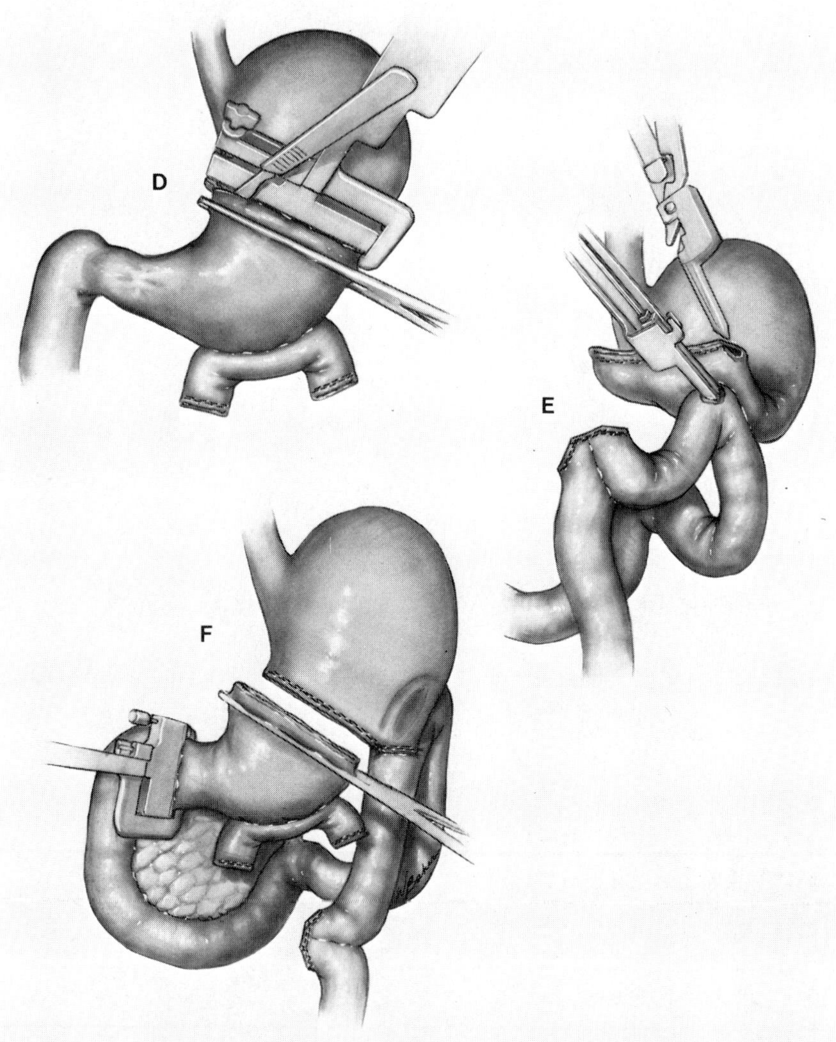

Fig V–21 (cont.).—D, the stomach is stapled and transected on the lower edge of a TA 90™ stapling instrument. **E,** one arm of the GIA™ instrument is inserted into the proximal jejunum and the other into the excised greater-curvature end of the gastric staple closure (see Fig V–10**F**). The drawing does not show the specimen which is still attached to the duodenum. **F,** the anastomosis thus created has its long axis more or less parallel to the greater curvature. Some operators choose to anchor the upper extremity of the jejunal loop to the stomach with a single silk stitch. The mucosa-to-mucosa TA 55™ closure of the GIA™ opening made for construction of the anastomosis crosses the staple line of the stomach and we often place a three-cornered stitch to reinforce this angle. The duodenum is closed with the TA 55™ instrument and amputated along the edge of the instrument. One must be careful either to be beyond the ulcer or, if one is proximal to the ulcer, to be certain that manipulation of the instrument does not crack the ulcer away from the pancreas, inviting a leak that subsequently may be interpreted as a "duodenal stump leak."

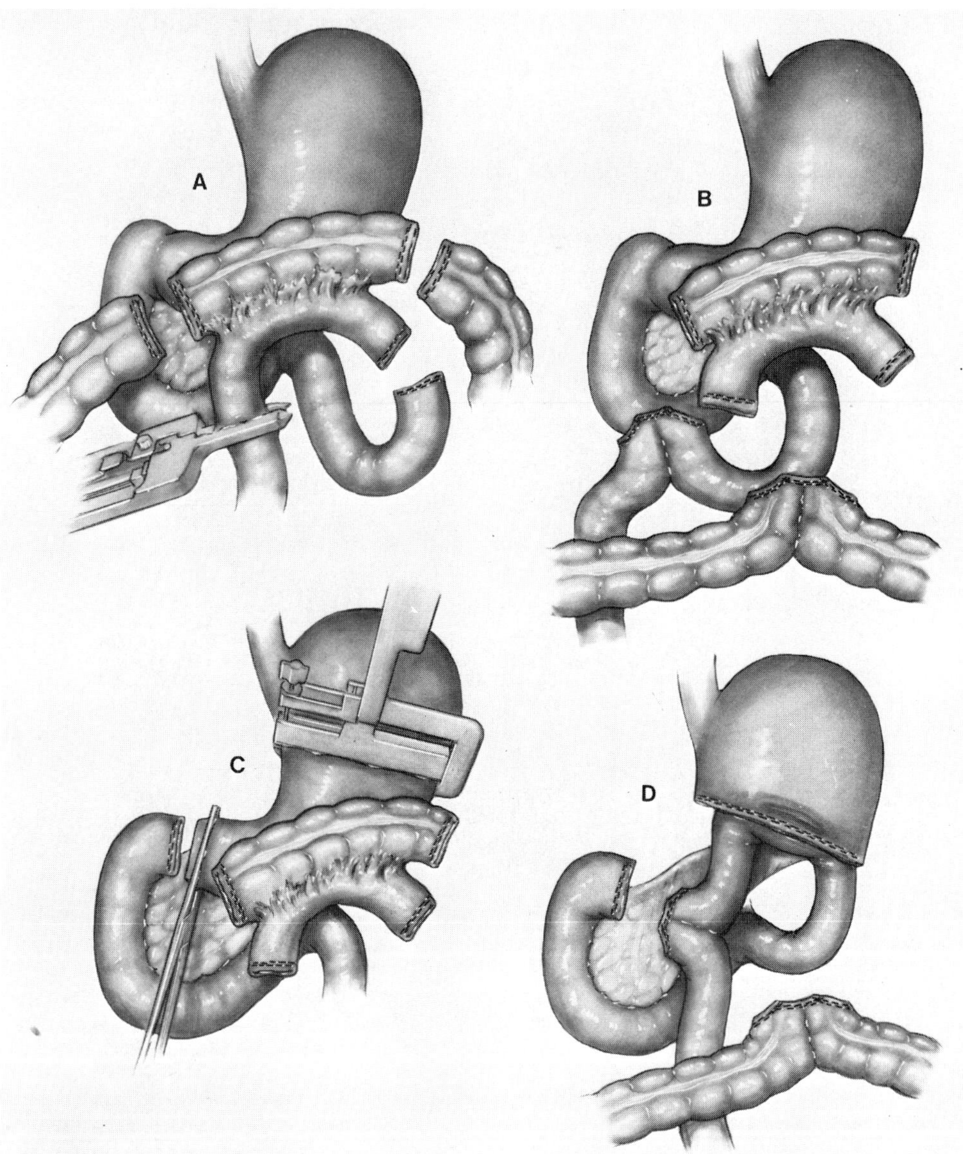

Fig V–22.—Application of the instruments to special problems in gastric surgery—Resection for gastrojejunocolic fistula. The swiftness, neatness, and freedom from bleeding or contamination permitted by the use of the instruments make them particularly useful in the resection of complicated compound lesions of this type, particularly when inflammatory adhesions add to the difficulty of the procedure. **A,** the colon proximal and distal to the lesion has been divided and sealed with the GIA™ instrument and the jejunum immediately proximal and distal is shown being similarly treated. This permits elevation of the stomach and the attached viscera and allows one good exposure for safe LDS™ division of the vessels supplying the segments being resected. **B,** the continuity of the colon and of the jejunum have been restored by the familiar functional end-to-end technique, and one can proceed to the gastrectomy (see Fig VIII–2). **C,** in this instance, because of the gastrojejunocolic fistula and attendant inflammatory mass, the duodenum is shown being divided first. In general, if we are dealing with duodenal ulcer, we divide the stomach first to provide better exposure of the duodenum. If we are dealing with carcinoma, we usually transect the duodenum first to provide better exposure of the stomach. **D,** the proximal stapling and transection of the stomach have been completed and a GIA™–TA 55™ gastroenterostomy has been performed on the posterior stomach wall (see Fig V–10**D,E,H,I,J**).

210

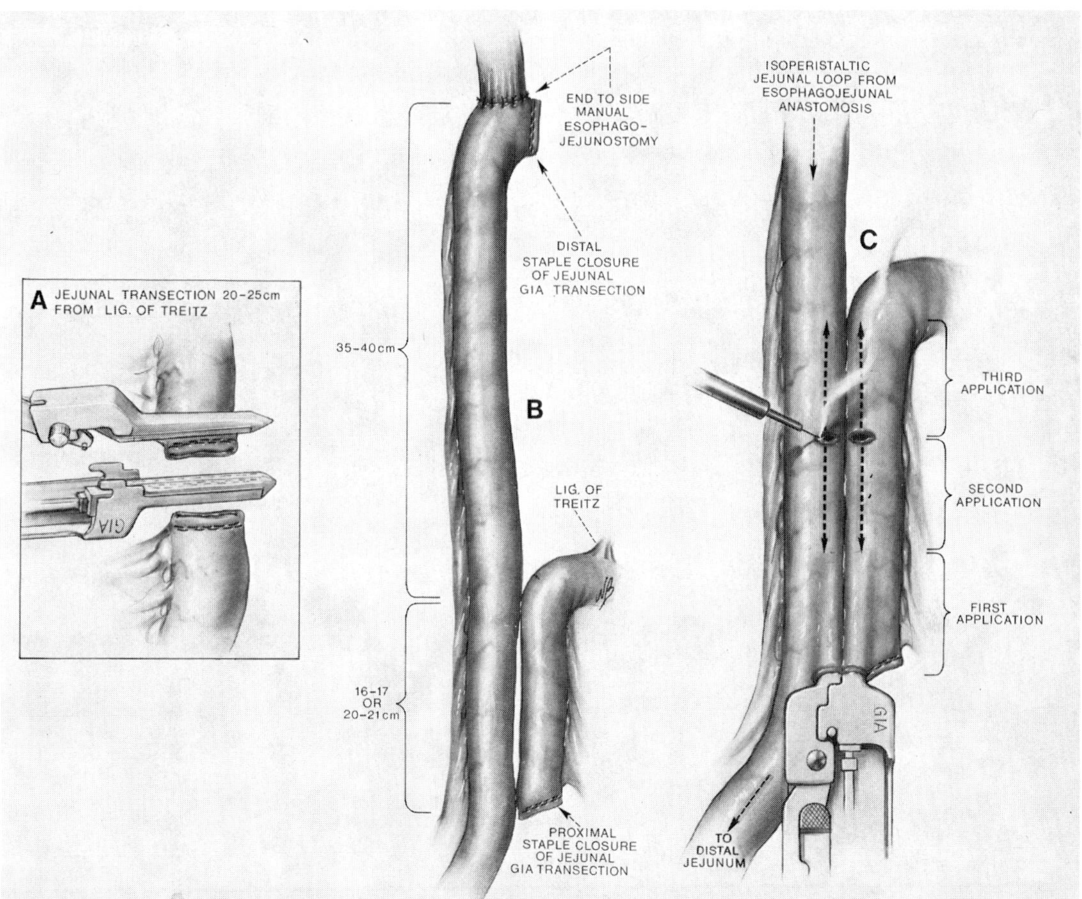

Fig V–23.—Total gastrectomy. Alternative techniques of reconstruction. The instruments lend themselves to almost every variety of reconstruction after total gastrectomy. The drawings show our preference for reconstruction by esophagojejunostomy with a pouch, usually of the Paulino type. The various combinations of the use of the GIA™, TA™, and EEA™ instruments shown make obvious other combinations and permutations that might be utilized. **A,** the jejunum is divided with the GIA™ instrument, 20–25 cm below the ligament of Treitz. This is our preferred mode of transection of the bowel, for whatever purpose, between the ligament of Treitz and the rectum, simultaneously sealing both ends. **B,** the proximal end of the distal jejunal loop is brought up to the esophagus. An open manual esophagojejunostomy is shown, attaching the esophagus to "the handle of the cane," which is the most cephalad portion of the loop brought up. Any excess jejunum is stapled off with a TA™ instrument. **C,** the duodenojejunal segment coming away from Treitz' ligament is apposed to the loop that has just been attached to the esophagus, so that there will be an isoperistaltic single limb of jejunum 35–40 cm from the esophagus before the beginning of the 15–20-cm jejunojejunostomy now being constructed as shown. The duodenojejunal segment can be stapled to the long, efferent jejunal limb either isoperistaltically or antiperistaltically, in this case isoperistaltically. The GIA™ instrument, inserted through a stab wound in the long jejunal limb and through the cutaway antimesenteric corner of the duodenojejunal limb, is passed upward and activated, creating a 5-cm anastomosis. Five centimeters above the end of this anastomosis, matching stab wounds are created in the two loops and the GIA™ instrument inserted first distally and then proximally, creating three connecting 5-cm anastomoses. *(continued)*

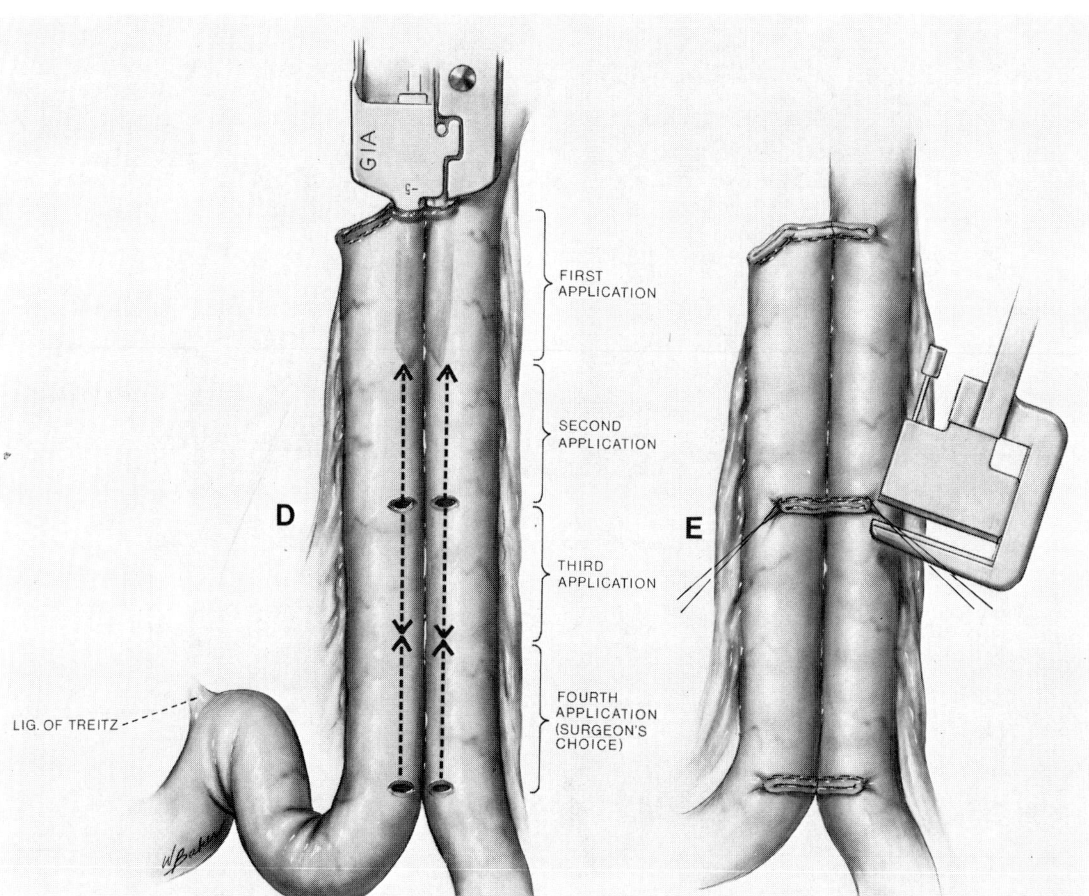

Fig V–23 (cont.).—D, the same technique can be utilized, with the duodenojejunal segment used antiperistaltically. If a larger pouch is desired, the GIA™ instrument is used four times. **E,** the openings left at the withdrawal of the GIA™ instrument are closed mucosa-to-mucosa with the TA™ instrument. Complicated reconstructions of this kind are performed much more swiftly with these instruments, with much less opportunity for soiling and bleeding and much less trauma to the bowel than with manual suture.

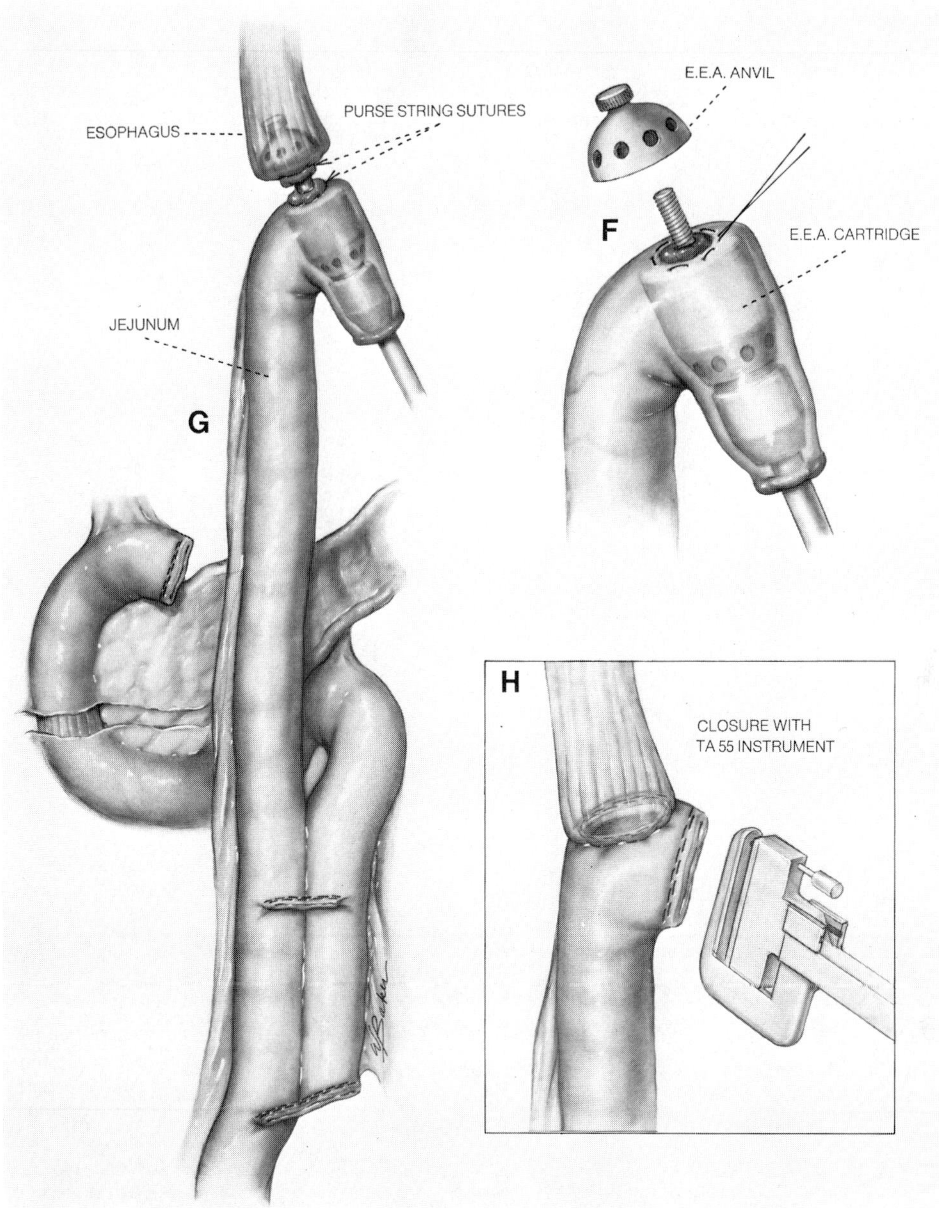

Fig V–23 (cont.).—F, the Roux-Y jejunojejunostomy has been constructed in a similar fashion, but the esophagojejunostomy is made with the EEA™ instrument. The EEA™ instrument, without the anvil-nose cone, is passed through the cut end into the jejunum, and the rod pushed through an antimesenteric stab wound, secured by a pursestring suture. **G,** the nose cone having been applied and passed into the esophagus, both pursestring sutures are tightly secured, the anvil and cartridge approximated, and the instrument fired. **H,** the circular minimally inverting anastomosis. The superfluous portion of the end of the jejunum has been stapled close to the anastomosis with the TA™ instrument and cut away.

A loop of jejunum can be brought up to the esophagus in continuity and an enteroenterostomy performed with the GIA™ instrument to create an omega loop (see Fig V–4). In that case, one can perform the esophagojejunostomy manually or, before completing the enteroenterostomy, pass the EEA™ instrument upward through the opening made for it, to the apex of the loop, and perform the esophagojejunostomy with the EEA™ instrument. *(continued)*

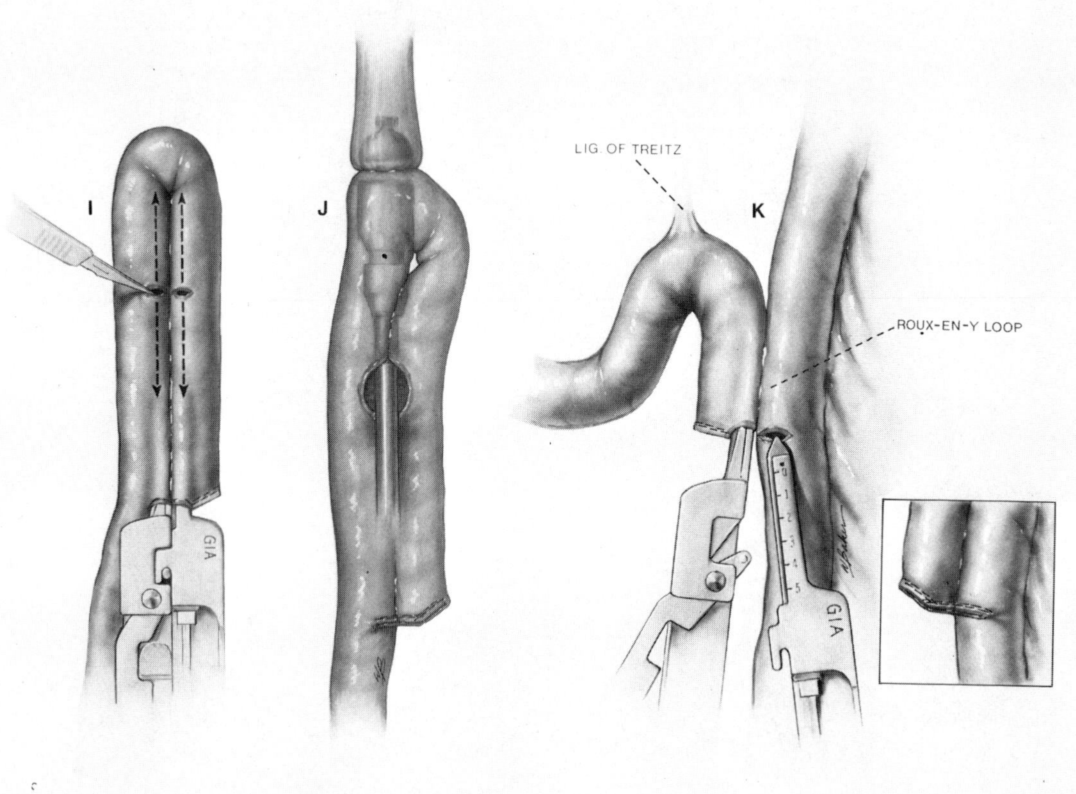

Fig V–23 (cont.).—**I, J,** and **K,** alternatively, the jejunum can be doubled back on itself, a 15-cm GIA™ jejunojejunostomy created, the EEA™ instrument passed upward through the GIA™ wound, and the inverting esophagojejunostomy constructed. After withdrawal of the EEA™ instrument, the GIA™ stab wound is closed mucosa-to-mucosa with the TA™ instrument. As shown in **K,** the proximal jejunum then is brought alongside the distal jejunum, some 35–40 cm below the pouch and the Roux-Y anastomosis performed. The antimesenteric corner of the staple closure of the proximal jejunum is cut away and matched with a stab wound in the distal jejunum. The serosa-to-serosa anastomosis is made with a GIA™ instrument, the lips of the GIA™ opening then held out and stapled mucosa-to-mucosa with a TA™ instrument. This technique for a Roux-Y anastomosis is the technique used in any end-to-side anastomosis, as in connecting the proximal end of a Roux-Y to the stomach or the distal end of a colonic esophageal replacement to the stomach. (**A–E** from F.M. Steichen, *American Journal of Surgery,* 1977, used by permission. **F–H** from F.M. Steichen and M.M. Ravitch, *Annals of Surgery,* 1980, used by permission.)

Barone (1979) reported the formation of a Hunt-Lawrence pouch after total gastrectomy with the use of the stapling instruments by the technique that we had been using for some time. At that time, he had used the Auto Suture® instruments in seven patients, with a substantial saving of time over his previous experience with the same operation performed manually. Neither in the manual nor the stapled cases were there any anastomotic leaks. The Lawrence pouch, constructed much as in Figure V–23*I* and *J*, was made with the staples and the esophagojejunostomy was performed manually.

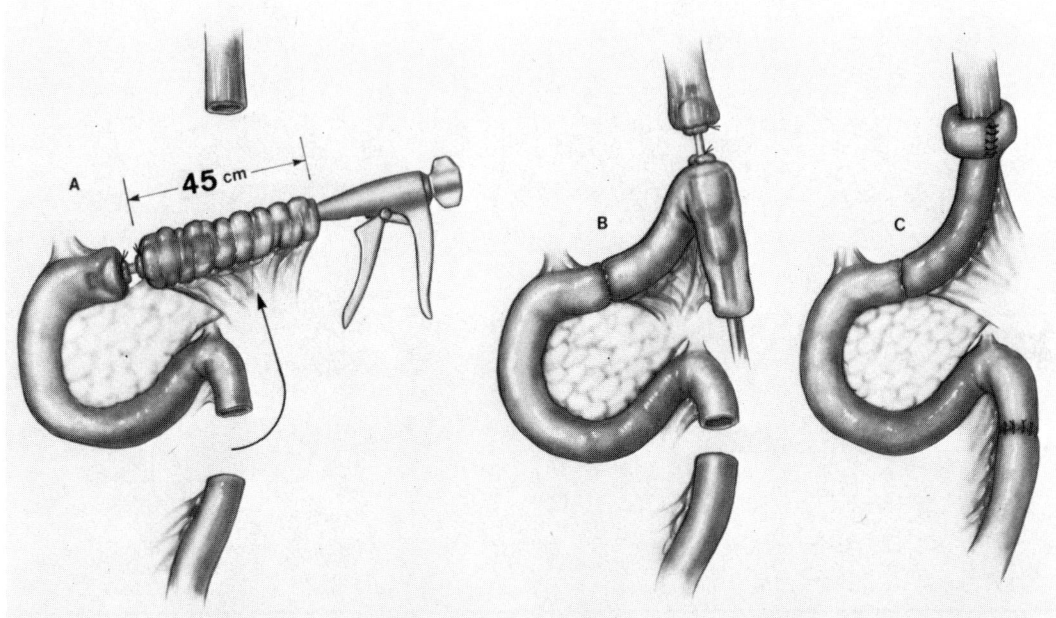

Fig V–24.—Jejunal loop interposition after total gastrectomy—technique of Fasching and Moritz (1980). Fasching and Moritz prefer, for reconstruction after gastrectomy, an interposed jejunal loop that they term "after Longmire-Gütgemann," and which they performed seven times with one fatal leak and one subphrenic abscess without fistula. The EEA™ instrument is inserted the length of the interposed loop from the proximal end, for end-to-end anastomosis with the duodenum, reloaded and inserted through the open proximal end partway into the loop for a side-to-end anastomosis between the jejunum and esophagus. The 15-cm-long redundant portion proximal to the anastomosis is wrapped around the esophagus to provide an antireflux mechanism. (From W. Fasching and R. Moritz, *Chirurg* 51:644, 1980, used by permission. In the published illustration, the extrapolated jejunal loop is indicated as being 30 cm long. In the illustration kindly sent us by Professor Fasching, this has been changed to 45 cm.)

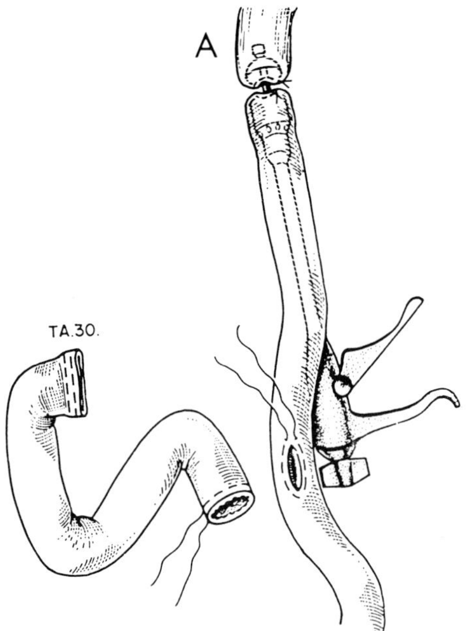

Fig. 2 bis — *Réalisation de l'anastomose œso-jéjunale termino-terminale*

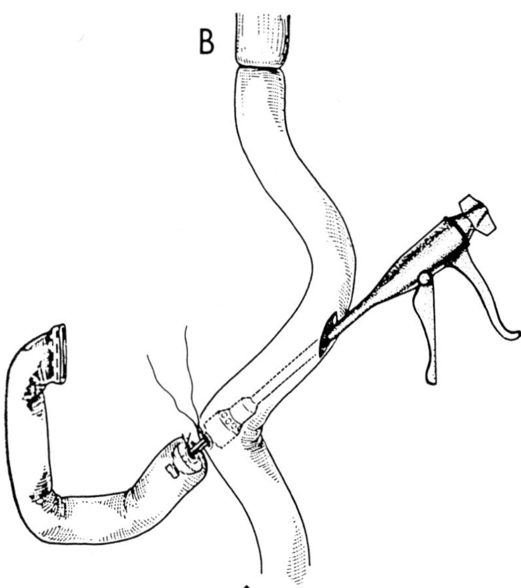

Fig. 3 — *Réalisation de l'anastomose jéjuno-jéjunale termino-latérale*

Fig V–25.—Total gastrectomy, EEA™ instrument in reconstruction—technique of Prémont and Clotteau (1981). The EEA™ instrument is inserted upward from the middle of the Roux loop for the esophagojejunostomy and downward for the Y anastomosis, the enterotomy being closed with the TA 55™ instrument. (From M. Prémont and J.E. Clotteau, *La Nouvelle Presse Médicale,* 1981, used by permission.)

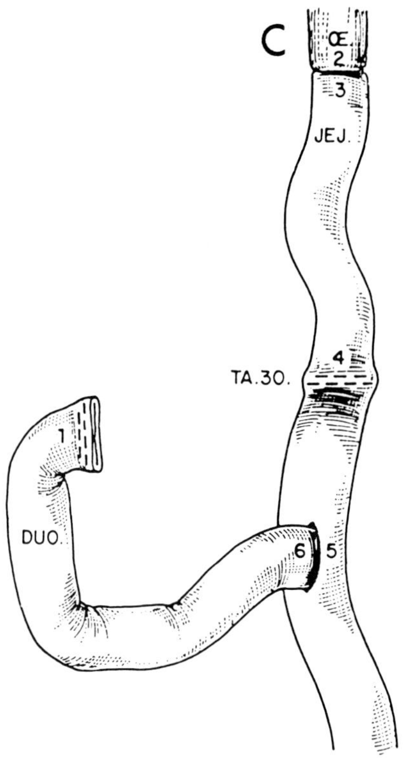

Fig. 4 — *L'intervention terminée (fermeture de la brèche latérale jéjunale à la T.A.)*

Prémont and Clotteau (1981) from France, reporting their technique of reconstruction after total gastrectomy, insert the EEA^{TM} instrument through an enterotomy in the distal jejunal loop after division of the jejunum below Treitz' ligament, pass the EEA^{TM} instrument upward for the esophagojejunostomy and downward for the Roux-Y side-to-end enteroenterostomy. The EEA^{TM} introduction site is closed with the TA^{TM} instrument. They state only that their experience over a number of years has been satisfactory and their complication rate reduced over that with their previous manual suturing techniques.

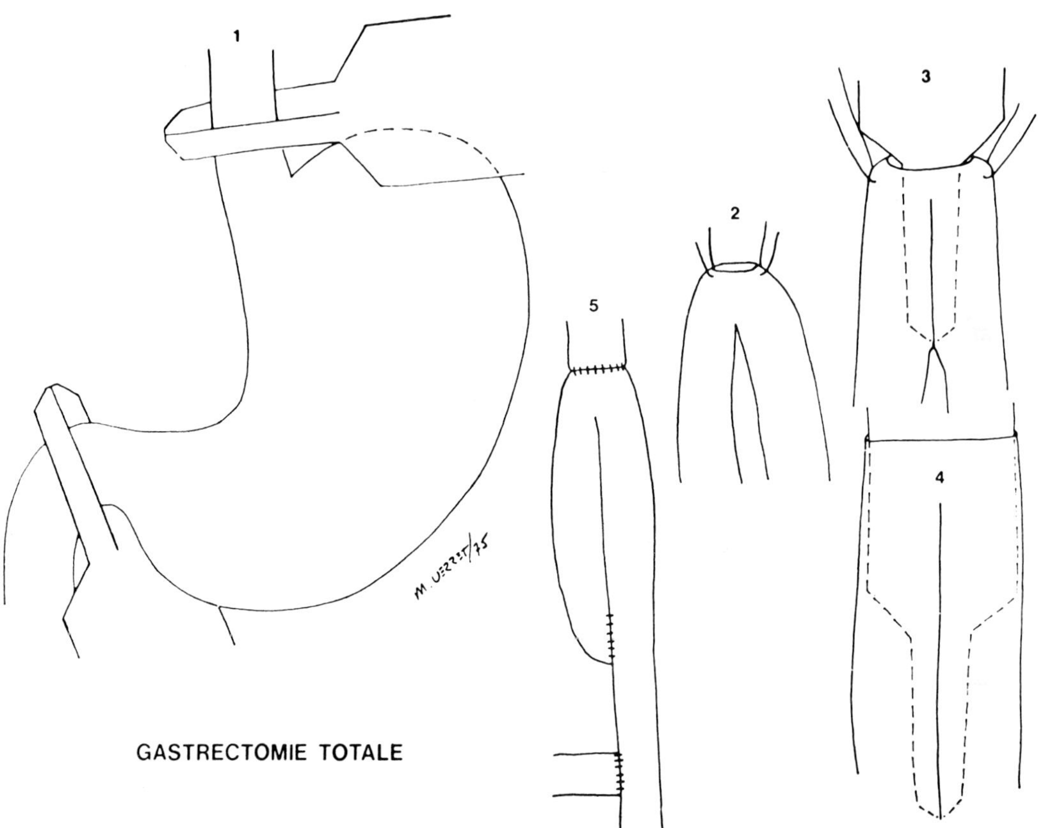

Fig V–26.—Total gastrectomy—technique of Dr. Wu Lu, Montreal, Quebec (unpublished illustration) (1981). (1) The esophagus and duodenum are transected by the GIA^{TM} instrument. The jejunum is divided (not shown). (2) The distal jejunal limb is doubled on itself and incised at the knuckle at the apex of the jejunal loop. (3 and 4) The GIA^{TM} instrument is inserted twice through this opening, creating a 10-cm division of the spur. The esophagojejunostomy is manually sutured. (5) The Roux-Y jejunojejunostomy is performed, the recurved end of the jejunum anastomosed to the pouch, and the opening at the knuckle of the jejunal loop anastomosed to the esophagus, all manually. Doctor Wu informs us that he has used this technique in a number of cases, with satisfaction. (From Dr. Wu Lu, used by permission.)

REFERENCES

Awe W.C., Loehden O.L.: Automatic stapling devices. *Am. Surg.* 39:475, 1973.
Barone R.M.: Reconstruction after total gastrectomy: Construction of a Hunt-Lawrence pouch using Auto Suture® staples. *Am. J. Surg.* 137:578, 1979.

Barrocas A.: The use of stapling devices in the management of postgastrectomy syndromes. *Am. Surg.* 45:656, 1979.

Charlier A.: Gastrectomie avec anastomose gastrojéjunale première intégrée—procédé mécanique original de Welter. Thèse de doctorat, Université René Descartes, Paris, 1981.

Cobb C.F.: Personal communication, September 14, 1981.

Dickman R.W.: Improved technics using the bowel stapling clamps in nineteen consecutive gastric resections. *Am. J. Surg.* 121:628, 1971.

Elliott T.E., Albertazzi V.J., Danto L.A.: Stenosis after stapler anastomosis. *Am. J. Surg.* 133:750, 1977.

Engelberg M., Lifschitz O.: Excision of villous adenoma of the rectum with a stapler. *Dis. Colon Rectum* 24:407, 1981.

Engelke B., Kamphausen U., vom Rath E.W.: Selektive proximale vagotomie (SPV). Erfahrungen und Technik mit dem LDS-Gerät. *Chirurg* 48:728, 1977.

Fasching W., Moritz R.: Zirkuläre Klammeranastomosen im Magen-Darm-Trakt mit den Klammernahtgeräten SPTU und EEA. *Chirurg* 51:644, 1980.

Fortin C.L., Poulin E.C., Leclerc Y.: Evaluation de l'utilisation des appareils d'autosuture en chirurgie digestive. *Can. J. Surg.* 22:580, 1979.

Freed J.S., Christodoulides G., Szuchmacher P.H.: A new technique for resection of gastric polyps. *Mt. Sinai J. Med.* 45:230, 1978.

Hardin W.J.: Evaluation of autosutures in gastrointestinal surgery. *South. Med. J.* 70:197, 1977.

Harrison M.R., Anderson J., Rosen M.A., Ross N.A., Hendricks A.G.: Fetal surgery in the primate I. Anesthetic, surgical, and tocolytic management to maximize fetal-neonatal survival. *J. Pediatr. Surg.* 17:115, 1982.

Hinchey E.J.: In discussion of Reiling R.B., Reiling W.A. Jr., Bernie W.A., Huffer A.B., Perkins N.C., Elliott D.W. *Am. J. Surg.* 139:147, 1980.

Hollender L.F., Meyer C., Blanchot P., Castellanos J.G.: Les sutures mécaniques en chirurgie gastrointestinale. *Bull. Acad. Natl. Med.* 164(3):260, 1980.

Hollender L.F., Blanchot P., Meyer C., de Silva e Costa J.M.: Erfahrungen mit der Anwendung von Nähapparaten in der Magen-Darm-Chirurgie. *Zentral. Chir.* 106:74, 1981.

Hunt T.K.: Personal communication, November 30, 1981.

Jacobs G., Ulrich B.: Einsatz der Klammernahtgeräte bei Eingriffen am Magen und Dünndarm. Abstrakt vom 98ten Kongress, Deutsche Gesellschaft für Chirurgie, Munich, April 22–25, 1981.

Jascalevich M.E.: The gastrectomy operation revisited with automated suturing devices. *Arch. Surg.* 105:524, 1972.

Knight C.D., Griffen F.D.: An improved technique for low anterior resection of the rectum using the EEA stapler. *Surgery* 88:710, 1980.

Korshunov A.V.: The risks of using certain suturing apparatuses in gastric surgery. *Klin. Khir.* (Kiev) 9:63, 1968.

Korshunov A.V.: The use of mechanical tantalum sutures in gastric surgery. *Vestn. Khir. Grekov* 103:129, 1969.

Korshunov A.V.: Use of the stapling instrument in ulcerative gastroduodenal hemorrhage. *Klin. Khir.* 9:58, 1973.

Lawson W.R., Hutchison J., Longland C.J., Haque M.A.: Mechanical suture methods in thoracic and abdominal surgery. *Br. J. Surg.* 64:115, 1977.

Moss G.: A simple technique for permanent gastrostomy. *Surgery* 71:369, 1972.

Nance F.G.: New techniques of gastrointestinal anastomoses with the EEA stapler. *Ann. Surg.* 189:587, 1979.

Pearce C.W., Jordan G.L. Jr., DeBakey M.E.: Intra-abdominal complications following distal subtotal gastrectomy for benign gastroduodenal ulceration. *Surgery* 42:447, 1957.

Pemberton L.B., Snider W.R.: Clinical applications of the end-to-end anastomosis (EEA stapler), American College of Surgeons Clinical Congress, 1979. ACS Film Library #1190.

Piksin I.N., et al.: Mechanical suture in operations on the gastrointestinal tract. *Klin. Khir.* 4:80, 1974.

Prémont M., Clotteau J.E.: Anastomoses à la pince automatique après gastrectomie totale. *Nouv. Presse Méd.* 10:331, 1981.

Ravitch M.M., Rivarola A.: Enteroanastomosis with an automatic instrument. *Surgery* 59:270, 1966.

Ravitch M.M., Rivarola A., VanGrov J.: Rapid creation of gastric pouches with the use of an automatic stapling instrument. *J. Surg. Res.* 6:64, 1966.

Ravitch M.M., Steichen F.M.: Technics of staple suturing in the gastrointestinal tract. *Ann. Surg.* 175:815, 1972.

Ravitch M.M., Steichen F.M.: Staples in gastrointestinal surgery, in Maingot R. (ed.): *Abdominal Operations,* 7th ed. New York, Appleton-Century-Crofts, 1979, pp. 2197–2210.

Ravitch M.M., Steichen F.M.: Mechanical sutures, in Shackelford R.T., Zuidema G.D. (eds.): *Surgery of the Alimentary Tract,* 2d ed. Philadelphia, W.B. Saunders Co., 1981, pp. 579–618.

Reichel K.: Nahtgeräte in der Bauchchirurgie. 16. Jahrestagung der Österreichischen Gesellschaft für Chirurgie, 5.-7. Juni, 1975.

Reuter M.J.P.: Les sutures mécaniques en chirurgie digestive et pulmonaire. Thesis, presented in 1982, at Université Louis Pasteur Faculté de Médecine de Strasbourg, France.

Reynolds W. Jr.: In discussion of Ravitch M.M., Steichen F.M. *Ann. Surg.* 175:836, 1972.

Reynolds W. Jr.: Personal communication, January 29, 1982.

Rignault D., Pailler J-L., Berthet A., Tardat M.: Les sutures mécaniques automatiques en chirurgie digestive. Appréciation de la méthode après 3 ans d'utilisation de l'appareillage américain. *Chirurgie* 102:945, 1976.

Rinecker H.: Operative Erfahrungen mit 100 maschinellen Nahtverschlüssen und Anastomosen am Duodenum. *Chirurg* 46:416, 1975.

Steichen F.M.: The creation of autologous substitute organs with stapling instruments. *Am. J. Surg.* 134:659, 1977.

Steichen F.M., Ravitch M.M.: Mechanical sutures in esophageal surgery. *Ann. Surg.* 191:373, 1980.

Waugh D.E.: A new technique for gastrotomy. *Surgery* 70:368, 1971.

Webster M.W. Jr., Carey L.C., Ravitch M.M.: The permanent gastrostomy: Use of the gastrointestinal anastomotic stapler. *Arch. Surg.* 110:658, 1975.

Welter R., Turbelin J.M., Charlier A.: Gastrectomie avec anastomose gastro-jéjunale "première" Technique originale d'emploi des procédés de suture mécanique. *Nouv. Presse Méd.,* 31 Janvier 1981, 10, n°4.

Wu Lu: Unpublished illustrations, 1981.

CHAPTER VI

Operations on the Esophagus

THE INSTRUMENTS lend themselves particularly to esophageal resection and reconstruction, because their precision and the decrease in the trauma from the manipulation required for multiple sutures is so important in this fragile organ, and because staples can be accurately placed at a distance, as at the apex of the thorax. The various anastomoses can be accomplished in a remarkable variety of ways with the GIA™–TA™ techniques or with the EEA™ instrument. A particular advantage of the instruments, in anastomoses performed to the intrathoracic esophagus, is that the remaining esophagus can essentially be left in its bed for the anastomosis, minimizing the risk of disrupting its vascular supply by the mobilization usually required for placement of manual sutures. The stapled terminal esophagus heals as well mucosa-to-mucosa as do other segments of the gastrointestinal tract, and the various anastomotic techniques shown have all been performed with satisfaction. We (Steichen, 1971; Ravitch and Steichen, 1972) and others (Chassin, 1978) have from the first used the GIA™ and TA™ instruments for esophageal resection and reconstruction, before the EEA™ instrument was available. Presumably because the inverting anastomosis produced by the EEA™ stapler does not challenge accepted surgical doctrine as the TA™ instruments had, there has been a flood of publications concerning its use. An additional explanation for the excitement with which the EEA™ instrument has been received lies in the fact that whereas the use of all the other stapling instruments results in neater, swifter, easier, and probably cleaner, drier, and more reliable operations, the EEA™ procedures in the esophagus and rectum have proved, in addition, to be decidedly safer than others and at times to enable the surgeon to do an operation that he could not safely have done manually. Nevertheless, other stapling techniques, and of course manual anastomoses, continue to have a place in the surgery of the esophagus. As experience with the EEA™ instrument accumulates, it becomes increasingly apparent that some of the earlier difficulties with it were the result of attempting to force too large a cartridge into a small esophagus. The 31-mm cartridge is too large for the esophagus in most patients. Féketé and associates (Féketé, Breil, and Ronsse, 1980; Féketé, Breil, Ronsse, Tossen, and Langonnet, 1981) have pointed out the necessity for gentle progressive dilatation of the esophagus with bougies or Hegar dilators before attempting insertion of the EEA™ instrument. Most exciting are the new experiences with the insertion of the EEA™ instrument through the mouth for anastomosis of the cervical esophagus to whatever structure has been brought up from below. If it is the stomach that has been brought up, it seems to us that the peroral technique would be preferable to insertion of the instrument from below through a gastrotomy with its additional suture line. The experience with the peroral insertion of the EEA™ instrument still is small and this technique is not always feasible. Pearson (1981), at least, feels that the superiority of the anastomosis produced warrants the careful manipulation required to pass the EEA™ instrument downward through the mouth and he has done so successfully in six patients. The new curved, and smaller caliber, disposable EEA™ instrument should lend itself particularly well to this use.

In our own attempts to place the EEA™ instrument through the mouth, we have so far not been successful in three cases, once because the 31-mm cartridge was definitely too large, in the early days when smaller cartridges were not available, and twice because even the 25-mm cartridge was too large and produced a longitudinal split of the muscle of the esophagus despite prior dilatation with Hegar dilators.

In the esophagus, rather than the modified Furniss clamp pursestring, we often prefer an over-and-over whipstitched pursestring, such as we use low in the rectum (see Fig VI–1).

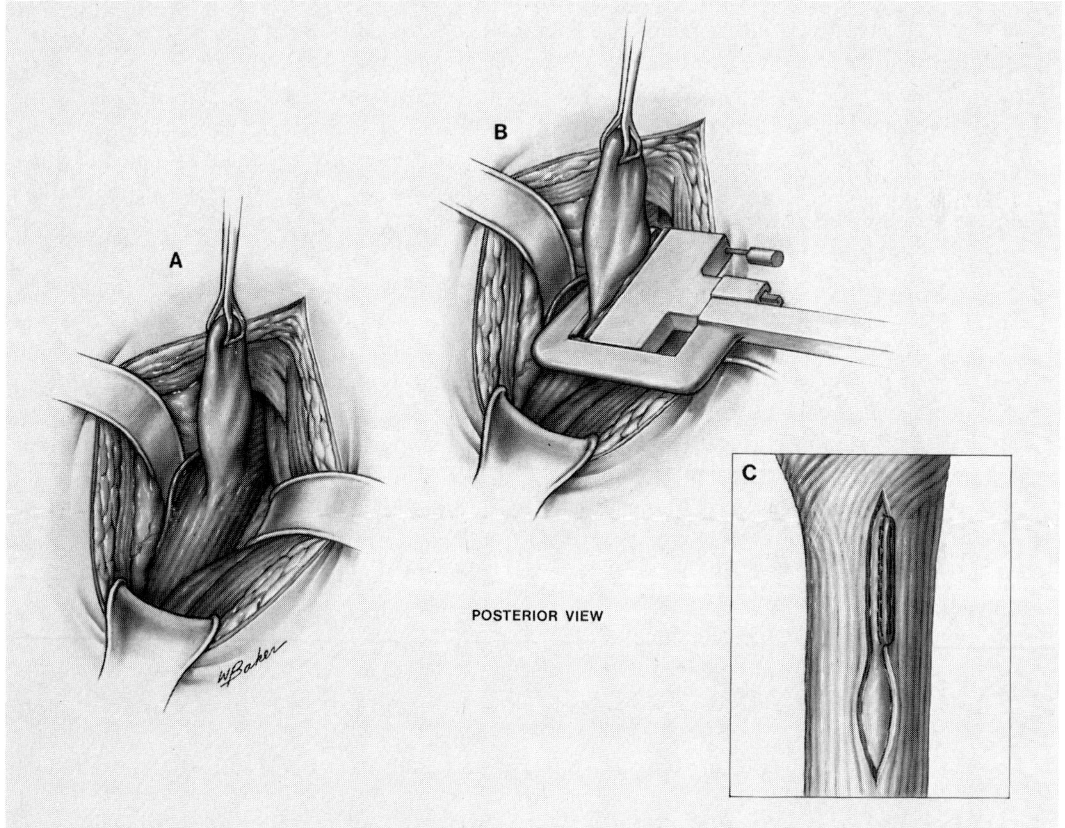

Fig VI–1.—Resection of Zenker's pharyngeal diverticulum. **A,** having been dissected out while a large tube is in the esophagus, the diverticulum is gently held up. As with other viscera, one should avoid stapling a structure being stretched by traction. **B,** the neck of the diverticulum is stapled with the TA 55™ instrument, so that the staple line will be parallel to the long axis of the esophagus, since that usually is the long dimension of the opening of the diverticulum from the pharynx [Payne (Hoehn and Payne 1969; Payne and Reynolds 1982) prefers to apply it transversely]. It may require a little manipulation to seat the TA 55™ instrument in those few patients in whom the neck of the diverticulum is too large for the TA 30™ instrument. As always, the TA™ instrument is brought down to the tissue to be stapled rather than the tissue being pulled up into the instrument. **C,** the staple line requires no reinforcement [Payne (Hoehn and Payne 1969; Payne and Reynolds 1982) sutures muscle transversely over it]. The usual myotomy is continued down 2 or 3 cm. (From M.M. Ravitch and F.M. Steichen, *Annals of Surgery,* 1972, used by permission.)

Payne (Hoehn and Payne, 1969) from the Mayo Clinic reported their initial experience with four Auto Suture® TA™ closures of the neck of Zenker's diverticula. Payne and Reynolds (1982), with a clinical experience of 888 patients undergoing one-stage pharyngoesophageal diverticulectomy since January 1, 1944, stated that, "During the past decade . . . we have utilized the TA 30™ stapling device to effect closure and prefer it in terms of both speed and accuracy of closure. . . ."

We have amputated 14 Zenker's diverticula at the University of Pittsburgh with the TA 30™ or TA 55™ instruments (Webster, 1982) with no leaks, fistulas, or strictures.

Epiphrenic diverticula have been amputated in the same way. Read of Little Rock, Arkansas (1970) reported two such cases and we have had two.

Another application of the staples to pharyngeal closure is the imaginative use of a Soviet instrument (UKL-60) (see Fig I–19*H,I*) of the TA™ type for closure of the pharynx in laryngectomy. Lukyanchenko (1971), in 15 laryngectomies, used the UKL-60 for closure of the pharynx, dividing the trachea distally and dissecting out the larynx, lifting the larynx forward, and applying the staples above the level of the hyoid bone. The larynx was amputated from the pharynx on the border of the stapler. Ten of the patients had had preoperative radiation. In operations done under local anesthesia, patients were urged to swallow, and in no case did saliva pass through the stapled closure. The staple line was closed over with adjacent muscles, with catgut. All of the tumors were limited to the larynx. There were no complications.

Sorokina (1971) used the UKB-25 (see Fig I–19*J,K*), which had been originally devised for bronchial closures, in the closure of the hypopharynx after laryngectomy. The staple suture line was oversewn with a layer of catgut sutures in the muscle. She had utilized the technique in 1970 on six patients. In four, the outcome was uncomplicated. Five patients had primary healing. One patient, who had been irradiated to a dose of 6,000 R preoperatively, developed dehiscence of the skin around the tracheostomy but there was no evidence of dehiscence of the pharyngeal closure. One patient had postoperative bleeding requiring reoperation 12 hours after the original procedure.

Paches, Ogoltsova, Tsibirne, Alekseyeva, and Ponomarkov (1972) reported their experimental studies of pharyngeal closure with a variety of the Soviet suturing instruments, finding that the UKL-60 gave the best results. The fact that Lukyanchenko and Sorokina already had reported their clinical experiences is not referred to in this paper and not cited in the bibliography.

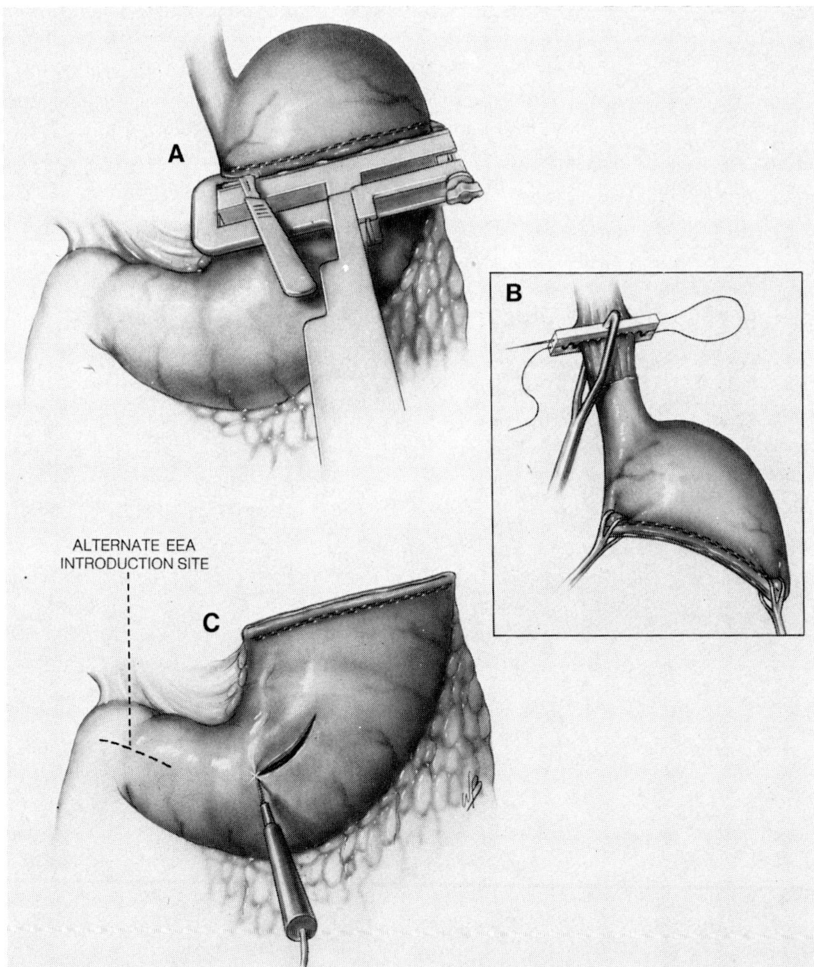

Fig VI–2.—Distal esophagectomy, EEA™ esophagogastrostomy. **A,** the fundus is divided after the second application of the TA 90™ instrument. If the GIA™ instrument is used, the distal gastric closure is oversewn. **B,** the modified Furniss clamp pursestring instrument is placed across the proximal limit of resection of the esophagus and the pursestring suture passed. **C,** the stomach is incised for passage of the EEA™ instrument into the midportion of the remaining stomach.

(continued)

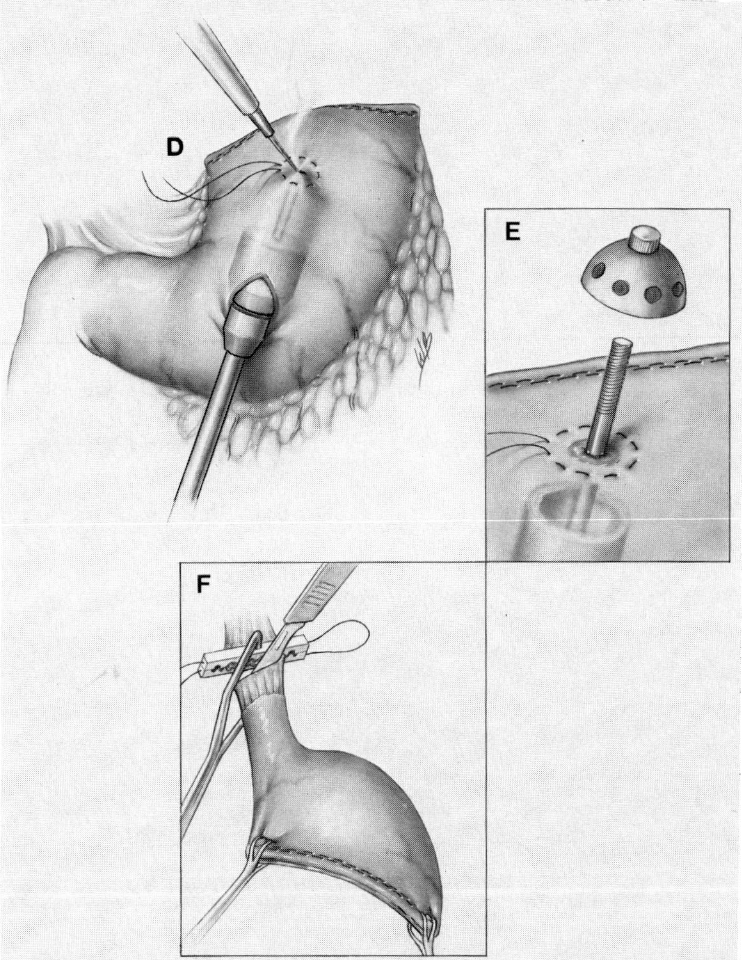

Fig VI–2 (cont.).—D, the EEA™ instrument is inserted through the gastrotomy, the center rod pressed up against the anterior gastric wall through a manually placed pursestring suture and an opening created with the cautery. If one is careful in making this incision small, for a tight fit, and manipulation is avoided in the creation of the anastomosis, one may dispense with the pursestring. **E,** the rod having been passed through anterior stomach wall, the anvil-nose cone is attached. **F,** the esophagus is transected on the lower edge of the pursestring instrument.

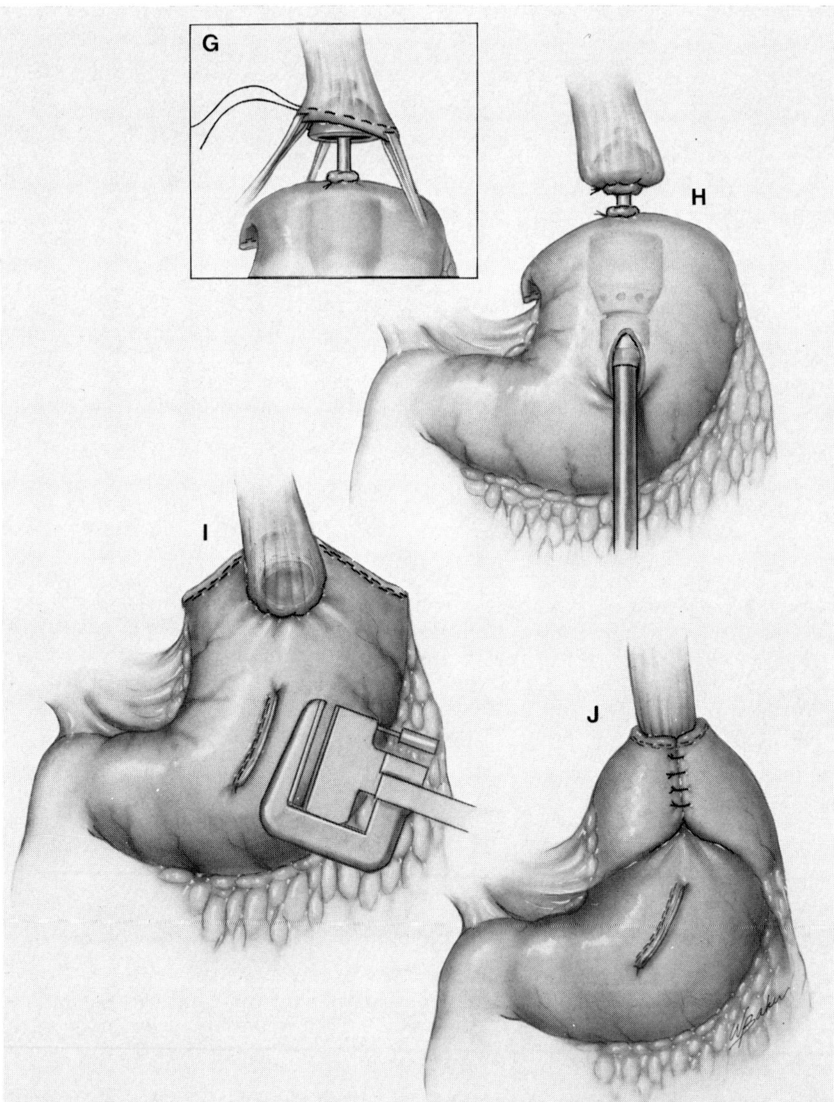

Fig VI–2 (cont.).—G, the anvil-nose cone is inserted into the esophagus. **H,** the two pursestrings have been tightly tied around the center rod and the esophagus and stomach are approximated by turning the wing nut on the instrument. **I,** the EEA™ instrument has been activated, achieving an end-to-end inverting esophagogastrostomy. The instrument is removed together with the two dough-nuts of tissue that represent the pursestringed ends. The TA™ instrument has been placed below the gastrotomy edges and the gastrotomy closed mucosa-to-mucosa. **J,** a gastric wrap, if possible, is manually sutured around the anastomosis for security and to provide an antireflux mechanism. (From F.M. Steichen and M.M. Ravitch, *Annals of Surgery,* 1980, used by permission.)

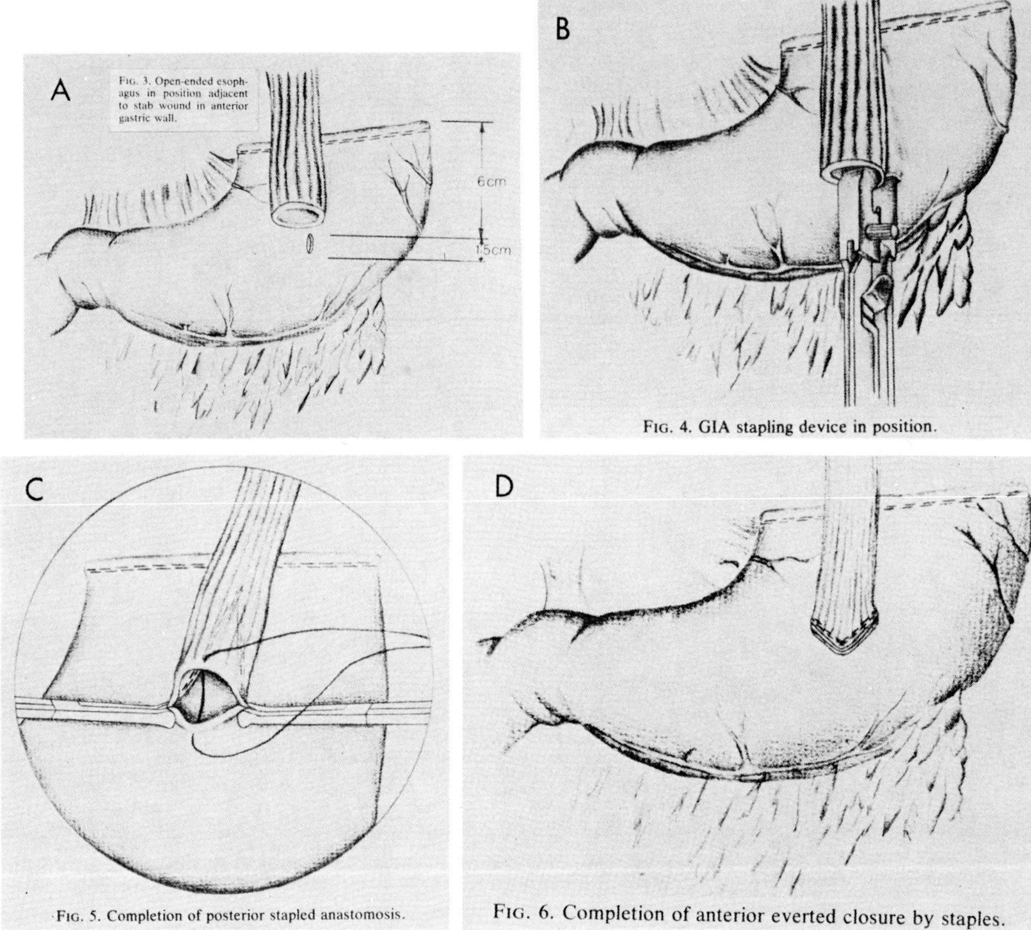

Fig VI–3.—Esophagogastrectomy—technique of J.L. Chassin, New York (1978). The esophagogastrostomy to the anterior wall is performed with the GIA™ instrument. The remaining open portions of stomach and esophagus are bisected with a traction suture and each half stapled mucosa-to-mucosa with the TA™ instrument, the two suture lines overlapping. (From J.L. Chassin, *Annals of Surgery,* 1978, used by permission.)

Chassin (1978, 1978) from Flushing, New York performed esophagogastrectomy by transecting the stomach with the Auto Suture® TA 90™ instrument and anastomosing the end of the esophagus well down on the anterior gastric wall in 12 cases, with the Auto Suture® GIA™ instrument, using two oblique overlapping TA 30™ lines to close the residual opening. There were no operative deaths, no hospital deaths, no overt fistulas, and no radiologic ''leaks.''

Shahinian and associates from Providence, Rhode Island (Shahinian, Bowen, Dorman, Soderberg, and Thompson, 1980) report use of the EEA^{TM} instrument in ten esophagogastrostomies, nine for carcinoma and one for ". . .achalasia with stricture," performed over a period of 15 months. There were no clinical or radiologic leaks in any of the patients and one minor stenosis that responded to dilatation.

Fasching and Moritz from the Second University Surgical Clinic in Vienna (1980) used the EEA^{TM} instrument in nine patients for esophageal anastomoses, inserting the EEA^{TM} instrument through a gastrotomy, the spindle perforating the posterior wall where the esophagogastrostomy was made. One patient developed an anastomotic leak and succumbed, autopsy disclosing a necrosis of the gastric wall between the TA^{TM} suture line and the stapled end of the stomach, which was only 1 cm away. Of the other eight patients, one had a stenosis of the anastomosis, which responded to two dilatations. They also performed eight anastomoses between the esophagus and the jejunum; one anastomosis high in the left chest, in a patient reoperated on after recurrence following total gastrectomy for cancer, leaked with fatal outcome. In another, subphrenic abscess developed, without fistula.

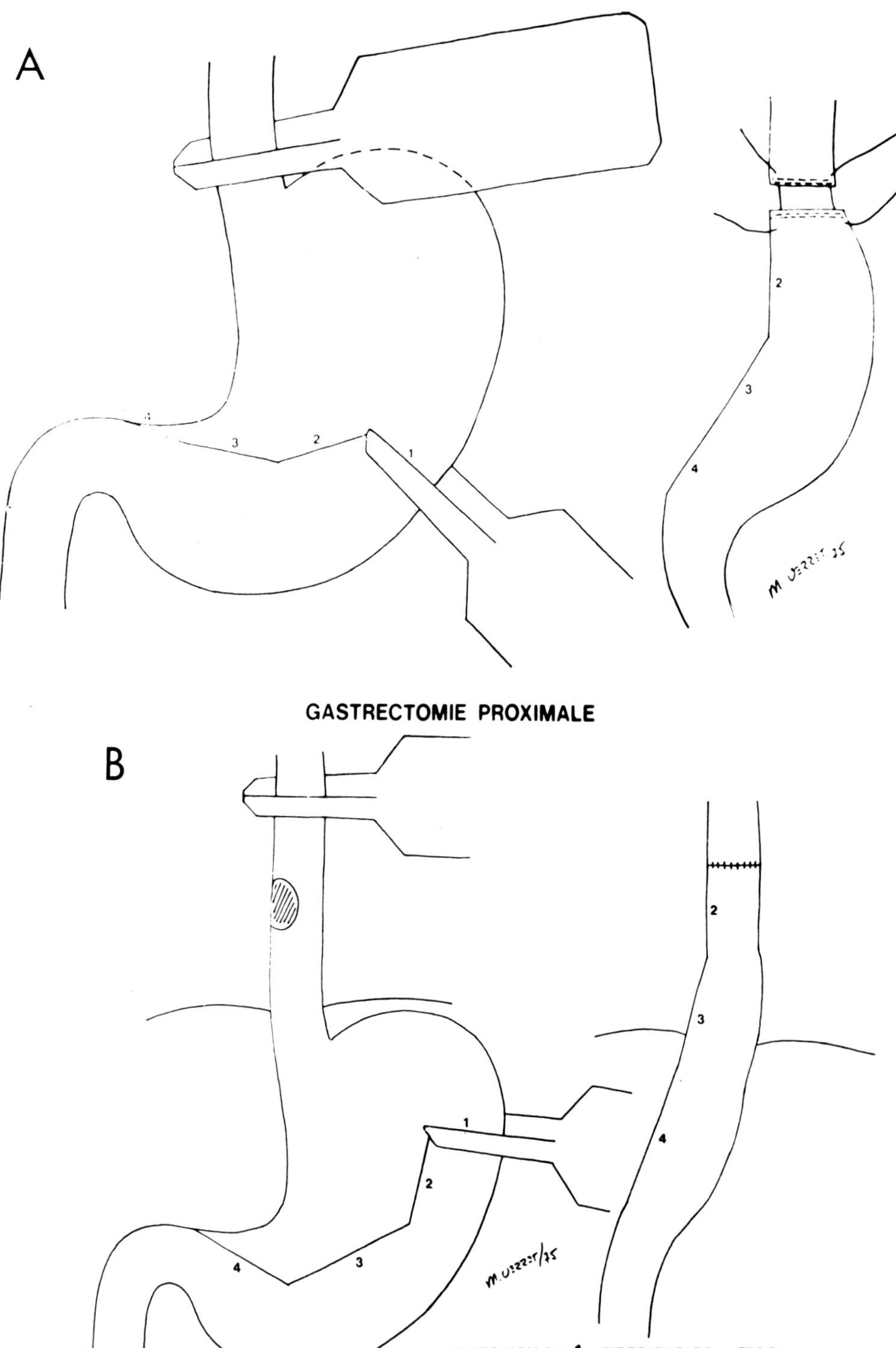

Fig VI–4.—Proximal gastrectomy and distal esophagectomy techniques of Dr. Wu Lu of Montreal, Quebec, 1981 (unpublished illustrations). The resections are done with the GIA™ instrument, serially applied, and a manual anastomosis performed of esophagus to the tubed distal stomach. (From Dr. Wu Lu, used by permission.)

Dr. Wu Lu of Montreal, Quebec (1981) uses the GIA™ instrument for an ingenious tailoring of the distal stomach ending up with a manual end-to-end esophagogastrostomy. As with his gastrectomy techniques, also unpublished, he provided no statistics.

Bérard and colleagues from Lyon (Bérard, Papillon, Jacquemard, Labrosse, Bigay, and Guillemin, 1981), reporting their first 104 gastrointestinal anastomoses with the EEA™ instrument, included 17 esophageal procedures: ten esophagojejunal anastomoses after total gastrectomy, two esophagogastric anastomoses after esophagogastrectomy, four annular resections for esophageal varices, and one colonic interposition. There was one esophagojejunal fistula, and that resulted fatally. They had no instances of bleeding in their entire series. There were no stenoses.

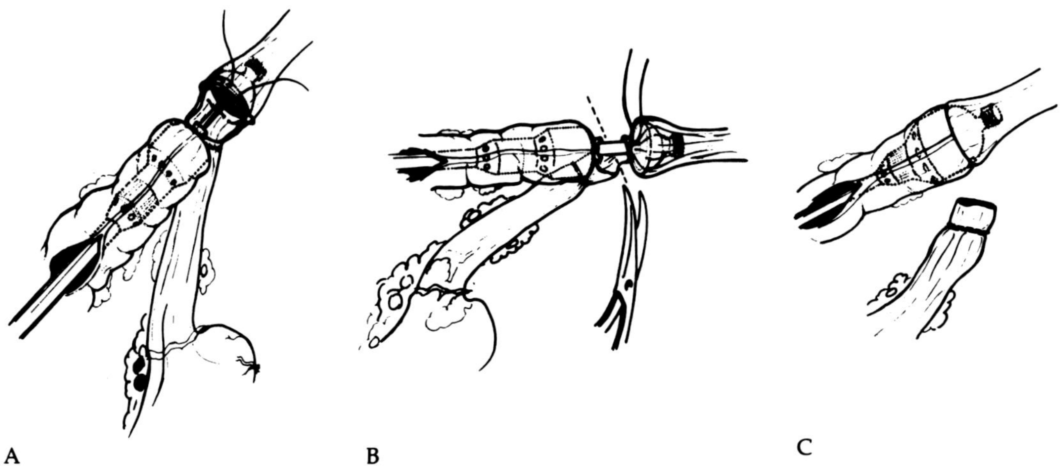

A   B   C

Fig 2. Thoracic stage of esophagocolonic anastomosis: (A) positioning of End-to-End Anastomosis unit in the esophagus; (B) resection of esophagogastric specimen; and (C) anastomosis completed.

Fig VI–5.—Esophagogastrectomy and esophagocolostomy technique of Molina of Minneapolis (Molina, Lawton, and Avance 1981; Molina, Lawton, Meyers, and Humphrey, 1982). For esophagocolostomy, Molina and associates, from Humphrey's clinic, describe insertion of the EEA™ instrument through a proximal colotomy, then passing into the proximal esophagus before the distal esophagus has been cut away posteriorly, obviously facilitating the esophagocolonic anastomosis. A similar technique for esophagogastric anastomosis was suggested to us by R. Wolsch (1979). (From J.E. Molina, B.R. Lawton, and D. Avance, *Annals of Thoracic Surgery*, 1981, used by permission.)

Molina, Humphrey, and colleagues (Molina, Lawton, and Avance, 1981; Molina, Lawton, Meyers, and Humphrey, 1982), in a total experience of 94 resections for adenocarcinoma of the cardia, reported 13 resections through simultaneous right thoracotomy and laparotomy, using the EEA™ instrument "with no extra stitches reinforcing the anastomosis." There were no leaks or fistulas. Full feeding was resumed in seven days. Reflux was a problem in all patients. "The use of a mechanical stapler is recommended since it will not only provide an adequate anastomosis and avoidance of leaks, but also will shorten the operative time."

Dorsey and associates (Dorsey, Esses, Goldberg, and Stone, 1980) from Toronto, in esophagogastrectomy transect the stomach with the GIA™ instrument, oversewing the distal end, insert the EEA™ instrument through a distal anterior gastrotomy, bring the central rod and anvil out again through a more proximal gastrotomy still at least 3 cm from the gastric suture line, and apparently close the distal gastrotomy manually. In only one of their 15 patients was it necessary to place an additional manual suture at the anastomosis. They had a total of nine patients with esophagogastrectomy, five patients with total gastrectomy, loop esophagojejunostomy in two, and Roux-en-Y in three. There were no anastomotic leaks, no postoperative deaths, and one fibrotic stricture at five months "treated successfully by a single bougienage."

From a large experience with cancer of the esophagus and gastric cardia, Kivelitz and Ulrich (1981) reported from Düsseldorf 18 manual intrathoracic anastomoses and 27 EEA™ intrathoracic anastomoses in the preceding two years. There were six leaks with the manual techniques and a 27% perioperative mortality. There was one leak with the EEA™ instrument and a 15% operative mortality. There were no radiologically demonstrated strictures in either group, but in the manual group, 25% had stenoses on endoscopy whereas a single patient in the EEA™ group had radiologically demonstrated strictures.

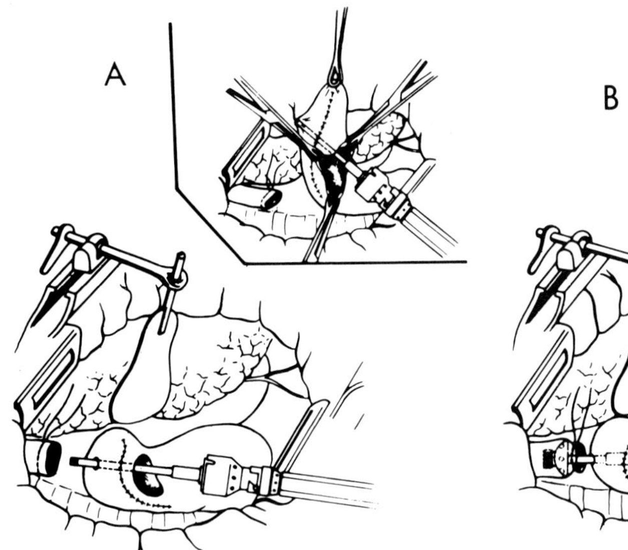

FIG. 1. Inversion of the EEA stapler through an anterior gastrotomy (right thoracotomy).

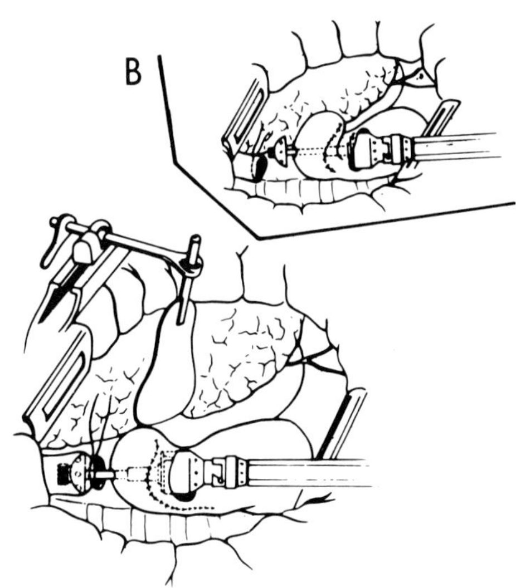

FIG. 2. The anvil is secured to the shaft and inserted into the esophagus.

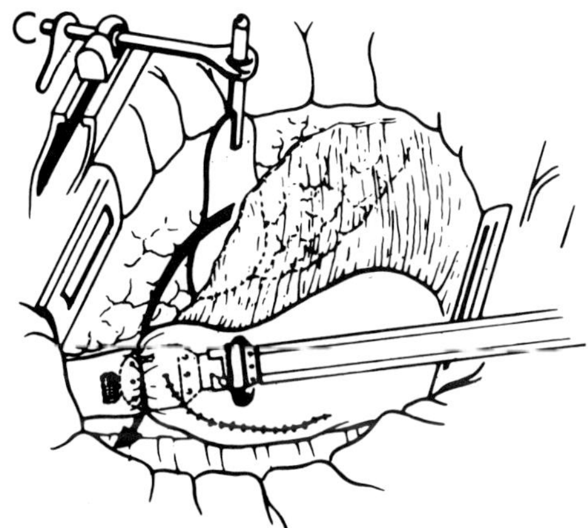

FIG. 3. Anastomosis course of the great omentum meant to wrap thoroughly the anastomosis and the gastric remnant.

Fig VI–6.—Esophagogastrectomy in right hemithorax, for middle third lesions—technique of Féketé (1981). **A,** through a laparotomy and a right intercostal incision, the distal esophagus has been resected and the stomach delivered into the chest. Inserting the EEA™ instrument through an anterior gastrotomy and out the posterior gastric wall solves the problem of using the rigid straight instrument inside the thorax. **B,** the anvil-carrying nose cone is secured to the central rod and passed into the pursestringed proximal esophagus. **C,** the instrument is closed and fired. Féketé lays great stress on utilizing the omentum as a wrap around the anastomosis—after the gastrotomy for the EEA™ instrument has been closed. Lower third lesions are attacked through a left thoracotomy and peripheral detachment of the diaphragm, the EEA™ instrument being used in the same way, placing the anastomosis on the posterior gastric wall. (From F. Féketé, Ph. Breil, H. Ronsse, J.C. Tossen, and F. Langonnet, *Annals of Surgery,* 1981, used by permission.)

TABLE VI–1.—EEA™ ANASTOMOSES IN ESOPHAGEAL RECONSTRUCTION
(F. Féketé—February, 1979–June, 1981)

	FISTULA		STENOSIS
PROCEDURES	Clinical	X-ray Only	
75 ESOPHAGOGASTRIC ANASTOMOSES			
64 Intrathoracic			
5 without omental wrap	2	0	1
59 with omental wrap	1	4	5
11 Cervical	1	0	1
19 ESOPHAGOJEJUNAL, INTRATHORACIC	1	0	0
6 ESOPHAGOCOLIC, CERVICAL	0	0	0

From the Beaujon Hospital in Clichy, France, Francois Féketé, successor to the great tradition in that hospital of Professor Lortat-Jacob, has reported (Féketé, Breil, and Ronsse, 1980; Féketé, Breil, Ronsse, Tossen, and Langonnet, 1981) his large and impressively successful series of esophageal reconstructions with the EEA™ instrument, and in June, 1981, sent us his updated figures as given in Table VI–1. The anastomoses were about equally divided between those done with the 25-mm cartridge and with the 28-mm cartridge. As in almost all experiences, the stenoses were more likely to be diagnosed radiographically or endoscopically than on the basis of symptoms, tended not to be rigid and to yield readily to dilatation—often a single dilatation.

H. Akiyama (1981) of the Toranomon Hospital in Tokyo was good enough to share with us his large experience with stapling in esophageal resection—at that time, 120 cases. His superb results with the Auto Suture® instruments are shown in Table VI–2.

TABLE VI–2.—ESOPHAGEAL ANASTOMOSIS
WITH EEA™ (H. Akiyama, 1981)

SITE OF ANASTOMOSIS		
Intrathoracic	26	
Abdominal	94	
TOTAL	120	
ORGANS ANASTOMOSED		
Esophagojejunostomy	118	
Esophagogastrostomy	1	
Esophagocolostomy	1	
TOTAL	120	
COMPLICATIONS		
Anastomotic leak		6 (6/120 = 5.0%)
Intrathoracic	4	
Subphrenic	2	
Anastomotic stricture		1 (1/120 = 0.8%)
Anastomotic bleeding		1 (1/120 = 0.8%)
OPERATIVE DEATH		0 (0/120 = 0.0%)

Although most place the EEA™ instrument through a separate stab wound in the organ brought up for anastomosis—most often the stomach—Pearson from the Toronto General Hospital has used a peroral insertion of the EEA™ instrument in six patients with esophagogastrostomy performed in the neck after total esophagectomy (1981). In two of the patients, a longitudinal split of the cervical esophageal musculature developed because the 30-mm cartridge was too large for a small esophagus in these patients, both women. In one of these patients, the mucosal anastomosis was complete and the muscular defect was closed satisfactorily after the stapler had been removed. In the second patient there was a mucosal defect also after the stapler had been removed and both the muscular and mucosal defects were manually sutured. This patient developed a minor leak and required one postoperative dilatation.

Gentili from the University of Sherbrooke in Quebec has used the EEA[TM] instrument in 15 transoral, cervical esophagogastrostomies (1981). Three minor anastomotic leaks developed and two stenoses occurred. Gentili also reports the occlusion of esophageal varices with the EEA[TM] instrument in six patients. There were no leaks and no strictures occurred. The one patient who bled postoperatively was treated nonoperatively. One patient in this group died two years after operation from carcinoma of the liver.

van Rensburg and associates from Stellenbosch University in South Africa (van Rensburg, Malherbe, Marais, Bouwer, and van Zyl, 1981) used the EEA[TM] stapler in eight esophagogastric and esophagojejunal anastomoses and 12 low rectal anastomoses. In esophagojejunostomy, they preferred to insert the EEA[TM] instrument through a separate jejunotomy rather than through the open end of the jejunum. They thought that the stapled gastrojejunal anastomosis was considerably wider than the usual manually sutured anastomosis. There was a single staple line leak. "In this particular case, the anastomosis was performed between the jejunum and the small cuff of stomach. We consider that this occurred because the stomach cuff did not permit an accurate enough closure with a pursestring suture, and that the blood supply to such a cuff is perhaps suspect."

In 39 esophagogastric anastomoses at the Barnes Hospital, West and associates (West, Marbarger, Martz, and Roper, 1981) used the EEA[TM] instrument in 31, and in eight a two-layer silk anastomosis, four of these because the stapler could not be used. The EEA[TM] instrument was inserted through a distal gastrotomy and the central rod and anvil brought out through a proximal gastrotomy remote from the proximal gastric closure. In three of the four patients, in whom staples "could not be used," the esophagus was too small for the 31-mm cartridge, which was the only one available at the time. In the fourth patient ". . .the circular knife failed to cut the central core of esophageal and gastric tissue. It was not clear whether this failure was due to improper loading of the device . . . inclusion of a metallic clip ligature within the staple line . . . or a defect in the cartridge. . . ." Two leaks were demonstrated immediately at operation and covered with Lembert sutures. Five anastomoses were ". . . in the extreme apex of the thorax. We would have considered these anastomoses extremely difficult to sew, even with the resection of an additional rib." One patient developed empyema and recovered after drainage and showed no leak on three successive barium examinations. Two patients had leaks from the TA[TM] staple line used to close the gastrotomy. Both patients recovered. There were no leaks from the EEA[TM] anastomoses.

For a traumatic perforation of the thoracic esophagus, Engelberg and colleagues from Kfar Saba, Israel (Engelberg, Jedeikin, Eschkol, Hoffman, and Reiss, 1981) performed a longitudinal stapled closure in the face of a grossly infected mediastinum, using the TA 55[TM] instrument with complete success.

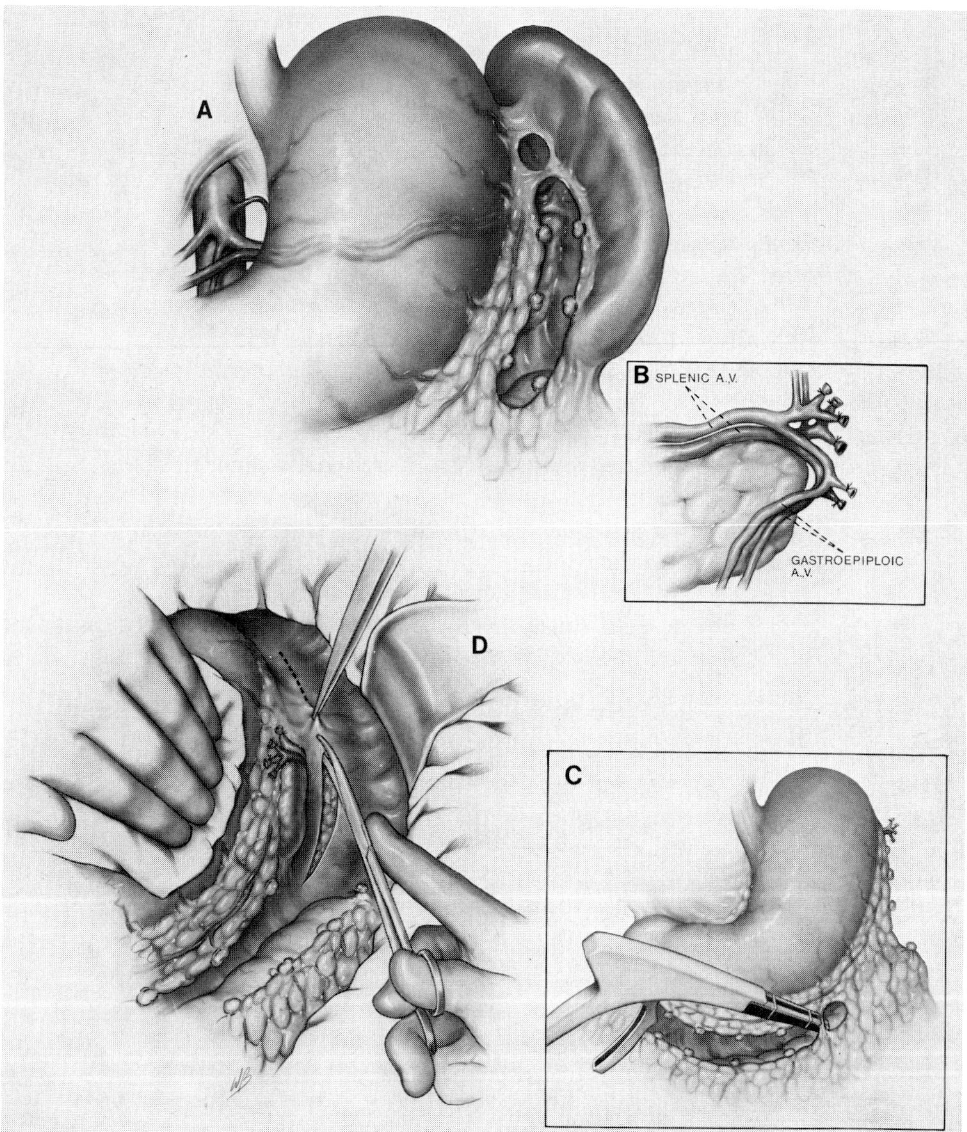

Fig VI–7.—Beck-Jianu-Gavriliu reversed gastric tube. **A** and **B,** the pertinent vascular anatomy is demonstrated. The gastroepiploic vessels are not always as beautifully continuous as they are shown in **B,** and in fact there usually is a gap well up on the fundus. The short gastric vessels are doubly clipped and divided with the LDS™ stapling instrument or manually divided and ligated. Splenectomy may be required **(B)** to permit development of a tube long enough to reach the desired level of cervical esophagus or pharynx. However, we make every effort to preserve the spleen even in adults and, in fact, generally succeed in doing this in children, where preservation of the spleen is an immunologic sine qua non. **C,** the gastrocolic omentum is serially divided and stapled with the LDS™ instrument just peripheral to the gastroepiploic vessels. The right gastroepiploic artery is divided at the level at which the tube is to be begun. **D,** the stomach is lifted forward and the loose posterior peritoneal attachments are divided, exposing the pancreas, as shown.

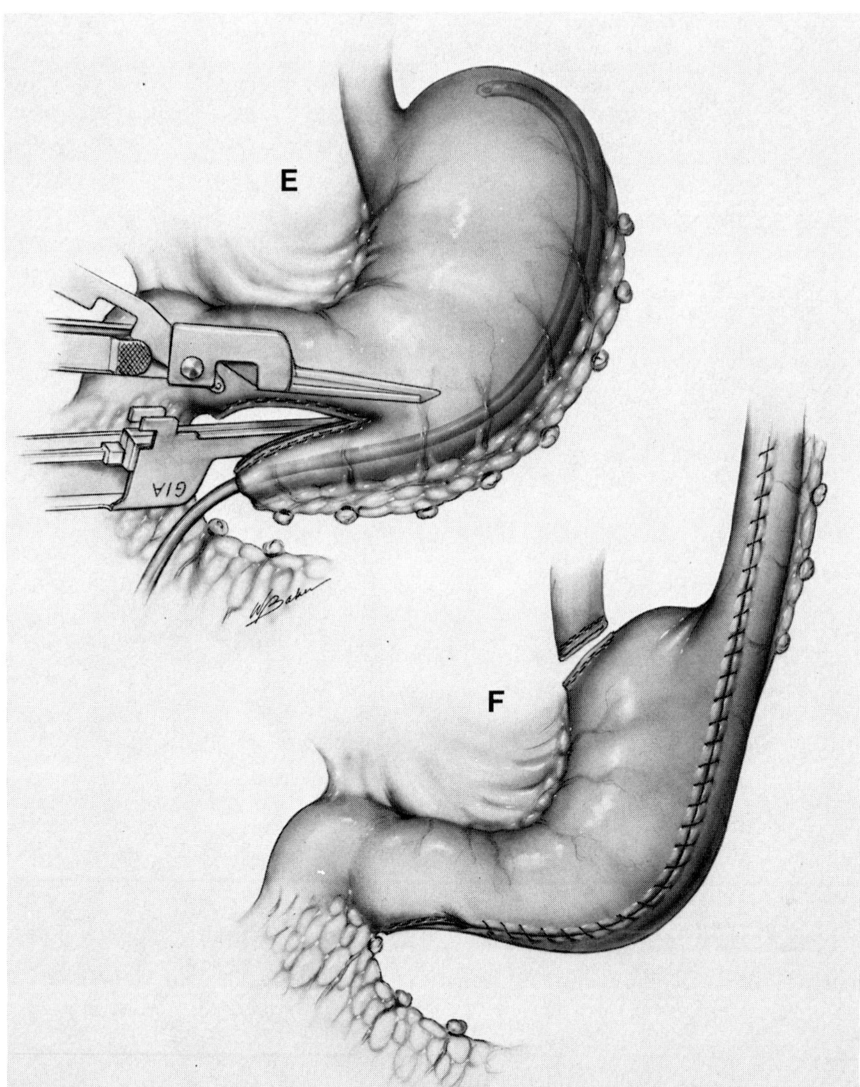

Fig VI–7 (cont.).—**E,** a No. 38–40 bougie or catheter is inserted into the stomach through a distal incision in the greater curvature some 2 cm proximal to the pylorus and the stomach serially divided longitudinally along the edge of this catheter with repeated applications of the GIA™ instrument. Each application produces a 5-cm tube. **F,** five or six applications quickly produce a tube that will easily reach above the clavicles. We oversew and invert the GIA™ closure of the stomach and tube because of the short length of the GIA™ staples in this suture of two thicknesses of gastric wall. Toward the end of the tube, the continuous oversewing suture is replaced by interrupted sutures so that if the tube requires to be shortened, one will not be dividing a continuous suture. If esophagectomy is part of the operation, the esophagus is divided from the stomach with the GIA™ instrument.   *(continued)*

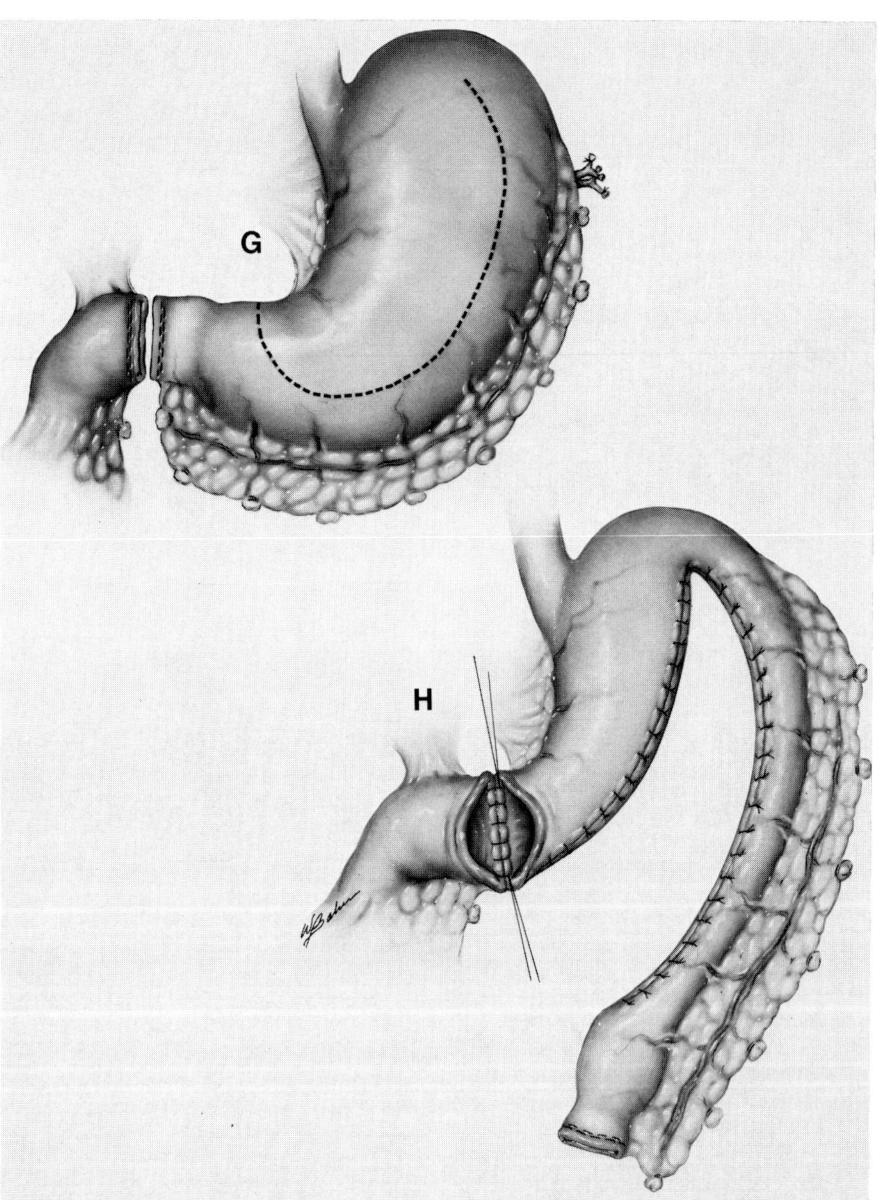

Fig VI–7 (cont.).—G, if additional length is required, as for direct anastomosis of the gastric tube to the pharynx, the gastric tube, instead of starting on the greater curvature, will follow the course shown by the dotted line, beginning on the lesser curvature, some 2 cm proximal to the pylorus, after the duodenum has been divided about the same distance beyond the pylorus, adding 4 or 5 cm to the length of the tube. **H,** the tube is shown completed. The new tubular gastric remnant is anastomosed manually to the duodenum, the GIA™ staples in the duodenum having been excised.

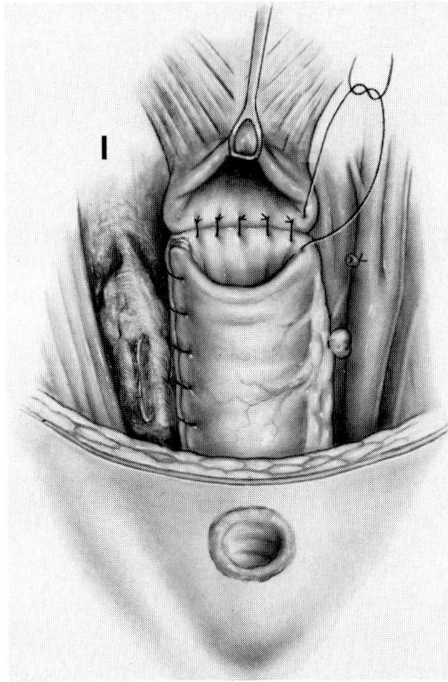

Fig VI–7 (cont.).—I, the reversed gastric tube, brought up in the anterior or posterior mediastinum, is shown being anastomosed manually, end-to-end, to the pharynx. Several thoracic surgeons have had success in performing an EEA™ anastomosis between esophagus or pharynx and the stomach, brought up in the neck, by passing the EEA™ instrument down through the mouth. It is possible that this technique already has been used for the anastomosis of the esophagus or pharynx to the end of a reverse gastric tube. (**A–D** and **G–I** from F.M. Steichen, *American Journal of Surgery,* 1977, used by permission.)

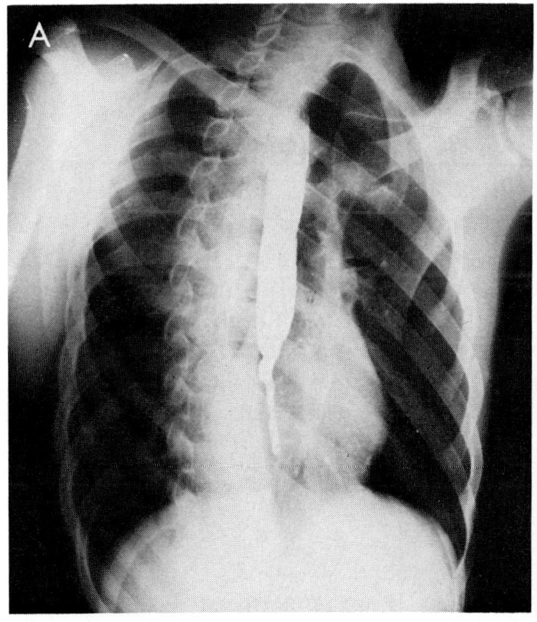

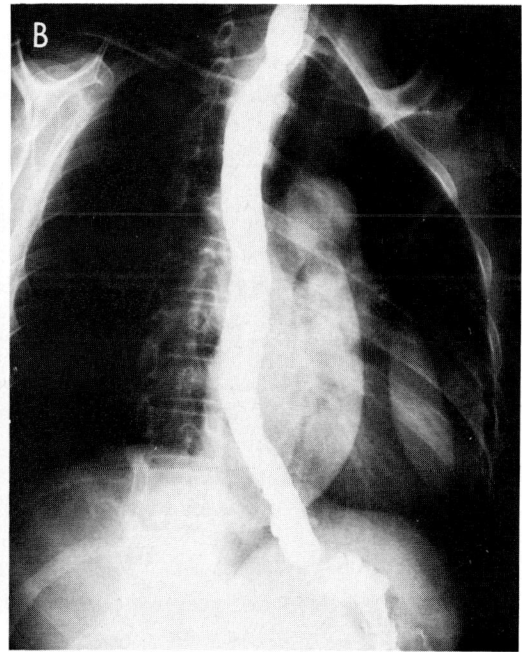

Fig VI–8.—Pre- and postoperative barium esophagograms—total esophagectomy and reverse gastric tube (one stage). The reverse gastric tube has a rich and dependable blood supply, takes little space, requires only a slender channel to pass through in either substernal or posterior mediastinal position, and readily reaches the neck. **A,** the carcinoma at junction of middle and lower thirds. **B,** the GIA™ constructed gastric tube in the posterior mediastinum, fills nicely and empties readily into the stomach. (Courtesy of Dr. Peter Weil.)

Kogan (1969) from Novosibirsk reported three patients with inoperable carcinoma of the esophagus and one with inoperable carcinoma of the cardia. He created a quite long greater-curvature Jianu tube by repeated applications of the UKL instrument (comparable in shape and function to the TA^{TM} series), so that the tube could be brought subcutaneously well above the costal margin to prevent leakage.

Skobelkin (1972) uses a TA^{TM}-type instrument with a slightly curved suture line, in which a knife simultaneously cuts through the tissue between the two staple lines at the moment of the driving in of the staples. This instrument, apart from the curve and the knife, is much like the UKL-60 (see Fig I–19*H,I*). It had been used clinically in construction of ten greater-curvature reverse gastric tubes, in 12 patients for wedge resection of the lesser curvature, and also in a variety of transections of stomach and colon. The instrument does not appear to have the retaining-aligning pin, and the published photograph suggests that its construction is accordingly substantially heavier than that of the UKL-60.

Cohen, Middleton, and Fletcher (1974) from the Royal Alexandra Hospital for Children in Sydney, Australia reported a series of 23 esophageal replacements in children with greater-curvature tubes, based on either the left or the right gastroepiploic artery, simply stating of the formation of the tube, "The Ravitch stapler is used to facilitate construction of the tube and gastric remnant which are further closed with two layers of sutures." There was a single complication related to the tube—a leak from the gastric tube into the chest producing empyema and ultimately resulting fatally.

Griffen and associates (Griffen, Daugherty, McGee, and Utley, 1976) from Lexington, Kentucky proposed the reverse gastric tube ". . . as a technique to be used in all patients who have carcinoma of the esophagus, whether the lesion is located in the upper, middle or lower esophagus." The reverse gastric tube was made with a GIA^{TM} stapler, reinforced by continuous manual suture. There were no staple line complications in their ten patients.

Skobelkin, Brechov, Ivanov, and Utkin (1977) from Moscow pointed out that, for reverse gastric loops, the straight instrument of the kind here described, or others that had been used, were awkward. They report a curved handleless instrument shaped much like the curved Japanese instrument (Uchiyama) (see Fig I–15*B*) but with staple slots and anvils of the delicate kind typical of the Russian instruments. On one limb is mounted a small housing that, as it is marched down the length of the instrument limb by turning a knob, drives in the staples and cuts down the middle, leaving a single staple line on each side of the cut. The instruments have removable cartridges that are, nevertheless, loaded by hand. The length of the instrument is not stated, except that the utilization of five magazines is said to leave a tube of 38–40 cm, so that it may, in fact, be as much as 8 cm long. After 88 animal experiments, the instrument was used in 20 patients for a reverse gastric tube and in 12 for a tube gastrostomy. The scanty description and the drawings suggest that the mechanism for driving in the staples is exactly like that in the Russian NZhKa instrument. In the operations there was good hemostasis in all cases and secure closure. Nothing is said of suture reinforcement of the single staple lines. There were no complications connected with the use of the apparatus.

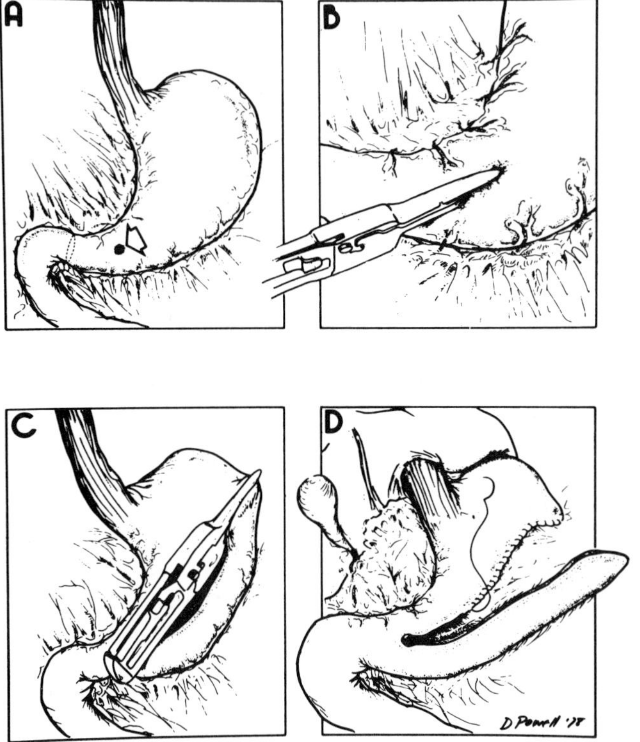

FIG. 1. A) After mobilization of greater curvature, a point is selected proximal to pylorus to begin tube. B) First application of stapler. C) Last application of stapler. D) Tube is formed, and staple row of stomach remnant is being closed with a continuous suture.

Fig VI–9.—Isoperistaltic gastric tube—Postlethwait of Durham, North Caroline (1979). The GIA[TM] instrument is inserted through a perforation in the antrum *(arrow)* and carried proximally as shown, coming across the greater curvature in the area of discontinuity of the left and right gastroepiploic vessels. The stapled edges are oversewn and the remaining portion of the initial perforation closed in two layers. One advantage of this technique is the fact that splenectomy is readily avoided. (From R.W. Postlethwait, *Annals of Surgery,* 1979, used by permission.)

Postlethwait (1979) of Durham, North Carolina, using the GIA[TM] instrument, prefers the isoperistaltic greater-curvature gastric tube based on the right gastroepiploic artery. The staple lines are oversewn with continuous synthetic suture. Isoperistaltic gastric tubes were constructed in 30 patients for a variety of indications. "Tube necrosis has not been seen, although in one patient who died postoperatively, autopsy showed a narrow rim of necrotic gastric mucosa."

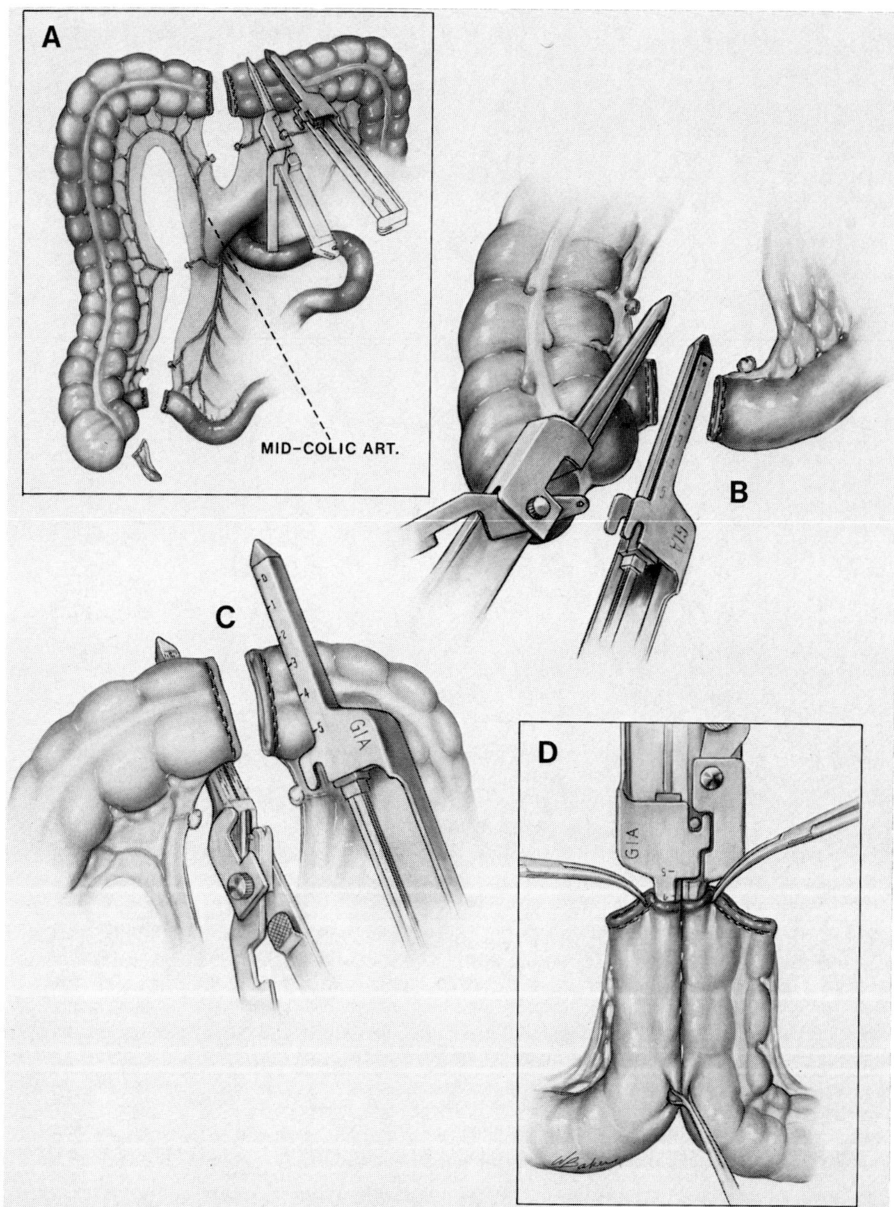

Fig VI–10.—Esophageal replacement with right colon. **A, B,** and **C,** the ileocecal and right colic vessels have been stapled and divided with the LDS™ instrument, the terminal ileum transected and stapled with the GIA™ instrument (as shown in detail in **B**), and the colon divided and stapled with the GIA™ instrument (as shown in **A** and **C**) to the left of the middle colic vessels, the left branch of which has been divided. The appendiceal vessels having been secured, the appendix has been amputated—with the GIA™ instrument, a bit of embroidery we do not usually indulge in. **D,** the ileo-transverse-colostomy is performed by the usual functional end-to-end technique (see Fig VIII–2), restoring intestinal continuity.

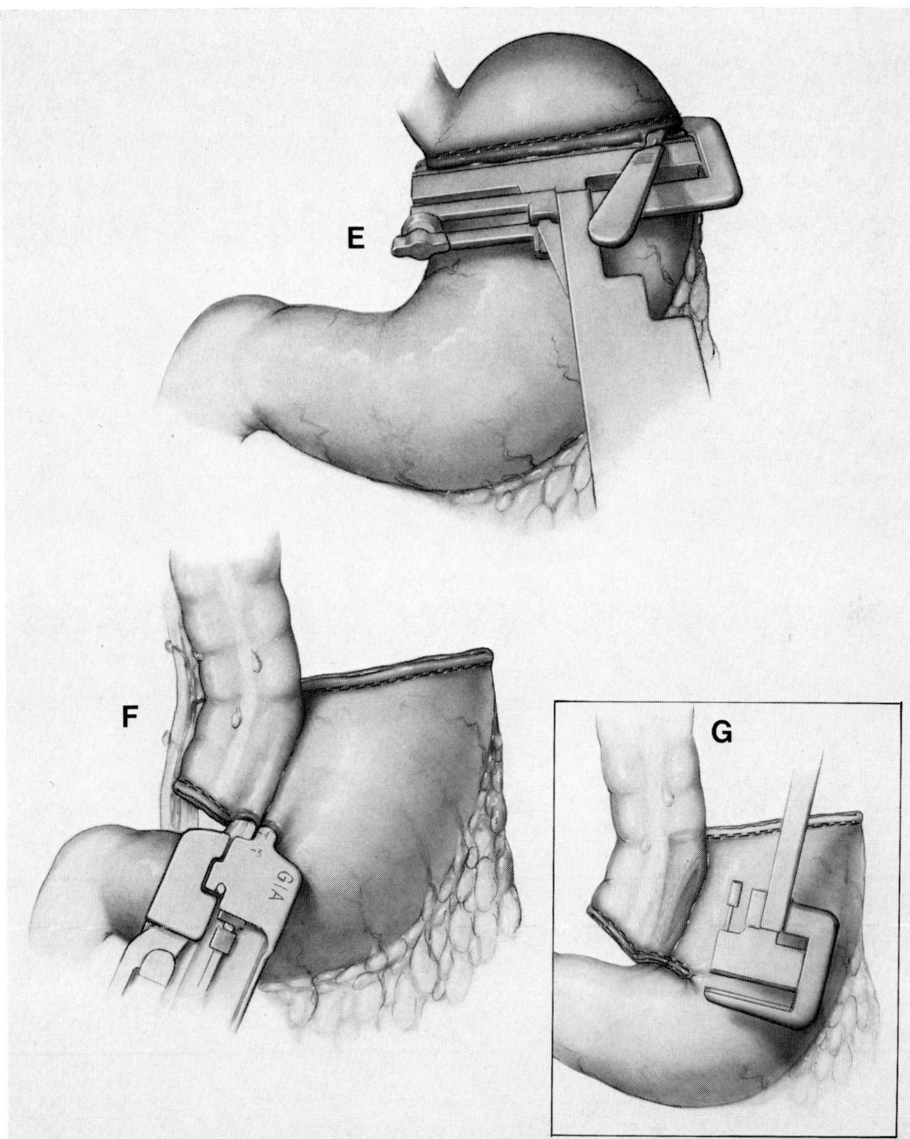

Fig VI–10 (cont.).—E, the gastric fundus is amputated, in this instance with two applications of the TA 90™ instrument, and the proximal double row of staples is seen still on the specimen side of the transection as it is begun. The GIA™ instrument could have served, the distal staple line then being inverted manually. **F,** the colon and its vascular pedicle have been brought up behind the stomach into the anterior or posterior mediastinum and the termino-lateral anastomosis is being performed between the colon and the stomach. The GIA™ instrument is inserted through the cutaway anti-mesenteric corner of the colon staple line and a stab wound in the stomach. **G,** the resultant single opening after withdrawal of the GIA™ instrument is closed mucosa-to-mucosa with the TA 30™ or TA 55™ instrument.   *(continued)*

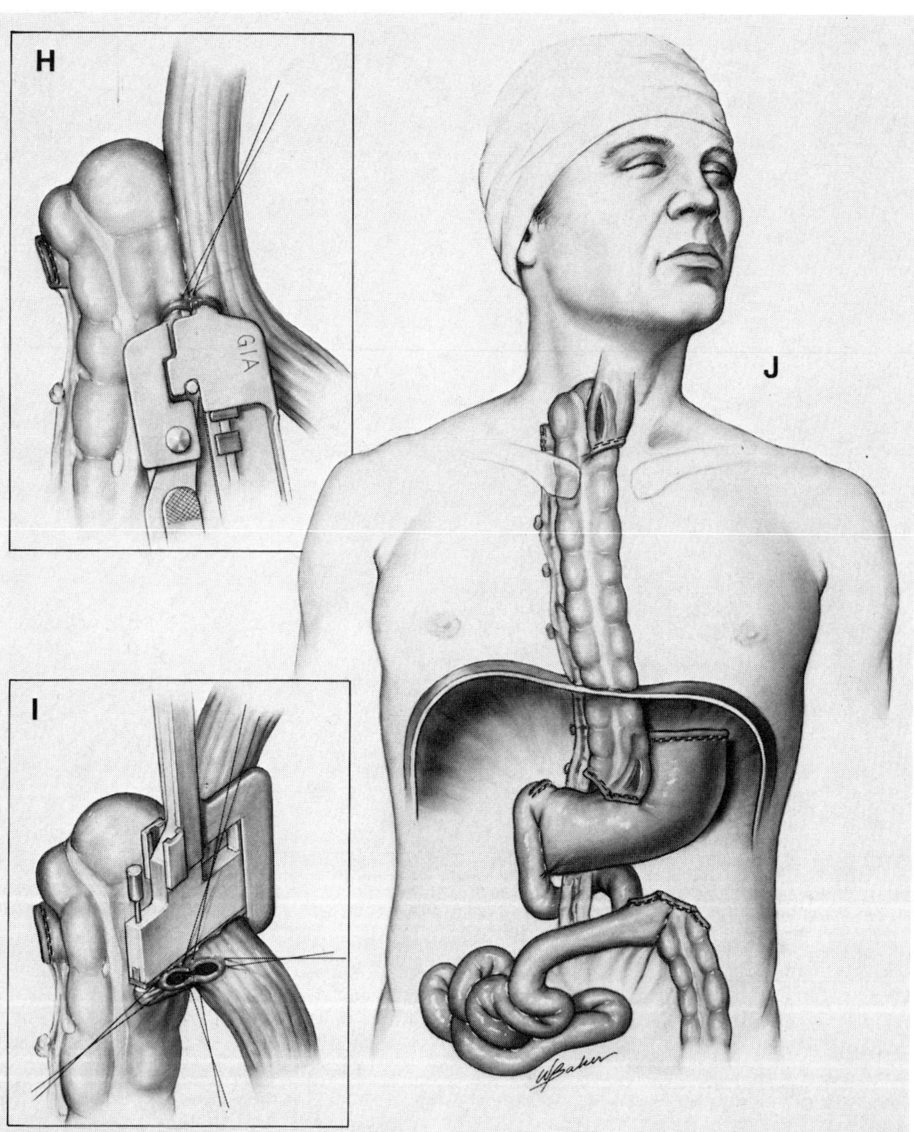

Fig VI–10 (cont.).—H, the cecum has been brought up into the neck, alongside the cervical esophagus, and the GIA™ instrument has been passed cephalad through stab wounds in the cecum and esophagus. **I,** with the GIA™ instrument withdrawn, an appropriate placement of the TA 55™ instrument permits one to staple off the esophagus obliquely, excluding the GIA™ opening (see NOTE below), so that when the esophagus and the open portion of the anastomosis are cut away with the scalpel on the border of the instrument, the anastomosis in effect is nearly end-to-end. This overlapping or bayonet-type reconstruction is applicable also to low rectal anastomoses (see Fig IX–2). **J,** the completed reconstruction, showing the Heineke-Mikulicz pyloroplasty (see Fig V–5), the division of the ileum, colon, and gastric fundus, the appendectomy, the ileocolostomy, the cologastrostomy, and the esophagocolostomy involve 13 residual suture lines. In general, we find that the great merit of the instruments lies in their precision and neatness, the decrease in the trauma inflicted on the tissues, and the lessened opportunity for bleeding or contamination. In operations as extensive as that shown in Figure VI–10, the time saved to the patient becomes a major factor indeed.

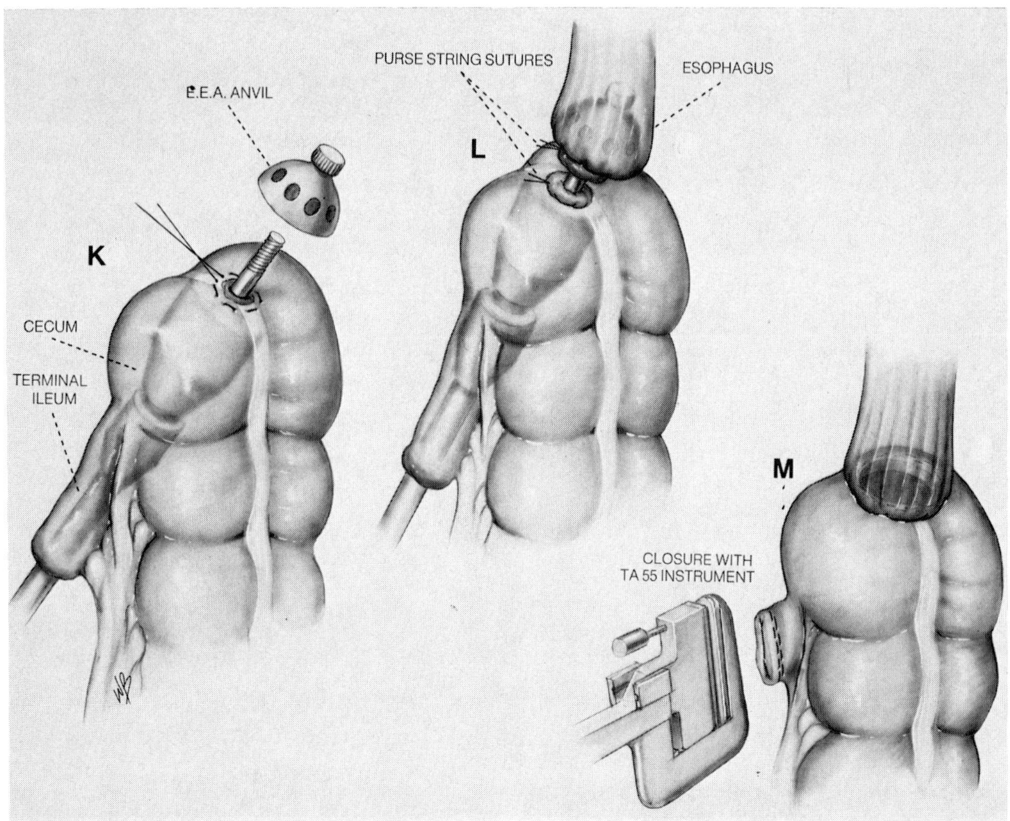

Fig VI–10 (cont.).—K and **L,** the use of the EEA™ instrument for the esophagocolic anastomosis in the neck. The EEA™ instrument with the anvil-nose cone unscrewed is slipped through the open terminal ileum, which may have to be dilated to accept the cartridge of the instrument. The center rod of the instrument is passed through the base of the appendix, which is, optionally, secured with a manually placed pursestring suture. The anvil-bearing nose cone is screwed onto the stem of the EEA™ instrument and passed into the esophagus, where it is secured with the pursestring made manually or with the pursestring instrument. **M,** the esophagus and colon have been brought together, the staples fired and the two rings of tissue cut out with the instrument's circular knife and the instrument withdrawn. The TA 55™ instrument now is used to staple and divide the ileum close to the cecum.

NOTE: The technique of stapling the esophagus and at the same time excluding the GIA™ orifice (Fig VI–10I) has been transposed by Welter, in the Billroth II reconstruction, simultaneously to close off the end of the stomach and to exclude the GIA™ opening made for the gastrojejunostomy (see Fig V–12), and is also shown by us in the Billroth I reconstruction (see Fig V–15). (**K–M** from F.M. Steichen and M.M. Ravitch, *Annals of Surgery,* 1980, used by permission.)

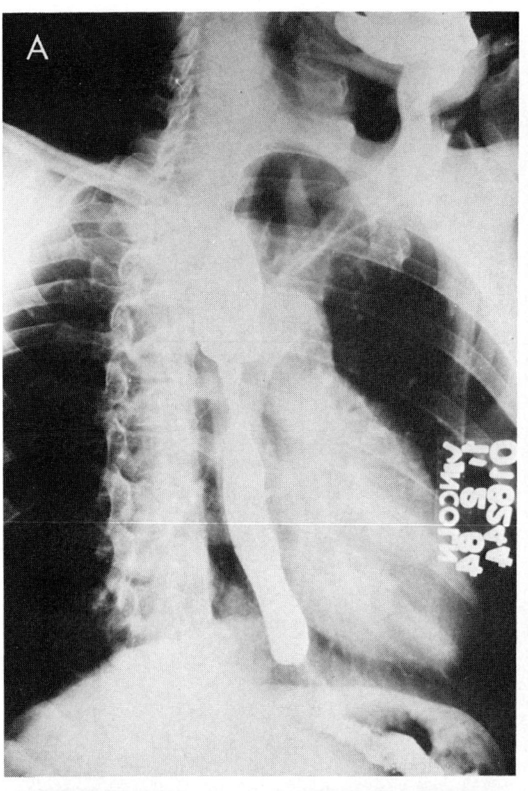

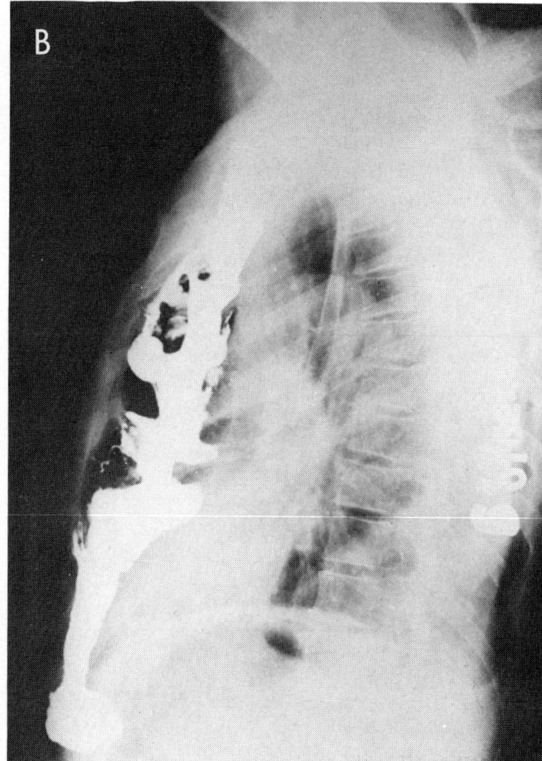

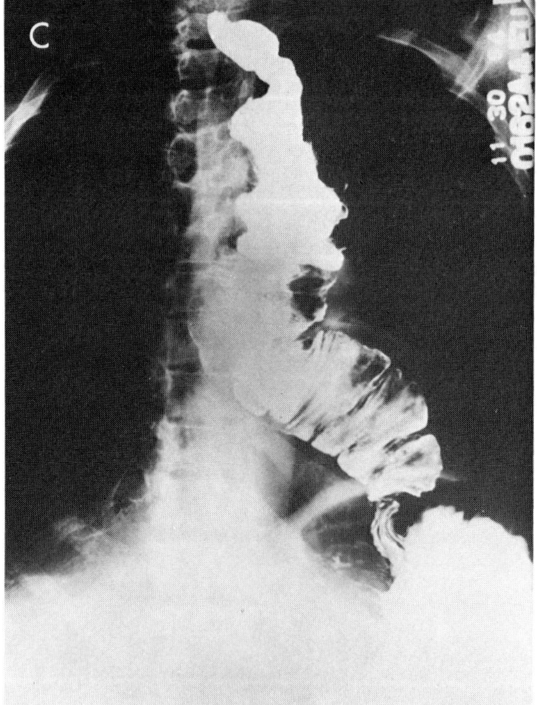

Fig VI–11.—Pre- and postoperative barium esophagograms—esophagocoloplasty. **A,** patient presenting with a constricting carcinoma of the mid-third of the esophagus. One-stage total esophagectomy with right colon replacement. All the steps involved in raising the colon are performed with the stapling instruments: transection of the proximal gastric fundus, transection and closure of terminal ileum and transverse colon, functional end-to-end ileocolostomy, Finney pyloroplasty, end-to-side cologastrostomy, end-to-side cervical esophagocolostomy (see Fig VI–7). **B** and **C,** postoperative barium study, showing the retrosternal esophagocoloplasty, extending from the cervical esophagus to the stomach.

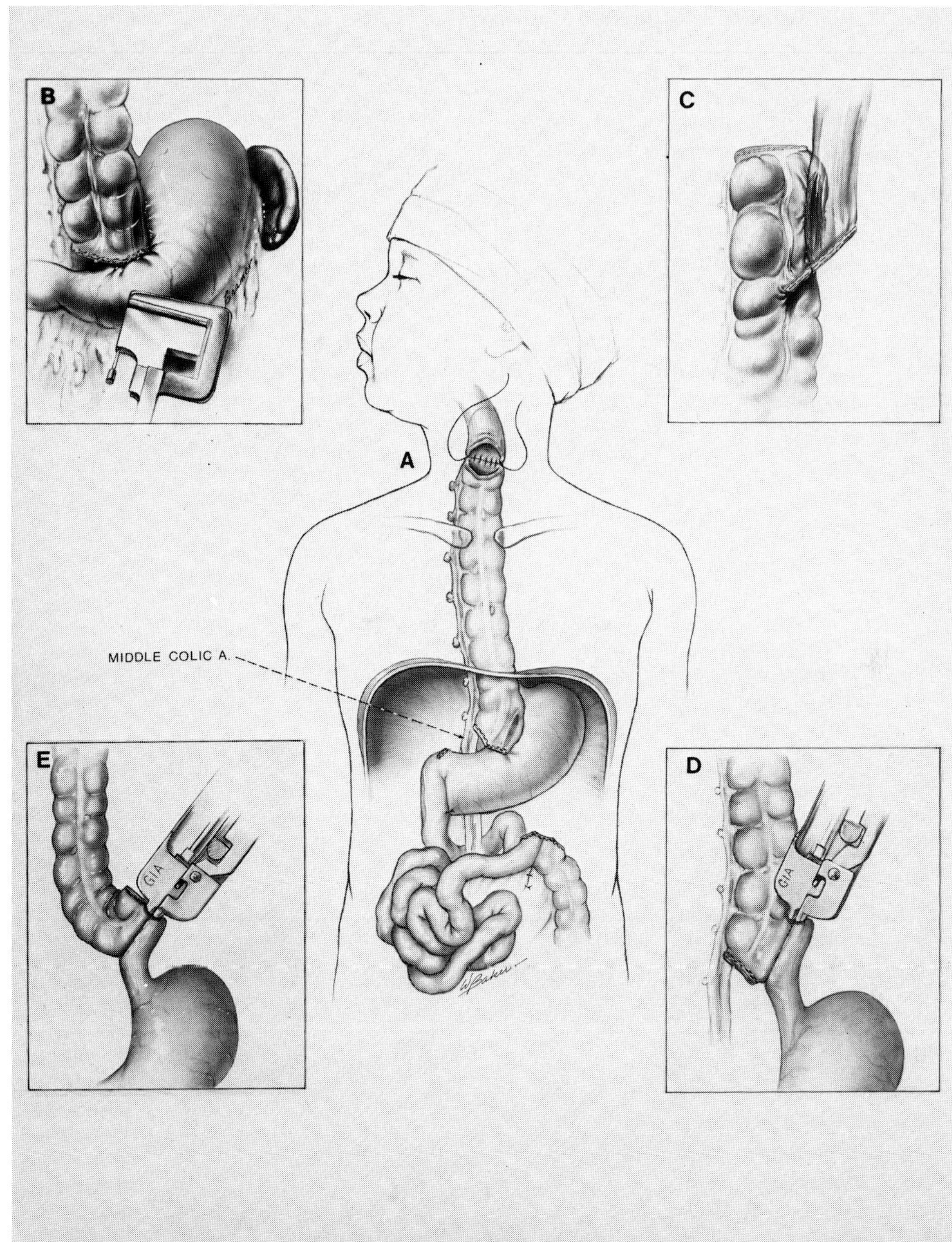

Fig VI–12.—Esophagocoloplasty in infancy. **A, B,** and **C,** the right colon has been mobilized on the middle colic artery (a procedure shown in Fig VI–10**A–E**) and brought up into the anterior mediastinum. The gastrocolic anastomosis is made with the GIA™ and TA™ instruments as in **B,** and the esophagocolic anastomosis made either manually in infants as in **A** or with the staples in larger children as in **C.**

D and **E,** the Waterston reconstruction in children with esophageal atresia, whether after a failed reconstruction or in the absence of tracheoesophageal fistula and with an excessive gap. The colon segment is brought up in the posterior mediastinum and the distal esophageal stump utilized for anastomosis to the distal end of the colon. Shown are two ways of using the GIA™ instrument to create the anastomosis. In a third option, with esophagus and colon held as in **D,** the GIA™ instrument would be passed upward, one blade through the cutaway corner of the colon and the other through a stab wound in the esophagus, much as in creating the cervical esophagocolic anastomosis in **C.** The current EEA™ instruments will not usually fit the infant or child esophagus (but see Fig VI–18**D**). (From F.M. Steichen, A.W. Dibbins, and E.S. Weiner, *Recent Advances in Paediatric Surgery,* 3d ed. New York, Churchill Livingstone, 1975, A.W. Wilkinson [ed.], used by permission.)

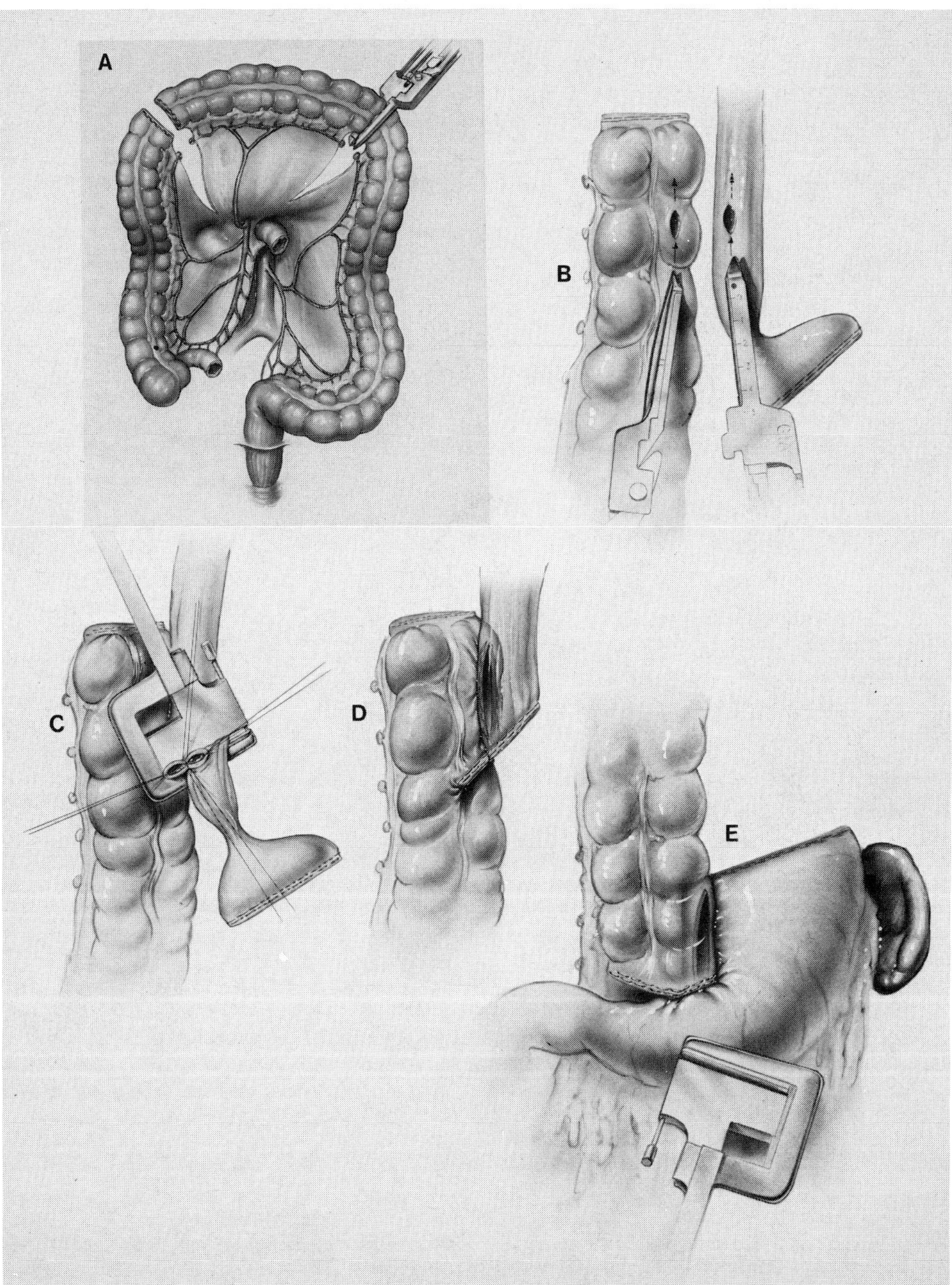

Fig VI–13.—Use of transverse colon to replace the distal esophagus. **A,** division and stapling of the colon at the flexures with the GIA™ instrument. The segment of colon required often is much shorter than that shown. **B,** the gastric fundus already has been stapled and divided, the esophagus freed and the colon brought up in the posterior mediastinum alongside the esophagus. The GIA™ limbs are inserted in the colic and esophageal openings as shown, passed upward, and the bayonet anastomosis made. **C,** much as in the esophagocolic anastomosis in the neck, an oblique placement of the TA 55™ instrument permits the staple closure of the esophagus and of the GIA™ wounds, with the result seen in **D. D,** an essentially termino-lateral but functionally end-to-end anastomosis. **E,** the colonic segment is anastomosed to the stomach, inserting the GIA™ instrument through the cutaway corner of the colic staple line and through a stab wound in the stomach and the GIA™ opening closed with the TA 55™ instrument.

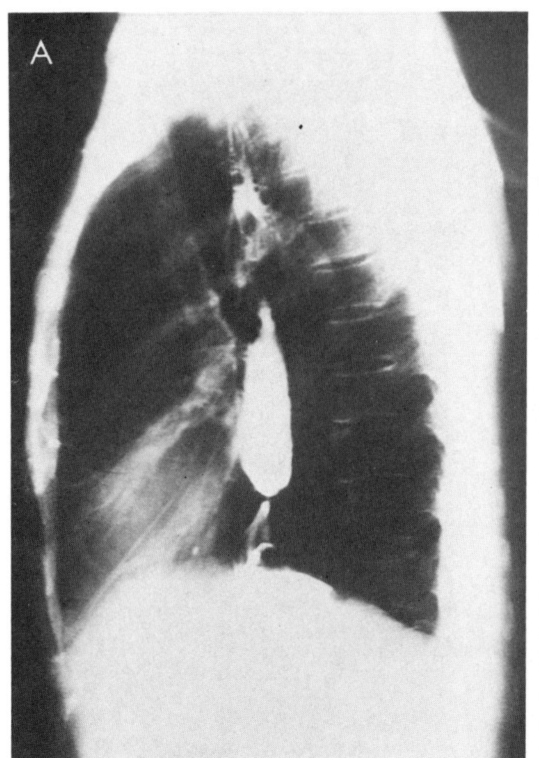
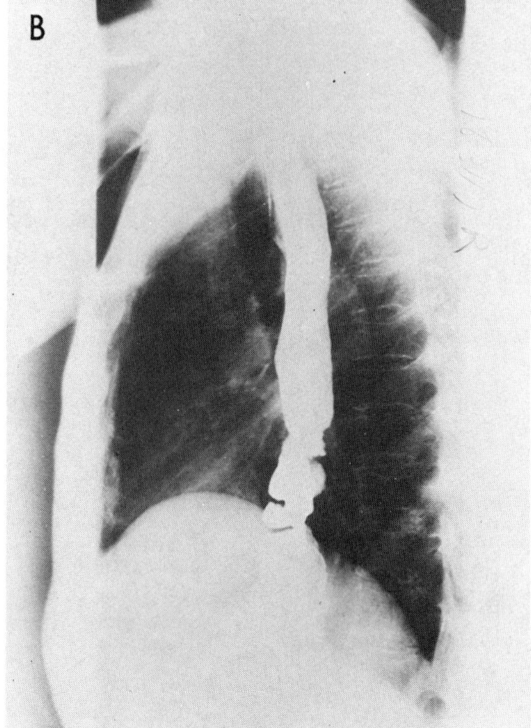

Fig VI–14.—Pre- and postoperative barium esophagograms—colon interposition. **A,** patient with a long, tight, fibrous stricture that could not be dilated preoperatively nor during operation when dilators were advanced under direct vision. **B,** barium swallow showing the result obtained with resection of the esophageal stricture and interposition of a segment of transverse colon. The approach was through a left thoracotomy and a separate upper midline abdominal incision.

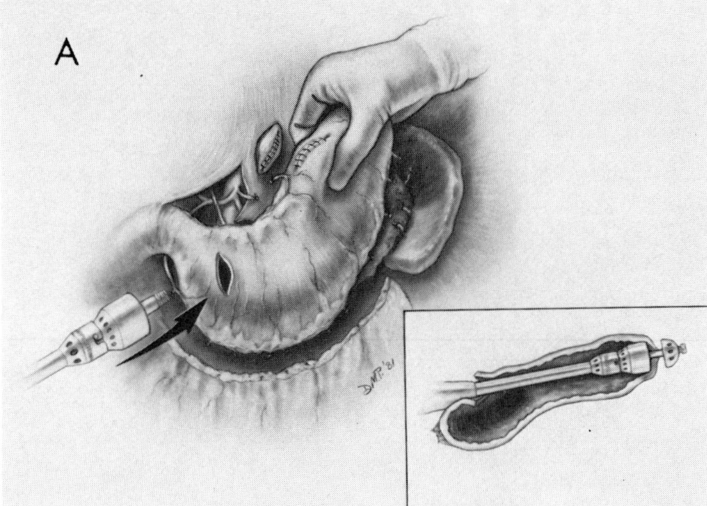

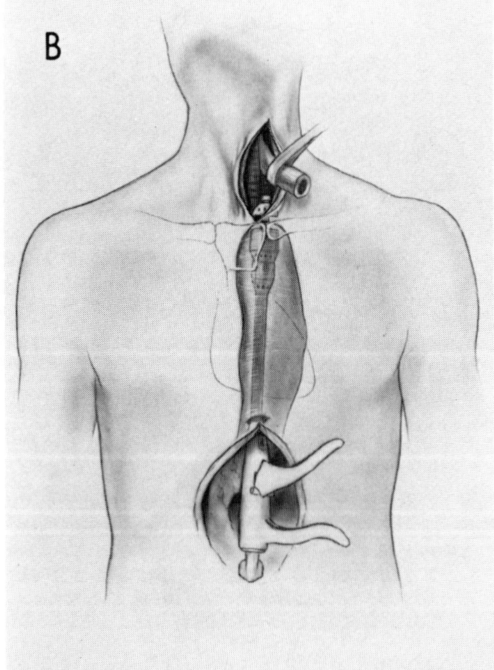

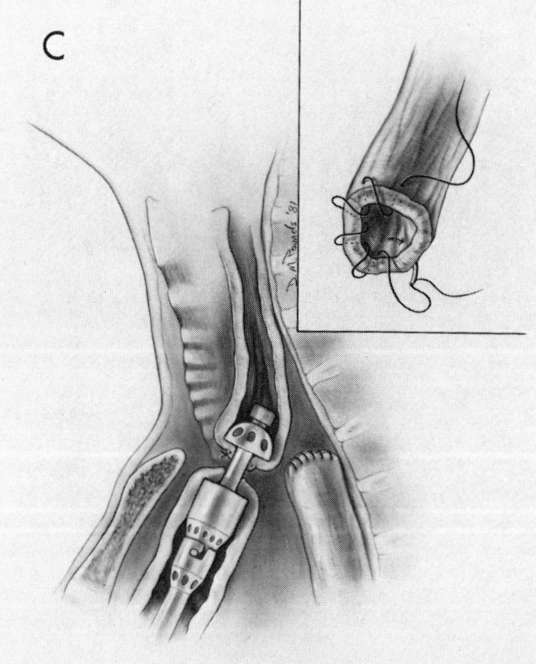

Fig VI–15.—Cervical esophagogastrostomy—technique of Mills (1981) for inoperable esophageal carcinoma and tracheoesophageal fistula. **A,** the esophagus has been transected at the stomach with the GIA™ instrument and both suture lines inverted. **B,** a substernal tunnel is created and the EEA™ instrument without the nose cone is inserted into the distal stomach through a gastrotomy and out the fundus. When the nose cone is screwed on, the EEA™ instrument carries the stomach up the tunnel and into the neck, the instrument being operated from within the abdomen. One patient required resection of clavicle and manubrium. The cervical esophagus is transected with the GIA™ instrument, the distal end dropped back, and the proximal end opened for the manually placed pursestring. **C,** details of pursestring and anastomosis. The EEA™ instrument is withdrawn and the gastrotomy closed manually. Two operations were performed as shown. In a third, enough stomach could be drawn into the neck to permit making the gastrotomy there for insertion of the EEA™ instrument. All three patients had primary healing of their anastomoses and were able to take nourishment by mouth. (From S.A. Mills, *Journal of Thoracic and Cardiovascular Surgery,* 1981, used by permission.)

From Winston-Salem, North Carolina, S.A. Mills reported (1981) his technique of substernal passage of the stomach, for palliative esophageal bypass. The EEA^{TM} instrument, inserted through a prepyloric gastrotomy, carries the stomach through the retrosternal tunnel to permit esophagogastrostomy in the neck. Two patients were successfully treated in this way. In a third, enough stomach was brought into the neck to permit inserting the EEA^{TM} instrument into that portion, also with success.

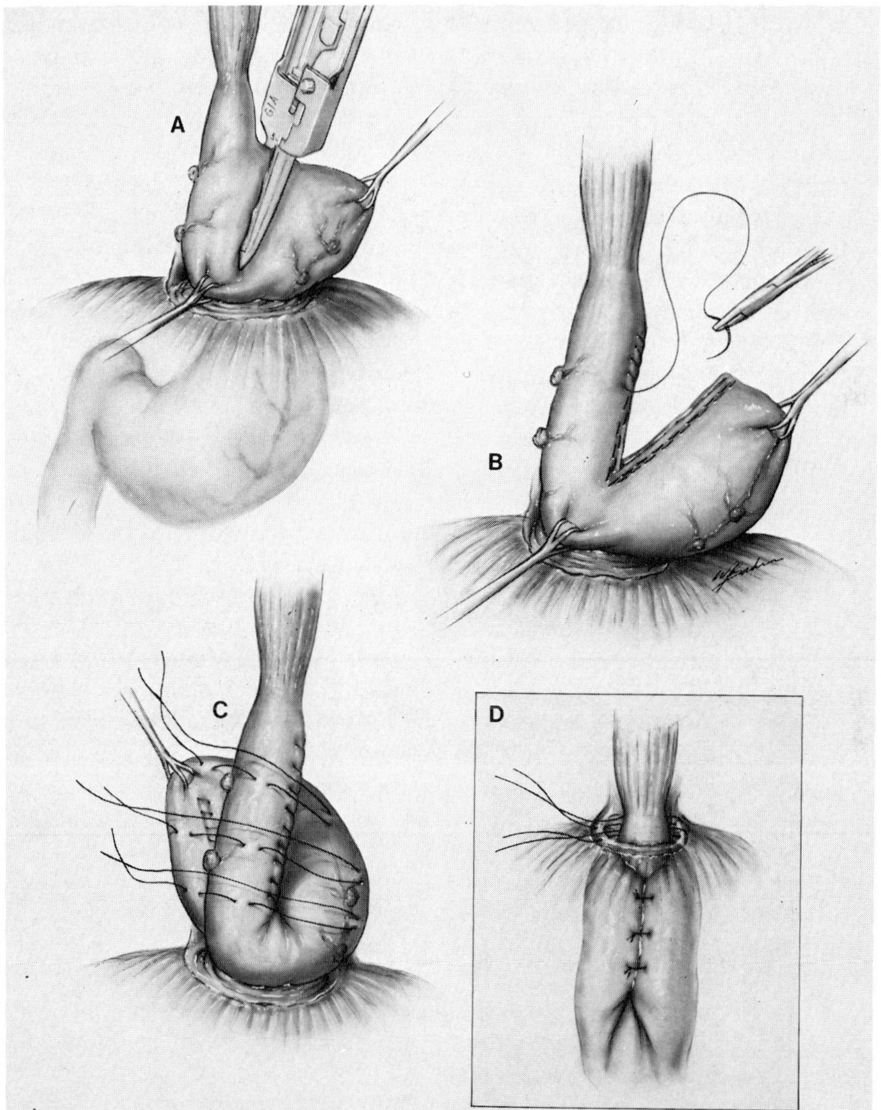

Fig VI–16.—Collis-Nissen gastroplasty. **A,** for fixed esophageal stricture due to esophageal reflux and esophagitis, with retraction of the abdominal esophagus into the mediastinum, the fundus of the stomach is pulled up through the hiatus and, with the GIA^{TM} instrument, a 5–6-cm gastric tube is created in continuity with the esophagus. **B,** as in all gastric uses of the GIA^{TM} instrument on a double thickness of gastric wall, the GIA^{TM} suture line is reinforced with a running suture. **C,** a Nissen wrap is performed, although generally this partakes more of the nature of swinging the dog-ear around the esophagus and suturing its tip to its base. **D,** the stomach has been replaced below the diaphragm and the hiatus closed around the tubed portion of the stomach, just distal to the stricture.

We had been looking for patients in whom to perform the Collis procedure with the GIA™ instrument. After Pearson's 1971 article (Pearson, Langer, and Henderson, 1971) on the Collis-Belsey procedure, we suggested to him (Ravitch, 1973) the applicability of the GIA™ instrument to the problem.

In fact, Orringer and Sloan (1974) first reported the use of the GIA™ stapler in creating the tubular gastric lengthening of the esophagus in the treatment of esophageal reflux by the Collis technique. The staple lines were covered with a continuous suture of 4–0 Prolene. At that point, Orringer was using the Belsey antireflux procedure. Orringer and Sloan by 1977 had used the GIA™ instrument in 83 Collis-Belsey procedures, with no complications from use of the GIA™ instrument.

By 1978, they (Orringer and Sloan, 1978) had abandoned the Collis-Belsey and had added Nissen fundoplication to the GIA™-Collis procedure as the antireflux measure. In 30 patients, they had one necrosis of the gastric tube, with salvage, and no other staple complications. By 1982 (Orringer, 1983), they could report 135 GIA™-performed Collis procedures with 89% two-year relief from reflux symptoms.

Pearson and his colleagues in 1977, from Toronto (Cooper, Gill, Nelems, and Pearson, 1977), published their physiologic studies of 11 patients in whom the Collis procedure was performed with the GIA™ instrument, without operative complications, not mentioning how many other patients might have been so operated on without having the detailed studies that were the subject of their report.

Urschel and Razzuk from Dallas (1979) used the GIA™ stapler in performing the Collis gastroplasty in 86 patients. "No patient had an esophageal leak or a wound infection, and there were no deaths."

Demos of Jersey City (1976), after animal experiments, created the Collis tube in 25 patients by a longitudinal partition of the stomach with the TA 55™ instrument, not dividing the tube from the stomach, and using a Nissen wrap. He reported good results and made no mention of complications.

Paris and Benages (Paris, Benages, Ridocci, Tarazona, Molina, Mora, Pastor, Lloret, and Garrido, 1977; Benages, Paris, Ridocci, Tarazona, Molina, Mora, Canto, Lloret, and Garrido, 1978) from Valencia, Spain, in 1977 similarly suggested that the American TA 90™ stapler or the Soviet UTL (see Fig I–19*L,P*) stapler could be used to partition off the Collis tube, without the necessity for dividing the tube from the stomach in most cases. If division was thought necessary, they reapplied the stapler and divided the stomach between the two double TA 90 ™ staple lines. In 34 cases, all done transthoracically, there were no fistulas and no leaks.

J.A.W. Bingham of Belfast (1977), also in 1977, reported transthoracic construction of a Collis gastroplasty with the TA 55™ instrument, without dividing the stomach, in 138 patients since 1971. A Nissen fundoplication was added. The single death was from fat embolism. There were no staple line problems other than the fact that eight patients developed "a side opening through the stapled partition" and one of these had continuing esophagitis requiring reoperation.

Evangelist, Taylor, and Alford from Charlotte, North Carolina (1978) report the use of the GIA™ stapler for the Collis procedure in 48 patients since 1973, and, like the groups from Spain and Ireland, did not divide the stomach, in their cases using the GIA™ stapler without the cutting blade. They considered that this much simplified the performance of the Nissen fundoplication. There were no staple line complications. All patients (17 with strictures) were relieved from the symptoms of reflux esophagitis. The patients were operated on between June, 1973 and July, 1977.

At the May, 1982 meeting of the American Association for Thoracic Surgery, Evangelist (1983) reported that 49 of his patients now had been followed eight to nine years. All patients had normal manometric and 24-hour pH studies. One patient had mild dysphagia and one had anatomical recurrence but no reflux. Henderson of Toronto (Henderson and Marryatt, 1983) commented that "Bingham, who originally reported having used an uncut tube, ran into problems of breakdown of the uncut tube and fistulas forming from the stomach through and into the gastroplasty tube. This may or may not be a problem, but I think it has to be sought in patients being treated by your operation."

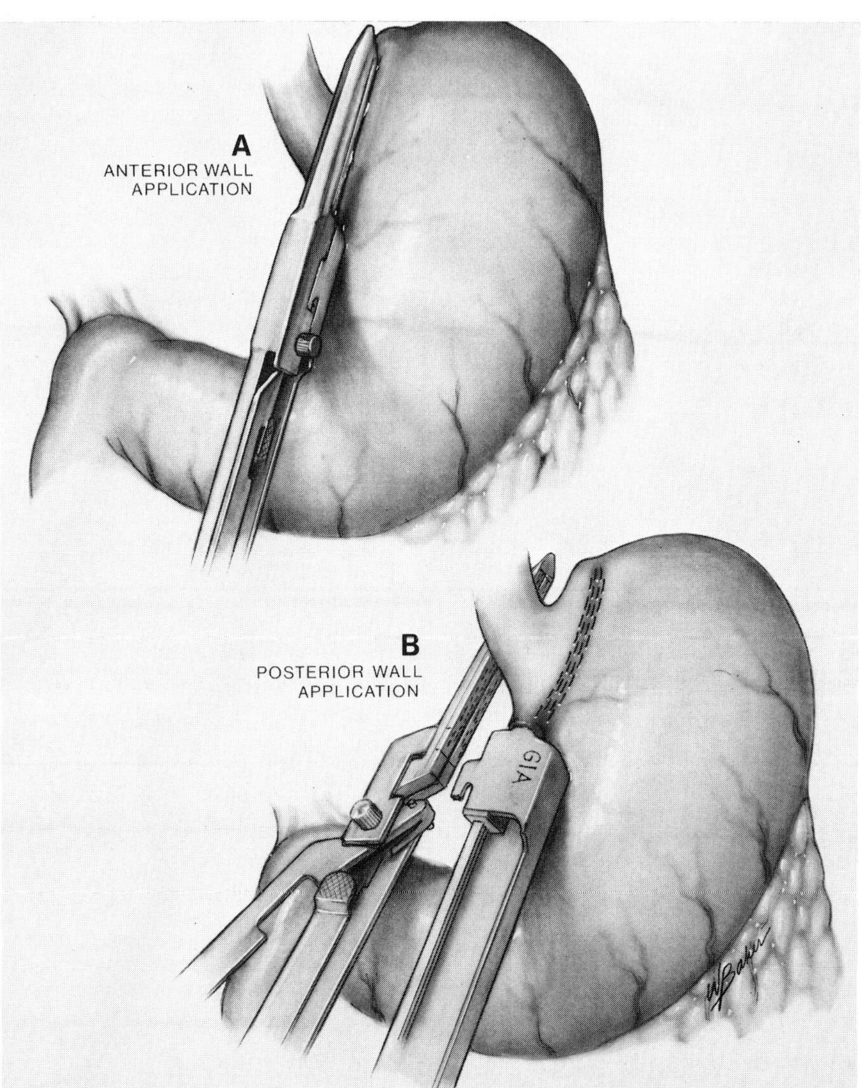

Fig VI–17.—Control of bleeding esophageal varices. Use of the GIA™ instrument. The GIA™ instrument with the special black cartridge (SGIA™), which inserts four rows of staples but does not have a knife (one can also simply break the knife out of the conventional standard GIA™ cartridge), is inserted twice through a lesser-curvature gastrotomy, once **(A)** stapling the anterior wall of the stomach and once **(B)** stapling the posterior wall of the stomach, with four rows of staples in each case. The opening made for the GIA™ instrument on the lesser curvature then is closed manually or with the TA™ instrument. (From F.M. Steichen and M.M. Ravitch, *Annals of Surgery*, 1980, used by permission.)

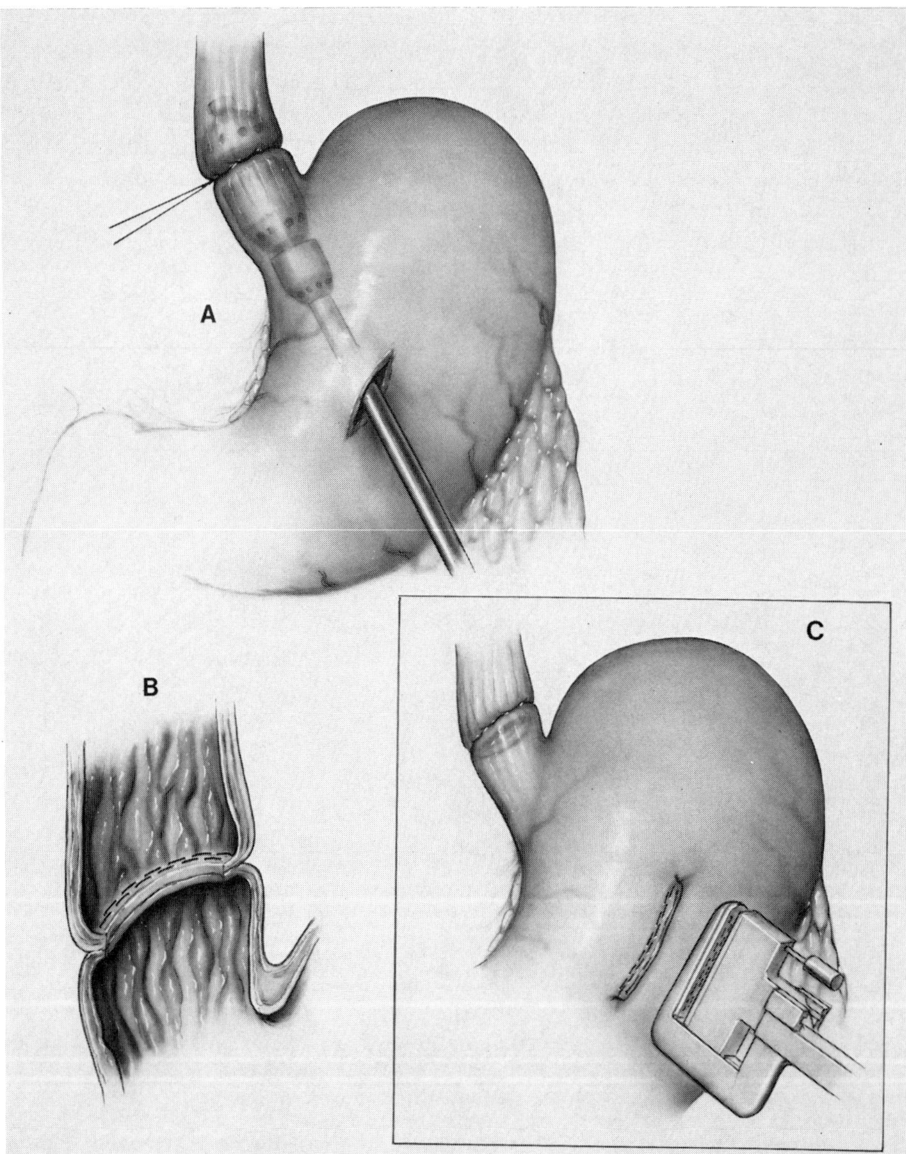

Fig VI–18.—Control of bleeding esophageal varices—Boerema operation (see Fig I–8U) with the EEA™ instrument. **A,** the collateral vessels along the esophagus having been appropriately ligated and divided, the fully assembled EEA™ instrument is passed upward through a gastrotomy into the abdominal esophagus. A ligature is passed around the esophagus, between the separated staple cartridge and anvil, and tied tightly, the instrument screwed shut and the handle squeezed, cutting out a short segment of the esophagus. **B,** there results a stapled anastomosis, the staples suturing full thickness of the esophagus. **C,** the gastrotomy has been closed mucosa-to-mucosa with the TA™ instrument. **D,** EEA™ annular resection of distal esophagus for bleeding varices. (case of Dr. Marc Rowe) An eight-month-old infant with liver failure from alpha-1-antitrypsin deficiency, severe portal hyperten-sion, gastric and esophageal varices, developed massive upper gastrointestinal hemorrhage while under consideration for liver transplantation. Transgastric insertion of the EEA™ instrument and annular resection of the distal esophagus stopped the bleeding immediately. There was no further bleeding during the child's short life, but decision was made against transplantation. Two other similar children have had their bleeding varices controlled by the same technique. The ring of staples is clearly seen at the lower end of the esophagus as well as the TA™ staple line marking the closure of the gastrotomy. Doctor Rowe's success with the EEA™ instrument in the gently dilated infant esophagus is thus far unique. (**A–C** from F.M. Steichen and M.M. Ravitch, *Annals of Surgery,* 1980, used by permission; **D** courtesy of M. Rowe, M.D.) →

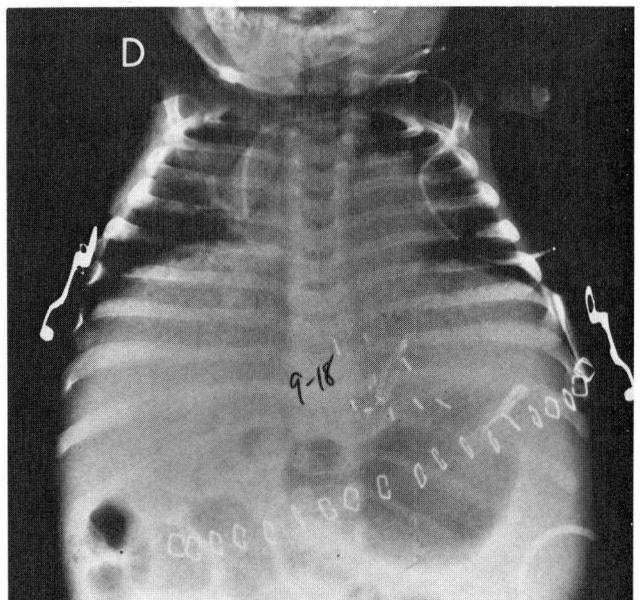

Fig VI–18 D.

The same result was achieved by the Boerema device (Boerema, 1954; Boerema, Klopper, and Holscher, 1970; Johnston and Kelly, 1976) (see Fig I–8*U*), essentially an esophageal Murphy button, which, by gradual necrosis of the inverted and compressed tissues, performed a full-thickness annular resection. It had the advantage that it could be inserted through the mouth and did not require a gastrotomy.

ESOPHAGEAL VARICES

Apparently there is a certain disenchantment with portosystemic shunting for portal hypertension and variceal bleeding, whatever the type of shunt, because of the late results—hepatic failure, and encephalopathy in particular—although control of bleeding has been reasonably satisfactory. In the search for "temporizing" measures to control bleeding, without unacceptable late effects, control of esophageal varices by sclerosing injection or by transection of stomach or esophagus have been reinvestigated. The GIA™ or PGIA™ instrument, without the knife blade, or the SGIA™ instrument, to staple first the anterior and then the posterior wall of the stomach, and the EEA™ instrument to perform a full-thickness annular resection and anastomosis of the distal esophagus, are both undergoing investigation. It would appear that the results by the two techniques are equivalent in control of bleeding. With the GIA™ technique, one must be certain that the closure of the gastrotomy is secure—we lost one patient from a failure in that. In patients operated on in emergency, the operative evacuation of blood from the stomach risks contamination. Johnston's comments (1981) about esophageal stenosis with the Russian instrument and his recommendations to prevent it should be noted (v.i.).

The first stapling attack on esophageal varices, which we have found was that by Kolesnikov (1969), who used the UKL-60 (see Fig I–19*H,I*) for what he called his modification of the Tanner operation. In fact, he inserted the UKL-60 instrument through a stab wound high on the lesser curvature, first stapling the anterior wall transversely and then the posterior wall. In the course of six years, he had performed seven such operations without any fatalities and presumably with control of bleeding, which is specifically stated only in the two case reports included.

Rinecker and Danek (1975) from Munich, apparently without any knowledge of Kolesnikov's prior use of the linear stapler—the UKL (see Fig I–19*H,I*)— in the transgastric control of bleeding varices, reported use of the GIA™ instrument, with the knife blade removed, for the same purpose. The GIA™ instrument inserted through a high lesser-curvature gastrotomy, first on the anterior wall, then on the posterior, placed four rows of staples on each wall whereas the UKL placed only two rows of staples. They reported a single case, with successful outcome.

Vankemmel of Lille, France (1976) used the Russian PKS (see Fig I–20*A-C*) and SPTU instruments, introduced into the esophagus through a gastrotomy, the esophagus tightly ligated and the instrument operated, excising an annular segment of esophagus and stapling the two ends together in the same procedure, which he recognized as an application of the Boerema principle, referring also to the prior work of Vosschulte (1957) and the subsequent work of Prioton (1973) (see Chapter I). At the time of his 1972 paper, Vankemmel had operated on 30 patients by this technique with the Russian cylindrical stapling instruments, eight times during massive hemorrhage with two deaths and 22 times subsequent to the hemorrhage with five deaths. Johnston (1981) cited a personal communication from Vankemmel in 1979 listing 52 stapling resections of the esophagus for bleeding varices. In the 37 patients operated on more than three years earlier there were ten operative deaths and six late deaths. There were six episodes of bleeding in the two years after operation as opposed to 162 in the two years before operation. In only three of the six instances was the recurrent bleeding due to varices.

Johnston (1977) of Belfast, adopting the annular resection—Boerema—technique with the Russian SPTU, reported 12 patients with one operative death from respiratory failure and four patients who required one to three esophageal dilatations for stricture. There were no anastomotic leaks. Persistent oozing in one patient was the only postoperative bleeding and there had been no late bleeding after seven months.

Booth, Criado, and Wilson (1980) from Baltimore reported a single successful use of the EEA™ instrument for control of variceal bleeding as suggested a year before (Ravitch and Steichen, 1979).

Carey (Cooperman, Fabri, Martin, and Carey, 1980), whose earlier experience was referred to by Booth, reported the use of the EEA™ instrument for annular resection of the esophagus in five patients with bleeding esophageal varices. One patient died of renal failure and there was one wound infection. There were no fistulas and there had been no recurrence of bleeding in patients followed up to 27 months.

From Montreal, Wexler (1980) reported a series of six patients with annular resection of the esophagus with the EEA™ instrument for variceal bleeding. Two patients were surviving at a year and a half and two years, respectively. One patient died approximately ten days after operation, one at 15 days with an ascitic leak, septicemia, and hepatorenal syndrome and DIC, one at 25 days with an ascitic leak, peritonitis, hepatic failure, and severe reflux, and one at ten days, of Pseudomonas septicemia. At the meeting of the Central Surgical Association at which Wexler presented his paper, F.M. Steichen (1980), in discussion, mentioned four cases in New York in which the Rinecker-Danek procedure had been done by him and 14 more by L.R.M. Del Guercio, both adding ligation of the coronary vein and its collaterals and of the splenic artery if it measured more than 0.9 mm in diameter.

Kuzmak (1981) of Irvington, New Jersey used the EEA™ instrument in the treatment of varices in three patients. One, who had had a LeVeen shunt removed at the same time, died nine days after operation of an autopsy-proved coronary occlusion. One died of liver failure six months later. Neither of these two patients rebled. The third patient was alive at 18 months, had not rebled, and his varices had diminished in size.

By 1981, Johnston had an experience with 60 patients using the SPTU, commenting only that the method was "equally applicable to the newer American EEA stapler." In 18 cases, the procedure, carried out as an emergency, resulted in six deaths. In the 42 patients operated on days or weeks after cessation of the bleeding there were five deaths. Two patients had leaks (all SPTU suture lines were reinforced), but there were no gross dehiscences. The one leak that was fatal was due to an unrecognized tear from dilatation of a stricture. The suture line itself was intact. Eight of his first 49 survivors developed strictures requiring dilatation—four of the first 12, four of the next 37. In the second group, he moved the transection from 1.5–2.5 cm above the cardia to "immediately above the esophagogastric junction."

REFERENCES

Akiyama H.: Personal communication, June 17, 1981.

Benages A., Paris F., Ridocci M., Tarazona V., Molina R., Mora F., Canto A., Lloret M., Garrido G.: Lesser curvature tubular gastroplasty with partial plication for gastroesophageal reflux: Manometric and pH-metric postoperative studies. *Ann. Thorac. Surg.* 26:574, 1978.

Bérard Ph., Papillon M., Jacquemard R., Labrosse H., Bigay D., Guillemin G.: Les anastomoses digestives à la EEA. A propos de cent quatre cas. *Ann. Chir.* 35:403, 1981.

Bingham J.A.W.: Hiatus hernia repair combined with the construction of an anti-reflux valve in the stomach. *Br. J. Surg.* 64:460, 1977.

Boerema I.: The technique of our method of transabdominal total gastrectomy in cases of gastric cancer. *Arch. Chir. Neerl.* 6:95, 1954.

Boerema I., Klopper P.J., Holscher A.A.: Transabdominal ligation-resection of the esophagus in cases of bleeding esophageal varices. *Surgery* 67:409, 1970.

Booth F.V. McL., Criado F.J., Wilson T.H. Jr.: Lower esophageal transection with the EEA stapler: An alternative method to control variceal bleeding. *Am. Surg.* 46:494, 1980.

Chassin J.L.: Esophagogastrectomy: Data favoring end-to-side anastomosis. *Ann. Surg.* 188:22, 1978.

Chassin J.L.: Stapling technic for esophagogastrostomy after esophagogastric resection. *Am. J. Surg.* 136:399, 1978.

Cohen D.H., Middleton A.W., Fletcher J.: Gastric tube esophagoplasty. *J. Pediatr. Surg.* 9:451, 1974.

Cooper J.D., Gill S.S., Nelems J.M., Pearson F.G.: Intraoperative and postoperative esophageal manometric findings with Collis gastroplasty and Belsey hiatal hernia repair for gastroesophageal reflux. *J. Thorac. Cardiovasc. Surg.* 74:744, 1977.

Cooperman M., Fabri P.J., Martin E.W. Jr., Carey L.C.: EEA esophageal stapling for control of bleeding esophageal varices. *Am. J. Surg.* 140:821, 1980.

Demos N.J.: A simplified, improved technique for the Collis gastroplasty for dilatable esophageal strictures. *Surg. Gynecol. Obstet.* 142:591, 1976.

Dorsey J.S., Esses S., Goldberg M., Stone R.: Esophagogastrectomy using the Auto Suture® EEA™ surgical stapling instrument. *Ann. Thorac. Surg.* 30:308, 1980.

Engelberg M., Jedeikin R.J., Eschkol D., Hoffman S., Reiss R.: Use of a stapling technique in closure of perforation of the esophagus. *Am. J. Surg.* 142:300, 1981.

Evangelist F.A.: In discussion of Henderson R.D., Marryatt G. *J. Thorac. Cardiovasc. Surg.* 85:81, 1983.

Evangelist F.A., Taylor F.H., Alford J.D.: The modified Collis-Nissen operation for control of gastroesophageal reflux. *Ann. Thorac. Surg.* 26:107, 1978.

Fasching W., Moritz E.: Zirkuläre Klammeranastomosen im Magen-Darm-Trakt mit den Klammernahtgeräten SPTU und EEA. *Chirurg* 51:644, 1980.

Féketé F.: Personal communication, June 17, 1981.

Féketé F., Breil Ph., Ronsse H.: Anastomoses mécaniques à la pince EEA en chirurgie oesophagienne. *Chirurgie* 106:659, 1980.

Féketé F., Breil Ph., Ronsse H., Tossen J.C., Langonnet F.: EEA® stapler and omental graft in esophagogastrectomy. *Ann Surg.* 193:825, 1981.

Gentili J.M.: Personal communication, June, 1981.

Griffen W.O. Jr., Daugherty M.E., McGee E.M., Utley J.R.: Unified approach to carcinoma of the esophagus. *Ann. Surg.* 183:511, 1976.

Henderson R.D., Marryatt G.: Total fundoplication gastroplasty. *J. Thorac. Cardiovasc. Surg.* 85:81, 1983.

Hoehn J.G., Payne W.S.: Resection of pharyngoesophageal diverticulum using stapling device. *Mayo Clin. Proc.* 44:738, 1969.

Johnston G.W.: Treatment of bleeding varices by oesophageal transection with the SPTU gun. *Ann. R. Coll. Surg. Engl.* 59:404, 1977.

Johnston G.W.: Bleeding oesophageal varices: The management of shunt rejects. *Ann. R. Coll. Surg. Engl.* 63:3, 1981.

Johnston G.W., Kelly J.M.: Early experience with the Boerema button for bleeding oesophageal varices. *Br. J. Surg.* 63:117, 1976.

Kivelitz H., Ulrich B.: Klammernahtgeräte am Oesophagus. Abstract from the 98th Kongress, Deutsche Gesellschaft für Chirurgie, Munich, April 22–25, 1981.

Kogan A.S.: The use of mechanical sutures in the Jianu gastrostomy. *Khirurg.* (Moskva) 45:128, 1969.

Kolesnikov A.I.: Use of tantalum clamp suture in Tanner's operation at the height of esophageal hemorrhage. *Klin. Khir.* (Kiev) 11:51, 1969.

Kuzmak L.I.: Use of EEA stapler in transection of esophagus in severe hemorrhage from esophageal varices. *Am. J. Surg.* 151:387, 1981.

Lukyanchenko A.G.: Suturing of the laryngeal defect in laryngectomy. *Vestn. Otorinolaringol.* 33:29, 1971.

Mills S.A.: Use of EEA stapler for substernal esophagogastric anastomosis in palliation of esophageal carcinoma. *J. Thorac. Cardiovasc. Surg.* 82:801, 1981.

Molina J.E., Lawton B.R., Avance D.: Use of circumferential stapler in reconstruction following resections for carcinoma of the cardia. *Ann. Thorac. Surg.* 31:325, 1981.

Molina J.E., Lawton B.R., Meyers W.O., Humphrey E.W.: Esophagogastrectomy for adenocarcinoma of the cardia. *Ann. Surg.* 195:146, 1982.

Orringer M.B.: In discussion of Henderson R.D., Marryatt G. *J. Thorac. Cardiovasc. Surg.* 85:81, 1983.

Orringer M.B., Sloan H.: An improved technique for the combined Collis-Belsey approach to dilatable esophageal strictures. *J. Thorac. Cardiovasc. Surg.* 68:298, 1974.

Orringer M.B., Sloan H.: Complications and failings of the combined Collis-Belsey operation. *J. Thorac. Cardiovasc. Surg.* 74:726, 1977.

Orringer M.B., Sloan H.: Combined Collis-Nissen reconstruction of the esophagogastric junction. *Ann. Thorac. Surg.* 25:16, 1978.

Paches A.I., Ogoltsova E.S., Tsibirne G.A., Alekseyeva S.I., Ponomarkov V.I.: Application of suture apparatuses during laryngectomy (experimental investigation). *Zh. Ushn. Nos. Gorl. Bolezn.* 32:61, 1972.

Paris F., Benages A., Ridocci M.T., Tarazona V., Molina R., Mora F., Pastor J., Lloret D., Garrido G.: Allongement oesophagien avec le "stappler" et valvuloplastie comme operation anti-reflux. *Ann. Chir. Thorac. Cardiovasc.* 16:335, 1977.

Payne W.S., Reynolds R.R.: Surgical treatment of pharyngoesophageal diverticulum (Zenker's diverticulum). *Surg. Rounds* 5:18, 1982.

Pearson F.G.: Personal communication, June 11, 1981.

Pearson F.G., Langer B., Henderson R.D.: Gastroplasty and Belsey hiatus hernia repair. An operation for the management of peptic stricture with acquired short esophagus. *J. Thorac. Cardiovasc. Surg.* 61:50, 1971.

Postlethwait R.W.: Technique for isoperistaltic gastric tube for esophageal bypass. *Ann. Surg.* 189:673, 1979.

Prioton J.B.: La ligature de l'oesophage sur bouton de Murphy dans les hemorragies par rupture de varices oesophagiennes. *Ann. Chir.* 27:343, 1973.

Ravitch M.M.: Personal communication to F.G. Pearson, May 17, 1973.

Ravitch M.M., Steichen F.M.: Technics of staple suturing in the gastrointestinal tract. *Ann. Surg.* 175:815, 1972.

Ravitch M.M., Steichen F.M.: A stapling instrument for end-to-end inverting anastomoses in the gastrointestinal tract. *Ann. Surg.* 189:791, 1979.

Read R.C.: In discussion of Hood R.M., Kirksey T.D., Calhoon J.H., Arnold H.S., Tate R.S. *Ann. Thorac. Surg.* 16:85, 1973.

Rinecker H., Danek N.: Operative Behandlung blutender Oesophagus-Varicen durch eine subkardiale Blutsperre mittels transmuraler maschineller Klammerung. *Chirurg.* 46:87, 1975.

Rowe M.: Personal communication, September, 1982.

Shahinian T.K., Bowen J.R., Dorman B.A., Soderberg C.H. Jr., Thompson W.R.: Experience with the EEA stapling device. *Am. J. Surg.* 139:549, 1980.

Skobelkin O.K.: Apparatus for simultaneous suturing and incising the stomach wall. *Med. Tekh.* 4:49, 1972.

Skobelkin O.K., Brechov E.I., Ivanov A.E., Utkin V.V.: Instrument for applying arciform sutures to the greater curvature of the stomach. *Khirurg.* (Moskva) 9:126, 1977.

Sorokina R.V.: Experience with the use of UKB-25 for suturing pharyngeal defects. *Zn. Ushn. Nos. Gorl. Bolezn.* 31:68, 1971.

Steichen F.M.: Clinical experience with autosuture instruments. *Surgery* 69:609, 1971.

Steichen F.M.: The creation of autologous substitute organs with stapling instruments. *Am. J. Surg.* 134:659, 1977.

Steichen F.M.: In discussion of Wexler M.J. *Surgery* 88:415, 1980.

Steichen F.M., Dibbins A.W., Weiner E.S.: Mechanical sutures in paediatric surgery, in Wilkinson A.W. (ed.): *Recent Advances in Paediatric Surgery,* 3d ed. New York, Churchill Livingstone, 1975, pp. 156–173.

Steichen F.M., Ravitch M.M.: Mechanical sutures in esophageal surgery. *Ann. Surg.* 191:373, 1980.

Urshel H.C. Jr., Razzuk M.A.: "Collis-Belsey" fundoplication for uncomplicated hiatal hernia and gastroesophageal reflux. *Ann. Thorac. Surg.* 27:564, 1979.

Vankemmel M.: Anastomoses oeso-gastrique et oeso-jéjunale par agrafes métalliques à l'appareil PKS 25. *Lille Méd.* 17:850, 1972.

Vankemmel M.: La résection-anastomose de l'oesophage sus-cardial a l'appareil PKS 25 ou SPTU 26 pour rupture de varices oesophagiennes. *Ann. Chir.* 30:187, 1976.

van Rensburg L.C.J., Malherbe E.B., Marais I.P., Bouwer E.L., van Zyl J.J.W.: Die gebruik van die end-aan-end (EEA) kraminstrument by anastomoses aan die esofagus. *S. Afr. J. Surg.* 19:43, 1981.

Vosschulte K.: Place de la section par ligature de l'oesophage dans le traitement de l'hypertension portale. *Lyon Chir.* 53:519, 1957.

Webster M.: Personal communication, July 8, 1982.

West P.N., Marbarger J.P., Martz M.N., Roper C.L.: Esophagogastrostomy with the EEA stapler. *Ann. Surg.* 193:76, 1981.

Wexler M.J.: Treatment of bleeding esophageal varices by transabdominal esophageal transection with the EEA stapling instrument. *Surgery* 88:406, 1980.

Wolsch R.: Personal communication, 1979.

Wu Lu: Unpublished illustrations, 1981.

CHAPTER VII

Operations on the Biliary Tract and Pancreas

BILIARY TRACT

THE APPLICATIONS of the stapling instruments in surgery of the biliary tract are not numerous. The LDS^{TM} instrument satisfactorily staples and divides the cystic duct. A number of surgeons have told us that the TA 90^{TM} instrument satisfactorily compresses and then staples portions of the liver, crushing through the parenchyma and then stapling the ducts and vessels. We have not attempted this. Obviously, any operative procedure in which a Roux-Y loop is created is facilitated by the stapling instruments. Cholecystojejunostomy is a method of diversion commonly used for common duct obstructions and, for this, the stapled anastomoses have been performed often. For ourselves, we prefer choledochojejunostomy. If the common duct in such situations is dilated enough and thick enough, the anastomosis is performed with the stapling instruments, either a side-to-end GIA^{TM}–TA^{TM} anastomosis with the Roux loop or, preferably, dividing and stapling off the lower end of the common duct and creating a functional end-to-end anastomosis with the hepatic end and the Roux loop. If the treatment chosen for a choledochal cyst is internal drainage, the staplers can be used for the entire procedure (Fig VII–1).

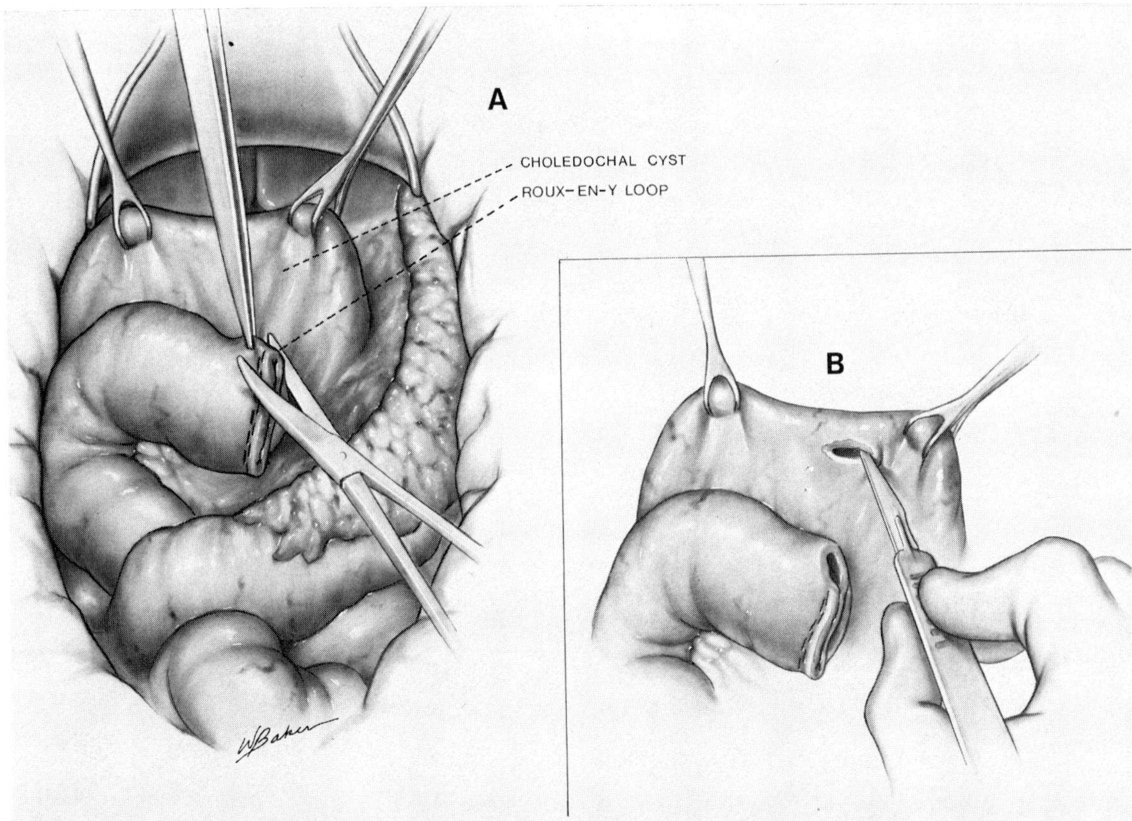

Fig VII–1.—Roux-Y drainage of choledochal cyst. **A,** the jejunum, having been divided with the GIA™ instrument beyond the ligament of Treitz, the proximal end of the distal segment is brought through the transverse mesocolon and laid alongside the choledochal cyst. **B,** the openings for the GIA™ instrument are through the excised antimesenteric corner of the staple closure of the jejunum and a small stab wound in the cyst. *(continued)*

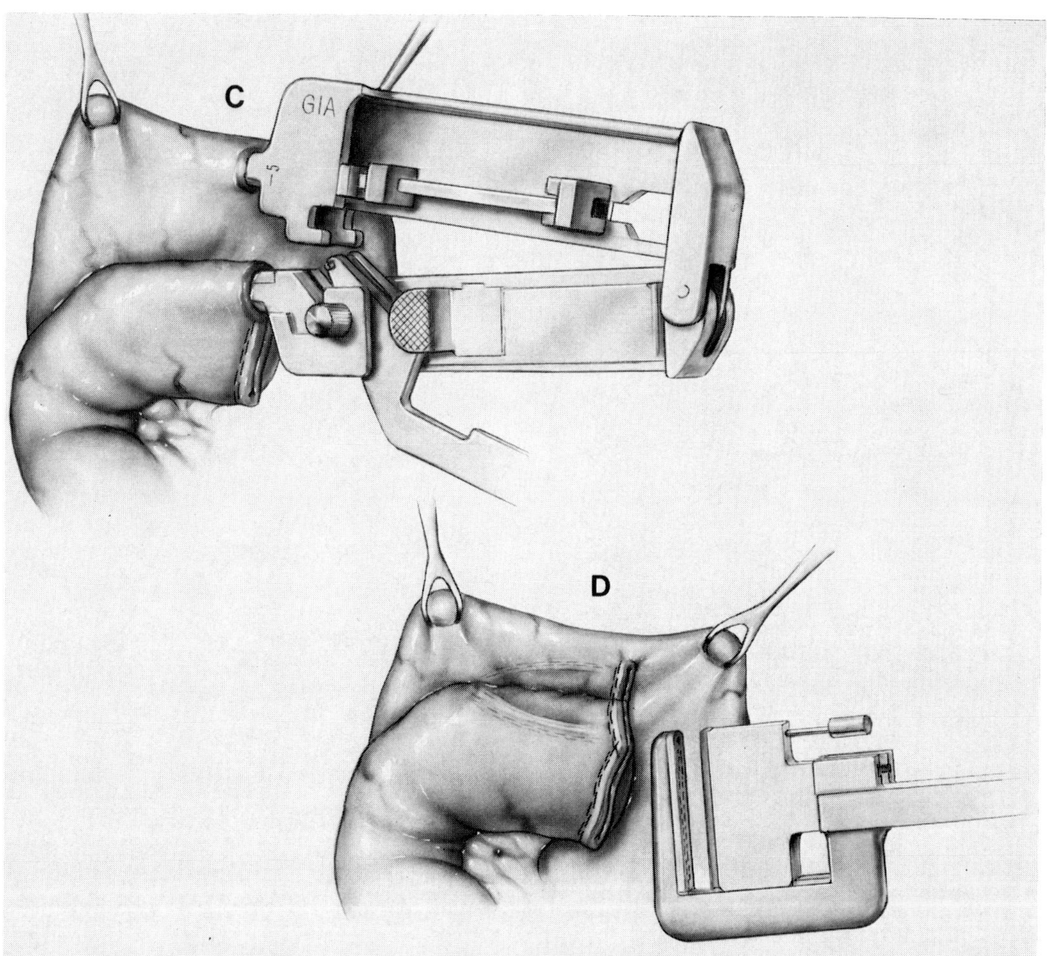

Fig VII–1 (cont.).—C, the usual GIA™ anastomosis is performed on the most dependent portion of the cyst (as shown, with the very bottom of the cyst elevated by Babcock clamps). **D,** after withdrawal of the GIA™ instrument, the remaining opening is stapled closed with the TA 55™ instrument.

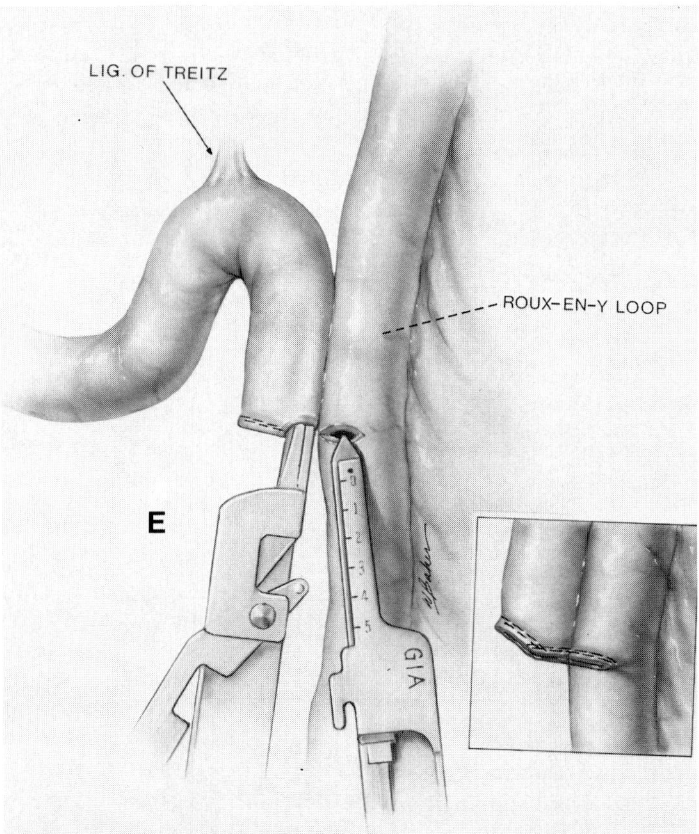

Fig VII–1 (cont.).—E, the end of the jejunum below the ligament of Treitz is anastomosed to the side of the Roux-Y loop coming away from the anastomosis to the choledochal cyst. The GIA™ limbs are inserted through the cutaway antimesenteric corner of the jejunal staple line and through a stab wound in the jejunal loop, the anastomosis created, and the GIA™ opening closed with a TA™ instrument in the usual way.

PANCREAS

In performing caudal pancreatectomy for whatever reason, we generally use the TA 55™ instrument. Beginning in the early 1960s with the Soviet UKL, we have not infrequently stapled and transected the pancreas in performing a caudal pancreatectomy, placing an additional suture if the pancreatic duct is obvious, often, in any case, whipping over the cut end of the pancreas with a continuous absorbable suture. We have not seen pancreatitis result nor have we had a pancreatic fistula from this procedure. Nagorney and Edis (1981) describe an imaginative technique for stapling the attachments of the uncinate process in proximal or total pancreatectomy (Fig VII–4). A pseudocyst, thick enough to sew manually, has a wall that will accept a stapled suture line satisfactorily, and our experience with this technique has been good (Taghizadeh, Bower, and Kiesewetter, 1979) (Fig VII–2).

In exposure of the papilla of Vater, the TA™ instruments facilitate closure of the duodenotomy (Fig VII–3). Although we have used the TA™ instruments with satisfaction for the excision and closure of pharyngeal and jejunal diverticula, we have not used the staples for duodenal diverticula. These tend to be so exceedingly thin-walled that we would be hesitant to do so.

The various vascular anastomotic instruments have been studied in their application to liver transplantation (Barron, Vogelfanger, and Waddell, 1975) and in reconstruction of the common duct (Klopper, Kelly, and Anton, 1968; Bornemisza and Furka, 1972; Barron, Vogelfanger, and Waddell, 1974), but we have not yet seen a report of their clinical use for such procedures.

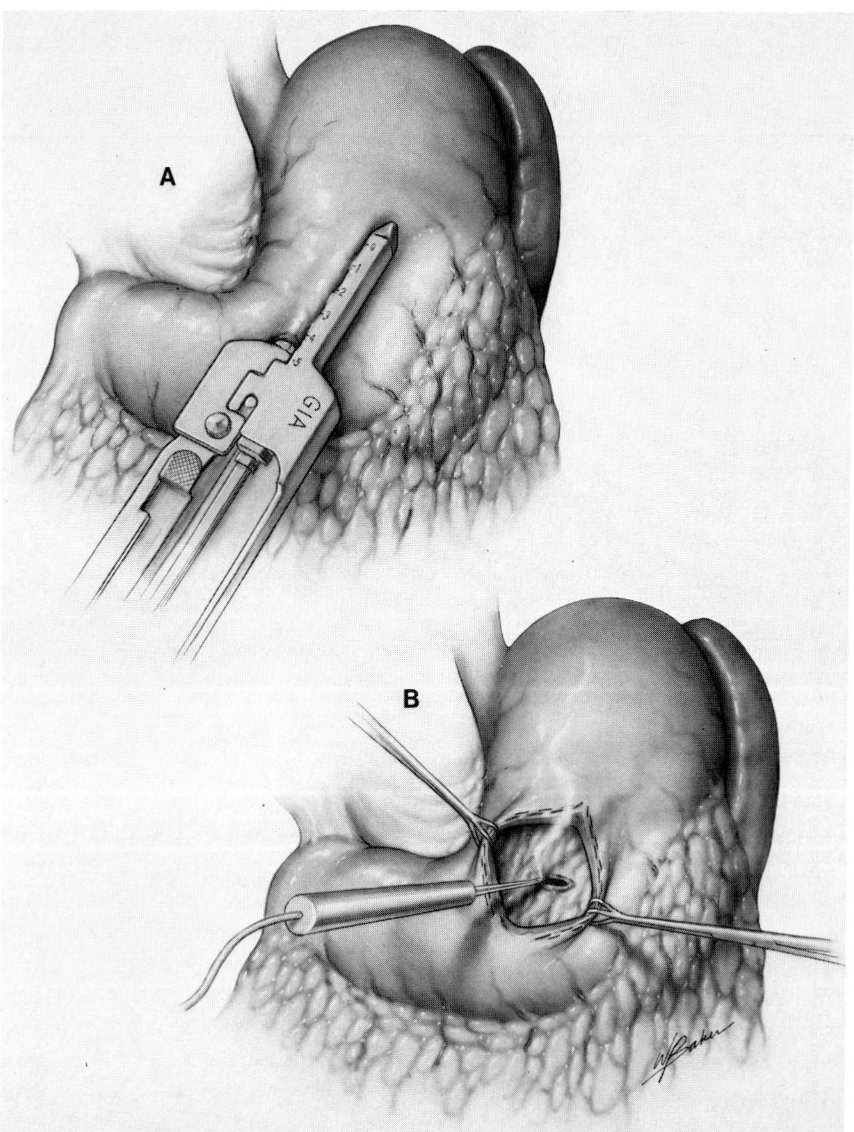

Fig VII–2.—Cystogastrostomy for pseudocyst of the pancreas. **A,** a gastrotomy is performed using the PGIA™ cartridge, which is hemostatic for a single thickness of gastric wall. **B,** the pseudocyst is identified on the posterior gastric wall by aspiration and an opening created with the cautery.

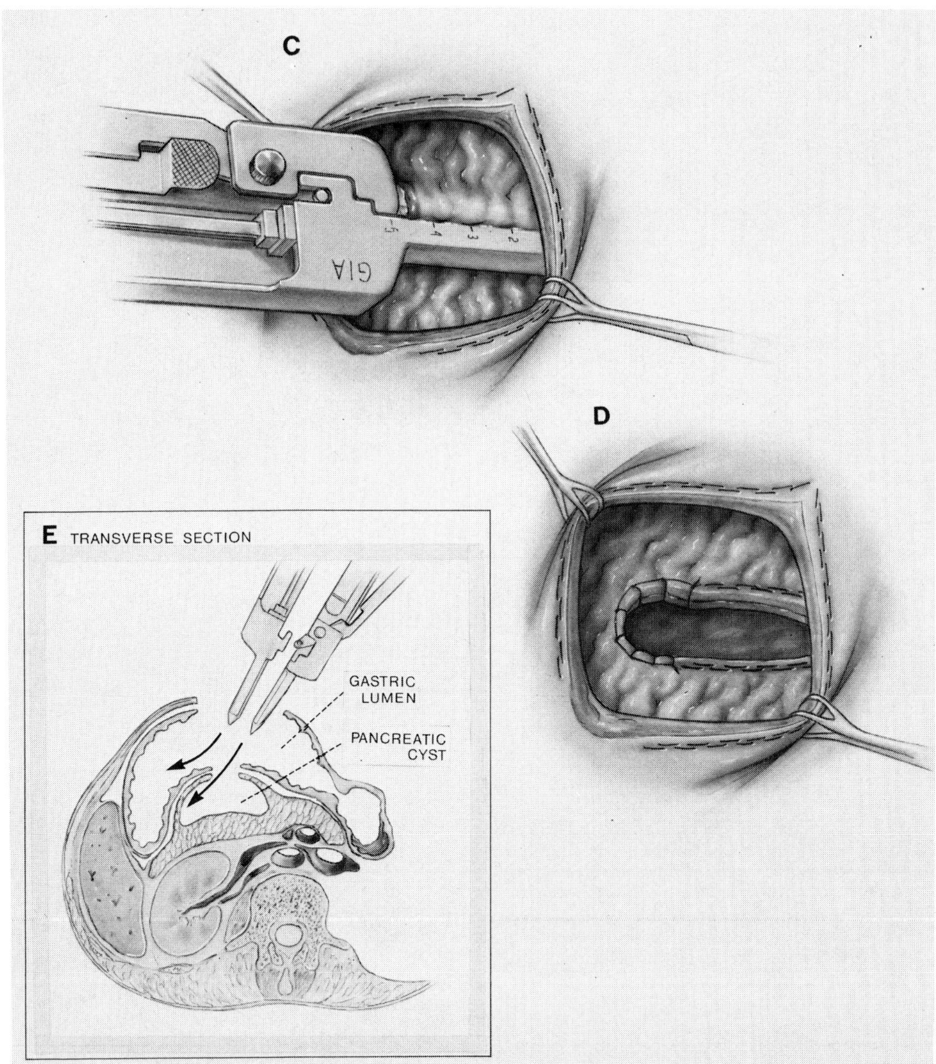

Fig VII–2 (cont.).—C, with one blade of the GIA™ instrument in the cyst and one in the stomach, an anastomosis is created between the two. **D,** a whipstitch or a lock stitch, as shown, may be used to suture the edges of the cystogastrostomy. **E,** sectional diagram of the stapled cystogastrostomy. The anterior gastrotomy will be closed mucosa-to-mucosa with a TA 55™ or a TA 90™ instrument, depending on the size of the gastrotomy. (From L.C. Gunn, *Archives of Surgery,* 1978, used by permission.)

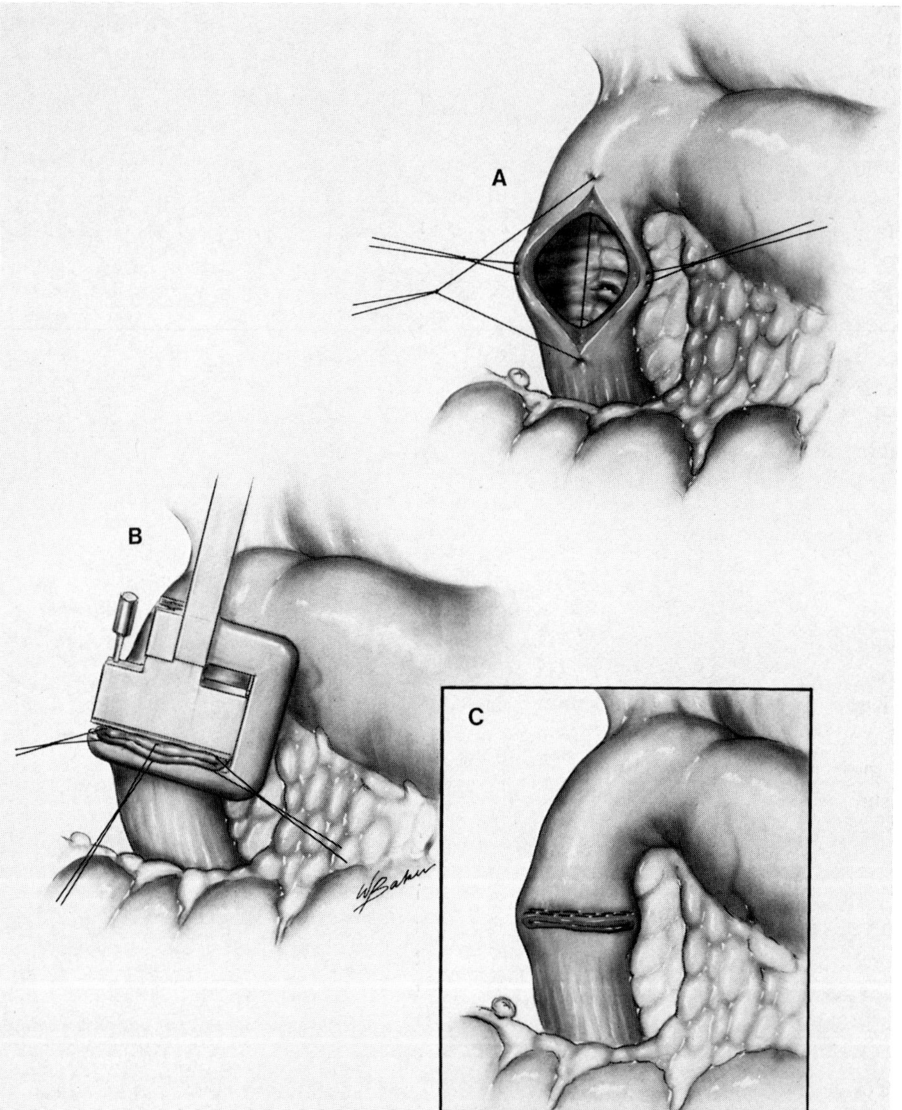

Fig VII–3.—Duodenotomy for exposure of the papilla of Vater. **A,** after completion of the intraduodenal manipulation, the longitudinal incision is shown drawn into a transverse opening by stay sutures. In point of fact, the duodenum is wide enough so that for short duodenotomies a longitudinal closure is satisfactory. **B,** the application of the TA 55™ instrument transversely stapling the duodenal opening mucosa-to-mucosa. **C,** the final result.

A review of the published material, some of which is referred to below, discloses a fairly wide and satisfactory use of the stapling instruments for bypass of biliary obstructions, repeated reference to stapled transection of the pancreas in distal pancreatectomy, and some experience, particularly Russian, with stapling of hepatic parenchyma in liver resection. Internal drainage of choledochal cysts and pancreatic pseudocysts by stapled anastomoses to the stomach or jejunum has been utilized by a number of individuals. In all of these procedures, the earlier experience is with the linear instrument. We can expect to see increasing use of the EEA[TM] instrument for cholecystojejunal and choledochocystojejunal anastomoses.

From the U.S.S.R., Garin, Gritsman, and Tanich (1957), reported use of the ULAV-5 (see Fig I–20*l*) for ligation of the cystic duct. It places two staples on the cystic duct, the division of the cystic duct with scissors being on the gallbladder side of these, so that the cystic duct and artery remain doubly ligated. The American LDS[TM] instrument, devised to overcome the inadequacies of the Russian instruments, simultaneously double staples and divides the cystic duct, between the two staples.

Ziarek (1969) from Poland reported the use of the UKL-60 for caudal pancreatectomy in 17 patients with pancreatitis of the tail or tail and body.

Kalinina (1972) showed the use of the Soviet tubular end-to-side anastomotic device, KTs-28, in the creation of experimental cholecystojejunal anastomoses, inserting the device through an enterotomy in the intact bowel. Twenty-eight dog experiments were performed. All dogs survived despite the fact that in 26 of them no manual sutures were used to reinforce the single row of staples.

Kulish and Burakov (1973) discussed the problem of liver resection with the UKL-60. In dogs this functioned well. However, they found that the instrument (analogous to the U.S. Auto Suture® TA[TM] instrument) was not secure for thicknesses of liver tissue greater than 3 cm. They were, however, able to utilize the UKL-60 clinically for wedge resections and five resections of the left lobe, and made suggestions concerning the general specifications for a liver stapler of this type.

Vinogradov, Ryneisky, and Zenonos (1975) reported a substantial experience with the use of the stapling instruments in biliary tract operations. They reported eight liver resections, both wedge resections and lobectomies, the wedge resections frequently being of segments large enough to include the gallbladder. In wedge resections, the liver was compressed and stapled with the UKL-60. In lobectomies, the UKL-60 was applied to the ducts and vessels exposed by digital fracture. In 25 cholecystectomies, the cystic duct and artery were secured with a linear double row of staples, without any complications. They performed 66 cholecystointestinal anastomoses for palliative relief from biliary obstruction, with anastomosis either to the stomach or to the small bowel, with the cylindrical end-to-end stapler (PKS-25). Fifty-five were cholecystogastrostomies and 11 were cholecystenterostomies. In 27 patients, they performed choledochoduodenal anastomoses with the SZhPDK, analogous to the GIA[TM] instrument, and designed a special modification of the instrument for that purpose. The advantage of the new instrument is that it is L-shaped, like our TA[TM] instruments. It places two rows of staples and simultaneously cuts between them.

Latimer, Doane, McKittrick, and Shepherd (1975) from Santa Barbara included one GIA[TM]–TA[TM] cholecystojejunostomy in their initial 104 stapling operations.

Wm. J. Hardin at the Scott and White Clinic in Temple, Texas, publishing his initial stapling experience (1977), reported transection of the pancreas with the stapler for distal pancreatectomy, stating only that no fistulas had developed and also reported performing stapled cholecystenterostomies.

Gunn from the University of Illinois (1978) illustrates the technique of GIA™ gastrotomy (Fig VII–2) and GIA™ cystogastrostomy, reporting two successful cases.

Pachter, Pennington, Chassin, and Spencer (1979) from New York University used the TA 55™ instrument with the 3.5 mm staples in 12 distal pancreatectomies, four for trauma and eight for elective indications. The single complication was a fistula in a man with a stab wound of the pancreas and vena cava and transection of the portal vein. This compared with a literature review of 12 publications reporting 234 distal pancreatectomies with an average fistula rate of 13% and individual reports of fistula rate as high as 25–30%.

Fortin, Poulin, and Leclerc (1979) from Quebec, in their total experience with stapling devices, included six cholecystojejunostomies and four distal pancreatectomies. The cholecystojejunostomies were the classic GIA™ anastomoses. The pancreas was simply transected with the TA 55™, usually in association with gastrectomy for cancer. They comment that "We must underline the security with which the six cholecystojejunal anastomoses were made in spite of the theoretic disadvantage posed by the difference in thickness of the walls of the two viscera."

From the Children's Hospital of the University of Pittsburgh, Taghizadeh, Bower, and Kiesewetter (1979) reported four children, ranging in age from four to six years, with stapled cystogastrostomy for pseudocyst of the pancreas. In three children, the course was uneventful. In the fourth, the serum amylase, having dropped, rose again, and endoscopy showed "closure of the cystogastrostomy stoma." At reoperation, the stoma was enlarged, and she recovered.

Rustamov, Shalimov, Zemskov, Diachuk, and Radzikovsky (1979) reported their experience with 30 liver resections between 1971 and 1977 using large and small sizes of the instruments comparable to the American TA™ series (UKL and UAP). Their experience included right and left hepatectomies. The portal structures were ligated and divided as needed, the capsule of the liver incised along the line of resection, and the UKL-60 applied repeatedly as seemed convenient, either from the edges or by inserting the lower jaw into the hepatic substance in an opening created by blunt dissection.

Reuter (1982) from the St. Thérèse Clinic in Luxembourg reported 28 cholecystoduodenostomies with the GIA™ instrument, no staple-related deaths, no hemorrhages, and no leaks.

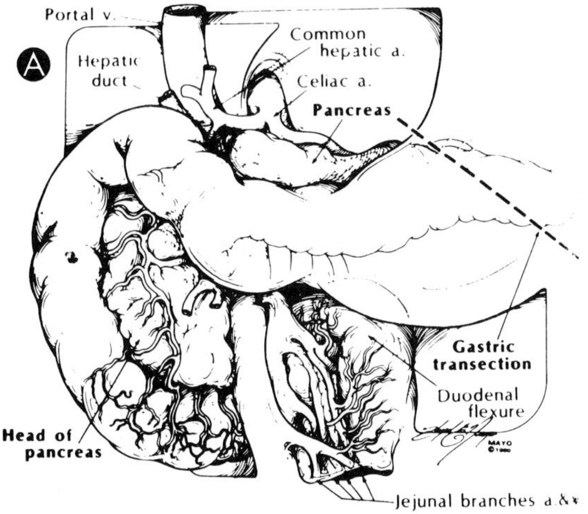

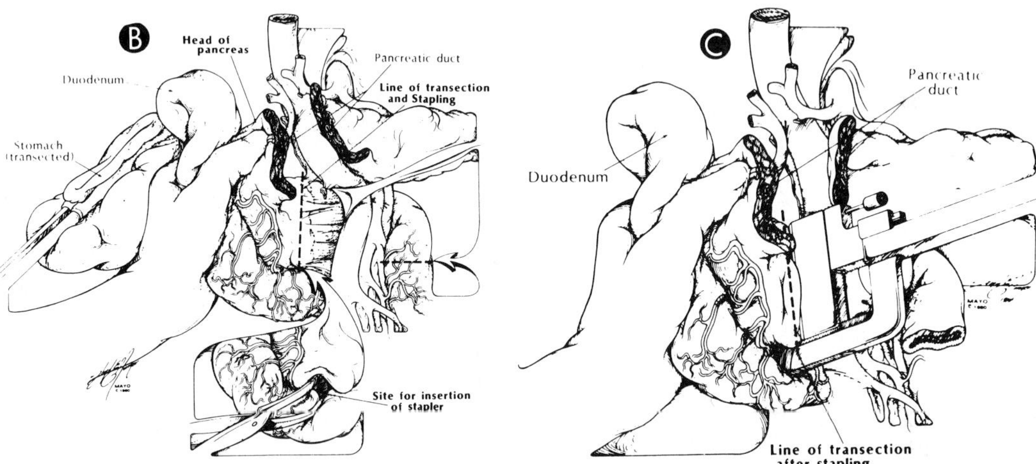

Fig VII–4.—Radical pancreaticoduodenectomy. **A,** basic regional anatomy of the pancreas and duodenum and the associated vasculature. **B,** preparation of uncinate process for stapler application. The head of the pancreas has been widely mobilized and the neck has been transected, and pancreatic head and the duodenum drawn to the right. A window (*lower arrow*) is made between the uncinate process and the duodenum for insertion of the stapler along the axis indicated by the dotted line. **C,** transection of uncinate process. The lower jaw of the TA 55™ stapler has been inserted through the window and positioned parallel to the portal and superior mesenteric veins. After firing of the stapler, the fibrous attachments of the pancreas are transected *(dotted line)* and the specimen is removed. (From D.M. Nagorney and A.J. Edis, *American Journal of Surgery,* 1981, used by permission.)

From the Mayo Clinic, Nagorney and Edis (1981) provide an imaginative use of the TA 55™ instrument. As they state, "One of the most difficult and tedious steps in performing radical pancreaticoduodenectomy, 95 percent distal pancreatectomy or total pancreatectomy, is the division of the uncinate process and the posterior vascular-areolar attachments of the pancreas to the portal and superior mesenteric veins." In ten patients, seven of them undergoing radical pancreaticoduodenectomy and three 95% distal pancreatectomy, at the appropriate stage in the operation, "A small window is made at the inferior border of the uncinate process between the short vasa recta supplying the third portion of the duodenum. Using the fingers of the left hand as a guide, the jaws of the TA 55™ stapling instrument (loaded with a 3.5 mm cartridge) are then inserted from below to encompass the uncinate process and the sheet of vascular-areolar tissue binding the head of the pancreas to the portal vein . . . the pancreas . . . is transected flush against the cartridge. . . . The stapled suture line across the uncinate process and its surrounding areolar attachments is usually. hemostatic, but on occasion minor bleeding will require suture ligation or cauterization."

From Denmark, Fahrenkrug and Clemmesen (1981), among their first 100 Auto Suture® operations, reported four cholecystojejunostomies.

For Oddi sphincteroplasty, Danilov, Strekopitov, Smirnov, and Ianzibaev from the Soviet Union (1981) reported their successful use of a new instrument shaped like the UKL series (Auto Suture® TA™) and called the TS-20. The anvil-containing lower jaw is made slender enough to fit through the ampulla of Vater. When the machine is closed and operated, it delivers a single row of staples on each side of a knife cut, thus dividing the papilla and suturing the two sides of the cut. After ten autopsy trials, they performed 16 operations in patients, with no deaths and no complications.

The economics of instrument manufacture in the Soviet Union are such as to permit the development and manufacture of special stapling instruments that have only a limited use.

REFERENCES

Barron P.T., Vogelfanger I.J., Waddell W.G.: Use of an automatic stapling instrument for the common duct anastomosis in experimental liver transplantation. *Eur. Surg. Res.* 6:301, 1974.

Barron P.T., Vogelfanger I.J., Waddell W.G.: Orthotopic liver transplantation utilizing a vascular stapling instrument. *Br. J. Surg.* 62:438, 1975.

Bornemisza Gy., Furka I.: End-to-end anastomosis of choledochal stumps by vessel suturing apparatus and adhesives. *Acta Chir. Acad. Sci. Hung.* 13:303, 1972.

Danilov M.V., Strekopitov A.A., Smirnov B.A., Ianzibaev Z.: Suturing machine for papillosphincteroplasty. *Med. Tekh.* 5:51, 1981.

Fahrenkrug L., Clemmesen T.: Anvendelse af et autosuturinstrument i gastroenterologisk kirurgi. *Ugeskr. Laeger* 143:263, 1981.

Fortin C.L., Poulin E.C., Leclerc Y.: Evaluation de l'utilisation des appareils d'autosuture en chirurgie digestive. *Can. J. Surg.* 22:580, 1979.

Garin N.D., Gritsman Yu Ya, Tanich L.F.: Mekanicheskaia pereviazka puzyrnovo protoka pri kholetsistektomii. *Eksp. Khir.* 2:21, 1957.

Gunn L.C.: Construction of pancreaticocystogastrostomy using an automatic stapling device. *Arch. Surg.* 113:298, 1978.

Hardin W.J.: Evaluation of autosutures in gastrointestinal surgery. *South. Med. J.* 70:197, 1977.

Kalinina T.V.: Anastomosis of the gallbladder or dilated bile duct with the intestine by means of a mechanical suture. *Eksp. Khir. Anesteziol.* 17:57, 1972.

Klopper P.J., Kelly K.A., Vos A.: Experimental anastomosis of the common bile duct. *Surgery* 63:459, 1968.

Kulish N.I., Burakov I.: Liver resection with stapling apparatus. *Klin. Khir.* 7:56, 1973.

Latimer R.G., Doane W.A., McKittrick J.E., Shepherd A.: Automatic staple suturing for gastrointestinal surgery. *Am. J. Surg.* 130:766, 1975.

Nagorney D.M., Edis A.J.: A use for the stapler in pancreatic surgery. *Am. J. Surg.* 142:384, 1981.

Pachter H.L., Pennington R., Chassin J., Spencer F.C.: Simplified distal pancreatectomy with the Auto Suture stapler: Preliminary clinical observations. *Surgery* 85:166, 1979.

Reuter M.J.P.: Les sutures mécaniques en chirurgie digestive et pulmonaire. Thesis, presented in 1982, at Université Louis Pasteur, Faculté de Médecine de Strasbourg, France.

Rustamov I.R., Shalimov S.A., Zemskov V.S., Diachuk I.S., Radzikovsky A.P.: Liver resection using mechanical suturing by means of the UKL and UAP apparatus. *Klin. Khir.* 9:50, 1979.

Taghizadeh F., Bower R.J., Kiesewetter W.B.: Stapled cystogastrostomy. A method of treatment for pediatric pancreatic pseudocyst. *Ann. Surg.* 190:166, 1979.

Vinogradov V.V., Ryneisky S.V., Zenonos A.: Application of a mechanical suture in operations on the liver and bile ducts. *Vestn. Khir.* 114:40, 1975.

Ziarek S., Szlachta E., Puzio J., Migas E., Pierzycki J.: Czesciowe wyciecie trzustki za pomoca aparatu UKL-60. *Pol. Przegl. Chir.* 41:1749, 1969.

CHAPTER VIII

Operations on the Small and Large Bowel

THE LINEAR STAPLING INSTRUMENTS of the TA^{TM} series lend themselves to rapid tangential resection of mural lesions—fibromas, leiomyomas, polyps, carcinomas, etc., much as in the excision of the gastric ulcer shown in Figure V–2. Penetrating wounds of the bowel, whether by missiles, knives, or scalpels, usually are closed transversely with the TA^{TM} instrument.

It has been a long time, 90 years of experience in some surgical clinics, certainly 75 years in others, since surgeons have had any concern about their ability to perform anastomoses with safety in the small bowel. The same can hardly be said for suture of the large bowel, the results with which still are not perfect, particularly below the pelvic floor. The stapling techniques present a number of specific advantages even in suture of the small bowel, quite apart from convenience and swiftness. Division and closure of the bowel, whether between a TA^{TM} instrument and a clamp, or as we usually prefer, with the GIA^{TM} instrument, requires only a minimal devascularization of the bowel, and often the instruments can, in fact, be inserted between the mesenteric edge of the bowel and a marginal vessel without dividing any vessels, except as subsequently may be needed for resection or mobilization. Perhaps most important is the fact that for the safe performance of manual anastomoses it is necessary to clear the mesentery back a bit from the transected end of the bowel, and yet this risks rendering the end ischemic. Such trimming is unnecessary for stapled anastomoses. Finally, the stapling techniques permit one to ignore disparity in the diameters of the proximal and distal bowel. We have commented before on the reluctance of surgeons to accept machine sewing instead of the more personal and artistic manual suturing. Even more difficult has it been for surgeons to accept two of the technical details of stapling by our techniques that run counter to traditional teaching, e.g., anatomical side-to-side anastomosis and the mucosa-to-mucosa closure, which transforms the anatomical side-to-side anastomosis into a functional end-to-end anastomosis. Some surgeons readily adapted to the new techniques, particularly on the experimental evidence and historical record that mucosa-to-mucosa closures are safe (Ravitch, Lane, Cornell, Rivarola, and McEnany, 1966; Ravitch, Canalis, Weinshelbaum, and McCormick, 1967; Ravitch, 1975). Others, although reluctantly accepting the fact that mucosa-to-mucosa staple closures would heal, were reluctant to accept what appeared to be a side-to-side anastomosis (Steichen, 1968), however clear it was that, in fact, this was simply a U-shaped end-to-end anastomosis: "functional end-to-end anastomosis." True end-to-end anastomoses made with the linear stapling instruments of the TA^{TM} series are feasible (Ravitch and Steichen, 1972) and satisfactory but considerably more difficult than any other anastomotic technique we know. Although McGinty and others (McGinty, 1970; Ferguson and Houston, 1975; Gautier-Benoit, 1976; McGinty, Kasten, Kinder, and Hunt, 1979) continue to be pleased with these, we see no justification for the use of this technique. We have accepted the principle of the functional end-to-end anastomosis (Steichen, 1968) (Figs VIII–2–4) as the basic technique for intestinal reconstruction, except in those situations to which the EEA^{TM} minimally inverting end-to-end anastomosis is better adapted. If the anastomosis is to be performed immediately on the resection of a loop of bowel, as in the jejunum in taking down a gastroenterostomy, as in an ileocolostomy after resection of the right colon, or after resection of any segment of bowel, including the descending colon when a colorectal anastomosis is to be performed, the modified functional end-to-end anastomosis reported in 1974 (Ravitch, Ong, and Gazzola) is used (Fig VIII–5). Whichever technique of functional end-to-end anastomosis is used, the end result, weeks or months later, is to all intents and purposes an end-to-end anastomosis. If one staples the bowel (see Fig VIII–2) at the outermost end of the GIA^{TM} staple line, one may leave an anastomosis that is larger in diameter than the bowel on either side. The aim is so to apply the TA^{TM} instrument that the diameter of the anastomosis will be the same as the diameter of the bowel on either side. This obviously is not possible in a functional end-to-end ileocolostomy, but that is offset by the advantage that the anastomosis can be performed without having to worry in the slightest degree about any disparity in caliber between the proximal and distal loops.

In an elegant study, Welter, Charlier, and Psalmon (1983) measured and compared anastomotic surfaces obtained by the triangulating end-to-end anastomosis using three everting TA^{TM} applications, by the inverting end-to-end anastomosis using the EEA^{TM} instrument and by the functional end-to-end anastomosis using the GIA-TA^{TM} instruments, separating the GIA^{TM} lines in an open V fashion. Their findings showed that the end-to-end everting triangulating technique creates an anastomosis almost equal to or only slightly smaller than the caliber of the original bowel. In the inverting end-to-end EEA^{TM} anastomosis, the diameter of the anastomosis is always smaller by the narrow margin of inverted tissue, but may be significantly smaller if a cartridge is used that does not comfortably fill the lumen of the bowel. With the functional end-to-end anastomosis, by contrast, the anastomotic surface can be increased by up to one-third of the original bowel lumen, if the TA 55^{TM} closing staple line is applied so as to hold the GIA^{TM} staple lines in an open V.

McGinty (McGinty, 1970; McGinty, Kasten, Kinder, and Hunt, 1979) of Cape Girardeau, Missouri reported a true end-to-end everting anastomosis (see Fig VIII–1*B–E*) made by triangulating the bowel and overlapping three TA 30^{TM} applications to the everted lips. In the laboratory in New York, Josefsen and Efron (1969) previously had demonstrated the feasibility in animals, and the satisfactory function, of a triangulated anastomosis, the posterior row inverting and the two sides of the triangle everting (see Fig VIII–1*A*), but we do not utilize this clinically because of the, to us, obvious superiority of the functional end-to-end anastomosis. McGinty's initial publication listed 38 anastomoses—13 ileocolostomies, 18 left colon anastomoses, and seven small bowel enteroenterostomies. There were two deaths in his entire series, neither from anastomosis-connected problems. A third patient went home apparently well on the tenth day after a right colon resection, was readmitted on the eighteenth day and was found to have an abscess around a leak at the ileocolic anastomosis. He recovered following drainage of the abscess and the fecal fistula closed spontaneously. The cases were all consecutive and a number of the operations were emergency procedures on unprepared, and at times obstructed, bowel. McGinty thought the technique to be superior to that of the functional end-to-end anastomosis.

Nine years later, McGinty's series (McGinty, Kasten, Kinder, and Hunt, 1979) had been extended to 445 triangulated everting end-to-end anastomoses. There was a total of five anastomotic complications: a radiologically demonstrated leak following low anterior anastomosis after resection for diverticulitis, clearing spontaneously; two chronic sigmoid cutaneous fistulas, in which the fistulas became involved with cancer; a leak after right colectomy and ileotransverse colostomy, which required operative closure on the sixth day and healed; a gross breakdown, the day after operation in a 74-year-old man with a bleeding, obstructing carcinoma of the sigmoid, and anastomosis " . . . on this edematous, tumor-beaded bowel." None of the other 16 deaths were anastomosis related.

Ferguson and Houston from Jacksonville, Florida (1975) reported their use of the TA^{TM} instrument in partially inverting, partially everting triangulating true end-to-end anastomoses of the rectum in 40 anterior resections. Thirty-three of the operations were for cancer, five for diverticulitis, one for procidentia, and one for endometriosis. All but four patients had either a cecostomy or diverting colostomy. There were no gross leaks. Two patients had visible dehiscences on proctoscopy. There were no deaths.

Gautier-Benoit (1976), reporting from France, described a true end-to-end totally everting anastomosis of the bowel utilizing three triangulating stay sutures and three overlapping staple lines with the TA^{TM} instrument (see Fig VIII–1F–H). He had used this five times in the small intestine and twice in the large intestine without leakage or fistula. He had used the TA 55^{TM} instrument, but thought that the TA 30^{TM} instrument would provide a long enough suture line. He thought that the stapling technique was particularly indicated in long procedures or in feeble patients for whom the appreciable saving in time would be desirable.

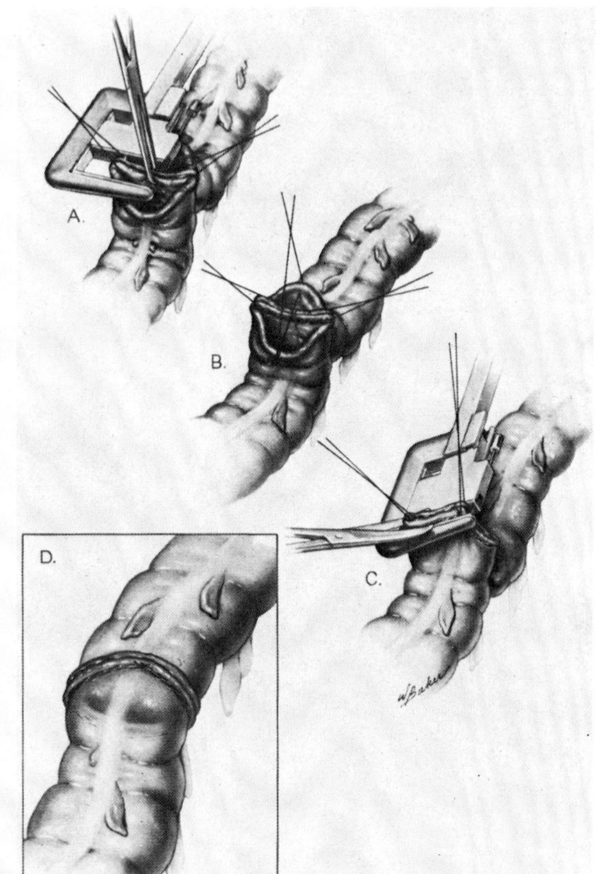

FIG. 1. *End-to-End Anastomosis of Intestine by Triangulation.* (A) The posterior row held by sutures at either end and an Allis clamp in the center, is drawn through the jaws of the TA instrument, the staples driven home and the excess tissue excised, between the stay sutures. (B) The posterior suture line is shown completed and a guy suture placed in the opposed anterior lips. (C) This allows one to place two more suture lines, the bowel edges being apposed mucosa-to-mucosa. (D) The completed suture line showing the overlapping of the staples from one suture line to the next.

Fig VIII–1.—Techniques of true end-to-end anastomosis with the TA™ instruments. They are included for their historical interest. We do not use any of these, considering them inferior to the functional end-to-end anastomosis or to the EEA™ end-to-end anastomosis. **A,** partially everting, partially inverting triangulated TA™ end-to-end anastomosis. *(continued)*

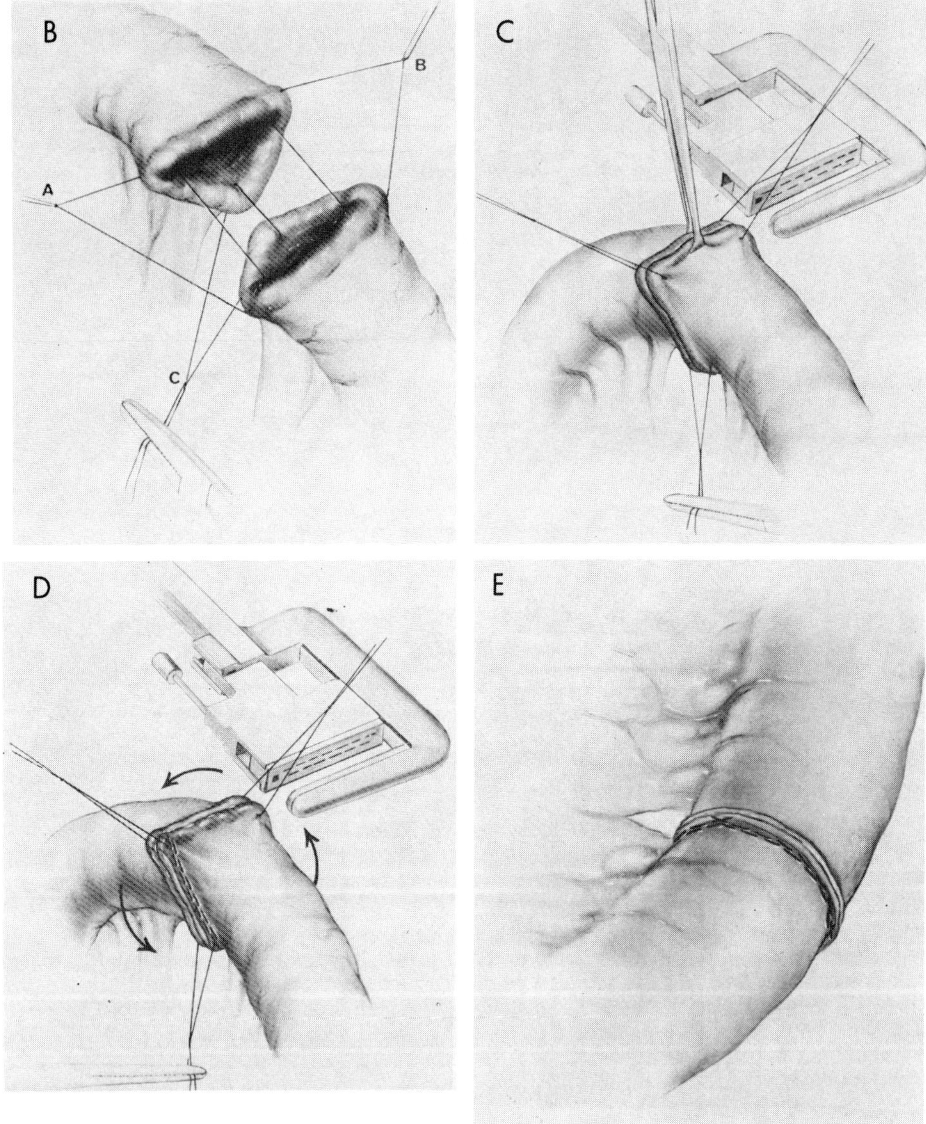

Fig VIII–1 (cont.).—B–E, McGinty's true end-to-end, everting anastomosis.

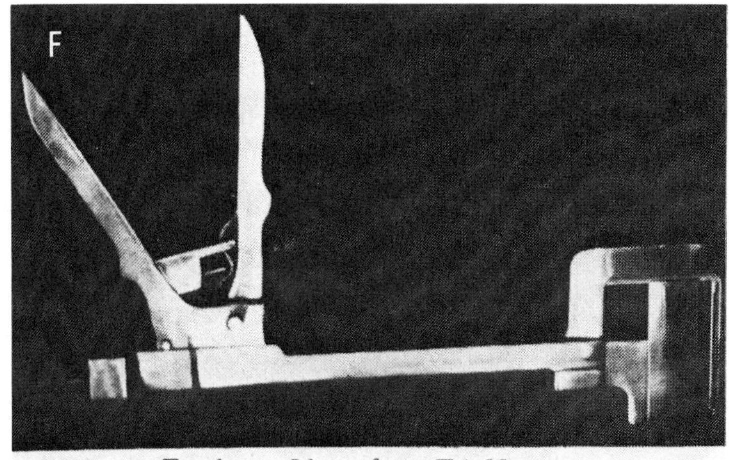

FIG 1. – *L'agrafeuse TA 55.*

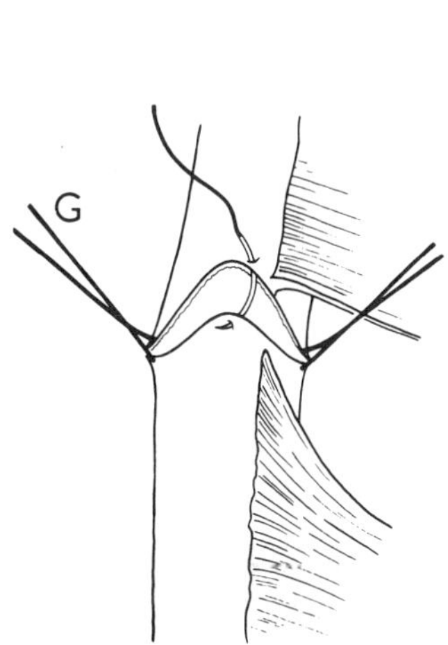

FIG. 2. – *Mise en place de trois points réalisant la triangulation.*

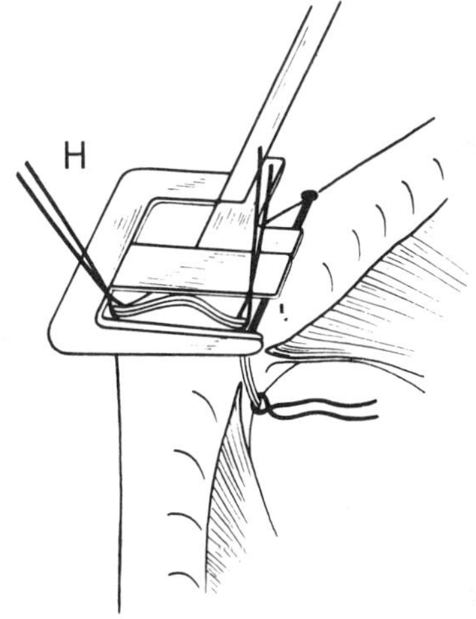

FIG. 3. – *Suture d'un des côtés du triangle au TA 55.*

Fig VIII–1 (cont.).—F–H, technique of Gautier-Benoit for everting true end-to-end anastomosis.

(**A** from M.M. Ravitch and F.M. Steichen, *Annals of Surgery,* 1972, used by permission; **B–E** from C.P. McGinty, M.C. Kasten, J.L. Kinder, and R.S. Hunt, *Missouri Medicine,* 1979, used by permission; **F–H** from C. Gautier-Benoit, *La Nouvelle Presse Médicale,* 1976, used by permission.)

The arrival of the EEA^{TM} instrument with its circular, minimally inverting anastomosis was greeted with enthusiasm by most surgeons, particularly those who had been unable to abandon true end-to-end anastomoses, and particularly those with atavistic distrust of mucosa-to-mucosa closures. We predicted from the first that as the stapling instruments were introduced, indications for them would appear, and techniques for their use would be developed, well beyond any originally envisioned. This has been particularly true of the EEA^{TM} instrument. We prefer to reserve the EEA^{TM} instrument for situations in which it can be introduced either through a natural orifice or through an orifice already created in the course of an operation (see Figs IX–3–6). Nance (1979), by making colotomies, enterotomies, or gastrotomies for the introduction of the instrument, had used it for essentially all gastrointestinal anastomoses. This is, of course, at the cost of having an additional bowel opening and the additional suture line that closes it. There is a considerable volume of reports in the North American and European literature with use of the original Auto Suture® instruments in intestinal anastomosis, and a rapidly growing number of publications worldwide dealing with the EEA^{TM} instrument. The material below, abstracted from this literature, indicates that stapled small bowel anastomoses can be done with close to absolute safety, that large bowel anastomoses are performed at least as safely as with manual techniques, and that the addition of the EEA^{TM} instrument has fortified one's optimism concerning the utility and safety of the instruments. In the chapter on gastric suture, we noted the occasional instances of anastomotic bleeding, possibly fewer than with manual suture. There is almost no experience with anastomotic bleeding in the small and large bowel. Anastomotic failures are rare. The EEA^{TM} instrument, used in the abdomen, has not been reported to cause bleeding, and the security of the anastomoses has been gratifying. Whereas stenoses of GIA^{TM} anastomoses have been reported with extreme rarity, some stenoses with the EEA^{TM} anastomoses have been reported in most series. In the esophagus and in the rectum, they appear, for the most part, to be asymptomatic, discovered by endoscopy or radiography, and yielding either to continued use of the gastrointestinal tract or to one or two dilatations. As a number of authors point out, stenotic anastomoses are not unknown in manual suturing experience. The fact that in a number of series such strictures occurred early in the experience of the individual surgeon suggests a technical problem, and it is clear from the review of the literature that the learning curve in the use of the EEA^{TM} instrument has a more gradual upward slope than the learning curve with the other stapling instruments. The best assumption is that significant stenosis with the EEA^{TM} instrument, rare though it is, results from inclusion of too much tissue to be compressed in the capsule of the anastomotic device, with enough consequent ischemia and resultant injury to invite fibrosis. A contained leak may produce the same result.

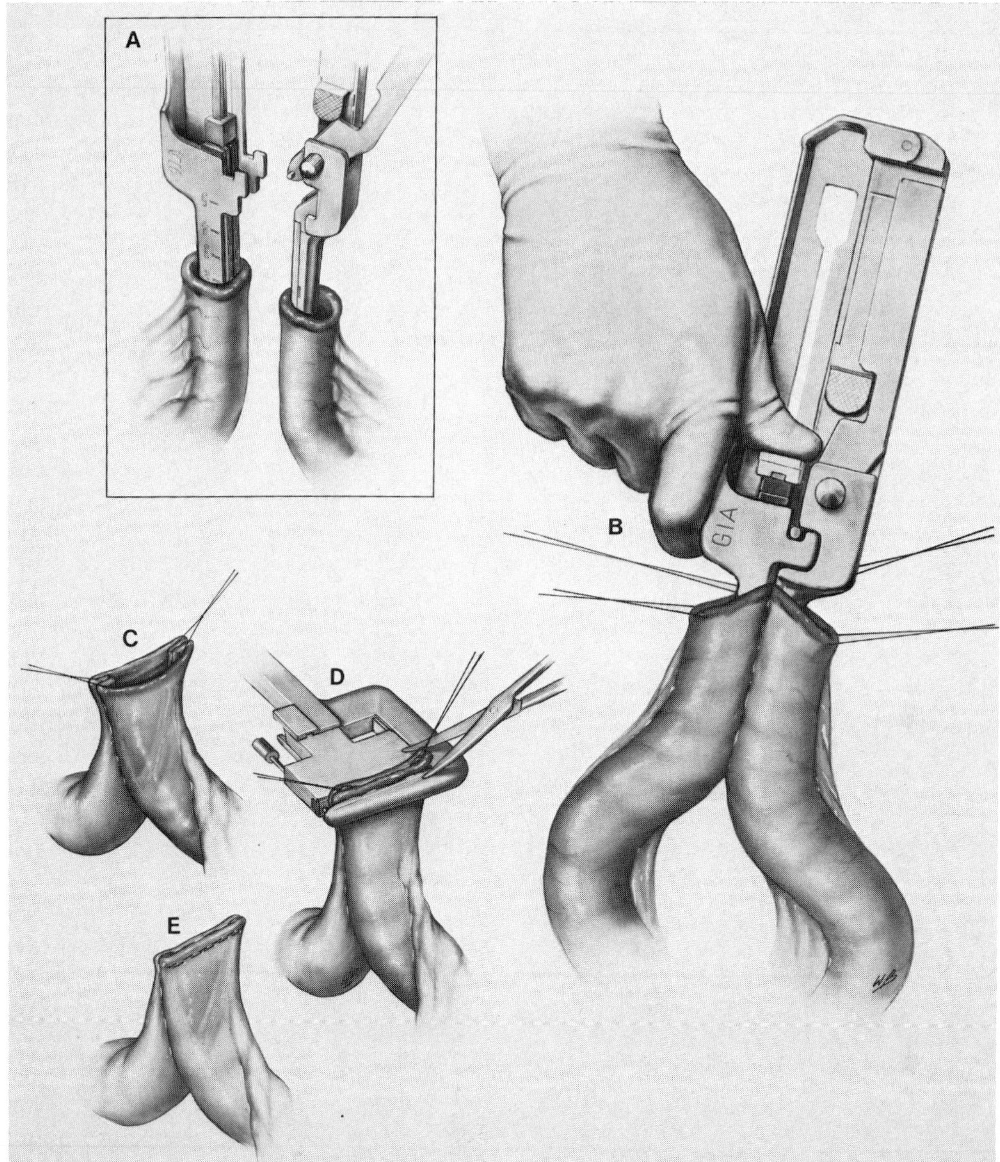

Fig VIII–2.—The functional end-to-end anastomosis—enteroenterostomy. More often than not, this is performed with bowel that already has been stapled earlier in the procedure (see Fig VIII–3), but shown here are two open loops of bowel. **A,** the GIA™ limbs are inserted into their respective loops, so that the instrument will close along the antimesenteric borders. The depth to which the calibrated instrument is inserted determines the size of the anastomosis. Allowance must be made for the amount to be amputated in **D.**

B, the instrument is operated, creating the stapled anastomosis. A hand grip on the instrument, as in operating a syringe, is preferred to that shown. **C,** the instrument having been withdrawn, the ends of the two staple lines are held apart so that when in **D** the bowel is clamped with the TA 55™ instrument, the cut edges of the GIA™ stapled bowel will be held widely apart. Since the cut edges of the bowel peripheral to the GIA™ staples are viable, it is theoretically possible, and has happened on rare occasions, that the cut edges will adhere if the TA™ instrument is applied at right angles to the plane shown here. In point of fact, we have not ourselves had that experience, but know that it has happened (Elliott, Albertazzi, and Danto, 1970). **D,** one must confirm that serosa and mucosa are visible completely around, beyond the TA™ stapler, guaranteeing a through-and-through closure of the opening. Scissors are used to cut away the lip of bowel beyond the instrument, since one will be cutting across the two GIA™ staple lines. **E,** the final result. Reoperation after some months will show the anastomosis looking for all the world like an end-to-end anastomosis, occasionally with a small bulge, if the application of the TA™ instrument in **D** has not been such as to make the length of the anastomosis equal to the diameter of the bowel on either side. One of the great advantages of staple transection and anastomosis is the fact that little or no devascularization of the bowel is necessary for transection, and none for anastomosis. Whereas in a manual anastomosis too little clearing of the mesentery may make anastomotic suturing insecure, too much may jeopardize the viability of the bowel end. In all the variations shown of the functional end-to-end anastomosis, one is careful to insert the GIA™ instrument on the antimesenteric surfaces and to be sure that no other loop of bowel—or mesentery—is caught between the two loops being anastomosed.

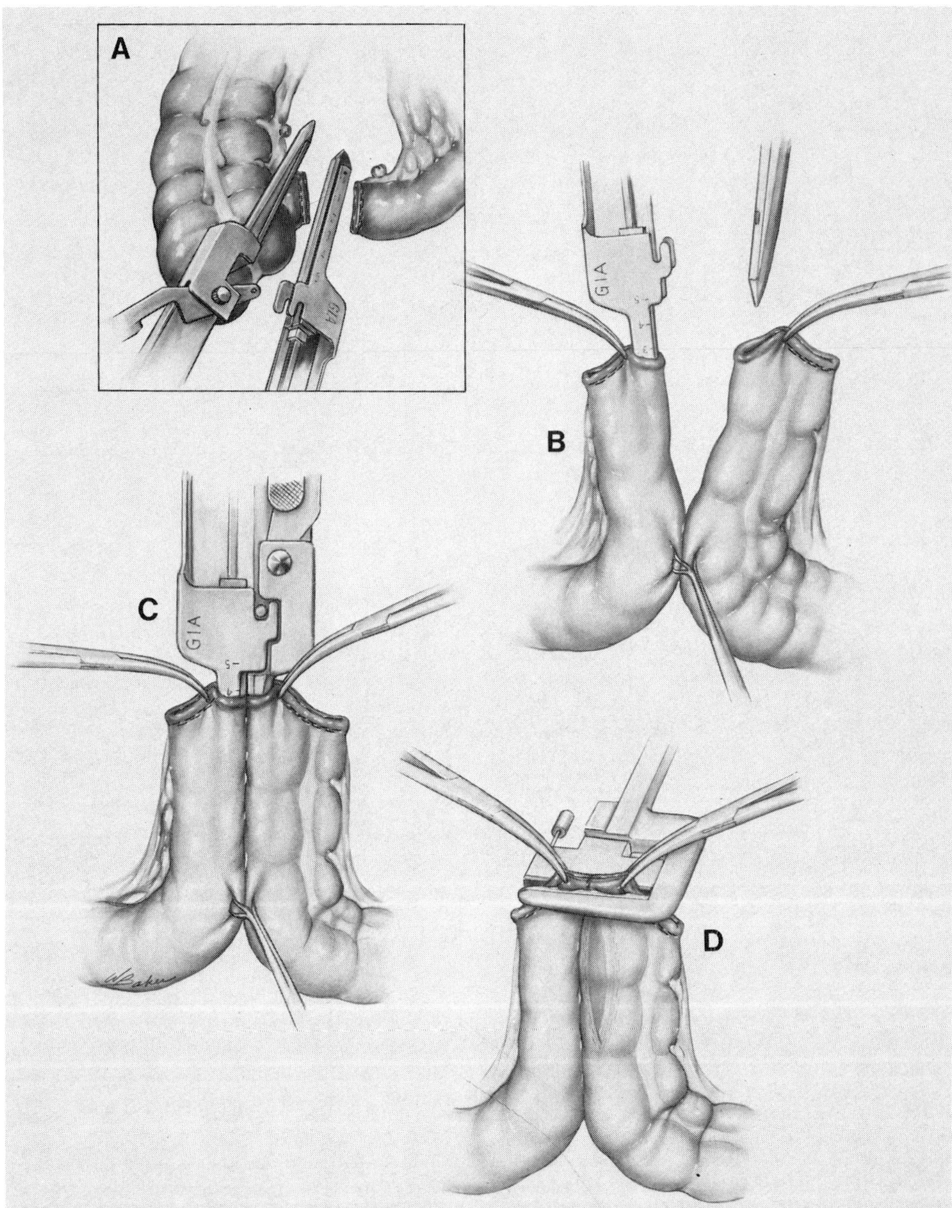

Fig VIII–3.—The functional end-to-end anastomosis—ileocolostomy. An attractive feature of the functional end-to-end technique is the fact that its performance is unaffected by any disparity in the diameter of the two loops. **A,** the terminal ileum is divided with the GIA™ instrument. The distal division of the colon is not shown. **B,** the ileum and colon are held in shotgun fashion and the GIA™ limbs inserted through the cutaway antimesenteric corners of the staple lines. **C,** the anastomosis is formed by operation of the GIA™ instrument. **D,** after the lumen has been inspected to be sure that there is no bleeding, the GIA™ opening is closed with the TA 55™ stapler. We generally prefer to hold the anastomosis apart with fine clamps on the two GIA™ staple lines, so that the anastomosis will be stapled wide open as in Figure VIII–2**C–E.** (From M.M. Ravitch and F.M. Steichen, *Abdominal Operations,* 7th ed. New York, Appleton-Century-Crofts, 1979, R. Maingot [ed.], with permission.)

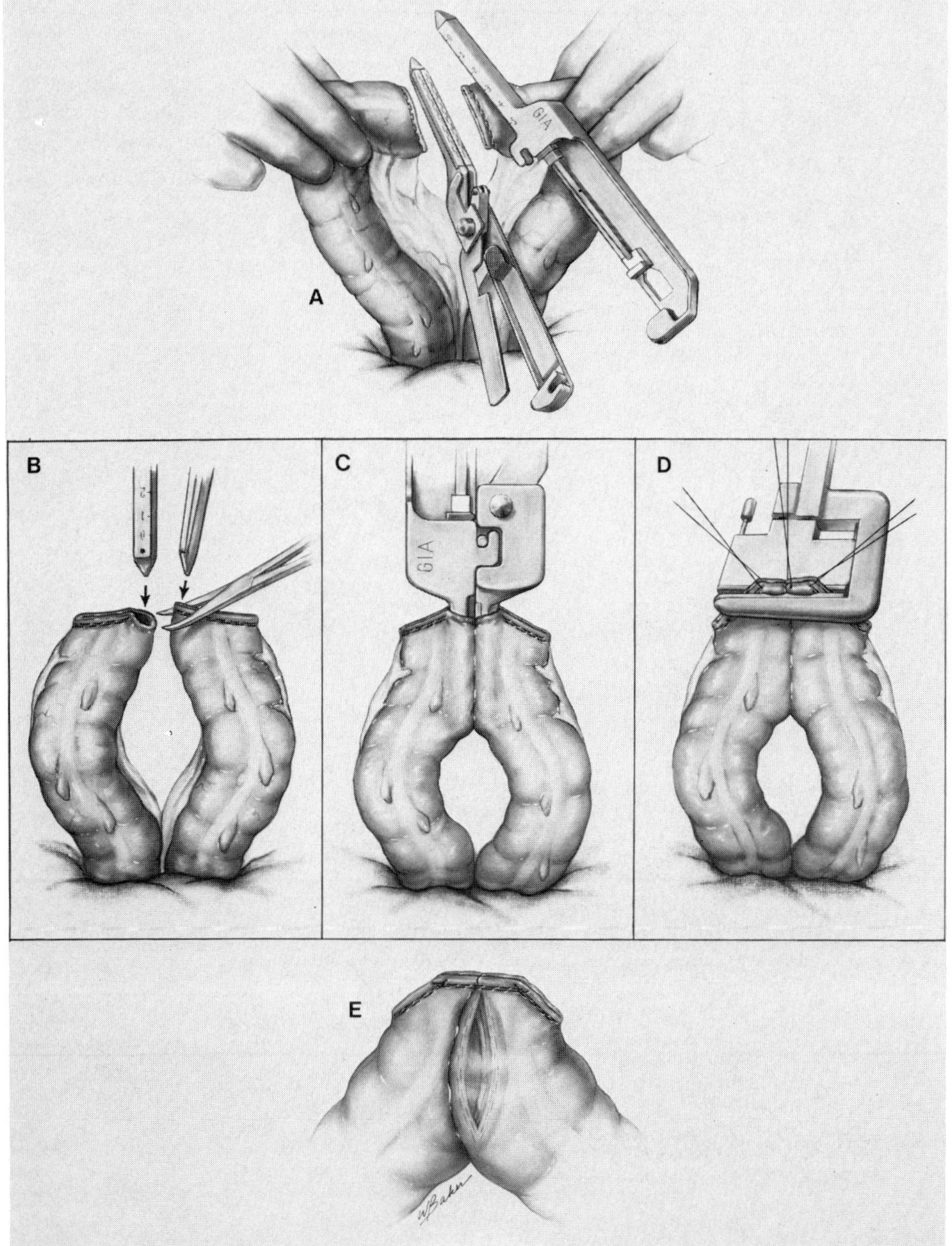

Fig VIII–4.—The functional end-to-end anastomosis—colocolostomy. **A,** the segment of colon is resected and stapled between two applications of the GIA™ instrument, so that the specimen always is sealed and risk of contamination is minimal. **B,** the antimesenteric corners of the staple lines in the proximal and distal ends are excised and the GIA™ limbs inserted. **C,** an anastomosis is created that ideally should be of the same length as the transverse diameter of the bowel. **D,** this is determined by the level at which the TA 55™ instrument is placed. The opening remaining when the GIA™ instrument is withdrawn is shown being closed mucosa-to-mucosa with the TA 55™ instrument. Once more, we point out that we usually prefer to apply the TA™ instrument at right angles to the position shown, to hold the anastomosis wide open. **E,** the final result. The transparency indicates an anastomosis that is of the same size as the diameter of the bowel on either side. (From M.M. Ravitch and F.M. Steichen, *Annals of Surgery,* 1972, used by permission.)

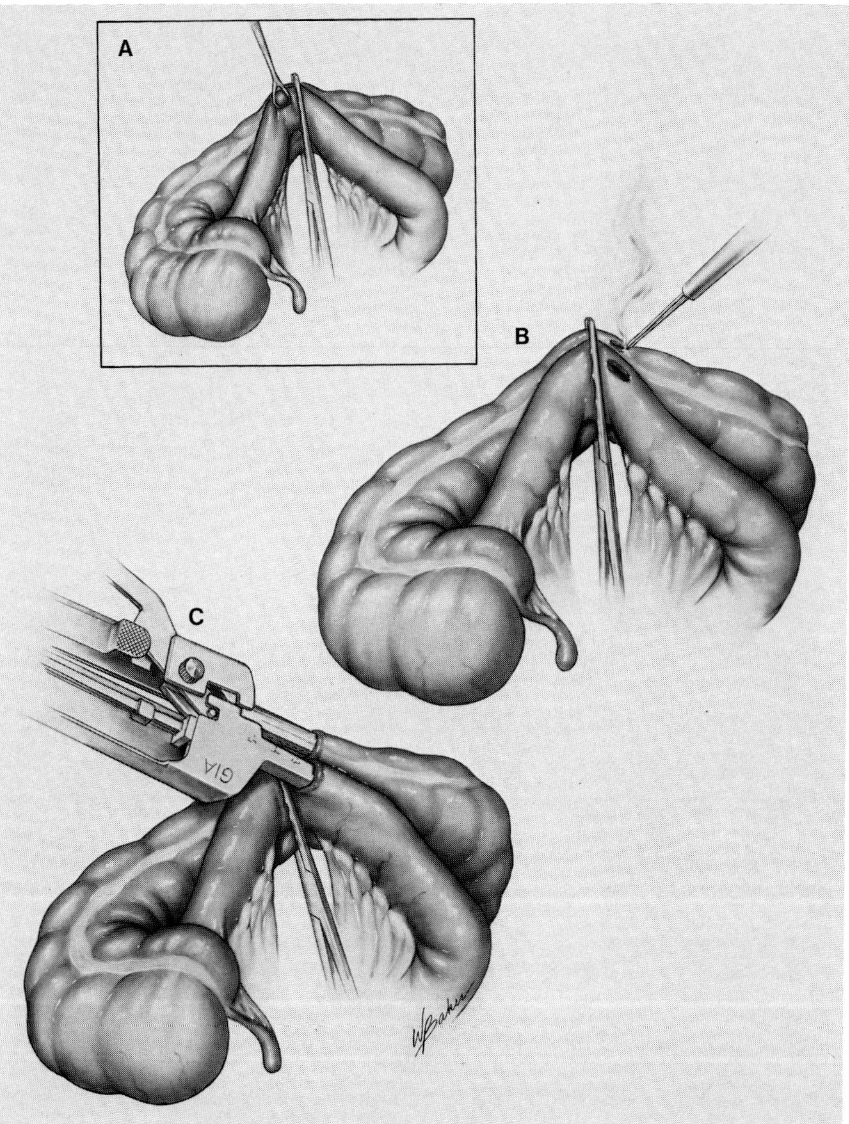

Fig VIII–5.—Modified functional end-to-end anastomosis. We have come to use this technique almost invariably if resection of bowel is to be followed by anastomosis of the divided proximal and distal ends. **A,** the terminal ileum and right colon have been devascularized. The antimesenteric borders are matched at the junction of viable and nonviable bowel, and fixed in that position with a Kocher clamp placed just barely on the specimen side. **B,** openings for the GIA™ instrument are made on the antimesenteric surface of the bowel just at the border of viability. **C,** the partially assembled limbs of the GIA™ instrument can be inserted simultaneously into the two openings, particularly if the bowel is held taut away from the Kocher clamp with a Babcock clamp or a traction suture (not shown).

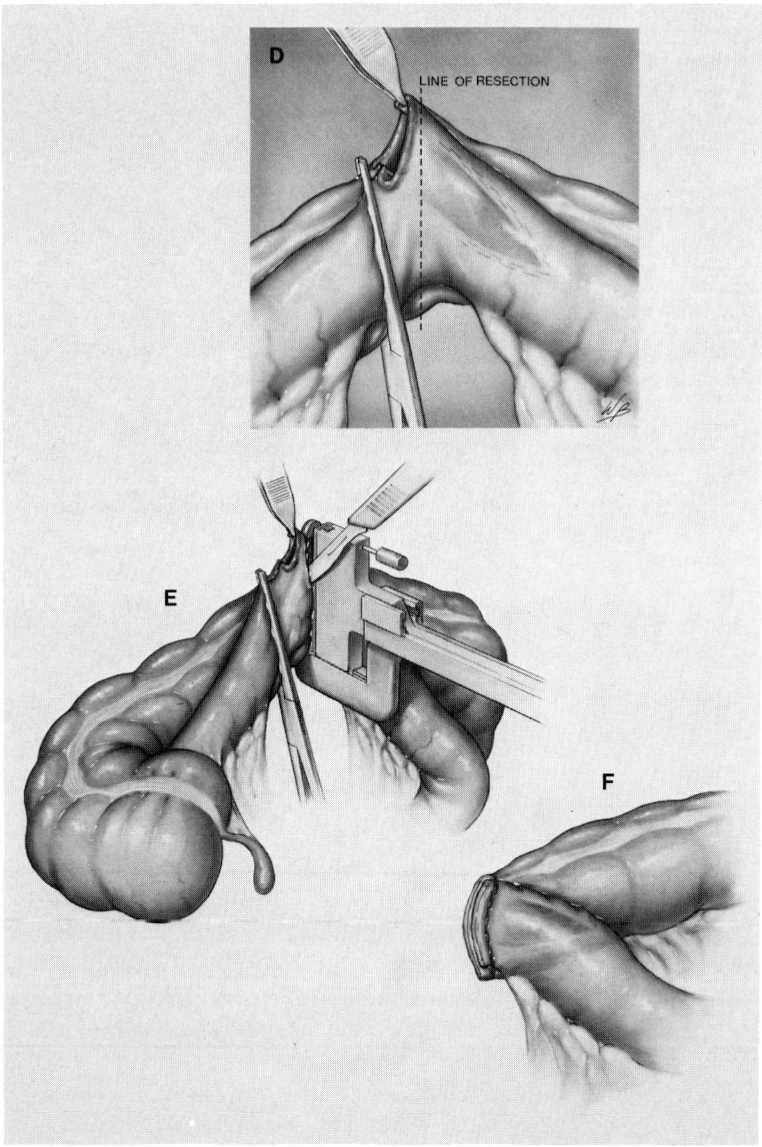

Fig VIII–5 (cont.).—The anastomosis having been completed and the GIA™ suture line inspected **(D)**, the TA55 ™ instrument **(E)** is placed across the two loops so as to exclude the GIA™ opening and the specimen is amputated, with the final result seen in **F.** This technique obviates the stapling and division of the bowel at either end of the resection and reduces to a matter of seconds the opportunity for possible contamination. We have used this technique in various resections of the small bowel, in segmental colectomies, and for low anterior resections. (From M.M. Ravitch and F.M. Steichen, *Abdominal Operations,* 7th ed. New York, Appleton-Century-Crofts, 1979, R. Maingot [ed.], used by permission.)

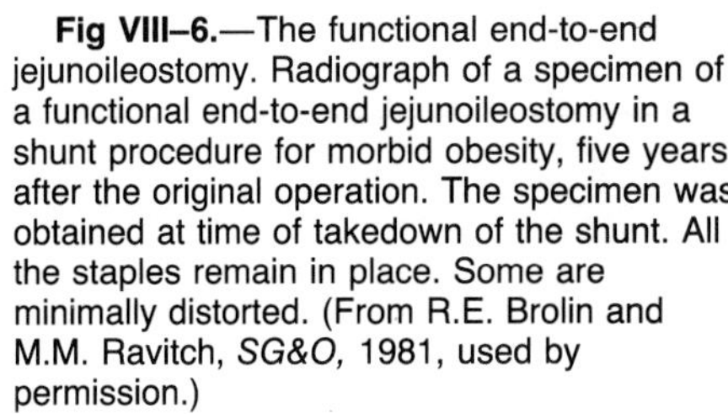

Fig VIII–6.—The functional end-to-end jejunoileostomy. Radiograph of a specimen of a functional end-to-end jejunoileostomy in a shunt procedure for morbid obesity, five years after the original operation. The specimen was obtained at time of takedown of the shunt. All the staples remain in place. Some are minimally distorted. (From R.E. Brolin and M.M. Ravitch, *SG&O,* 1981, used by permission.)

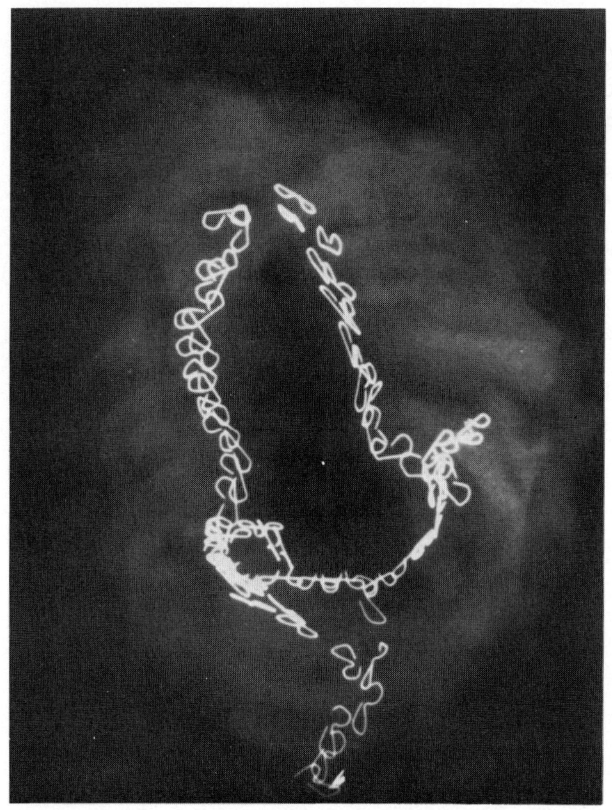

In this country and abroad, we have seen a repeated pattern as surgeons first risk the TA^{TM} and the GIA^{TM} instruments for bowel closures, then progressively adopt the techniques of anastomosis. In the discussion below, all anastomoses are of the functional end-to-end variety unless otherwise stated.

Weber (1972), from Rudler's Clinic in Geneva, reporting their first 16 months of use of the TA^{TM} and GIA^{TM} instruments, performed six right hemicolectomies and seven sigmoid resections, and anastomoses of the small bowel or colon, with no fistulas or abscesses and a single death from renal insufficiency in a man of 86 years.

From Putnam, Connecticut, Painter, Park, and Hochberg (1974) reported their initial experience with the staplers in 87 cases from November, 1971 to November, 1972. Their use of staples included seven small bowel and 28 large bowel applications with a single fistula in a functional end-to-end ileocolostomy, which was resected and a new stapled anastomosis successfully constructed.

Pediatric surgeons have found some special applications for the staplers. The ineffective propulsion of succus entericus in the hugely dilated blind jejunum proximal to an atresia is appreciated to result in functional obstruction when only a simple anastomosis is made after resection of the atretic zone. Resection of a substantial segment of the blind end before anastomosis has been the standard corrective measure. Thomas (1969), Howard and Othersen (1973), and others have tapered the dilated jejunum by excising a long strip of the antimesenteric wall. As DeLorimier (1973) said in discussion of Howard's paper, "This can be a very long and tedious procedure." Barbara of Hackensack, New Jersey (1973), in the further discussion, stated that he had ". . . used the GIA stapling machine with the pediatric clip. That took the entire antimesenteric margin off very quickly and saved blood loss. I then just ran a seromuscular stitch over the top and tapered it rather quickly." Grosfeld (1979) used the same technique.

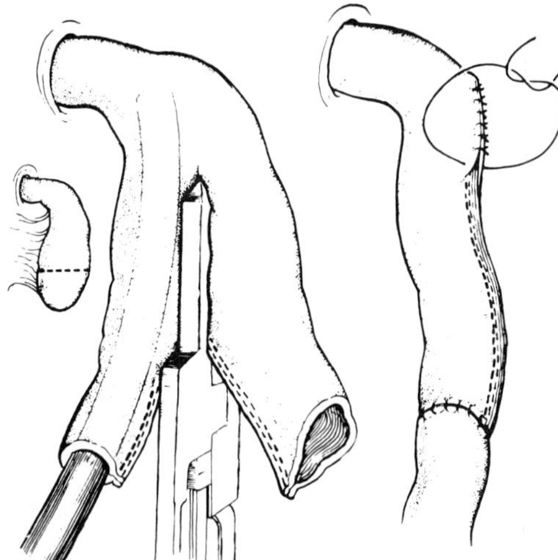

Fig VIII–7.—Grosfeld's technique for a tapering jejunoplasty when there is "significantly foreshortened bowel" so that resection of all of the dilated proximal bowel is inadvisable. (From J.L. Grosfeld, in *Pediatric Surgery,* 3d ed., M.M. Ravitch, et al. [eds.], Year Book Medical Publishers, Chicago, 1979, used by permission.)

TAPERING JEJUNOPLASTY

Latimer and colleagues (Latimer, Doane, McKittrick, and Shepherd, 1975) from Santa Barbara, reporting their experience with the TA^{TM} and the GIA^{TM} instruments from July, 1972 to December, 1974, performed 23 enteroenterostomies, 27 ileocolostomies, and 15 colocolostomies. They had one fistula after closure of an enterotomy, one "intramural hematoma with abscess" after sigmoid colotomy-polypectomy, and no other complications.

Lawson and associates (Lawson, Hutchison, Longland, and Haque, 1977) from the Royal Infirmary, Glasgow performed 20 colon resections and four colon bypasses. The single death—after a colon bypass—related to a stapled GIA^{TM} anastomosis, under great tension, which pulled apart under the operator's eyes and then was replaced by a manual anastomosis, which leaked. There was a late, temporary, leak in one ileocolic anastomosis. There were no other complications.

Rinecker (1977) of Munich used the instruments in 300 cases, including 16 Braun loops or Roux anastomoses, 19 small bowel resections, 14 closures of jejunotomy or amputation of Meckel's diverticulum, seven ileotransversostomies, 17 right hemicolectomies, 13 low colon resections, and ten Hartmann procedures. In 16 side-to-side small bowel anastomoses there were no deaths and no complications. In 19 small bowel resections there was one fatal leak. In 15 closures of small bowel ends there were no leaks. In 14 ileotransversostomies there were two questionable temporary leaks. In 13 low colon resections there were three fatal leaks and three questionable temporary ones. In ten side-to-side colon anastomoses there was one questionable leak. The six fatal staple-related complications represented a 2% mortality in the 300 cases. Rinecker believed stapling to be the preferred technique for gastrointestinal closures and anastomoses.

Fortin, Poulin, and Leclerc (1979) from Quebec used the TA[TM] and GIA[TM] instruments on the small bowel 66 times and in the colon 118 times. They had a 4.5% fistula rate in their small bowel cases with no deaths and a 5% fistula rate with the large bowel, three of the fistulas in patients who died, a 2.5% mortality. None of the deaths was attributed to the stapling procedure.

Brodman and Brodman from the Albert Einstein College of Medicine (1981) reported their experience with 88 consecutive stapled colonic anastomoses above the pelvic floor done by the functional end-to-end GIA[TM]–TA[TM] technique. There were no deaths, one subphrenic abscess in a patient with an associated splenectomy, and one abscess, requiring drainage, after sigmoid resection. Neither these nor any of the other patients had fistulas or other evidences of anastomotic leak. The wound infection rate was 9.5%. There was no bleeding from any anastomosis.

Reynolds (1970) of Anniston, Alabama used the TA 30[TM] instrument in appendectomy on four patients, covering the stump with silk sutures, and the GIA[TM] instrument in ten, again inverting the closure by silk sutures. There were no complications in either group.

Others report appendectomy with the GIA[TM] instrument, but only as an incidental procedure in a major laparotomy. We, too, occasionally have succumbed to the temptation to divide and staple the appendix with the GIA[TM] instrument.

Reuter's Strasbourg doctoral thesis, based on the St. Thérèse, Luxembourg experience (1982), includes 69 colocolic or ileocolic anastomoses, with two staple-related deaths. One was in an 80-year-old man with Crohn's disease for which terminal ileum and a portion of right colon were resected—death with "multiple fistulae." The other was a septic death after sigmoidectomy. There were no instances of bleeding. There were six anastomotic fistulas, four requiring reoperation, and in two of these "one found the fistula at the point of a nylon suture which was used to close the GIA introduction site."

We have not used the EEA[TM] instrument for intestinal anastomoses in the segments between the ligament of Treitz and the sigmoid, except to the esophagus. We prefer the simpler and quicker functional end-to-end technique and have, in addition, not wished to make the additional enterotomy or colotomy required for most EEA[TM] techniques in colon or rectum. However, it must be acknowledged that beginning with the enthusiastic report by Nance (1979) there has been increasing use of the EEA[TM] instrument for intestinal and colonic anastomoses, largely, we suspect, because of an atavistic preference for inverting anastomoses, although the same authors close the site of introduction of the EEA[TM] instrument, with the TA[TM] instrument, mucosa-to-mucosa.

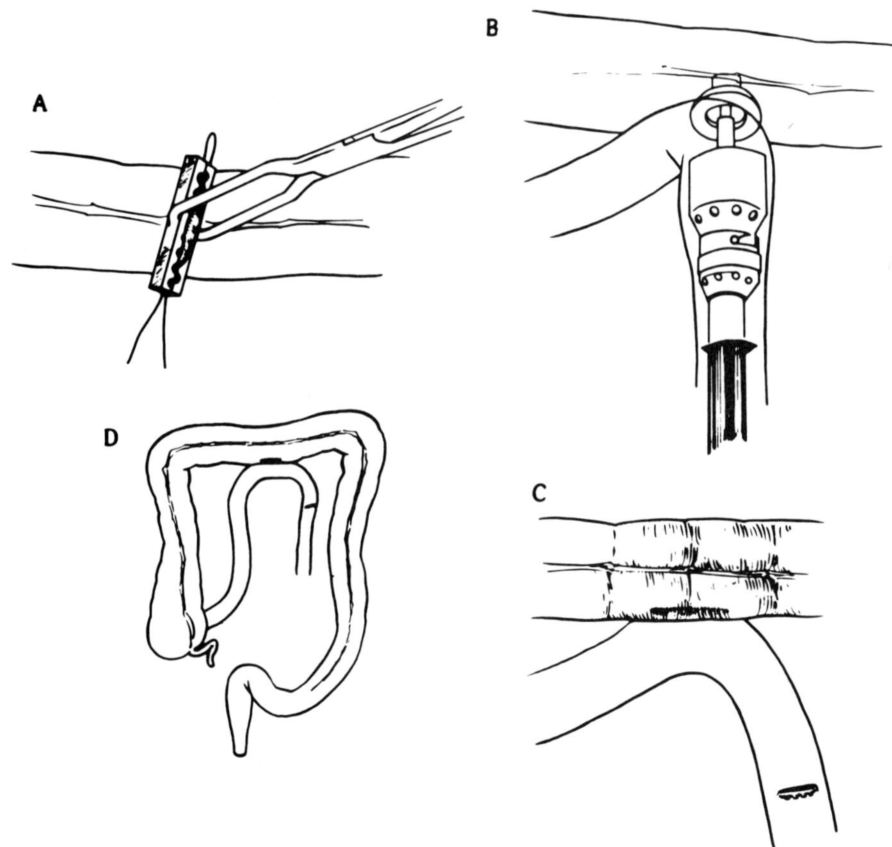

Fig VIII–10.—Side-to-side ileocolostomy with the EEA™ stapler—technique of Nance (1979). **A,** a transversely oriented pursestring suture/enterotomy is placed at the proposed site of the anastomosis In the colon, using the pursestring instrument. Excising the tit of bowel that protrudes through the clamp opens the colon. **B,** the EEA™ instrument, *without* the anvil-nose cone, has been inserted into the ileum through a proximal enterotomy. The spindle of the EEA™ instrument is brought through a small stab wound at the site of the anastomosis, without a pursestring. The anvil-nose cone is attached and inserted into the pursestringed colotomy, which is tied snugly over the spindle. The instrument is closed and fired. **C,** completed anastomosis. The proximal enterotomy has been stapled closed with the TA™ instrument. **D,** completed ileocolic bypass in continuity. (From F.C. Nance, *Annals of Surgery,* 1979, used by permission.)

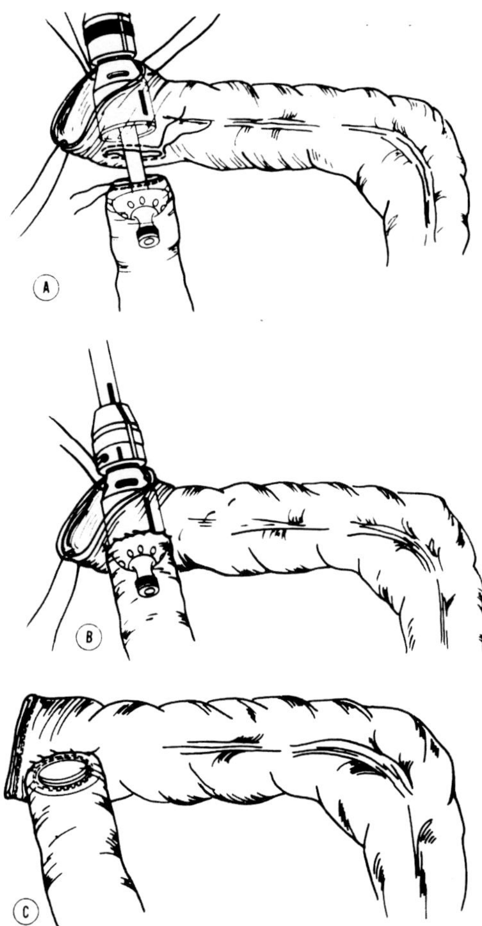

Fig VIII–11.—Ileocolostomy with EEA™ stapler inserted through open end of colon—technique of Mittal and Cortez (1980). **A,** with the pursestring instrument, a pursestring suture is inserted in the distal ileum. The EEA™ stapler is inserted without the anvil through the open distal line of resection of the colon and the central rod passed through the colon wall and the opening pursestringed. The anvil is attached and the two pursestrings tied. **B,** the EEA™ stapler is closed and fired. **C,** the distal line of colonic section is closed mucosa-to-mucosa with the TA 50™ stapler. The end-to-side ileocolostomy is complete. The identical technique was pictured by Gautier-Benoit (1976) and Fasching and Moritz (1980). (From V.K. Mittal and J.A. Cortez, *Surgery,* 1980, used by permission.)

Nance (1979), using the EEA™ instrument, performed 17 end-to-end colocolostomies, five end-to-end ileocolostomies, one side-to-side ileocolostomy, five end-to-end small bowel anastomoses, and seven Roux-en-Y jejunojejunostomies. There were no leaks (see Figs VIII–8–10).

Hollender and colleagues (Hollender, Meyer, Blanchot, and Castellanos, 1980) from Strasbourg reported their five-year experience with the use of the staplers, including the EEA™ instrument, in the gastrointestinal tract. They did not indicate the number of individual operations performed in the various sections of the gastrointestinal tract, analyzing their experience, as others have done, by the number of closures (217) and the number of anastomoses (173). There were 12 additional staple lines—pyloroplasties, greater-curvature tubes, etc. Two of their deaths were from attempts to bypass intestinal fistulas with the GIA™ instrument: one death from a new fistula remote from the intact anastomosis, one from a dehiscence in the anastomosis. In addition, they had two radiologically demonstrated colocolic fistulas in defunctionalized bowel.

Mittal and Cortez (1980) from Detroit describe performing an end-to-side ileocolostomy inserting the EEA™ instrument through the open end of the colon, which then is stapled closed with the TA 55™ instrument (see Fig VIII–11). They performed three such procedures in their first 30 anastomoses in all parts of the gastrointestinal tract. They had one leak in their entire experience, but do not say from which type or location of anastomosis. This is the technique that we at times use for low rectal anastomoses (see Fig IX–4), jejunoesophageal anastomoses (see Fig V–23), and for cervical anastomoses of esophagus to cecum (see Fig VI–10*K*).

Fahrenkrug and Clemmesen (1981) from Denmark reported their experience with the EEA™ instrument, having performed two ileoileostomies, ten ileotransversostomies, 41 colocolostomies, and 35 low anterior resections. In the two ileoileostomies there were no leaks. There was one clinical leak and one radiologic leak in ten right hemicolectomies. There were no leaks in the 17 colocolostomies above the sigmoid, one in the 24 sigmoid resections, and two in the 35 low anterior resections. There was one death in a sigmoid resection and two deaths in low anterior resections.

Marti, Fiala, and Rohner (1981) from Geneva report their experience with 98 EEA™ anastomoses, 79 of them in the large bowel, 23 right hemicolectomies, 19 left hemicolectomies or sigmoid resections, 28 colorectal anastomoses, and 12 reconstructions after Hartmann procedures. Their single catastrophe was in a patient who developed a postoperative rectovesical fistula resulting from interposition of the bladder in the colorectal staple suture line, death occurring despite emergency operation. There were three patients who developed clinical colocutaneous fistulas without evidence of abscess or sepsis and seven patients in whom there was only radiologic evidence of an anastomotic leak, requiring no operation, drainage, or treatment.

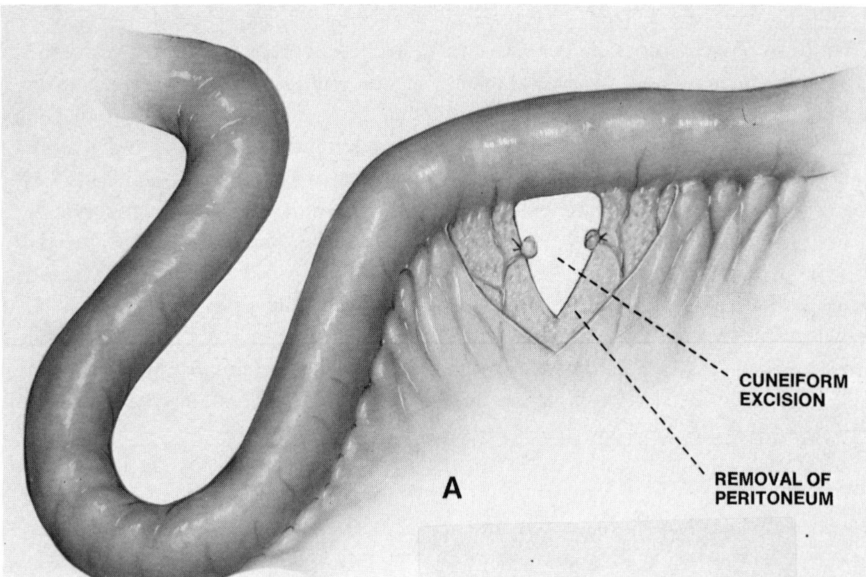

Fig VIII–12.—Continent ileal reservoir (Kock). This is an operation that still is evolving, but the principles of the use of the instruments in the rapid construction of the pouch and in maintaining the ileostomy nipple are basic. **A,** an avascular spot on the mesentery of the terminal ileum, 8–10 cm proximal to the distal cut end, is chosen and a triangular section of mesentery excised in preparation for the fashioning of the nipple valve. On either side of the opening thus created, the serosa is stripped from the mesentery for a short distance on either face. The actual construction of the nipple valve is undertaken later in the procedure. The mesenteric window step is taken early, to provide time in the course of the operation to determine that the viability of the bowel has not been jeopardized.

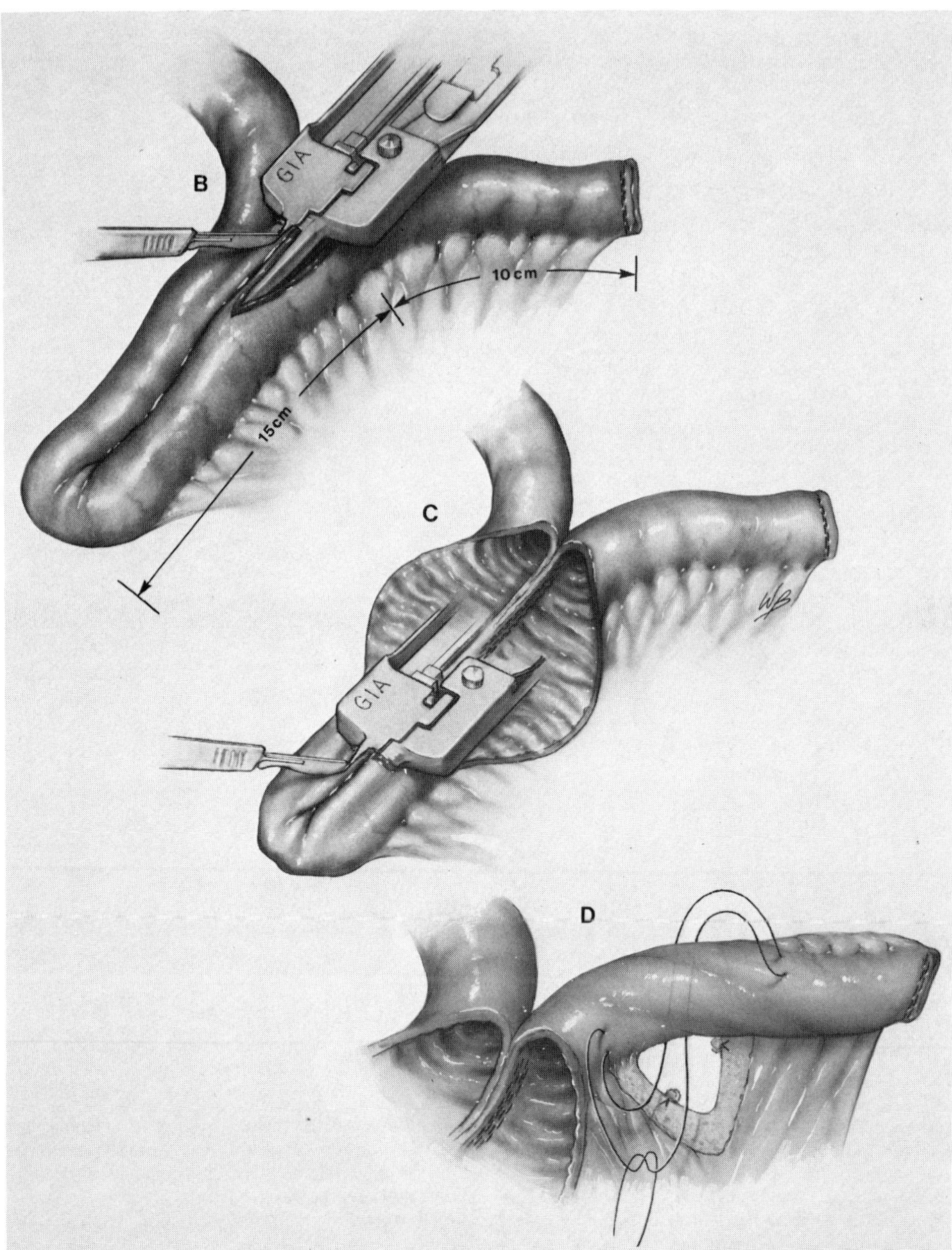

Fig VIII–12 (cont.).—B, the bowel has been measured as indicated so that each arm of the loop doubled on itself is 15 cm and there is a 10-cm free segment of distal ileum beyond the doubled segment. The GIA™ instrument with the special cartridge *without a knife* (SGIA™) is inserted through stab wounds and fired, stapling the two limbs together with four rows of staples. Incision now of each loop just alongside the crevice between the two blades of the GIA™ instrument begins to free up the serosa-to-serosa stapled union of the two loops. **C,** repeated application of the special GIA™ instrument (SGIA™) and division of the anterior wall of the two loops opens up a large flat paddle of the two joined loops. **D,** at this point, the special suture devised by Kock is inserted as illustrated to produce a small degree of torsion, which minimizes the amount of mesentery caught in the intussusception to be made for construction of the nipple. Not shown is the abrasion of the peritoneum of the bowel to be intussuscepted to encourage adherence.   *(continued)*

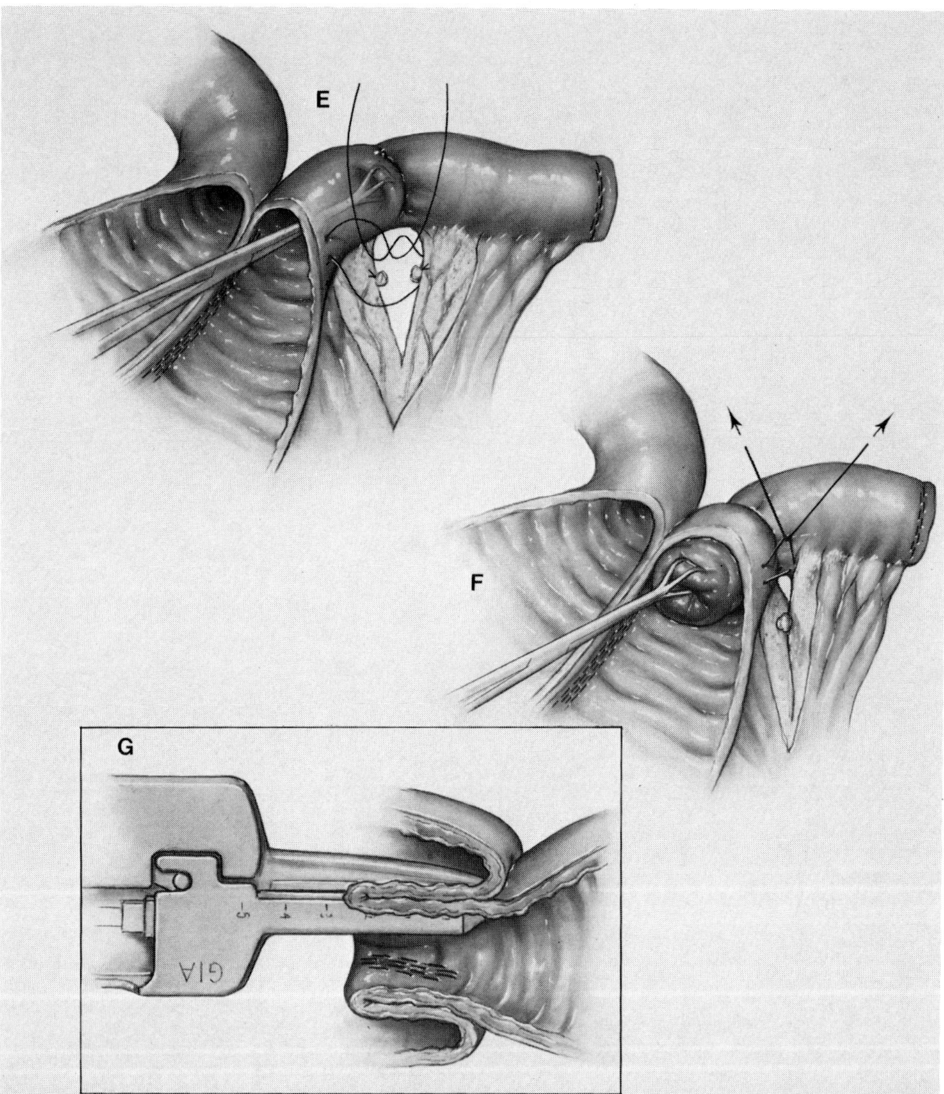

Fig VIII–12 (cont.).—**E,** a Babcock clamp is passed up the efferent limb into the terminal ileum, the wall of which is grasped at the preselected point, 8 cm or 10 cm from the end. **F,** traction on the Babcock intussuscepts the nipple valve at the same time that gradual tension on the rotating suture achieves its purpose, after which the suture is tied. **G,** the SGIA™ instrument, which has no knife blade, is inserted as shown and applied four or five times to fix the nipple and prevent sliding. We have done this quite close to the mesenteric border of the bowel and thus far have observed no problems with hematoma formation, bleeding, or ischemia.

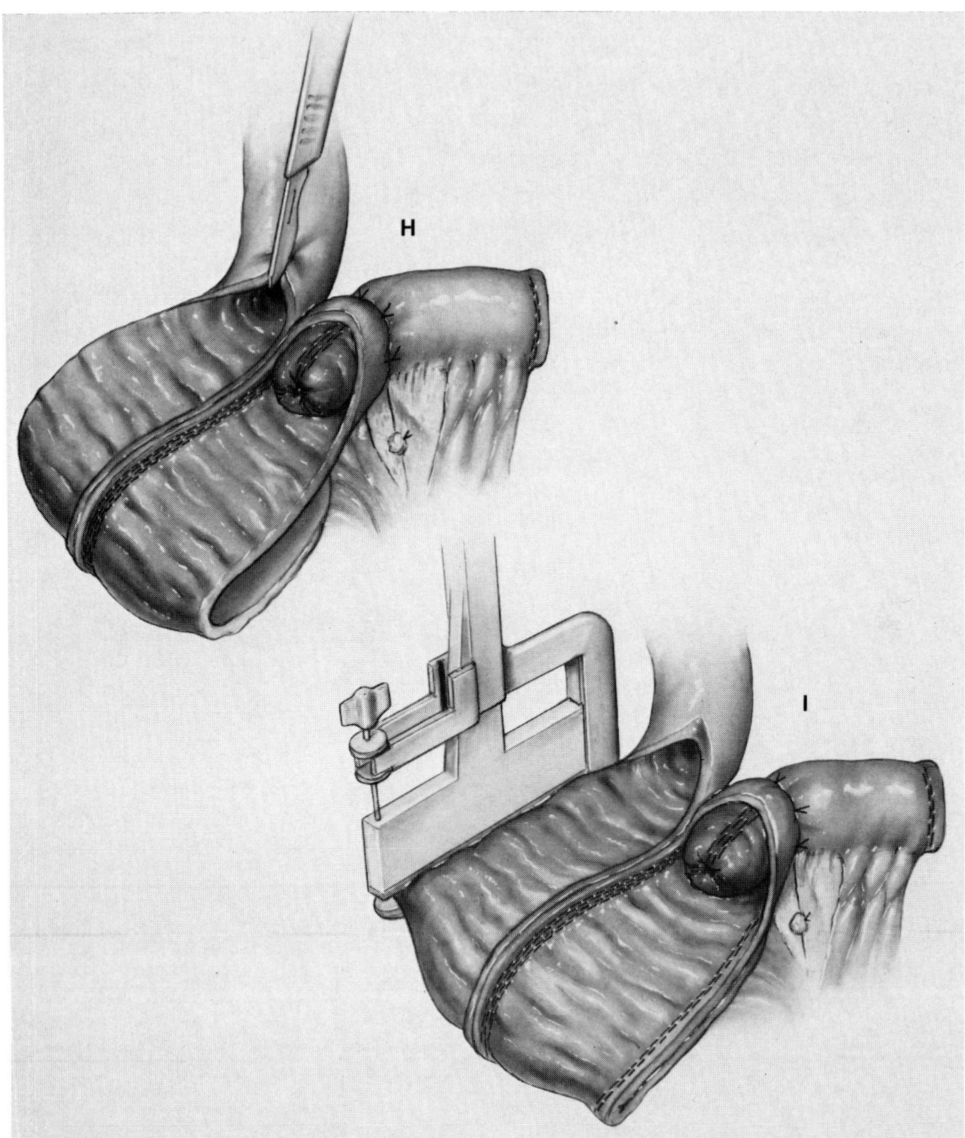

Fig VIII–12 (cont.).—H, the paddle of bowel lies doubled back on itself. An incision of 4 cm is being made into the afferent loop so that when the pouch is closed, the openings into the afferent and efferent loops will be staggered and not lie opposite each other. Sliding of the nipple is the single most troublesome complication, and a number of interrupted sutures are taken in the bowel wall externally to help discourage this tendency. **I,** using the TA 90™ instrument, the edges of the everted pouch are stapled from their mucosal surfaces, producing a serosa-to-serosa union. *(continued)*

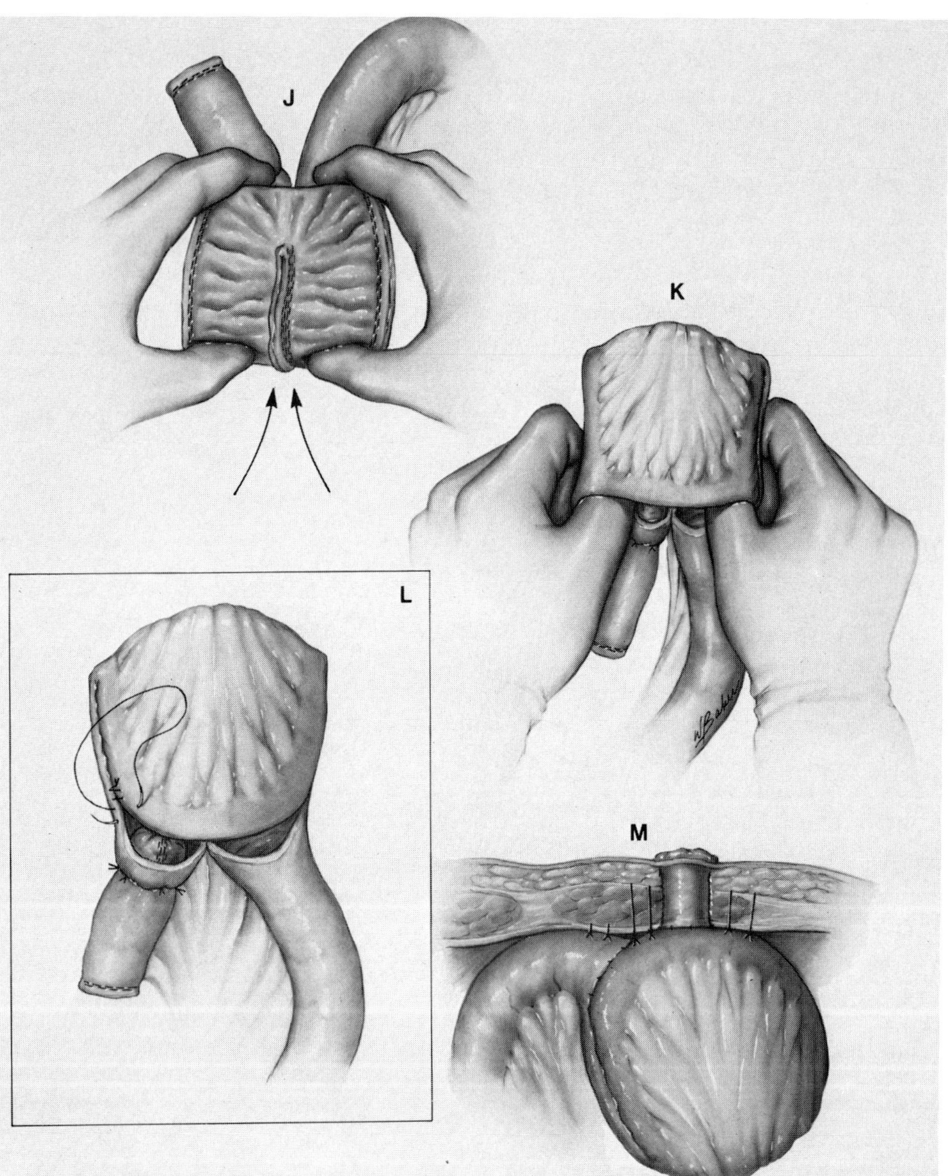

Fig VIII–12 (cont.).—J and **K,** the everted pouch now is turned right side out by the manual maneuver shown. **L,** the final portion of the closure of the pouch is completed manually. To staple a suture line like this, with its double curve and sharp angulation, would require placing the TA™ instrument as a chord across an arc with resultant loss of tissue that one would not wish to sacrifice. **M,** the pouch itself is firmly sutured to the abdominal wall, the ileal spout brought out through the abdominal wall and sutured to the orifice made in the skin. Except for the skin sutures, the efferent loop is not anchored to the abdominal wall, to prevent the weight of a filled pouch from pulling at a rigidly fixed efferent loop, thought to be one mechanism of nipple loss. To prevent kinking and obstruction to inflow, the afferent loop is sutured to the abdominal wall in the same plane as the pouch. (From F.M. Steichen, J.M. Loubeau, and J.F. Stremple, *Surgical Rounds,* September, 1978, used by permission.)

We have described the formation of the Kock pouch with staples (Steichen, 1977; Steichen, Loubeau, and Stremple, 1978), using the TA 90^{TM} instrument for the construction of the pouch itself, either mucosa-to-mucosa (by applying the TA 90^{TM} instrument with the paddle of bowel flopped mucosa-to-mucosa) or serosa-to-serosa, and using the GIA^{TM} instrument without the knife (SGIA^{TM}) for the application of four or five radial staple lines in the nipple, to discourage reduction. In an experience up to July, 1982 of 19 cases with stapled pouches, we have had no leaks, one perforation by a catheter, and no wound infections and consider the neatness and timesaving to be well worthwhile. In an experience with 13 nipples stapled to discourage reduction we have had two failures. We have not encountered any other descriptions in the literature of the use of the staplers for formation of the pouch itself, although we understand that a number of surgeons have used them. There are a number of references to the use of the GIA^{TM} instrument without the knife (SGIA^{TM}) in through-and-through stapling of the nipple.

Loygue and colleagues from the Hôpital Saint-Antoine in Paris (Loygue, Salmon, Amand, and Levy, 1978) varied the technique of staple fixation of the nipple valve by stapling it longitudinally with two applications of the TA 55^{TM} instrument. They had used this technique in their last four patients with great satisfaction. They stated that they were planning to begin making the pouch with the staplers.

Westbrook of Little Rock, Arkansas (1979), at the Southwestern Surgical Congress in Las Vegas, Nevada, with an experience of " . . . approximately 12 Kock pouches . . . ", said he had constructed half of the pouches with the staplers with satisfactory results, but that the use of the modified GIA^{TM} cartridge for stapling the nipple had not been satisfactory. "We have used this cartridge for nipple formation and the staples pulled through, causing nipple failure."

On the other hand, Cohen and Stone from Toronto (1980), in an experience with 17 patients, stapled the nipple with three or four applications of the SGIA^{TM} instrument, commenting also that they were using the stapling technique of Nils Kock himself, which in fact he adopted after a visit to Pittsburgh.

From the Mayo Clinic, Dozois and colleagues (Dozois, Kelly, Beart, and Beahrs, 1980), with a total experience of 199 Kock pouches, apparently indifferently used either nonabsorbable sutures or stainless steel staples in fixing the nipple. The pouches all appear to have been made manually.

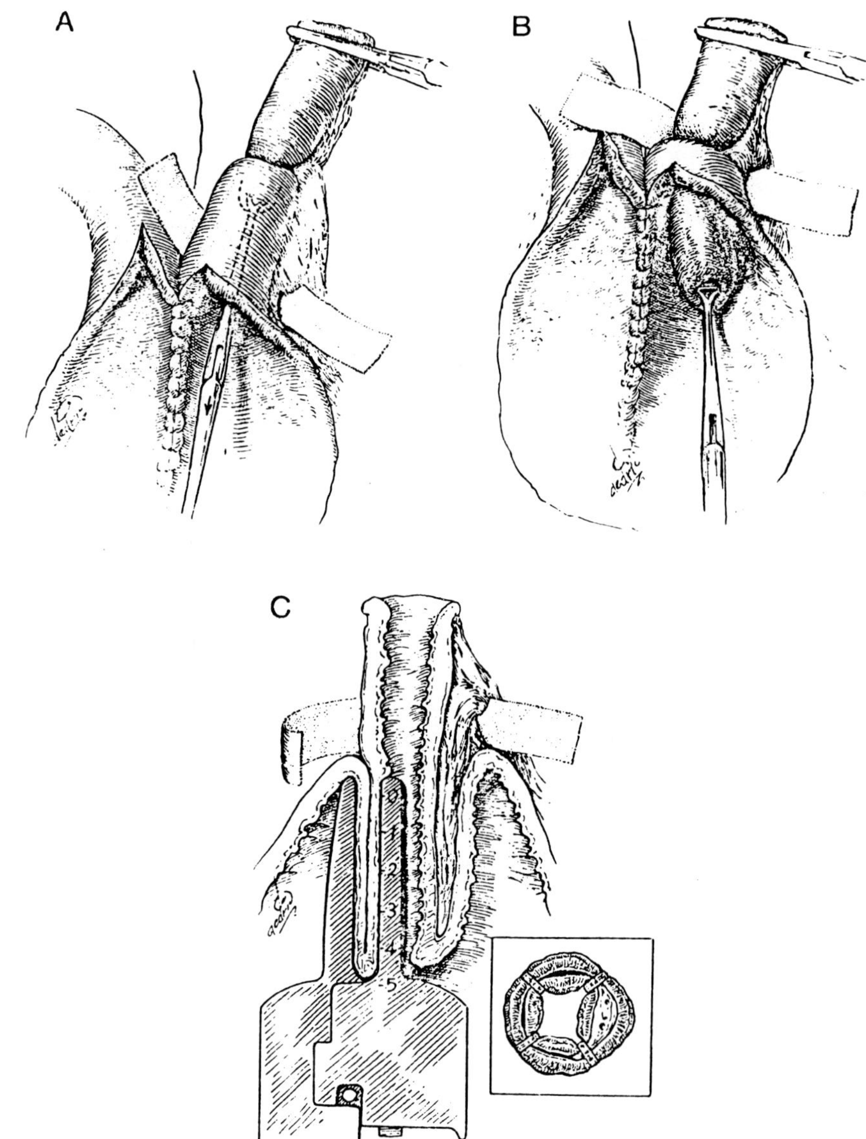

Fig. 7. Construction of the nipple valve.

Fig VIII–13.—Kock's technique of stapling the nipple valve and a collar of Marlex around the emerging ileal spout. With the SGIA™ instrument, "Four such applications are performed, two of them partly involving the mesentery. The total length of the arms of the GIA-instrument should be utilized when applying the staples." In 32 patients they saw no injury to the blood supply of the nipple and in no case did the nipple slide. (From N.F. Kock, H.E. Myrvold, L.O. Nilsson, and C. Åhren, *Annales Chirurgiae et Gynaecologiae,* 1980, used by permission.)

Kock and associates (Kock, Myrvold, Nilsson, and Ahrén, 1980) illustrated the use of the SGIA^TM instrument for stapling the nipple, placing also a collar of Marlex or fascia around the emerging ileum just at the level of the abdominal wall (see Fig VIII–13). Kock commented that in 32 patients operated on in this way there had not been a single instance of slipping of the valve. With respect to the danger of interfering with the blood supply of the nipple valve by the several applications of the SGIA^TM instrument, Kock said, "In the present [clinical] experiments, staples were placed so that large areas of the mesentery were involved, but the blood supply was never seriously disturbed by the staples." The following year, Kock (Kock, Myrvold, Nilsson, and Philipson, 1981) stated that they were continuing to use this technique with satisfaction.

Also in the same year, from the Sloan-Kettering in New York, Papachristou (1981) experimented with an SGIA^TM stapled nipple valve in dogs, without a pouch, and thought that the procedure might be applicable in humans. The ileum was intussuscepted and the SGIA^TM instrument inserted from outside the bowel, one blade in the serosal pocket between intussusceptum and intussuscipiens and the other blade outside the intussuscipiens.

Cranley and McKelvey (1981) from Belfast undertook to examine the stapling of the nipple valve experimentally and claimed that they had found " . . . that the use of staples, apart from saving considerably on operating time, did not prevent extrusion of the mesenteric border." They had not used the technique clinically.

Recently, Sohn, Weinstein, Robbins, and Steichen (1983) have used the GIA^TM instrument in the construction of the J-ileal pouch for the ileo-anal pull through after total colectomy and rectal mucosa stripping, using two applications of the GIA^TM instrument and creating an ileal pouch similar to the jejunal Hunt-Lawrence reservoir. The curved bottom of the J, 5 cm, below the GIA^TM side-to-side anastomosis, is used for the end-to-side ileo-anal anastomosis after endorectal pull through, employing Goligher's EEA^TM technique for low "anterior" colorectal anastomosis. Preliminary results in 17 patients have been very encouraging, but must wait for the test of time.

ILEAL LOOP URINARY DIVERSION

The isolation of a segment of terminal ileum for an ileal loop urinary diversion is an obvious application of the staplers, so far as handling the intestine itself is concerned. A large part of its appeal may well be that urologists, not frequently dealing with the intestine, have found the functional end-to-end anastomosis to be a safe and secure technique.

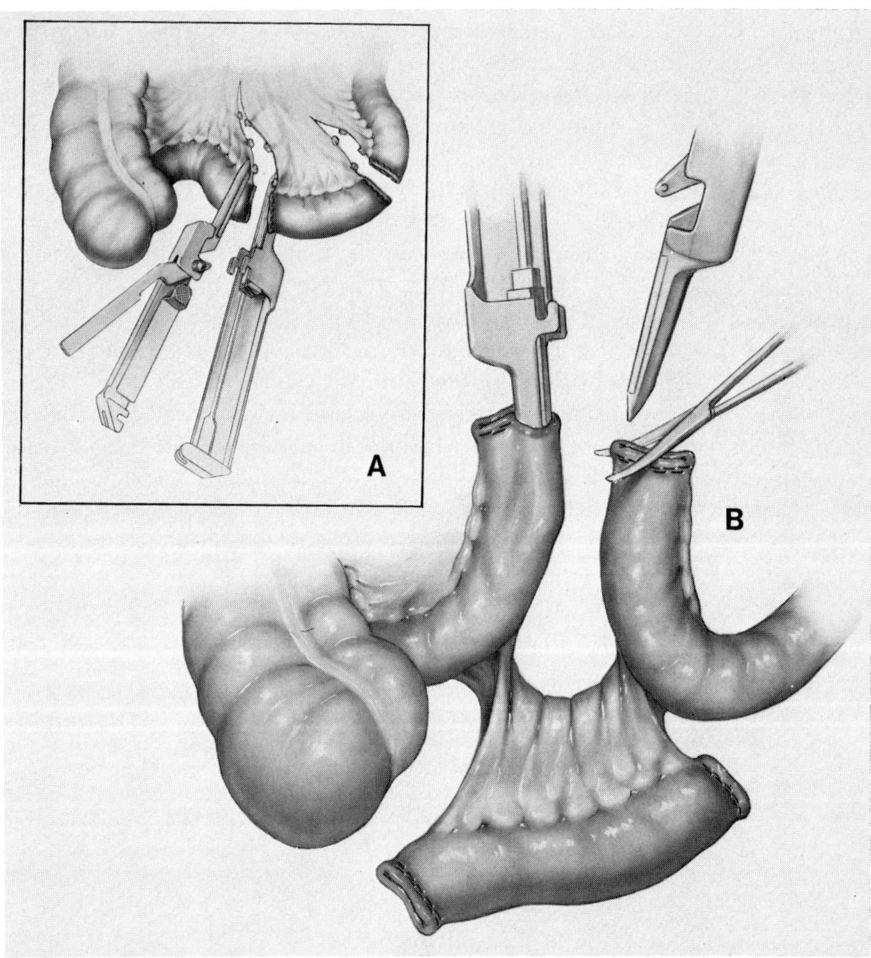

Fig VIII–14.—Ileal loop for urinary diversion. **A,** the ileum is stapled and divided twice with the GIA™ instrument, 8–10 cm apart, at relatively avascular spaces in the mesentery. **B,** the GIA™ limbs are inserted through the cutaway antimesenteric corners of the staple closures of the proximal and distal ends of the ileum.

C, the limbs approximated, the instrument locked, and the staple and knife assembly driven home. **D,** the application of the TA™ instrument to the opening left after withdrawal of the GIA™ instrument completes the functional end-to-end anastomosis as the excess tissue beyond the staple jaw is cut away, restoring intestintal continuity. **E,** the ureters have been implanted into the proximal end of the loop, the mesenteric defect closed, and the ileal loop is ready to be brought up through the abdominal wall, then to be opened. (**A** and **D** from F.M. Steichen, *American Journal of Surgery,* 1977, used by permission.)   →

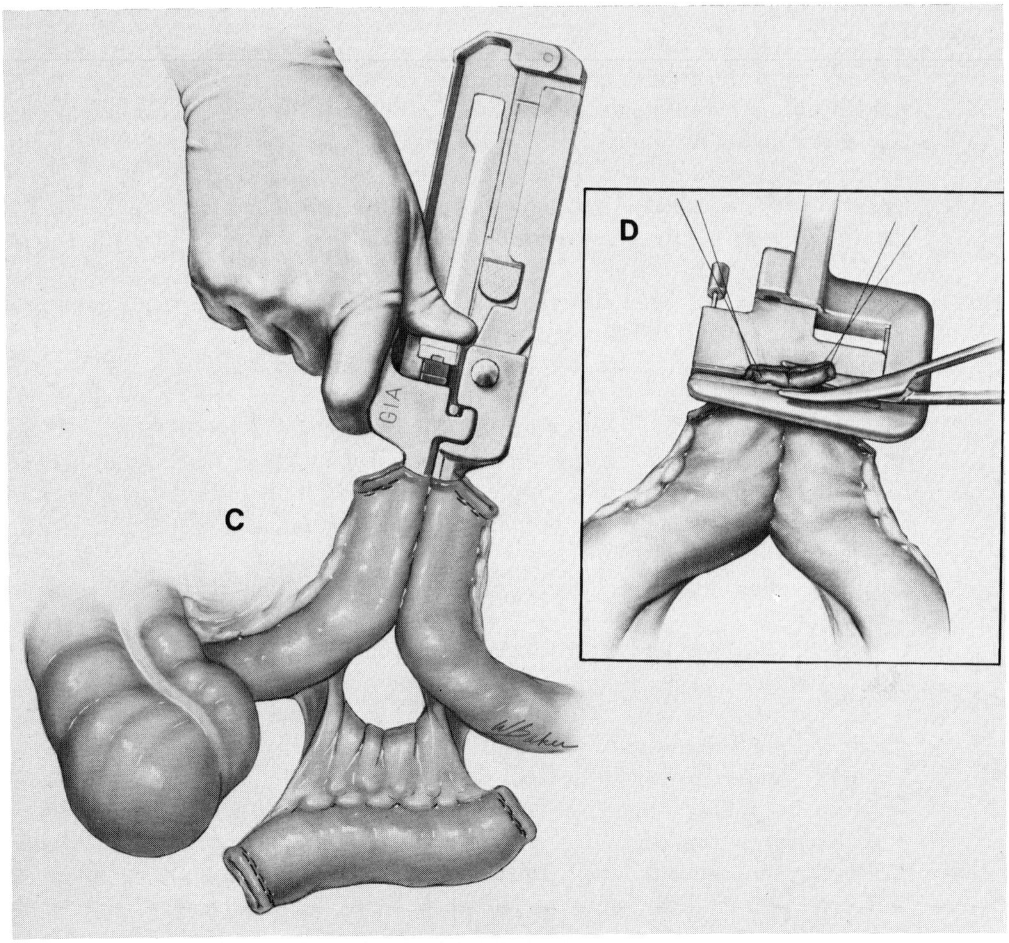

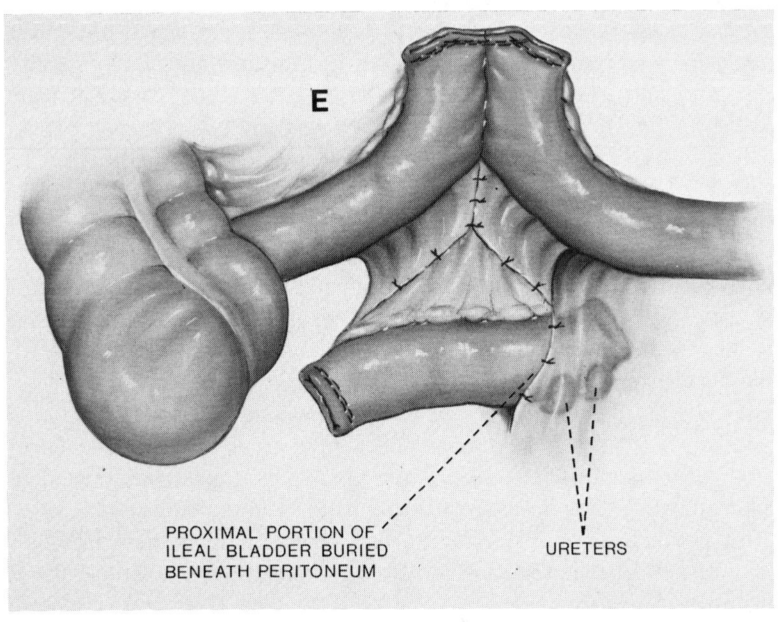

Fig VIII–14 C–E (cont.)

We began performing ileal loops for urinary diversion in 1971 (Karamcheti, O'Donnell, Hakala, Schwentker, and Steichen, 1978). In fact, the first published report of the use of staplers in the formation of ileal conduits was from Hamot Hospital in Erie, Pennsylvania (Assadnia, Lee, Petre, and Lyons, 1972). Between May, 1968 and September, 1970, after total cystectomy, they had constructed five ileal conduits with the stapler. They reported that subsequently two patients passed stones from the loops and staples were found embedded in the stones. Apart from the discharge of calculous material there were no symptoms. Their conclusion was that "The stapling instrument probably has no place in urologic operations."

From the M. D. Anderson Hospital in Houston, Johnson and Fuerst (1973) reported 24 consecutive ureteroileal cutaneous urinary conduits. They used the TA 30^{TM} instrument to close the proximal end of the ileal loop and performed a functional end-to-end anastomosis between the two open ends of the ileum. "There were no postoperative deaths and no case of intestinal obstruction. The only postoperative complication directly related to the auto suture technique was the development of a small enteroanastomotic leak in 1 patient who underwent operation early in the series . . . healed spontaneously within a week." Operative time was shortened and postoperative ileus was much briefer.

Turnbull and Weakley (1975) of the Cleveland Clinic, writing in a urologic text, describe the stapling ileal loop technique in detail but provide no statement of experience, remarking only that, "With the use of the auto suture instruments, bowel can be closed and divided and anastomoses made in a fraction of the time these maneuvers take with conventional suture material . . . bowel lumen . . . is exposed to the operative field for a much shorter period of time than is the case for a conventional, open type of suture anastomosis." Our own experience with the first 110 cases of ileal conduit construction with the Auto Suture® staplers was reported in 1978 (Karamcheti, O'Donnell, Hakala, Schwentker, and Steichen, 1978), the series having begun in 1971. Almost all of the procedures were done by the resident urologic staff. During the same period, 55 ileal loops were performed by manual suture techniques, principally early in the period and at the operator's preference. There was a substantial difference in operating time, calculated to be more than an hour less in stapled patients, and the duration of postoperative ileus was thought to be shorter by two to three days with stapling. The postoperative hospital stay was five to six days shorter in the stapled patients. There were no fistulas or cases of peritonitis with either group and there was one case of ". . . subacute intestinal obstruction . . ." in each group. Formation of stones in the ileal loops in any of the patients was not reported.

However, by 1980, Bennett and Taylor (1980), continuing the University of Pittsburgh study, reported two patients who had conduit calculi with embedded staples. They proposed using the pursestring instrument to place a pursestring suture just beyond the line of staples in the pouch, excising the staple line and inverting the cut end with the absorbable pursestring suture.

A report from the Surgery Branch of the National Cancer Institute (Bergman, Sears, and Javadpour, 1978) describes one patient in a series of two with stapled ileal loops who " . . . began passing ileal loop stones containing staples one year after creation of the ileal conduit." They discussed the association and importance of " . . . residual urine in the conduit, metabolic acidosis, and chronic urinary tract infection. . . ." They had inverted their stapled closure of the proximal end of the ileal loop and cautioned against that practice.

From the Massachusetts General Hospital, Heney and colleagues (Heney, Dretler, Hensle, and Kerr, 1978) reported 41 urinary intestinal conduits made with the Auto Suture® devices—12 colonic, 25 ileal, and four jejunal. "There were no urine or bowel leaks, although in one postoperative gastrointestinal bleeding occurred in association with a partial small-bowel obstruction probably related to the stapled enteroanastomosis. Use of the instruments reduced peritoneal contamination and facilitated conduit manipulation. Operating time was reduced. Four patients have passed stones composed of struvite and apatite with staples imbedded within." Their technique was illustrated by reproduction of our illustrations and they considered the stones a " . . . moderate complication. . . ."

Bisson, Vinson, and Leadbetter (1979) from the University of Vermont expressed themselves as delighted with the Auto Suture® technique for preparation of the loop and reconstitution of continuity of the bowel, but had three patients out of an unstated total number who passed stones with staples embedded in them " . . . despite our separating the metallic sutures from the urine by a running suture of chromic catgut." They subsequently excised the staples from the ileal segment and either closed it with catgut or anastomosed the ureters into the opened end of the loop.

Bredael, Kramer, and Anderson (1980), reporting from Duke University but writing in the *Acta Urologica Belgica,* reported 22 consecutive ileal conduit urinary diversions made by the technique illustrated in Figure VIII–14. No major complications occurred, only one patient having a delay in the restoration of bowel action. One intraoperative mechanical failure required a second placement of the staple line. Nothing is said about stones.

From Rush-Presbyterian-St. Luke's Medical Center in Chicago, Gottesman (1981) reported 35 urinary stapled intestinal loop diversions, 11 with the colon and 24 with terminal ileum. For the colon, they used the true end-to-end technique for reconstruction and for the ileum the functional end-to-end anastomosis. There were no enteric leaks and " . . . most observers felt that bowel function returned more quickly with stapled anastomoses than with conventional techniques." They had closed the blind end of the urinary conduit with staples in six of the cases, and thus far had seen no stone.

Wheeless and Dorsey (1981) constructed 52 intestinal loops with the staplers in women with pelvic malignancy. There were no operative complications. No stone formation was seen in the conduits.

In general, it would seem that the formation of calculi in the ileal loop is relatively infrequent and is subject to the usual influences promoting the formation of calculi—stasis, infection, acid urine, and foreign bodies. A number of the reported instances certainly have been associated with the unnecessary inversion of the stapled closure by manual sutures. Given the large size of the opening of the enteric loop in relation to the size of the stones, and the fact that the stones form in the loop and not in the ureters and so do not cause obstruction, they would seem to represent a minor complication, largely preventable by eliminating stasis and totally avoidable by following the suggestions of those (Bennett and Taylor, 1980) who excise the stapled end and invert the bowel by pursestring suture.

USE OF THE LINEAR STAPLING INSTRUMENTS IN SPECIAL SITUATIONS IN INTESTINAL SURGERY

We have referred to the applicability of the TA 55™ or GIA™ instruments in the exclusion of portions of the bowel wall containing mural nodules, cysts, polyps, or diverticula. We have chosen not to demonstrate the technique of jejunoileal bypass, since we consider that operation in the treatment of obesity no longer justified, and in the treatment of the lipidemias as still being experimental. However, for some years to come there will be a substantial population of patients with jejunoileal bypasses who will require restoration of normal intestinal continuity. The stapling instruments find great use in these procedures with their multiple disconnections and reconnections. The techniques illustrated here are applicable to many other situations in which rearrangements of intestinal continuity are required.

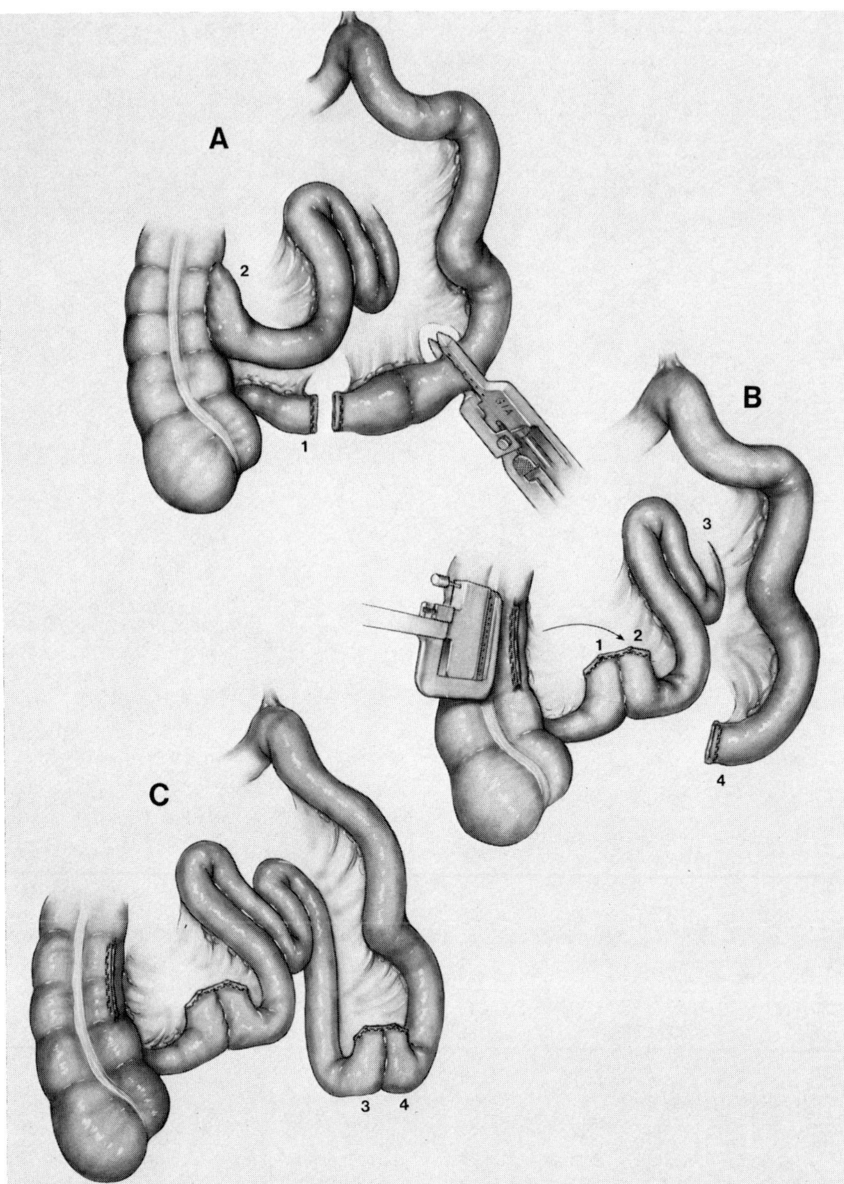

Fig VIII–15.—Scott jejunoileal shunt—restoration of alimentary continuity. **A,** the region of the old end-to-end jejunoileostomy in which the bowel tends to be dilated and thickened, and frequently inflamed, is resected with two applications of the GIA[TM] instrument, sometimes going a little farther proximally if a short segment of the bowel is much thickened. **B,** the ileocolostomy draining the terminal end of the bypassed bowel is taken down by a single application of the TA 90[TM] instrument placed along the border of the colon, carefully excluding the ileum. (The GIA[TM] instrument could be used for the same purpose.) A clamp on the distal end of the bypassed bowel prevents soiling. The terminal ileum for several inches just proximal to this anastomosis is likely to be so thickened as to justify excision by application of the GIA[TM] or the TA[TM] instrument. The newly stapled distal end of the bypassed bowel[2] now is placed alongside the terminal ileum[1] in shotgun fashion and a functional end-to-end anastomosis made. **C,** the blind, closed-over proximal end of the bypassed bowel[3] is laid alongside the stapled end of the proximal jejunum[4] in shotgun fashion. The GIA[TM] instrument is inserted through the cutaway antimesenteric corner of the jejunal staple line, and through a stab wound in the long-closed bypassed loop, and a functional end-to-end anastomosis completed. Such patients usually have had stools in 24–72 hours.

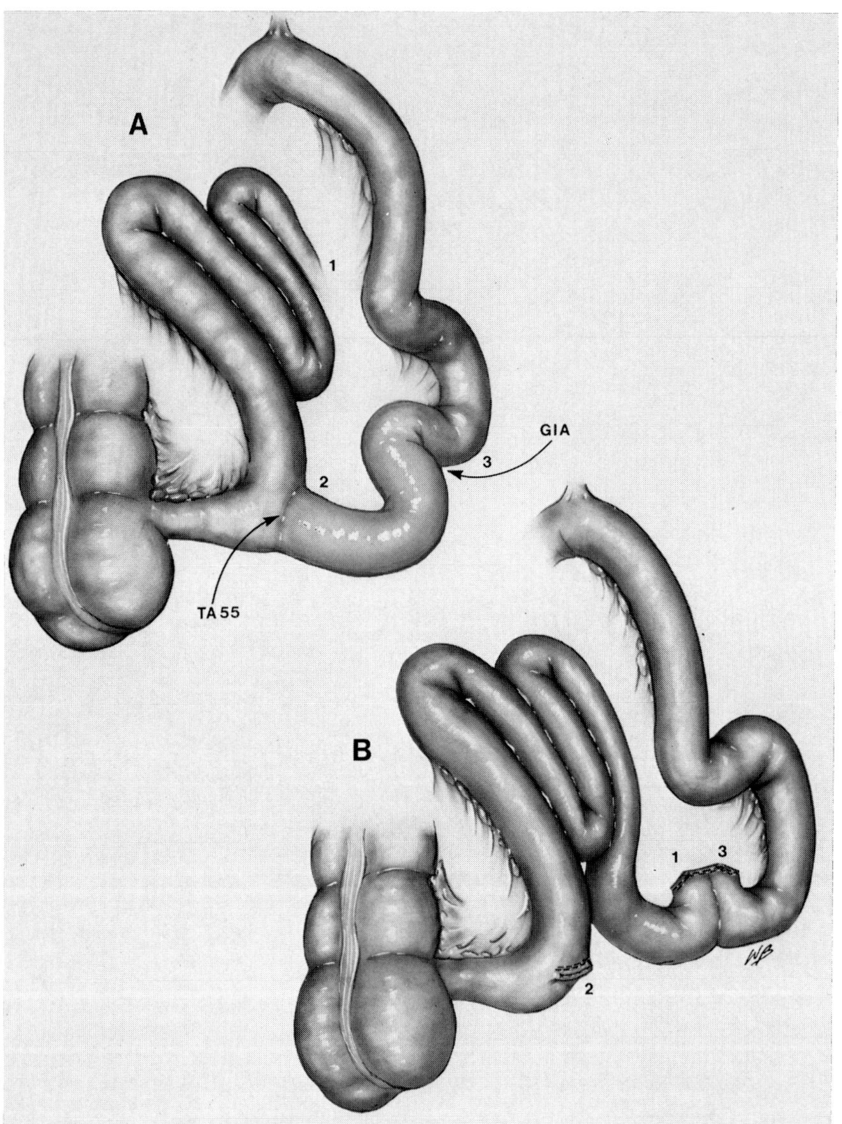

Fig VIII–16.—Payne shunt—restoration of alimentary continuity. **A,** the *arrow* indicates the point at which the TA 55[TM] instrument will be applied to close the opening in the terminal ileum and transect the jejunum, the instrument being so placed that the closure will be transverse on the ileum, thus avoiding the risk of constriction. The proximal jejunum will be divided with the GIA[TM] instrument several inches above the anastomosis to resect the short, distended, hypertrophied segment of jejunum. **B,** the proximal, long-closed end of the bypassed bowel[1] is held alongside the freshly stapled distal end of the proximal jejunum[3] in shotgun fashion and a functional end-to-end anastomosis is constructed. Distally, in the terminal ileum, one can see the transverse stapled closure[2] of the original jejunoileostomy.

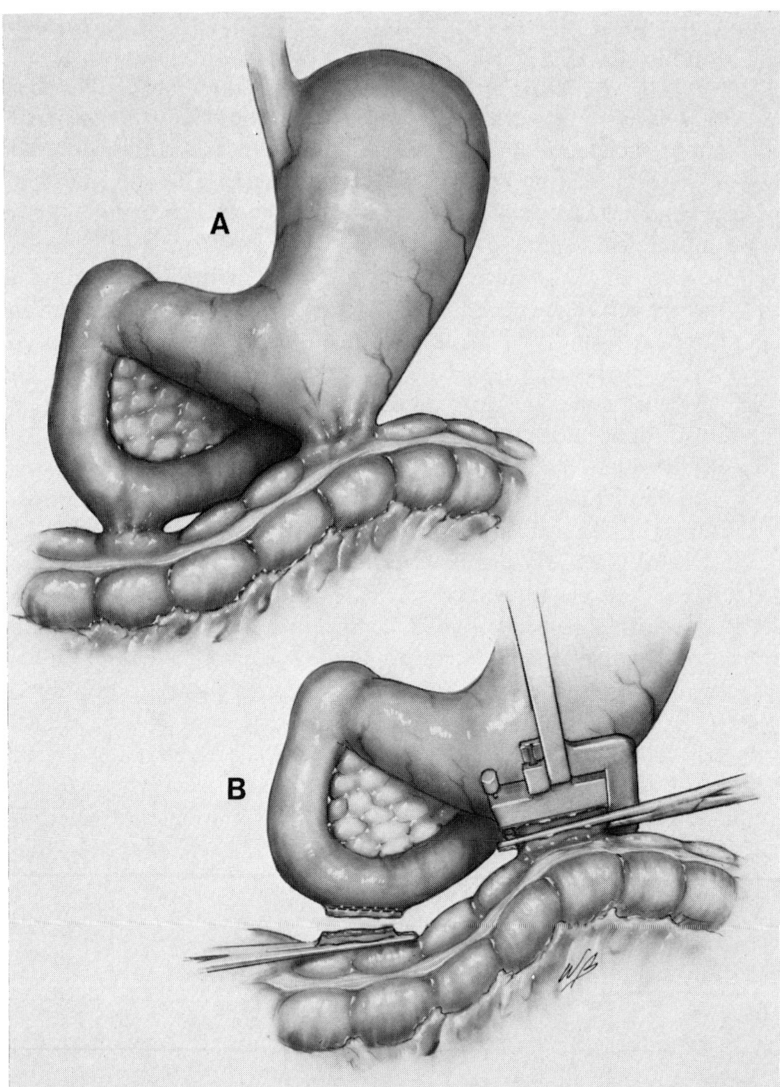

Fig VIII–17.—Pancolectomy for granulomatous colitis with duodenocolic and gastrocolic fistulas. **A,** the attempt to mobilize the transverse colon was hampered by an intimate connection between the inferior angle of the duodenum and the colon as shown to the left and of the stomach and the transverse colon as shown more to the right. The extensive inflammation and, for the duodenum, the considerable depth of the lesion, might have posed some problems for conventional excision and closure. In this instance, it was possible simply to pass a finger around the duodenocolic connection until enough of the duodenum had been freed up so that the lower blade of the TA 55™ instrument could be inserted behind it. The staples were placed tangentially on the duodenum without significantly narrowing it. A clamp on the colon prevented leakage. **B,** the same technique was used on the stomach. The specimen showed a small fistula in each site, the existence of which had not been demonstrated by the preoperative roentgenographic studies. Particularly in hard-to-reach situations of this sort, and in cases of inflammatory disease, the staplers make it possible to liberate the specimen, securely closing the attached normal portion of the gastrointestinal tract without risk of bleeding or soiling. The stapled closures healed uneventfully.

We have said relatively little of the matter of securing mesenteric or omental vessels. The LDS^{TM} instrument, in our hands, and the new, disposable, powered LDS^{TM} instrument, satisfactorily secure individual vessels, and since a single operation doubly clips the vessel and divides it between the two clips is a substantial convenience. If the vessels need not be skeletonized as for serial individual application of vessel clips, they nevertheless do need to be exposed. Neither clips nor the LDS^{TM} instrument, therefore, are useful in patients with fat, heavy mesenteries or in those in whom the mesentery is thickened by inflammatory disease. It was tempting from the first to experiment with use of the linear stapling instruments for rapid control of the splenic hilus or of the mesentery to substantial segments of bowel, the appealing thought being that a single application of the TA^{TM} or GIA^{TM} instrument might be all that was required to control the entire vascular supply requiring division. In dogs, at least, the hope proved to be illusory, and even with the fine 30V staples, division and stapling of mesentery, or splenic hilus, did not regularly achieve secure hemostasis. Bleeding occurred through the cut end of the tissues, as well as into the stapled tissue. The problem was solved (Ravitch, Hirsch, and Noiles, 1972) by applying a strip of compressed Gelfoam$^{®}$ over cartridge and anvil of the loaded TA^{TM} clamp. This method, combining a standard stapling cartridge with use of a double layer of hemostatic material through which the staples were driven, gave safe hemostasis. The technique shown in Figure VIII–18 was used, without event, in splenectomy in six consecutive patients. The application of the Gelfoam$^{®}$ to the clamp jaws, or alternatively to the splenic hilus before the clamp was placed, proved to be a bit awkward and time-consuming, partially offsetting the time saved by stapling. The neatness and absolutely perfect hemostasis were attractive. The use of Gelfoam$^{®}$ in the upper quadrant, for splenectomy, seemed not objectionable. Its use on bowel mesentery might invite adhesions. At the time, we were unsuccessful in arranging for Gelfoam$^{®}$ coating of the packaged cartridges. It is to be anticipated that a successful technique for linear stapling of omentum, mesentery, or splenic hilus will be developed.

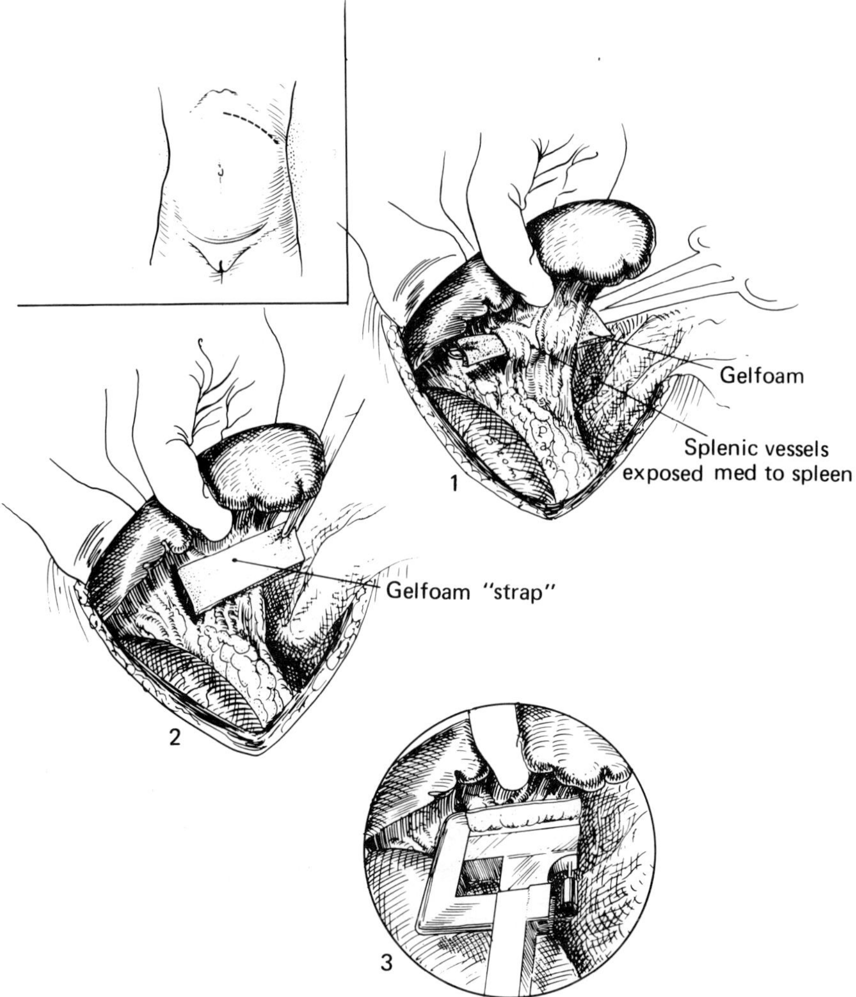

Fine vascular staples applied with TA-30

Fig VIII–18.—Technique of splenectomy applied in six patients using a staple closure through a hemostatic (Gelfoam®) sponge. *(1)* portions of the splenic pedicle of a length to fit easily within the 3-cm jaw of the TA 30™ instrument are isolated. Since the tissues are to be compressed, and the mechanism of the jaw prevents them from being extruded beyond the instrument, a somewhat longer segment can be taken *(1, 2).* A strip of compressed Gelfoam® is passed around the isolated portion of the pedicle in a flat U, and *(3)* compressed between the jaws of the TA 30™ stapling instrument. *(continued)*

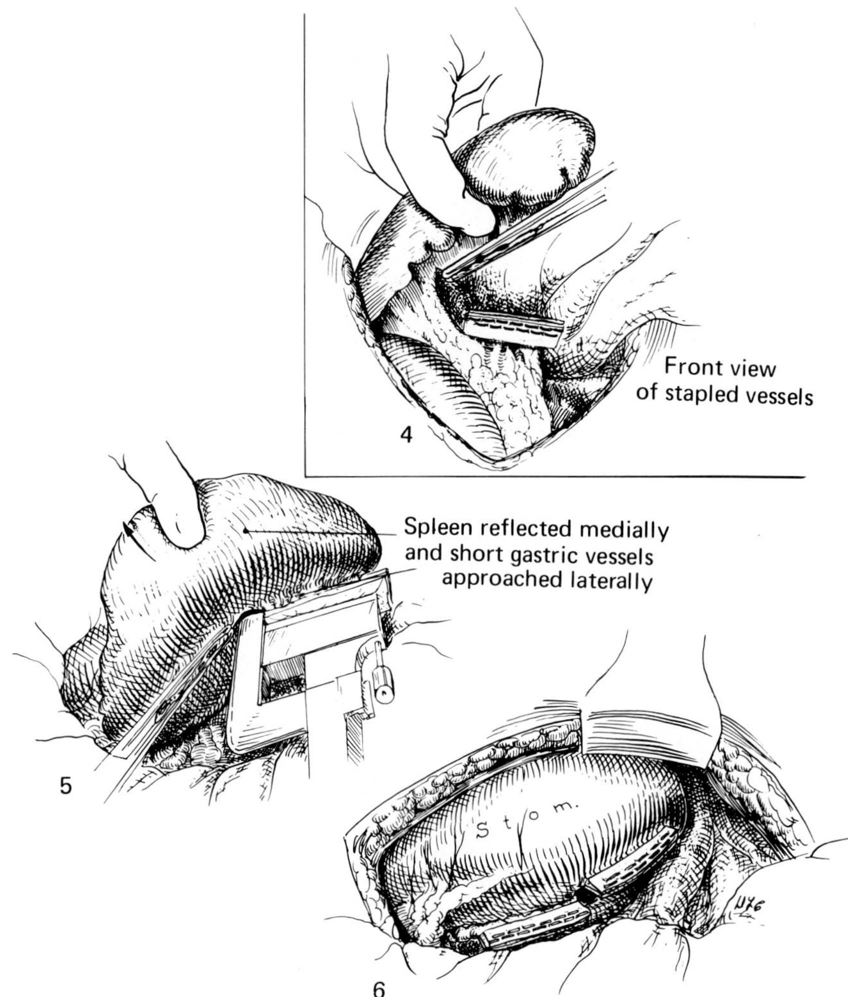

Fig VIII–18 (cont.).—*(4)* after the instrument has been closed, the staples have been driven in, and the tissues have been divided between a hemostat and the stapling instrument (half the pedicle in this instance is seen to have been divided), the narrow strip of Gelfoam® is held down by the double line of fine, staggered staples. These are the fine, short, closely spaced staples of the white cartridge (30V) for vascular use. *(5 and 6)* a second application of the stapler completes the division of the pedicle and the short gastric vessels now are taken in the same way. (From M.M. Ravitch, L.C. Hirsch, and D. Noiles, *Surgery,* 1972, used by permission.)

REFERENCES

Assadnia A., Lee C.N., Petre J.H., Lyons R.C.: Two cases of stone formation in ileal conduits after using staple gun for closure of proximal end of isolated loop. *J. Urol.* 108:553, 1972.

Barbara A.C.: In discussion of Howard E.R., Othersen H.B. Jr. *J. Pediatr. Surg.* 8:685, 1973.

Bennett A.H., Taylor R.J.: Purse-string closure of ileal loop in stapler surgery. *Urology* 16:297, 1980.

Bergman S.M., Sears H.F., Javadpour N.: Complication with mechanical stapling device in creation of ileoconduit. *Urology* 12:71, 1978.

Bisson J., Vinson R.K., Leadbetter G.W. Jr.: Urolithiasis from stapler anastomosis. *Am. J. Surg.* 137:280, 1979.

Bredael J.J., Kramer S.A., Anderson E.E.: Ileal loop urinary diversion by the auto suture stapling technique. *Acta Urol. Belg.* 48:498, 1980.

Brodman R.F., Brodman H.R.: Staple suturing of the colon above the peritoneal reflection. *Arch. Surg.* 116:191, 1981.

Cohen Z., Stone R.M.: Continent reservoir ileostomy: 1. Early experience and evolution of the surgical technique. 2. Current surgical technique. *Can. J. Surg.* 23:259, 1980.

Cranley B., McKelvey S.T.D.: The Kock ileostomy reservoir: An experimental study of methods of improving valve stability and competence. *Br. J. Surg.* 68:545, 1981.

deLorimier A.A.: In discussion of Howard E.R., Othersen H.B. Jr. *J. Pediatr. Surg.* 8:685, 1973.

Dozois R.R., Kelly K.A., Beart R.W. Jr., Beahrs O.H.: Improved results with continent ileostomy. *Ann. Surg.* 192:319, 1980.

Elliott T.E., Albertazzi V.J., Danto L.A.: Stenosis after stapler anastomosis. *Am. J. Surg.* 133:750, 1977.

Fahrenkrug L., Clemmesen T.: Anvendelse af et autosuturinstrument i gastroenterologisk kirurgi. *Ugeskr. Laeger* 143:263, 1981.

Fasching W., Moritz E.: Zirkuläre Klammeranastomosen im Magen-Darm-Trakt mit den Klammernahtgeräten SPTU und EEA. *Chirurg* 51:644, 1980.

Ferguson E.F. Jr., Houston C.H.: Simplified anterior resection: Use of the TA stapler. *Dis. Colon Rectum* 18:311, 1975.

Fortin C.L., Poulin E.C., Leclerc Y.: Evaluation de l'utilisation des appareils d'autosuture en chirurgie digestive. *Can. J. Surg.* 22:580, 1979.

Gautier-Benoit C.: Anastomoses intestinales termino-terminales par suture mécanique. *Nouv. Presse Méd.* 5:1639, 1976.

Gottesman J.E.: Use of the surgical staple for bowel anastomoses in urology. *Br. J. Urol.* 53:18, 1981.

Grosfeld J.L.: Small intestine, in Ravitch M.M., et al. (eds.): *Pediatric Surgery,* 3d ed. Chicago, Year Book Medical Publishers, 1979, pp. 939–940.

Heney N.M., Dretler S.P., Hensle T.W., Kerr W.S. Jr.: Autosuturing device in intestinal urinary conduits. *Urology* 12:651, 1978.

Hollender L.F., Meyer Chr., Blanchot Ph., Castellanos J.G.: Les sutures mécaniques en chirurgie gastrointestinale. *Bull. Acad. Natl. Méd.* 164:260, 1980.

Howard E.R., Othersen H.B. Jr.: Proximal jejunoplasty in the treatment of jejunal atresia. *J. Pediatr. Surg.* 8:685, 1973.

Johnson D.E., Fuerst D.E.: Use of auto suture for construction of ileal conduits. *J. Urol.* 109:821, 1973.

Josefsen T., Efron G.: Personal communication, 1969.

Karamcheti A., O'Donnell W.F., Hakala T.R., Schwentker F.N., Steichen F.M.: Autosuture ileal conduit construction: Experience in 110 cases. *J. Urol.* 120:545, 1978.

Kock N.G., Myrvold H.E., Nilsson L.O., Ahrén C.: Construction of a stable nipple valve for the continent ileostomy. *Ann. Chir. Gynaecol.* 69:132, 1980.

Kock N.G., Myrvold H.E., Nilsson L.O., Philipson B.M.: Continent ileostomy. *Acta Chir. Scand.* 147:67, 1981.

Latimer R.G., Doane W.A., McKittrick J.E., Shepherd A.: Automatic staple suturing for gastrointestinal surgery. *Am. J. Surg.* 130:766, 1975.

Lawson W.R., Hutchison J., Longland C.J., Haque M.A.: Mechanical suture methods in thoracic and abdominal surgery. *Br. J. Surg.* 64:115, 1977.

Loygue J., Salmon R., Amand Ph.St., Levy E.: L'iléostomie continente. Expérience de 17 cas. *Chirurgie* 104:512, 1978.

McGinty C.P.: A new method of bowel anastomosis. *Cape County J.* (Missouri) November, 1970.

McGinty C.P., Kasten M.C., Kinder J.L., Hunt R.S.: Update on stapled bowel anastomosis. *Mo. Med.* 76:145, 1979.

Marti M-C., Fiala J-M., Rohner A.: EEA stapler in large bowel surgery. *World J. Surg.* 5:735, 1981.

Mittal V.K., Cortez J.A.: New techniques of gastrointestinal anastomoses using the EEA stapler. *Surgery* 88:715, 1980.

Nance F.C.: New techniques of gastrointestinal anastomoses with the EEA stapler. *Ann. Surg.* 189:587, 1979.

Painter R.L., Park S., Hochberg D.T.: One year's experience with the auto-suture stapling device at the Day Kimball Hospital. *Conn. Med.* 38:59, 1974.

Papachristou D.N.: A simplified method of continent ileostomy: Experimental observations. *Am. Surg.* 47:548, 1981.

Ravitch M.M.: Observations on the healing of wounds of the intestine. *Surgery* 77:665, 1975.

Ravitch M.M., Canalis F., Weinshelbaum A., McCormick J.: Studies in intestinal healing: III. Observations on everting intestinal anastomoses. *Ann. Surg.* 166:670, 1967.

Ravitch M.M., Hirsch L.C., Noiles D.: A new instrument for simultaneous ligation and division of vessels, with a note on hemostasis by a gelatin sponge-staple combination. *Surgery* 71:732, 1972.

Ravitch M.M., Lane R., Cornell W.P., Rivarola A., McEnany T.: Closure of duodenal, gastric and intestinal stumps with wire staples: Experimental and clinical studies. *Ann. Surg.* 163:573, 1966.

Ravitch M.M., Ong T.H., Gazzola L.: A new, precise, and rapid technique of intestinal resection and anastomosis with staples. *Surg. Gynecol. Obstet.* 139:6, 1974.

Ravitch M.M., Steichen F.M.: Technics of staple suturing in the gastrointestinal tract. *Ann. Surg.* 175:815, 1972.

Ravitch M.M., Steichen F.M.: Staples in gastrointestinal surgery, in Maingot R. (ed.): *Abdominal Operations,* 7th ed. New York, Appleton-Century-Crofts, 1979, pp. 2197–2210.

Reuter M.J.P.: Les sutures mécaniques en chirurgie digestive et pulmonaire. Thesis, presented in 1982, at Université Louis Pasteur, Faculté de Médecine de Strasbourg, France.

Reynolds W. Jr.; Techniques of total appendectomy. *Surg. Gynecol. Obstet.* 130:891, 1970.

Rinecker H.: Indikationsbereiche maschineller Nahtmethoden am Gastrointestinaltrakt. Operationsergebnisse bei 300 Fallen. *Chirurg* 48:241, 1977.

Sohn N., Weinstein M.A., Robbins R.D., Steichen F.M.: Personal communication, 1983.

Steichen F.M.: The use of staplers in anatomical side-to-side and functional end-to-end enteroanastomoses. *Surgery* 64:948, 1968.

Steichen F.M.: The creation of autologous substitute organs with stapling instruments. *Am. J. Surg.* 134:659, 1977.

Steichen F.M., Loubeau J-M., Stremple J.F.: The continent ileal reservoir. *Surg. Rounds,* pp. 10–18, September, 1978.

Thomas C.G. Jr.: Jejunoplasty for the correction of jejunal atresia. *Surg. Gynecol. Obstet.* 129:545, 1969.

Turnbull R.B. Jr., Weakley F.L.: Special intestinal procedures, in Stewart B. (ed.): *Operative Urology.* Baltimore, Williams & Wilkins Co., 1975.

Weber M.: Utilisation de l'autosuture par agrafes en chirurgie digestive. Technique et résultats. *Helv. Chir. Acta* 39:263, 1972.

Welter R., Charlier A., Psalmon F.: Personal communication, 1983.

Westbrook K.C.: In discussion of Flake W.K., Altman M.S., Cartmill A.M., Gilsdorf R.B. *Am. J. Surg.* 138:851, 1979.

Wheeless C.R. Jr., Dorsey J.H.: Use of the automatic surgical stapler for intestinal anastomosis associated with gynecologic malignancy: Review of 283 procedures. *Gynecol. Oncol.* 11:1, 1981.

CHAPTER IX

Operations on the Rectum

We HAVE BEEN PLEASED with our long experience with the linear stapling instrument of the TA™ and GIA™ series in the performance of rectal anastomoses by any of a variety of techniques, including the elegant modified functional end-to-end, and these have been rather widely accepted. With the arrival of the EEA™ instrument, almost at once it was demonstrated in the experience of many surgeons that colorectal anastomoses below the peritoneal reflection could be performed with greater safety than manually sutured anastomoses, and much more quickly. Particularly striking was the general agreement that anastomoses could be safely performed 3 cm or 4 cm from the anal verge, thus sparing a considerable number of patients from abdominoperineal resections and permanent colostomies. With the EEA™ instrument, as with the linear stapling instruments, a surprising variety of techniques have come to be utilized in performing low rectal anastomoses, and new techniques still are being evolved and evaluated. Particularly attractive has been the extraordinary simplification that the EEA™ instrument has brought to the re-establishment of bowel continuity after the Hartmann procedure, essentially eliminating any dissection in the pelvis around the rectal stump.

In the Duhamel operation for Hirschsprung's disease, the division of the spur, creating a long linear anastomosis between the rectal pouch and the proximal ganglionated bowel brought down for anastomosis, has eliminated the major cause for dissatisfaction with that operation. In a single reported instance, the EEA™ instrument has been successfully used for what amounts to a State operation, with a quite low anastomosis (Hugh and Ihrahim, 1979).

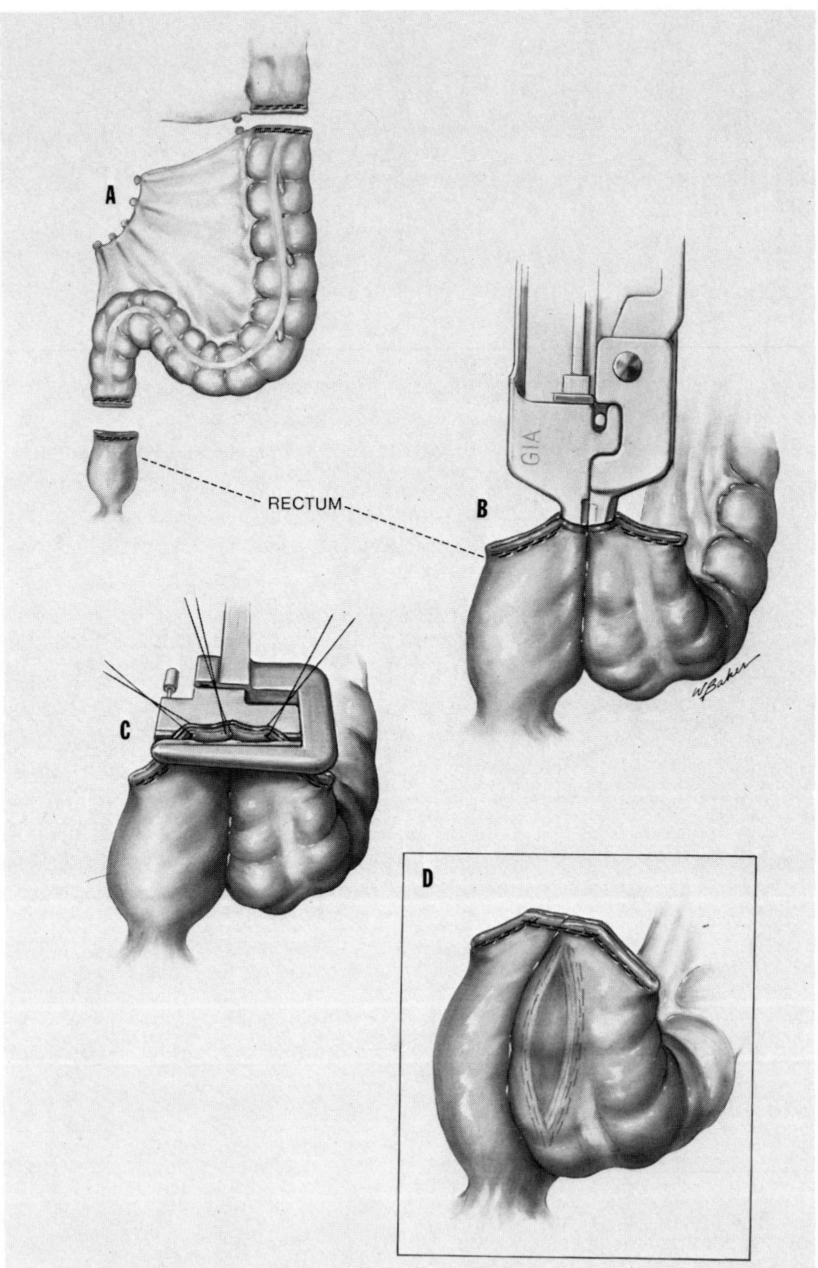

Fig IX–1.—Low anterior resection—functional end-to-end anastomosis. **A,** with the GIA™ or TA™ instrument, the bowel has been transected at either end and stapled. **B,** the ends of the descending colon and rectum are held in shotgun fashion as shown. The GIA™ instrument is inserted through the cutaway corners of the staple lines. The rectal stump need not be dissected out or delivered up into the wound. At this point, before removing the GIA™ instrument, we usually place a single suture in the lowest point of the approximation between the two loops to protect against any possible tension at the close of the operative procedure. **C,** the anastomosis having been made, the GIA™ opening is stapled shut and the protruding tissue removed. **D,** the final result. In the functional end-to-end anastomosis, although the anastomosis is made side-to-side, the effect is of an end-to-end anastomosis and, in fact, in follow-up endoscopy or barium enema, it is not possible to discern that this was anything other than an end-to-end anastomosis. In many cases, usually with the higher anastomoses, the anatomical situation is such as to permit the elegant, *modified* functional end-to-end anastomosis (see Fig VIII–5) of colon to rectum. (From M.M. Ravitch and F.M. Steichen, *Annals of Surgery,* 1972, used by permission.)

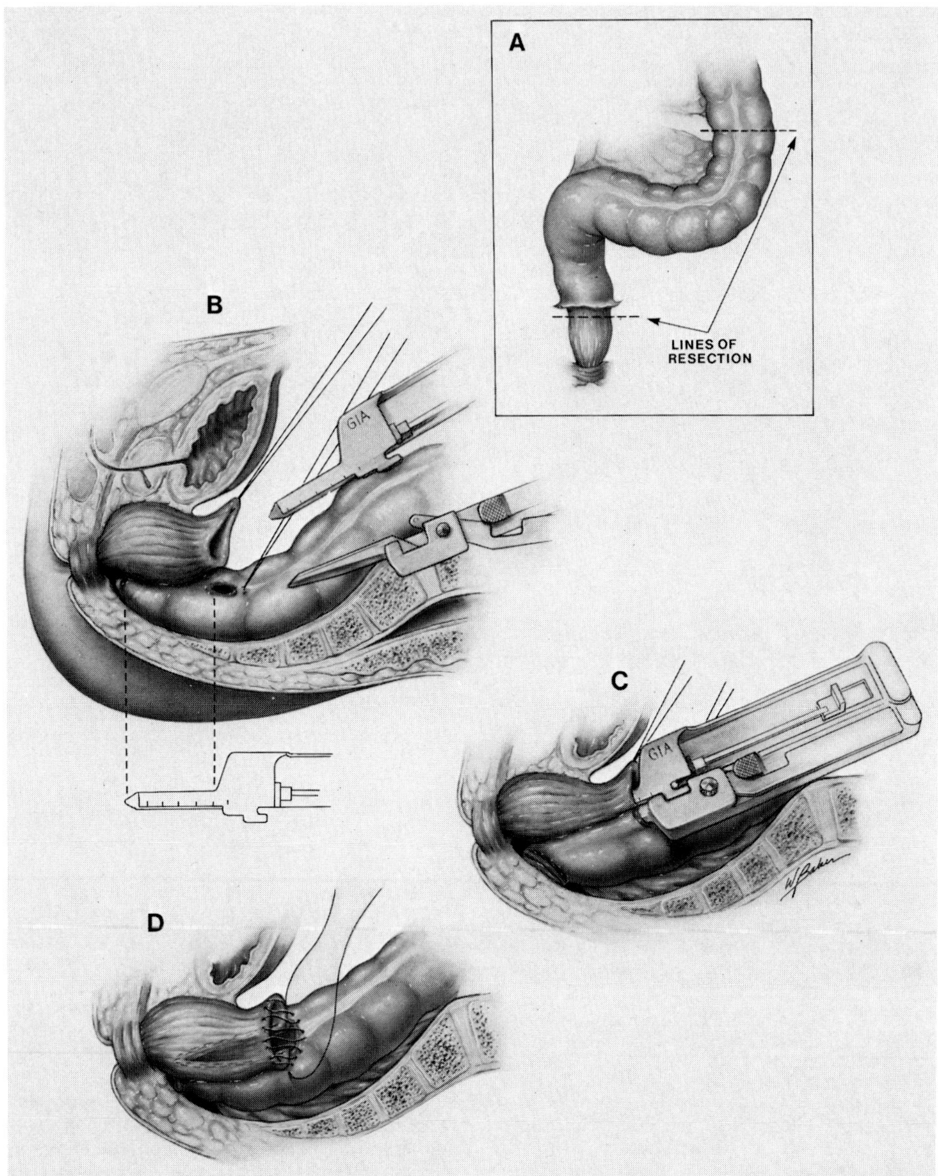

Fig IX–2.—Low anterior resection—GIA™ bayonet anastomosis. **A,** the bowel is divided at the appropriate points with the GIA™ instrument or on the edge of the TA™ instrument. For an extremely low anastomosis, as shown, the splenic flexure usually must be taken down for full mobilization of the left colon. **B,** the distal end of the rectum is shown open for insertion of the one blade of the GIA™ instrument, while the other is inserted through a stab wound in the colon, placed some 4–5 cm (the length of the GIA™ blade) proximal to the colon closure. The *dotted lines* show the length of the anastomotic opening produced, which leaves initially only a minimal pouch on the colonic side and subsequently, with contraction and healing, none at all. **C,** the GIA™ instrument fully inserted. Usually we prefer to staple the rectum and to insert the GIA™ instrument through the cutaway corner of the staple closure line, as in Figure IX–1**B.**

D, in extremely low anastomoses of this kind, it may not be feasible to close the GIA™ introduction sites with the stapler, in which case, the continuous Connell suture shown is used, reinforced by a few interrupted sutures.

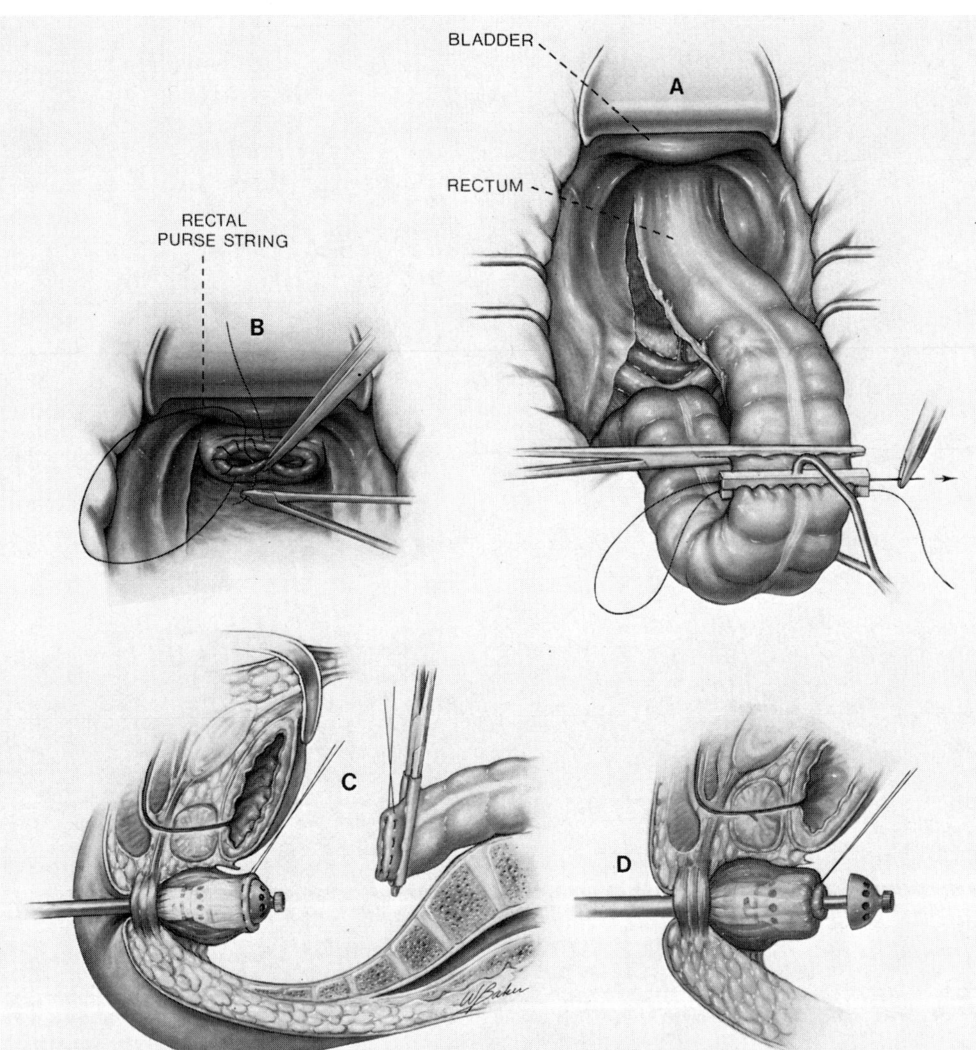

Fig IX–3.—Low rectal anastomosis—transanal insertion of the EEA™ instrument. **A,** the modified Furniss pursestring clamp is shown applied to the descending colon. The needle being passed through one channel and out the other completes the pursestring suture and the bowel then may be divided along the distal face of the pursestring clamp. **B,** particularly with a low anastomosis in a male pelvis there may not be room for both the Furniss clamp and the long straight needle, and one then preferentially uses a manual pursestring suture that begins outside the bowel, whips around the circumference of the bowel including all coats, and emerges once more outside the bowel. This takes a little longer than the use of the pursestring clamp, but even in situations in which there is room for the clamp pursestring suture technique, we are inclined to find this manually placed whipstitch pursestring suture more secure and more satisfactory. In either case, 2–0 or heavier monofilament suture is used to provide easy sliding for a tight and secure closure about the central rod. **C,** the EEA™ instrument is inserted through the rectum and as the anvil-bearing nose cone emerges, the wing nut on the instrument is turned to separate the nose cone from the staple cartridge, allowing the purse-stringed end to slip in below the nose cone and **(D)** to be tied tightly around the central rod. The EEA™ instrument may be inserted blindly by an assistant working under the drapes or, as we prefer, the patient may have been initially placed in the lithotomy-Trendelenburg position with wide abduction and minimal flexion of the hips, the anus and perianal region draped out for easy manipulation. At times, we have performed the operation with a patient in the Sims lateral decubitus position, which again makes it easy to insert the EEA™ instrument. As in many other situations, the curved model of the disposable EEA™ instrument greatly facilitates the manipulation of the instrument, in this case allowing it to curve upward in the pelvis.

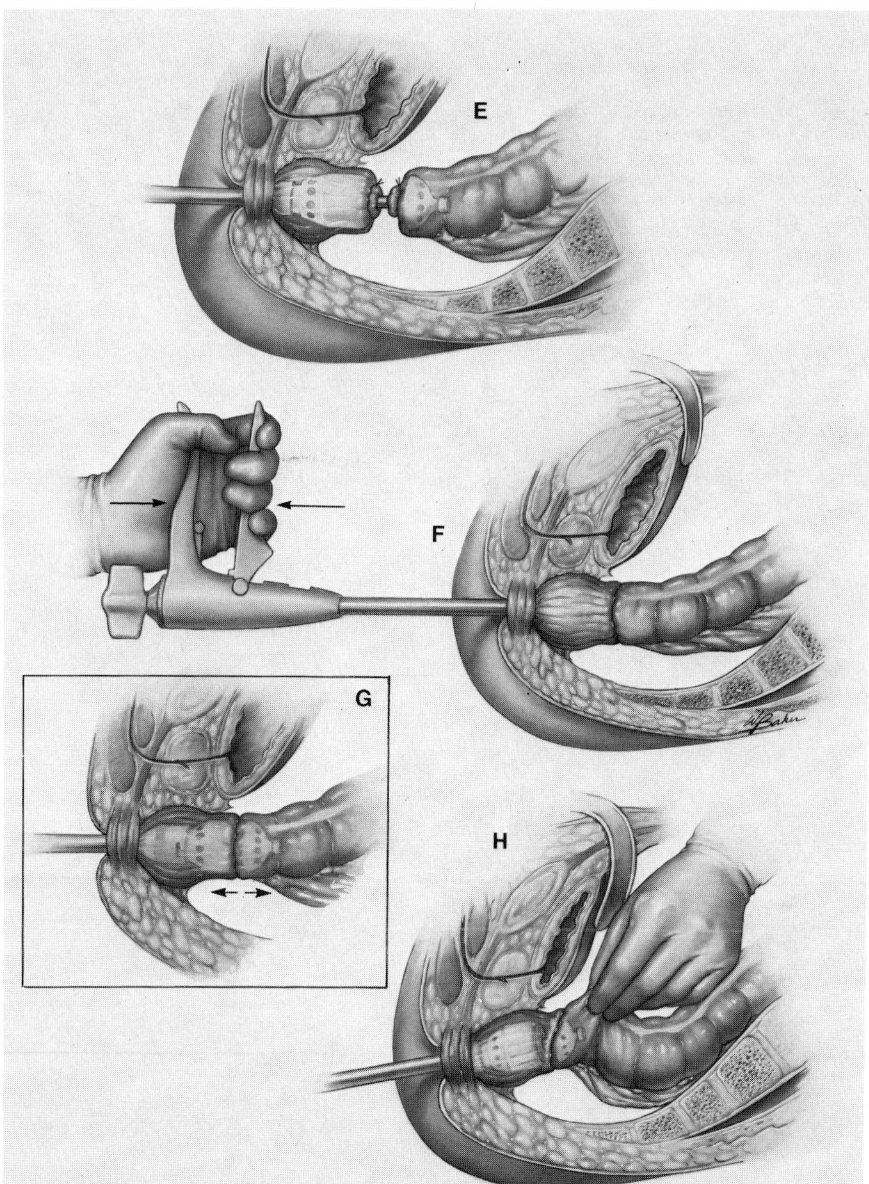

Fig IX–3 (cont.).—E, the nose cone has been inserted into the proximal bowel and the proximal pursestring securely tied around the central rod. **F,** the wing nut, having been turned until, as shown by the vernier marks, the instrument is properly closed, the handle is operated, driving in the two rows of staples and the circular knife, which cuts out the abutting pursestringed ends. **G** and **H,** the *arrows* indicate the necessity for separating the anvil and the cartridge by counterclockwise rotation of the wing nut, so the instruments can be withdrawn by spiral twisting. It may be necessary to steady the proximal end with the fingers on a sponge and, in rare instances, it may be necessary to place a traction suture through the bowel anteriorly at the anastomosis to steady the bowel. If the patient is in the lithotomy-Trendelenburg position, it is convenient for the operator to steady the anastomosis with one hand and to extract the instrument himself with the other.

(continued)

Fig IX–3 (cont.).—I, the completed anastomosis. We do not ordinarily use reinforcing or security sutures. The double rings of excised bowel still inside the cartridge always must be carefully inspected while their orientation is maintained. If there is a deficiency in either ring, sutures are placed at that point. We do not ordinarily use oversewing or "security" sutures, nor do we test the anastomosis with saline, antiseptic solution, or gas any more than we ever did in a manual anastomosis, although a number of authors report such techniques. (From M.M. Ravitch and F.M. Steichen, *Annals of Surgery,* 1979, used by permission.)

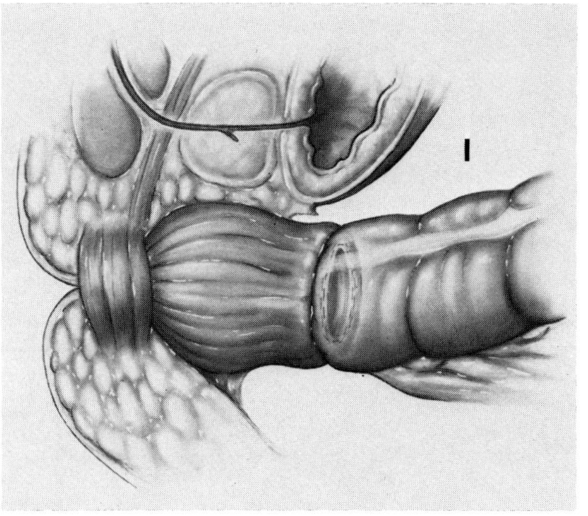

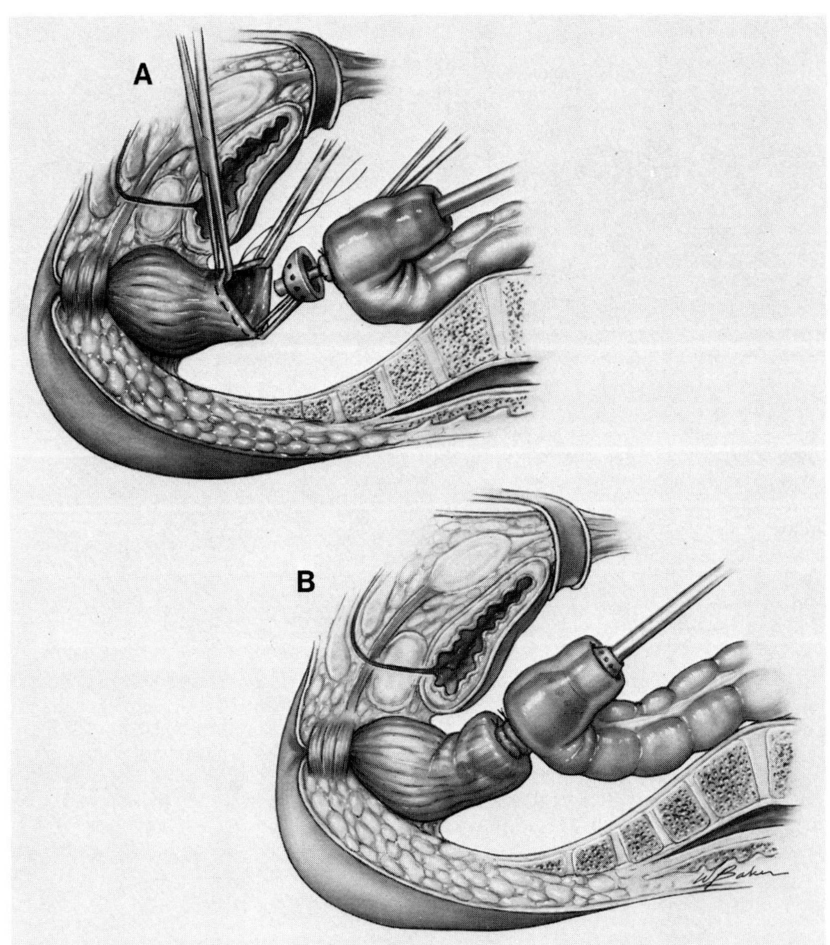

Fig IX–4 A–B. →

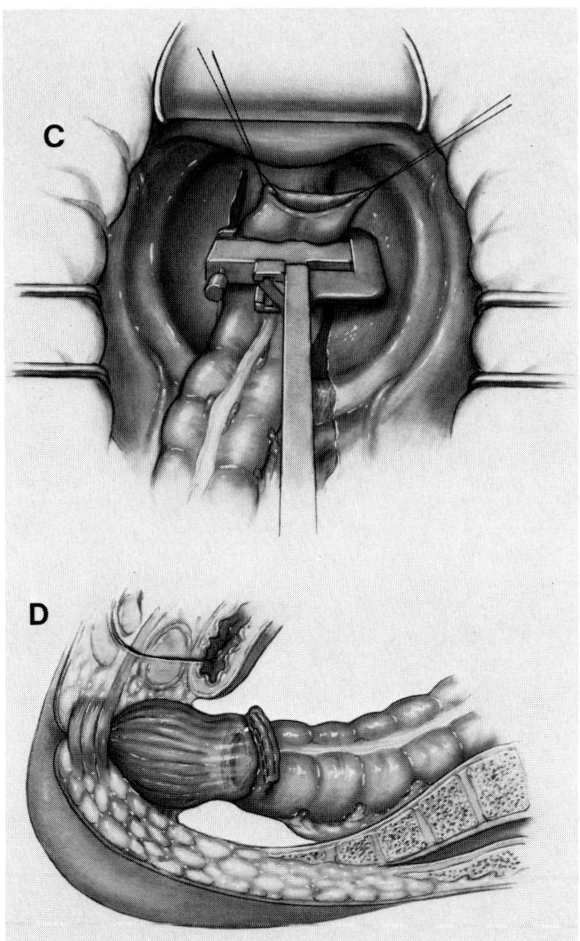

Fig IX–4.—Low rectal anastomosis—insertion of EEA™ instrument through open end of proximal bowel. **A,** the EEA™ instrument, without the nose cone, has been inserted through the open distal end of the proximal bowel, the central rod emerging through a pursestring in the antimesenteric border and the anvil-nose cone then screwed on and passed into the distal segment through the pursestring suture, which will be tightly tied about the center rod. **B,** the wing nut is being turned to approximate the segments of the EEA™ instrument. Activation of the instrument produces the usual minimally inverting anastomosis. **C,** the EEA™ instrument having been opened and withdrawn, the redundant stump of proximal bowel is stapled conveniently close to the anastomosis with the TA 55™ instrument and the excess excised. **D,** the end result is an end-to-end anastomosis that has been made from above and without the necessity for a proximal colotomy, although there are indeed two suture lines.

←

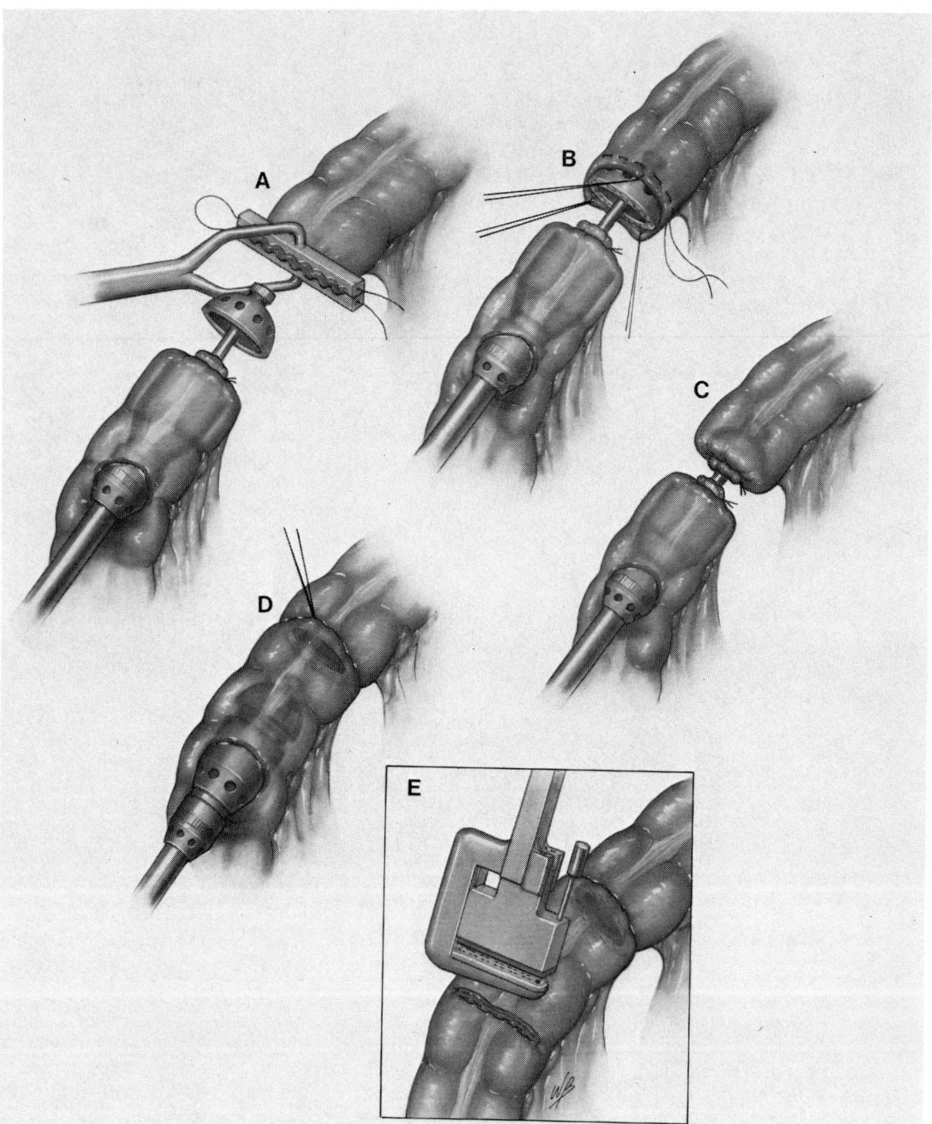

Fig IX–5.—Low rectal anastomosis—EEA™ instrument inserted through proximal colotomy. **A,** the pursestring is shown being placed on the distal rectum and the EEA™ instrument inserted through a colotomy in the proximal colon, the pursestring already tied about the stem. **B,** the anvil-nose cone is inserted into the distal lumen. **C,** the distal pursestring has been tied tightly around the spindle. **D,** the EEA™ instrument, having been fired, is opened and withdrawn. A suture is shown across the anastomosis, to aid in withdrawal of the opened EEA™ instrument. **E,** the procedure is completed by transverse TA 55™ closure of the colotomy made for insertion of the EEA™ instrument. The proximal colotomy or enterotomy technique for insertion of the EEA™ instrument obviously permits end-to-end or end-to-side anastomoses anywhere in the intestinal tract, and this technique has many advocates. In general, we prefer to utilize a natural orifice, or an opening necessarily made in the bowel for purposes of the resection, rather than to make a proximal enterotomy with its additional suture line and perhaps increased opportunity for intraoperative soiling.

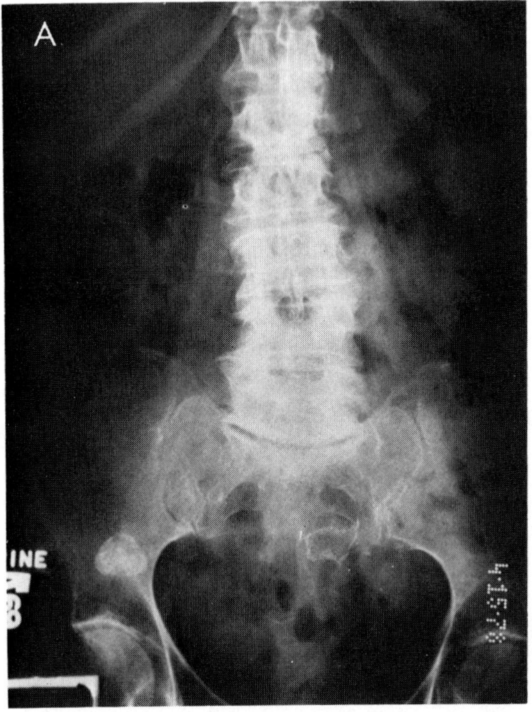
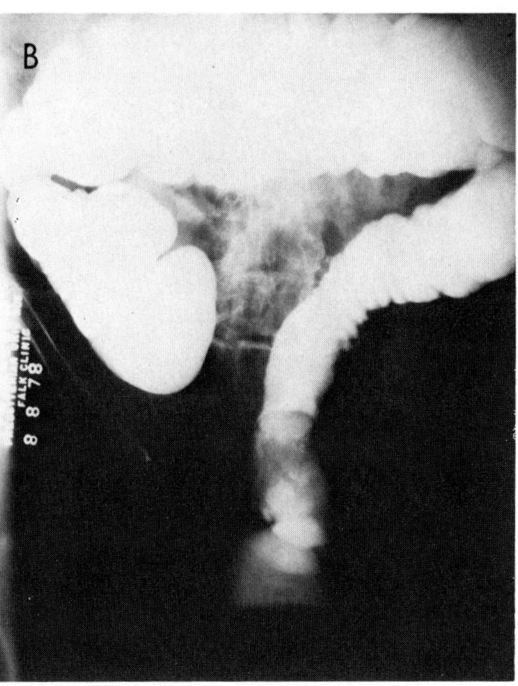
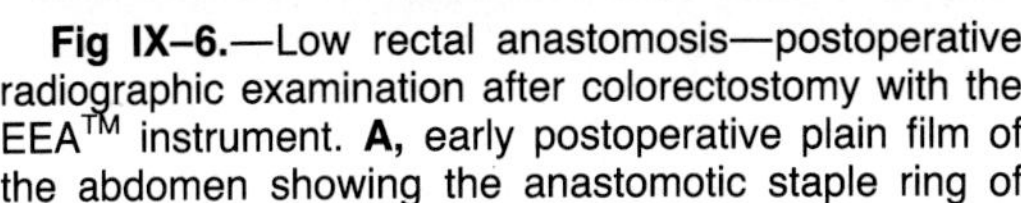

Fig IX–6.—Low rectal anastomosis—postoperative radiographic examination after colorectostomy with the EEA™ instrument. **A,** early postoperative plain film of the abdomen showing the anastomotic staple ring of the EEA™ instrument. **B,** postoperative barium enema on the same patient. The area of the anastomosis is barely discernible as a crease in the barium column.

Ferguson and Houston (1975) from Jacksonville, Florida reported their use of the TA™ instruments for the triangulating true end-to-end anastomosis of the rectum in anterior resection in 40 cases. Thirty-three of the operations were for cancer, five for diverticulitis, one for procidentia, and one for endometriosis. All but four patients had either cecostomies or diverting colostomies. There were no gross leaks. Two patients had visible dehiscences on proctoscopy. There were no deaths.

Otte, Kestens, and Pringot (1975) from Louvain in Belgium, referring to our 1968 paper on the use of the GIA™ instrument for eliminating the spur in the rectocolic anastomosis in Duhamel's operation for Hirschsprung's disease, used precisely the same technique in restoration of continuity after the Hartmann operation in a single case, with success.

Reynolds (1972) from Anniston, Alabama described the functional end-to-end anastomosis for low rectal anastomosis in two patients in 1972.

Kalinina (1966) at the Scientific Research Institute for Experimental Surgical Apparatus and Instruments in Moscow, in one of the earlier Russian papers on the use of the tubular instrument (model KTs-28) in animal (dog) studies, published sketches (Fig IX–7) of the techniques she had used. The Russian legend states that the drawings illustrate six of the 37 variations they had tried. Many of these have come into clinical use with the EEA™ instrument, reinvented independently by operators in the United States and Western Europe, innocent of any contact with the Russian literature.

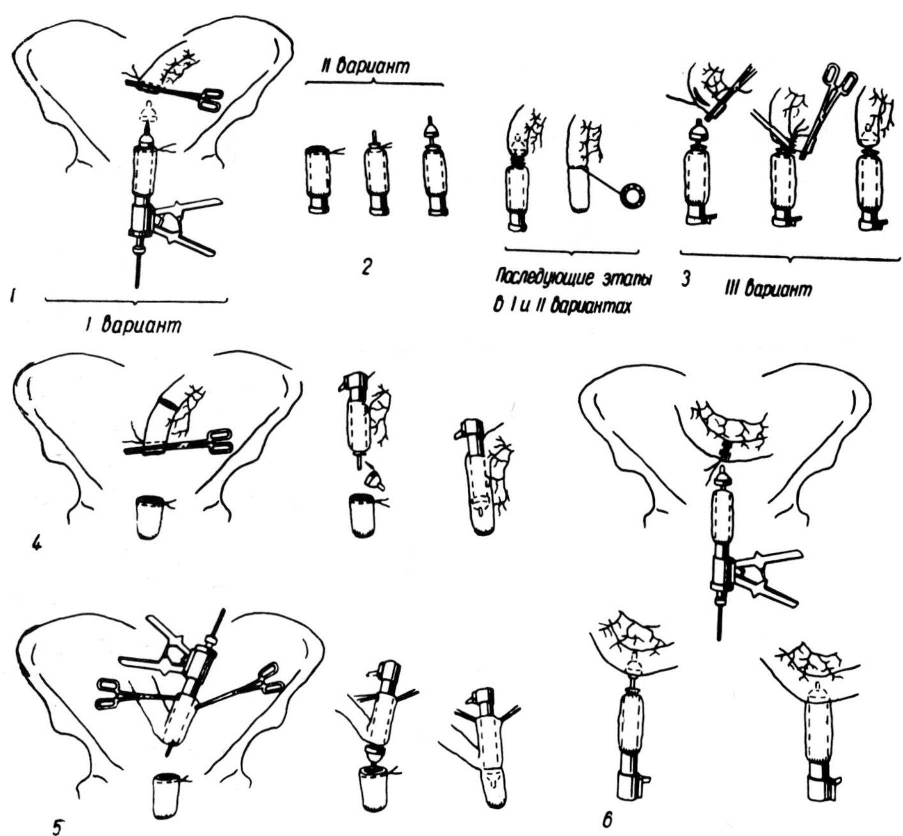

Рис. 2. Методика применения аппарата КЦ-28 (6 вариантов из 37).

Fig IX–7.—Techniques of use of the circular inverting stapler for end-to-end anastomoses—Kalinina, 1966. Most of these techniques have been rediscovered with the EEA™ instrument in the Western literature. (From T.V. Kalinina, *Klin. Khir.* (Kiev), 1966, permission requested.)

From Mercadier's Clinic in Paris, Cady (Cady, Godfroy, Sibaud, and Mercadier, 1980) reported a comparison of 64 manual colocolic or rectocolic anastomoses and 84 stapled anastomoses, 64 of these with the GIA™–TA™ functional end-to-end technique and 21 with the EEA™ technique. In all types of anastomoses, the fistula rate was greater with the manual suture, except—surprisingly—after anterior resection, where only one of eight manually sutured anastomoses leaked and six of 12 stapled anastomoses leaked. No patients in either group died. Apart from the fact that the study was not randomized, its value is somewhat clouded by the high overall fistula rate. For instance, there were four fistulas in 11 right colectomies with manual suture and two in 16 with stapled suture, resulting in six deaths in the manual group and one in the stapled group.

Fratkin of Vancouver (1981), from 1973 through 1979, performed 67 colon resections with the functional end-to-end GIA™–TA™ technique, many of them by the modified functional end-to-end variant. There were five leaks, all in the early days, none ending fatally.

From Luxembourg, Reuter (1982) reports 22 rectosigmoid anastomoses by the bayonet TA™–GIA™ technique. There were no staple-related deaths, no instances of bleeding, two fistulas that healed spontaneously, and two "radiologic" fistulas.

The GIA™–TA™ instruments were fairly widely accepted for rectal anastomoses, but the EEA™ instrument was at once enthusiastically accepted for rectal anastomoses and there now is a quite large overall experience. Whereas some operators find no difference in security of most colorectal anastomoses, whether done manually or with the EEA™ instrument, all agree that with particularly low anastomoses, the EEA™ instrument is safer and makes possible anastomoses at a level at which manual anastomoses might not be attempted. This fact carries with it its own potential hazard: there may be the temptation to perform an EEA™ anastomosis for a tumor that is so low that it ought to be treated by an abdominoperineal resection. As we have pointed out a number of times, the scalpel may be used as inadvisedly as the stapler.

In 1979, in a panel discussion (Steichen, Richards, Chassin, Weakley, and Welter, 1979), Weakley said that in his first 537 stapling procedures on large and small bowel, he had one self-terminating postoperative bleeding episode and six fistulas (the GIA™ openings were closed manually). The context of the discussion suggests that a substantial proportion of the anastomoses were colorectal. In a panel before the American Society of Colon and Rectal Surgeons, Weakley (Weakley, Beart, Bubrick, and Smith, 1981) indicated the general thinking of the group by stating that the panelists had used "the previous line of instruments—the GIA, TAs and the LDS. . ." in more than 3,000 cases, but now would confine themselves to their "over 250" cases of EEA™ instrument use.

Our own early experience with the EEA™ instrument is given in Table IX–1.

TABLE IX–1.—STATISTICS OF EEA COLORECTOSTOMIES

TRANSRECTAL EEA ANASTOMOSIS		DIAGNOSIS	
Oct. 1977–Dec. 1979		CA rectum	14
33 pts., 17M, 16F		CA sigmoid	12
Age—40–84, average—64		Villous adenoma	1
Complications—4 (12.1%)		Diverticulitis	2
Deaths—none		Rectovesical fistula	2
		Crohn's disease	1
		Trauma	1

SURGICAL TECHNIQUE		MECHANICAL FEATURES	
Colorectal anastomosis	30	Cartridge size	31 mm—25
Ileosigmoid anastomosis	3		28 mm—7
End-to-end anastomosis	32		25 mm—1
Side-to-end anastomosis	1	MECHANICAL FAILURES	
Intraperitoneal anastomosis	9	Wide rectum	2
Extraperitoneal anastomosis	24	Poor pursestring	1
Level of anastomosis	4–20 cm	EEA assembly	1
Colostomy	3		

COMPLICATIONS

TOTAL	4/33 (12.1%)	
Intraperitoneal anastomosis	0/9 (0%)	
Extraperitoneal anastomosis	4/24 (16.6%)	

INTRAOPERATIVE
Anvil-bowel discrepancy—2
(Leak, colostomy, stricture—1)
(Abscess, stricture—1)
POSTOPERATIVE
Late fecal fistula—1, healed
Retrorectal abscess—1, drained spontaneously

Fain (1980), who had had a large experience in Russia with the cylindrical end-to-end stapler, reported his first several cases operating in this country with the EEA[TM] instrument for low anterior resections in seven patients without complications (Fain, Patin, and Morgenstern, 1975). In his personal series of 165 patients in Russia with the Russian instrument, the tumors were located between 7 cm and 16 cm from the anal verge. Without making direct comparisons, he commented that the EEA[TM] instrument would ". . .be very useful for creating a very low colorectal anastomosis and will eliminate in many cases a permanent colostomy." He seemed reassured by the double row of staples in the American instruments as opposed to the single row in the Russian ones.

Kirkegaard from Roskilde, Denmark (1978) used the EEA[TM] instrument for low anterior resection for rectal cancer in 15 consecutive patients. There were two radiologic leaks and no clinical leaks. It was Kirkegaard's opinion that "At least six patients in the series would have been subjected to abdominoperineal resection with permanent colostomy if they had been operated on before the stapling technique was adopted."

By January 29, 1979, Kirkegaard (Kirkegaard, Christiansen, Lauritzen, Henrichsen, and Jörgensen, 1979) could report a total of 20 patients with low anterior resections for carcinoma with the EEA[TM] instrument, operating on patients in the lithotomy-Trendelenburg position and passing the instrument through the anus. There were three radiologically demonstrated leaks and one clinically demonstrated leak consisting only of fecal secretions along the drain, which ceased within two days, the subsequent course being uneventful. All patients were continent at the time of discharge. Three patients, with anastomoses at 4 cm and 5 cm, had ten to 15 stools per day, which decreased to three to four over the ensuing three months.

Dorsey and Stone (1979) of Toronto said that in the first eight months of 1978 they had performed anastomoses with the EEA[TM] instrument in 20 patients after low anterior resections. There were ten clinically apparent anastomotic leaks, three requiring transverse colostomies, all of them closed and all 20 patients ultimately were continent.

J.C. Goligher of Leeds (1979) has of course written abundantly on cancer of the rectum and has had large experience first with the Russian rectal stapling instrument, the SPTU model, and then with the American EEA[TM] instrument. He operates with the patient in the lithotomy-Trendelenburg position, inserting the instrument through the anus. He compared his results with 62 cases of stapled anterior resections of the preceding two years with the results in 135 manual anastomoses made in the four years before that. In the stapled anastomoses, he had two clinically evident leaks and four demonstrated only radiologically, 3.2% and 6.5%, respectively, and in the hand-sutured anastomoses, nine evident clinically and 39 detected radiologically, 6.7% and 28.9%. "As can be seen, there were fewer anastomotic dehiscences after the use of the gun. What makes the achievements with the stapler all the more creditable is that the group of 24 patients given low resection with its aid includes a number with exceptionally low anastomoses . . . In at least 6 cases anterior resection with a hand-sutured anastomosis would have been quite impossible." He pointed out that since the pursestring inversion of the distal end resulted in a resection of another 1.0–1.5 cm, one could plan on this in choosing the level of transection ". . . by taking in the original operative specimen a distal margin of clearance of only 3.5 cm instead of 5 cm." For extremely low anastomoses, he placed the lower pursestring from below and tied the lower pursestring either from below or from above (Fig IX–8).

In a paper published more or less simultaneously in the United States on the same 62 anterior resections, Goligher (1979) mentioned three patients with bleeding, one with an ileorectal anastomosis, and two with low anterior resection, two of them requiring blood transfusion and none of them endoscoped. All three proved to have intact anastomoses on Gastrografin® enema study. Anastomoses lying between 7.5 cm and 10.0 cm from the anal verge resulted in normal control of feces and flatus and anastomoses below 7.0 cm produced variable functional results with at least temporary incontinence with the lower anastomoses. Two patients developed stenosis, one requiring dilatation and the other not. These patients all were operated on using the ''Russian 249 suture gun.''

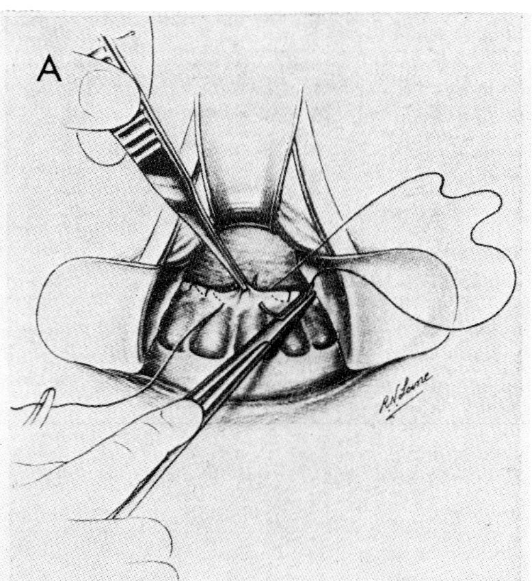

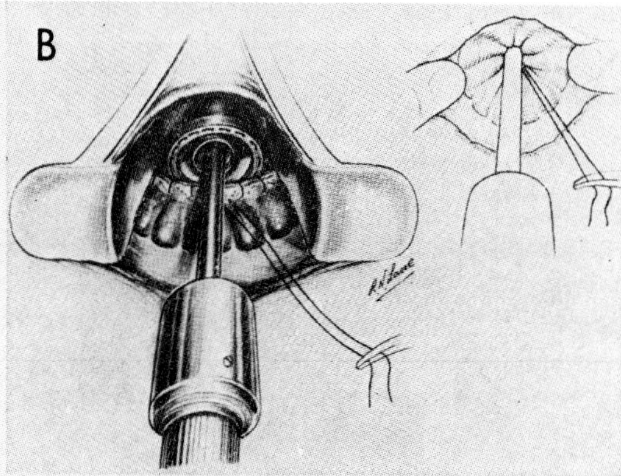

Fig. 1. View obtained of interior of anorectal remnant with anal speculum in position. The 2/0 monofilament Prolene suture has been inserted along the top of the remnant starting in the midline posteriorly and continuing as an over-and-over stitch from inside the lumen 4 mm or so from the cut edge, the retractor having been rotated to expose each sector of the bowel in turn. The stitch has now reached the posterior sector again and is approaching the starting point.

Fig. 2. The third blade of the anal retractor has been removed and the separation of the other two blades reduced somewhat, whilst the head end of the opened suture gun is inserted through the anal canal to beyond the top of the anorectal remnant. (Inset) The anal retractor has been removed and the anorectal purse-string suture has been tied from below on the central shaft.

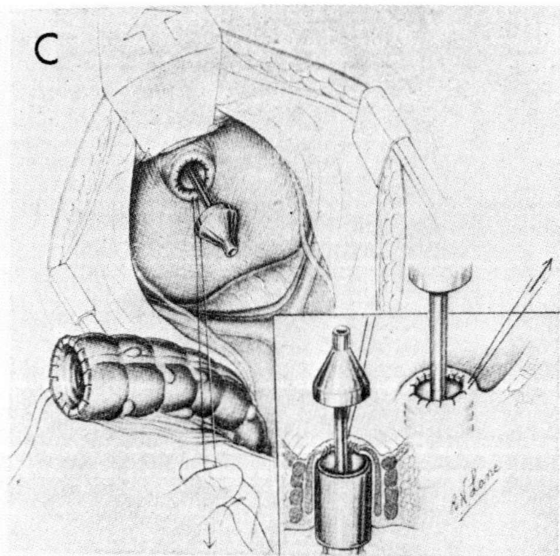

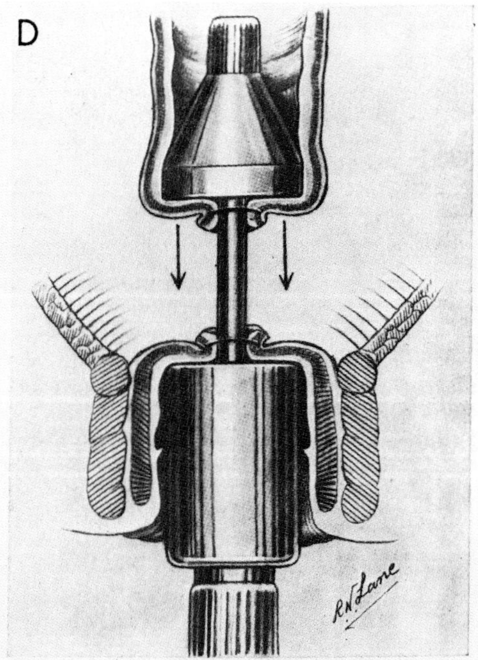

Fig. 3. Alternative method of tying anorectal purse-string suture from above. The tails of the suture have been passed up through the anal canal to the abdominal operator. Whilst the bladder and prostate are retracted strongly forwards to expose the top of the anorectal remnant held up by the purse-string suture, the suture gun is inserted from below by an assistant and opened to carry the head into the pelvis beyond the edge of the anorectal stump, whilst the distal edge of the shoulder-piece still lies in the remnant (*see* inset). The purse-string suture is then tied on the central shaft just above the shoulder-piece.

Fig. 4. Diagrammatic view of the 'opened' suture gun in position with the purse-string sutures in both anorectal and colonic stumps tied and the instrument about to be 'closed' preparatory to 'firing' the staples.

Fig IX–8.—Low rectal resection—technique of J.C. Goligher (1979). Goligher, after a large experience with the Russian stapling instruments, was even more enthusiastic about the American instruments. The illustrations show his technique of placing the distal purse-string through the anus for the extremely low resections. His initial experience with such low anastomoses—always accompanied by transverse colostomy—suggested that increased frequency of stools resulted but that the initial incontinence was gradually overcome. (From J.C. Goligher, *British Journal of Surgery,* 1979, used by permission.)

In a paper devoted solely to the extremely low anastomoses (1979), Goligher illustrates the technique in detail (Fig IX–8), reporting four patients operated on by this technique, all men, two of them "decidedly obese." All were given transverse colostomies. In one, radiologic studies showed "moderate anastomotic dehiscence," which healed satisfactorily. The anastomoses proved to be at 5 cm, 4.5 cm, 4.5 cm, and 4.0 cm. Three patients whose colostomies already had been closed had increased frequency in stools; two had overcome their incontinence and one still was not fully continent.

From Helsingborg, Sweden, Ling and associates (Ling, Broomé, and Rydén, 1979) reported their experience with 21 patients, 18 with carcinoma of the rectum and three with diverticulitis of the colon, treated by anterior resection and EEA™ anastomosis. All patients had a temporary colostomy. Anastomoses were made as low as 4 cm above the anus and all patients were continent. Twelve patients had no leaks, six patients had a small leak without clinical signs, one patient had a "medium" leak with rectovaginal abscess, and two patients had a considerable leak with resultant stenosis. There were no deaths. In their own prior experience with manual anastomosis, they had a 10% mortality rate from anastomotic insufficiency.

Wheeless of Baltimore (1979) reported with enthusiasm his technique with the use of the EEA™ instrument in extremely low anastomoses in six patients with carcinoma of the cervix or ovary, two of them with "total" exenterations (Fig IX–9). Three of the patients had had extensive irradiation for carcinoma of the cervix. Two of them had rectovaginal fistulas and one had an ileorectal fistula. Four patients had the anastomosis heal completely, their proximal colostomies were closed, and the women were continent. One patient was only two months after the low anastomosis and still had her colostomy. There was one suture line dehiscence. Wheeless considered that the EEA™ instrument made possible anastomoses that otherwise would not be undertaken, and spared the patients permanent colostomy.

Wheeless' series now extends to 72 cases (Wheeless, 1982) involving three groups, surgical debulking procedures for advanced malignancy (ovarian), exenteration for recurrent cervical carcinoma, and patients with rectovaginal fistulas following extensive irradiation. "In none of the patients have we performed a permanent colostomy. We have had one breakdown of the stapler anastomosis with resultant rectovaginal fistula . . . diverting colostomy, reoperation at 3 months . . . successful result . . . almost all of our anastomoses are extremely low, at the levator sling or below, some as low as 2–3 cm from the anal verge . . . these women are not universally incontinent . . . we have had 2 patients out of the 72 who suffer some degree of incontinence only when they developed a rapid intestinal transit time for some other reason." Wheeless tests staple suture lines with rectal air injection and the pelvis filled with saline solution. "If we find a leak, we take down the entire anastomosis and repeat it. We have avoided placing Lembert sutures to cover defects as we feel these techniques lead to postoperative complications that are described by others as fallacies in the EEA stapler system." In patients with pelvic irradiation, he always performs a protective colostomy and failed to do that in the one patient mentioned with a rectovaginal fistula.

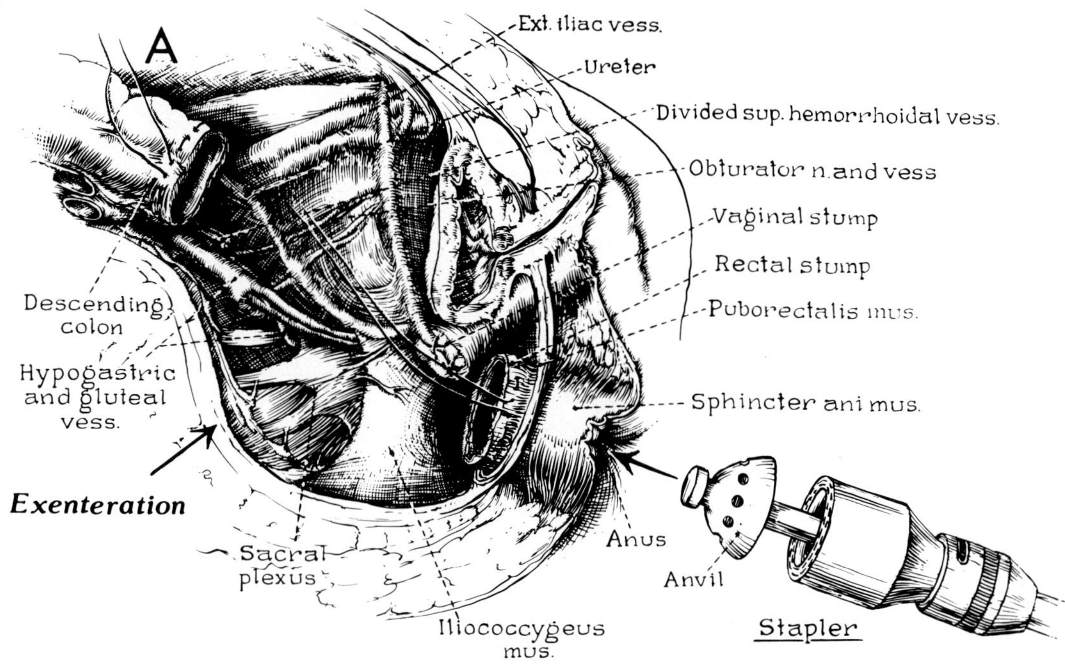

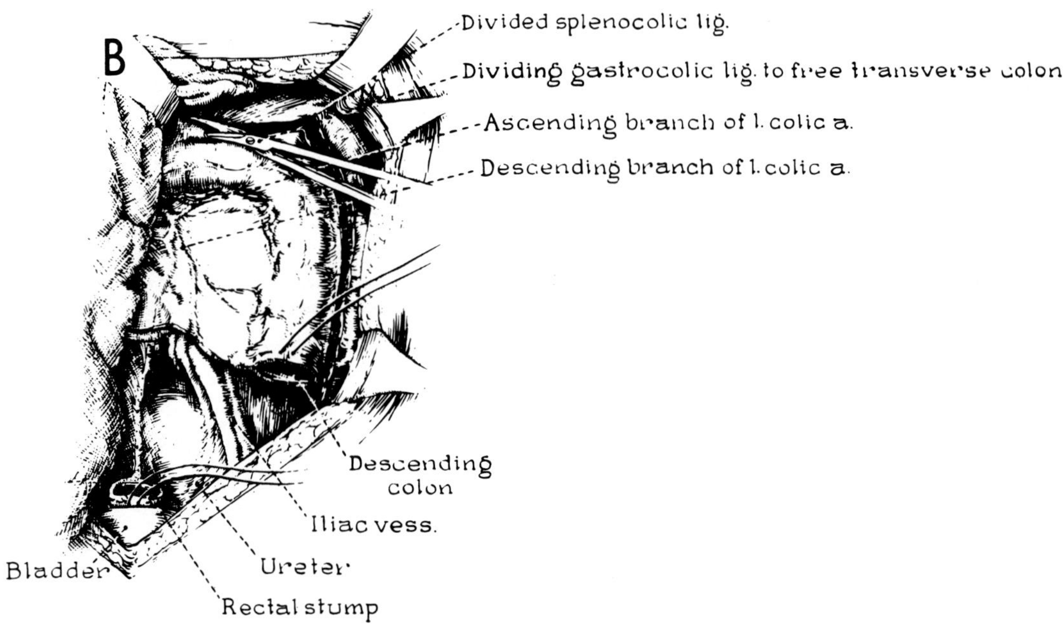

Fig IX–9.—Low EEA™ colorectal anastomosis after exenteration—technique of C.R. Wheeless Jr. (1979). Wheeless' initial experience with extremely low EEA™ colorectal anastomosis after exenteration, in four patients with carcinoma of the cervix, and two of the ovary, led him to believe that not only could EEA™ anastomoses be made when anastomosis was scarcely feasible by hand, but that healing in the irradiated tissue was more secure with the stapled anastomosis. (From C.R. Wheeless Jr., *Obstetrics and Gynecology,* 1979, used by permission.)   →

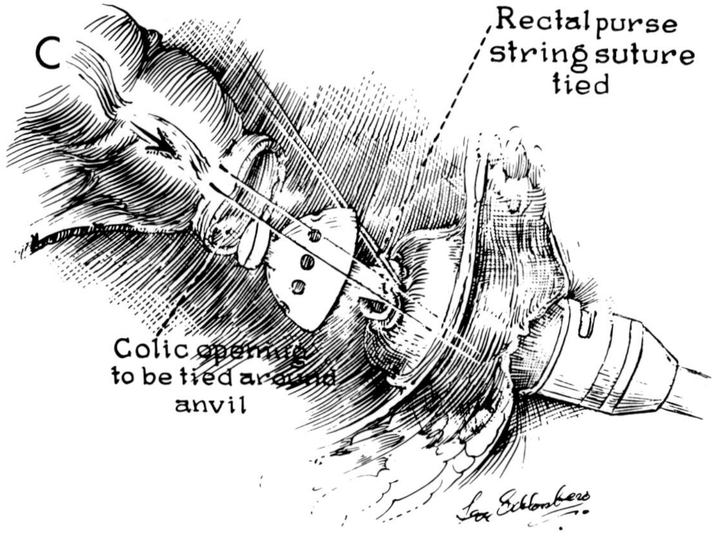

Fig IX–9 (cont.) C.

In general, there has not been much difficulty in inserting even the largest, 31 mm, EEA™ cartridge in an adult rectum and the sizers or dilators that commonly are used in the esophagus frequently are ignored for the rectum. Occasionally, what appears to be spasm of the rectal stump interferes with passage of the instrument from the anus. Harford from Wilford Hall USAF Medical Center, Lackland Air Force Base, Texas (1979) found that glucagon, 2 mg, given intravenously to relax the rectum, facilitated passage of the instrument.

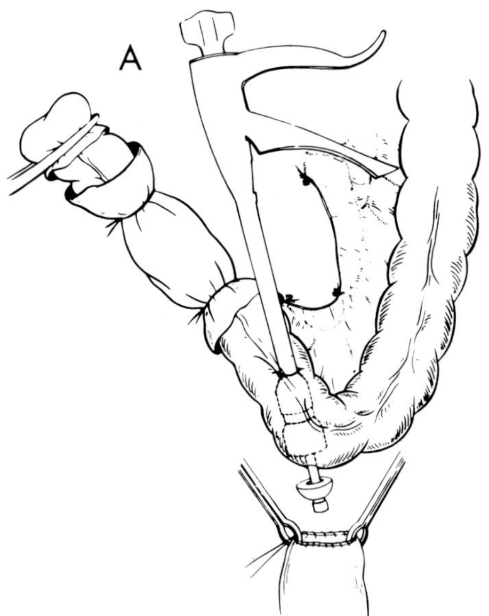

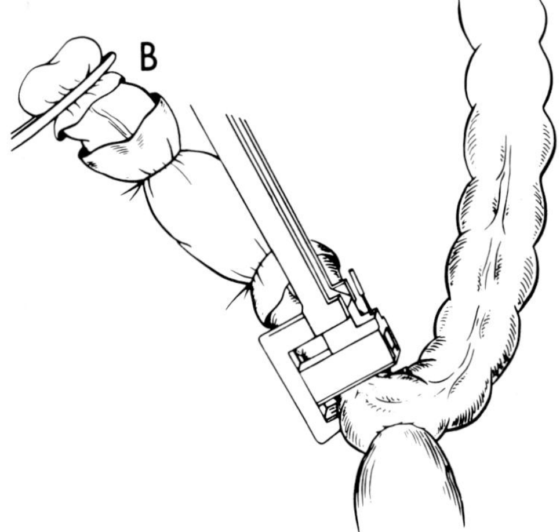

Fig. 1. The EEA stapling device is introduced without the anvil into the bowel through a small colotomy. The spindle of EEA is brought out through a small stab wound at the site of colic anastomosis. After 180° rotation toward the rectal section, the anvil is attached to the spindle, inserted into the rectum, and the purse-string is tied down against the spindle. The instrument will now be closed and fired.

Fig. 2. The distal diseased colon is closed below the colorectal anastomosis with a TA 55 stapler.

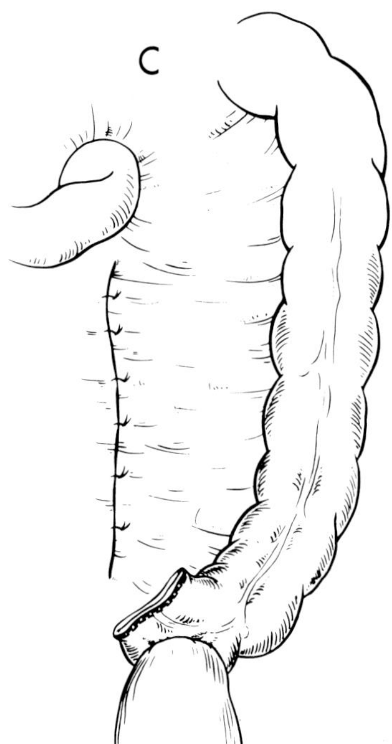

Fig IX–10.—Strasbourg technique of side-to-end low rectal anastomosis with the EEA™ stapler—Adloff, Arnaud, Beeharry, and Turbelin (1980). The Strasbourg technique combines the proximal enterotomy technique seen in Figure IX–5 with the introduction of the stapler through what is a part of the specimen, seen in Figure IX–4, permits transecting the bowel proximally only once, and leaves no proximal colotomy closure. (From M. Adloff, J.P. Arnaud, S. Beeharry, and J.M. Turbelin, *Diseases of the Colon and Rectum,* 1980, used by permission.)

Fig. 3. Completed side-to-end anastomosis.

Adloff and colleagues (Adloff, Arnaud, Beeharry, and Turbelin, 1980) described their technique of side-to-end low anterior anastomosis (Fig IX–10). They divided the bowel below the tumor, inserted the EEA™ instrument from above through a colotomy in a portion of the bowel to be resected, stapling off the bowel with a TA 55™ instrument after completion of the EEA™ anastomosis, the colotomy thus being excluded with the specimen. They had performed 17 anastomoses of this kind, 16 colorectal and one ileorectal. There was one wound infection, no instances of anastomotic dehiscence, fistula, peritonitis, or abscess, and no stenoses. They point out that this technique permits one to ignore the difference in size between the rectum and the descending colon.

Adloff (1982) subsequently writes that he has done 104 colorectal EEA™ anastomoses, 47 of them terminoterminal, seven terminolateral, and 50 lateroterminal—the technique illustrated in Figure IX–10—and had only two deaths, neither of them directly related to the anastomosis. They had had two leaks resulting in mild discharge for four to five days, three that lasted up to three weeks, and 14 that were discovered only radiologically and were without clinical manifestations.

From Frankfurt, Becker and associates (Becker, Probst, and Ungeheuer, 1980) reported their experience with 26 low rectal EEA™ anastomoses of the traditional type, by five operators. They had no anastomotic failures or leaks, no bleeding or stenoses—a good performance for a group of surgeons being introduced to the instruments.

At St. Martin's Hospital in Bath, England, Bolton and Britton (1980) performed ten conventional two-layer low rectal anastomoses with cecostomy, ten EEA™-stapled anastomoses protected by tube cecostomy, and ten stapled anastomoses without fecal diversion. There was one anastomotic leak in the ten hand-sutured patients and one anastomotic leak in the 20 stapled patients. There were two strictures in the hand-sutured group and none in the others. There were two wound infections in the ten hand-sutured cases and four in the 20 stapled cases. The stapled anastomoses were somewhat lower and the patients left the hospital on the average of four or five days earlier, ". . . due partly to the relative absence of trauma of the stapling technique and partly to the fact that the instrument is designed to excise the damaged cut ends of the bowel, thus encouraging reliable anastomotic healing. . . . Protection of a stapled anastomosis by a tube caecostomy was found to be unnecessary. The ability of the stapler to produce a low extraperitoneal anastomosis in the pelvis is unique. This technique has almost certainly reduced the incidence of permanent colostomies over the past year. . . ."

At Senning's Clinic in Zürich, Buchmann and associates (Buchmann, Uhlschmid, and Hollinger, 1980) performed 35 sigmoid or low anterior resections and anastomoses, 13 sutured and 22 with the EEA™ instrument. The 13 manually sutured anastomoses immediately preceded the 22 EEA™ anastomoses. There were no clinical anastomotic leaks in the stapled group but three in the manual anastomoses. There were two radiologically demonstrable leaks in the stapled group and one in the manual anastomoses.

Berthold, Alexander-Williams, and others (Berthold, Alexander-Williams, Hänni, and Eckmann, 1980) from Birmingham, England performed 14 low rectal anastomoses with the EEA™ instrument. During one of their operations, two of the bowel rings were incomplete and the anastomoses required suture reinforcement. A single patient had a minute radiologic dehiscence but no clinical signs.

From the General Hospital in Birmingham, England, from the service of J. Alexander-Williams, 50 EEA™ rectal anastomoses performed by five consultant surgeons were reported (Dorricott, Baddeley, Keighley, Oates, and Alexander-Williams, 1980): 28 anterior resections, 11 sigmoid colectomies, three left hemicolectomies, six total colectomies, and two reconstructions after the Hartmann procedure. As in many initial series, there were some instances of inability to use the instruments, the anastomoses being sutured by hand—five cases in this series. In the first 25 cases there were clinical leaks in three patients, with one death, and radiologic leaks in ten. They thought that the instrument would permit a more rapid anastomosis and that the leakage rate was ". . .lower than in most reported handsewn series. Successful anastomoses with the instrument increased with experience of the operator. The instrument allowed very low anastomoses and avoided the need for permanent colostomy in some patients with consequent decrease in morbidity and cost."

The same year, from Bern, Switzerland, Hänni, with J. Alexander-Williams as co-author (Hänni, Berthold, Alexander-Williams, and Eckmann, 1980), reported 100 EEA™ sigmoidorectal anastomoses, 74 performed in Birmingham and 26 in Bern. There were two radiologic but no clinically evident leaks in the Bern cases and none in the (last 24?) Birmingham cases.

From Oulu in Finland, Laitinen and associates (Laitinen, Huttunen, Ståhlberg, Mokka, Kairaluoma, and Larmi, 1980) reported their experience in 39 patients with EEA™ anastomoses after anterior resection or left hemicolectomy. There was a temporary fecal fistula in one patient, and another patient, discharged on the ninth day after a low anterior resection, returned to the hospital a week later with fever and a posterior dehiscence in the anastomosis. He recovered without operation. There were no wound infections. They thought that the anastomosis was more reliable than a hand-sutured anastomosis and commented that three or four of their patients would have required abdominoperineal resection and permanent colostomy had the instrument not been available.

Fasching and Moritz at the Second Surgical Clinic in Vienna (1980) performed 23 low rectal anastomoses with the SPTU and 18 with the EEA™ instrument, with a single death in each group. Of the 41 low anastomoses, 38 were performed by the usual transanal introduction of the EEA™ or SPTU instrument, but two were performed by Localio's abdominal-transsacral approach and one by an entirely posterior approach for villous adenoma. Unlike Kirkegaard, Christiansen, and Hjortrup (1980), they stated, and we agree, that "Since application of these staplers may be difficult, this, like any other surgical technique, must be specially learned."

From Rohner's Clinic in Geneva, Switzerland, Fiala and colleagues (Fiala, Marti, Meyer, and Rohner, 1980) reported using the EEA™ instrument in 35 sigmoid resections and low anterior resections, 18 right colectomies, and ten reconstructions after a Hartmann procedure. They were especially pleased with the facility of using the EEA™ instrument in anastomoses after Hartmann procedures, calling it ". . .particularly seductive." In their total, they had a single death due to a technical error not recognized at operation (a fold of the bladder was caught in the stapler in making an anastomosis after a Hartmann procedure). There were two anastomotic leaks that healed spontaneously and one that required operation. There were six radiologically demonstrated sinuses that were clinically occult.

A year later (Marti, Fiala, and Rohner, 1981), their 63 anastomoses had increased to 98—23 right hemicolectomies, 19 left hemicolectomies and sigmoid resections, 28 colorectal anastomoses, and 12 reconstructions after a Hartmann procedure. There were no more deaths, one more clinical leak and colocutaneous fistula without abscess or sepsis, and one more radiologically demonstrated leak.

From São Paulo in Brazil, Cutait, Raia, and their associates (Cutait, Cutait, da Silva, Manzione, Lourencão, Calache, Nahas, and Raia, 1980), beginning in November, 1978, performed stapled anastomoses in 38 patients with colorectal resections, 20 of them for cancer of the rectosigmoid or rectum and ten for the megacolon of Chagas disease. They performed the standard end-to-end EEA™ anastomosis, inserting the instrument through the anus. Thirty-one of the patients had colorectal anastomoses and those with pancolectomy for polyposis had ileorectal anastomoses. There were three anastomotic dehiscences with spontaneous recovery and one with fecal peritonitis and fatal outcome—the only death in the series. One patient had a presacral infection, three patients had stenosis, two of them detected only by digital rectal examination and the third requiring dilatation.

The following year, Cutait (Cutait, Cutait, da Silva, Manzione, Kiss, Lourencão, and Calache, 1981) reported 49 ileorectal or colorectal anastomoses with the EEA™ instrument. There were four leaks with anterior resection, three of which healed spontaneously, the fourth resulting in a fatal peritonitis. In one ileorectal anastomosis after total colectomy there was a leak requiring reoperation and ileostomy. One patient had a presacral infection that cleared with antibiotic treatment alone. Of three patients with mild stenosis, only one needed dilatation. They had no bleeding.

At Basingstoke in England, Heald (1980) performed 40 low anterior resections in a year with the EEA™ instrument in patients ". . .who would otherwise have undergone an operation involving a permanent colostomy. . . ." Two-thirds of the anastomoses were between 3 cm and 6 cm from the anal verge and 15 were at 6–8 cm. Six of the 40 patients had anastomotic leaks, three of the first four and three of the next 36. He used both the EEA™ instrument and the Russian SPTU. The single leak causing peritonitis was with the SPTU gun, as was the single hemorrhage—in the first postoperative hour. There were, in addition, three radiologically demonstrated sinuses. It is not clear how many of the anastomoses were done with the SPTU and how many with the EEA™ instrument.

The following year, Heald with Leicester (1981) reported an experience with 100 stapled low rectal anastomoses, the first ones done with the SPTU Russian stapler. With those, they had two ". . .brisk 500 to 1000 ml bleeds. . . .No hemorrhage has been seen with the American EEA™ stapler with its double row of staples." Fifty-two of their anastomoses were 2.5–5.0 cm from the anal margin, 17 were 5.5–7.0 cm, and the others higher. Only one of their patients developed symptoms and a palpable stricture, and the symptoms "passed off spontaneously. Some narrowing was invariable in the period between three and eight weeks after surgery, particularly in defunctioned cases, but dilatation occurred quickly and spontaneously after this and only one patient in this series has required a single manual dilatation at the time of colostomy closure." In a stricture referred to them, they performed ". . .a resection of the stricture with the EEA gun itself, this being effected by passing the stem through the stricture and the anvil through a small proximal colotomy, so that no purse strings were required." They ventured it as their "personal opinion," with which we agree, ". . .that permanent stricturing occurs only as a result of failure of healing by first intention with granulation tissue formation and consequent fibrosis. . . .A stricture specific to the gun dilates easily because it follows crushing of the narrow inverted ring of tissue that holds the staples. . . .It is perhaps relevant in this respect that the excised fibrous ring from the patient just mentioned contained only two staples. . .the remainder having presumably sloughed away. By comparison, the perfectly healed anastomosis shows a complete ring of staples almost permanently present on roentgenogram. . . ." They had 13 leaks, four that resulted in peritonitis, four that produced an external fistula, one that produced a vaginal fistula and an abscess, and four asymptomatic x-ray sinuses. They gave it as their opinion that ". . .the usual cause of 'primary failure' is that too much of the rectal muscle has been taken in the gathering stitch, so that longitudinal splitting is started or an excess 'turn-in' is eccentrically squeezed outwards by closure of the gun." They used an over-and-over 0-Prolene manually placed pursestring. They recommend complementary colostomy for all the extremely low anastomoses.

From the Boskilde Hospital in Copenhagen, Kirkegaard, Christiansen, and Hjortrup (1980) reported 30 patients undergoing anterior resection with reconstruction of the rectum at levels of 7–12 cm, with the EEA^{TM} instrument introduced transanally. Three patients had leaks demonstrated only radiologically and two had clinical leaks. There were two with wound infections. The one death was from multiple lung abscesses in a patient with chronic pulmonary disease and an intact anastomosis. The two clinically diagnosed anastomotic leaks closed spontaneously within three days. Digital and sigmoidoscopic examination of all patients disclosed defects only in the two with radiologically demonstrable leaks. All patients were continent for feces and gas. Four of the five patients with clinical or radiologic leaks had strictures that responded to dilatation. They considered that the EEA^{TM} instrument made possible anastomoses lower than usually were feasible, saved time, and did not ". . .require the same degree of training as low anterior resection with conventional suture anastomosis." This is an almost unique opinion, most surgeons pointing out that the instrument requires its own special skills and understanding and that there is a learning curve with technical problems and complications occurring early in a surgeon's EEA^{TM} experience.

Shahinian and others (Shahinian, Bowen, Dorman, Soderberg, and Thompson, 1980) from Providence, Rhode Island reported 29 anterior EEA^{TM} resections, four of them within 4 cm of the dentate line. There were two wound infections and one intra-abdominal abscess requiring drainage. Two patients had temporary incontinence for four or five months. Slight stenosis in one patient responded to dilatation. The single anastomotic dehiscence was recognized when a rectovaginal fistula developed eight weeks after operation ". . .in an elderly diabetic who had received radiation to the pelvis 15 years earlier."

From the University of British Columbia in Vancouver, Stoller, Dowell, and Atkinson (1980) reported 19 colorectal anastomoses with the EEA^{TM} instrument passed up through the anus—their initial experience. The patients were operated on in the Lloyd-Davies combined lithotomy-Trendelenburg position. Two patients developed minor leaks that required no treatment and one patient developed a fecal fistula that closed spontaneously. There were two minor wound infections. It was thought that "In 12 of the 19 patients a permanent colostomy was certainly avoided while another 5 might have needed a permanent colostomy."

From Kiel in West Germany, Thiede and his colleagues (Thiede, Troidl, Poser, Jostarndt, and Hamelmann, 1980) reported their initial experience with the EEA^{TM} instrument in 14 colon resections and 16 low anterior resections. They had a single death, from myocardial infarction, on the fifth day. Autopsy showed an intact anastomosis. Two of the low anterior resections required suture reinforcement at the time of operation. One patient had massive bleeding from the anastomosis after resection for diverticulitis. The anastomosis was resected and a new EEA^{TM} anastomosis performed successfully. Five of the low anterior resections showed radiologic "dehiscences" without clinical signs. One of the low anterior resections resulted in a fecal fistula. Like a number of others, they favor transanal distention of the rectum with fluid to test for a possibly inadequate anastomosis. They recommended a controlled prospective comparison of stapled and manual anastomoses.

By the time of the Munich Symposium on Colorectal Surgery in June, 1980 (Thiede, Jostarndt, Troidl, Poser, and Hamelmann, 1980), their series had increased to 60 anastomoses overall. They claimed no anastomotic dehiscences attributable to the apparatus and had performed anastomoses as low as 3.5 cm and 4 cm from the anocutaneous junction, but gave no detailed statistics.

By 1981, Thiede et al. of Kiel (Thiede, Jostarndt, Troidl, Poser, Bertz, and Hamelmann, 1981) had a total of 91 low rectal EEA^{TM} anastomoses, 17 at 3–5 cm, 24 at 6–8 cm, and 50 at 9 cm or higher. They had no deaths due to anastomotic failure. In the 50 anastomoses above 9 cm there were four radiographic leaks, no clinical leaks, and no fistulas. In the 24 cases at 6–8 cm there were five radiologic leaks and one clinical leak (fistula). In the 17 cases at 3–5 cm there were seven radiologic leaks and four clinical leaks (two fistulas). There were, in all, ten radiologic stenoses, ". . .none of them of clinical significance."

From the Royal Victoria Hospital in Belfast, Northern Ireland, Graham and associates (Graham, Johnston, McKelvey, and Kennedy, 1981) reported performing 42 anterior resections over a period of five years, the earlier ones with the SPTU and the later ones with the EEA^{TM} instrument, inserted transanally. They had two leaks, four strictures, and two deaths. Three of the anastomoses were at 3.5 cm and seven of them at 4–6 cm. They tested the suture line with injection of povidone-iodine transanally. One of the two deaths was due to pulmonary embolism, the other in a 95-year-old woman, after six weeks, from dehiscence of a low anastomosis. Four patients were found on rectal examination to have a ". . .tight anastomosis. . . .These required only gentle manual dilatation without anaesthetic." Most of their cases appeared to have been done with the SPTU.

Among those who test the anastomoses by injection of fluid, Engelberg and associates (Engelberg, Reiss, and Saba, 1981) from Israel inject povidone-iodine solutions into the rectum through a Foley catheter with distended balloon, the operator pinching off the colon proximally within the abdomen. They performed this technique in ten anterior resections and 11 total gastrectomies and found no leaks in any.

Schaeffer and Giordano (1981) from the George Washington Medical Center in Washington, D.C. reported 19 low anterior EEA^{TM} anastomoses performed by five surgeons, with four stenoses, three anastomotic dehiscences, one anastomotic line bleed, one anastomotic line recurrence, one split of the bowel, and one colocutaneous fistula, perhaps reinforcing Fasching's (q.v.) suggestion that stapling techniques require learning as well as do manual techniques. As the authors said, "The high incidence of complications noted in this series contrasts sharply with the previous reported experience of other surgeons. Lack of experience with the EEA stapler explains this. For the most part the surgeons surveyed were using the EEA stapling device for the first time. Surgeon D had four complications in ten patients, but all complications occurred in his first three patients. This supports Nance's statement that 'there is a definite learning curve associated with its [EEA] use.'"

We have referred to the prospective comparison by Beart and Kelly from the Mayo Clinic (1981) of low anterior anastomoses performed manually or with the stapler. Eighty patients were entered into the study, but in ten of them it was judged not feasible to perform a manual anastomosis and these, therefore, were removed from the study and had stapled anastomoses. In the randomized staple anastomosis group and the randomized manual anastomosis group there was a pelvic infection in each group and an anastomotic dehiscence in each group, resulting fatally in the stapled anastomosis. The time required for the anastomosis was significantly shorter in the stapled group (11 minutes versus 19 minutes). It is noteworthy that most other time studies include the time for the entire operation and not solely the time for the anastomosis. The ten "excluded" patients, who had stapled anastomoses, resulted in one anastomotic dehiscence with subsequent colostomy and one incomplete anastomosis recognized at operation and covered by a simultaneous colostomy. The mean level of the anastomosis in the ten "excluded" patients, determined postoperatively, was 3 cm, ranging from 2 cm to 6 cm from the dentate line. Beart concluded that, "A rectal anastomosis can be done more rapidly with a stapling device than with the hand-sewn technique. . . .The saving in morbidity, however, is probably minimal. Our study confirms Goligher's conviction that a lower anastomosis can be done with the stapler than with the hand-sewn technique. Approximately 12 percent of such patients had the rectum preserved when otherwise it might have been sacrificed." The single death was in a patient in whom x-rays taken after operation demonstrated that the ring of staples was not intact.

Bérard and colleagues from Lyon (Bérard, Papillon, Jacquemard, Labrosse, Bigay, and Guillemin, 1981) reported their first 50 EEA^{TM} low rectal anastomoses, 3–10 cm from the anal verge, the operations performed between April, 1978 and April, 1980. In this period, the use of the EEA^{TM} instrument diminished the frequency of abdominoperineal resections and of Hartmann operations. The patients were in the lithotomy-Trendelenburg position, the EEA^{TM} instrument introduced through the anus, and pursestrings fashioned with the pursestring clamp. Like a number of others in their initial experiences, they had one injury to the rectum by the tip of the instrument. A number of authors reporting a single instance of this kind in their early experience were able to close the perforation manually and proceed with the anastomosis. Bérard abandoned that patient to a Hartmann procedure. In two cases, an incomplete anastomosis required suture reinforcement. They used proximal colostomy 12 times. Three patients died, all with autopsy-proved intact anastomoses. In the 47 survivors there were no fistulas and no abscesses, two wound infections. Seven anastomoses were determined by digital examination to be stenosed. Two "stenoses" cleared after the colostomy was closed, two were asymptomatic, and in three the stenoses indicated recurrence of the malignancy; in two of those, the stricture occurred only after intracavitary irradiation.

Athanasiadis, Barry, Gandji, and Girona (1981) from the Prosper Hospital in Recklinghausen reported a successive series of 82 manual colorectal anastomoses, 65 SPTU (Russian) anastomoses, and 253 EEA^{TM} anastomoses. The abstract of their remarks at the Munich Congress of the German Surgical Society in April, 1981 states only that the radiologic anastomotic insufficiency was 11.8% in the EEA^{TM} anastomoses, 12.2% in the manual anastomoses, and 17.1% in the SPTU anastomoses. When one compares their earlier paper (Athanasiadis, Barry, and Girona, 1981), it is seen that they began using the SPTU in 1978 and the EEA^{TM} instrument in 1979, but continued to use the SPTU, since the earlier paper lists 35 SPTU anastomoses and 225 EEA^{TM} anastomoses and the later abstract 65 SPTU anastomoses and 253 EEA^{TM} anastomoses. The basis on which the choice of SPTU, EEA^{TM}, or manual anastomosis was made is not stated, but much of the SPTU experience was prior to the EEA^{TM} experience. The earlier paper mentions a clinical dehiscence rate of 4.6% for the stapled anastomoses.

At the Groote Schuur Hospital in Cape Town, Brown and associates (Brown, Gasson, and Brown, 1981) performed EEA™ colorectal anastomoses in 37 patients between August, 1979 and September, 1980. They thought that ten of the patients otherwise would have required abdominoperineal resection. They advise freeing the splenic flexure in all cases, so that if the distal descending colon is narrow, the anastomosis can be done at a higher level in the colon. They preferred the manual over-and-over pursestring to the modified Furniss clamp pursestring. There were no clinically demonstrated anastomotic leaks. In one patient with a complementary colostomy there was a radiologically demonstrated leak. There were no instances of bleeding. There had been ". . .2 cases of 'hold-up' requiring postoperative dilatation." They had two wound infections. There were two deaths, one from pulmonary embolism and one from heart failure. They commented of the EEA™ stapler that ". . .an anastomosis performed in this manner is equal to any hand-sewn high anterior resection in the upper rectum, and superior to any other method in the lower rectum. It saves many patients with carcinoma of the lower rectum from having abdominoperineal resections and reduces the number of temporary colostomies needed. . .and at least 1 hour, if not 2 hours, of operating time is saved in a difficult case."

Cade and colleagues (Cade, Gallagher, Schofield, and Turner, 1981) from Manchester, England analyzed their complications in 50 patients with anterior resection and end-to-end anastomosis with the EEA™ instrument. There was a single death, from a massive pulmonary embolus on the seventeenth day in a patient who at autopsy had a well-healed anastomosis. Two patients who had had colostomies passed blood and mucus per anum in the second week and were found to have defects in their anastomoses, but did well. One patient after five days developed a small intestinal obstruction. A loop of small bowel was found adherent to a defect in the back of the anastomosis. A colostomy was performed and the anastomotic defect was sutured per anum. The patient did well. Thus, 46 of 49 patients showed a perfect union. There were ten wound infections. Two patients at three months developed paradoxical diarrhea and were found to have strictures that were readily dilated. They had four anal fissures that they thought were due to stretching of the anus in inserting the device and they now always dilate the anus before the device is inserted.

Detry and associates (Detry and Kestens, 1981; Detry, Otte, and Kestens, 1981) from Brussels, between March, 1979 and November, 1980, performed 45 left colectomies and 55 "anterior sigmoidorectal" resections, performing the anastomoses in all with the EEA™ stapler. The rectal anastomoses ranged from 2 cm to 11 cm above the anal margin and 17 of the rectal anastomoses ". . .would have been difficult, and seven quite impossible, without the stapling gun." There was a single death, from leukemia. The instrument was inserted through the anus with the patient in the lithotomy position. There was one fecal fistula that closed within four days and ten minimal dehiscences detected radiographically. One of those patients developed a tight stricture. There was one instance of bleeding. No patient required reoperation.

Fahrenkrug and Clemmesen (1981) from Denmark performed 17 colonic resections, 24 sigmoid resections, and 35 low anterior resections with the EEA™ instrument. In the 41 colonic and sigmoid anastomoses there was a single clinical anastomotic leak and three radiologic anastomotic leaks. The single death was in a patient with a cardiac problem. Two of the 35 low anterior resections resulted in fatal leaks and six showed only radiologic evidence of leak.

Kirwan (1981) from Cork in Ireland analyzed his first 30 low rectal EEA™ anastomoses. The splenic flexure was mobilized in all, the sigmoid colon resected completely. "After anastomosis, the pelvis was filled with saline, and air insufflated into the colon through a sigmoidoscope so as to confirm the absence of leakage." Gastrografin® enema was performed ten days after operation. In the first group of ten cases there were four radiologic subclinical leaks, in the next group, two, and in the last ten, none, which indicates, he says,". . .that with experience a leakage rate approaching zero can be achieved." Toward the end of this series they stopped performing complementary colostomies, but still advised them for extremely low anastomoses ". . .between columnar epithelium of the colon and squamous epithelium of the anal canal."

From Brussels, Lantin and associates (Lantin, Lantin, and Vandeperre, 1981) reported 24 consecutive cases of low rectal anastomoses with the EEA™ instrument between October, 1978 and September, 1980, the instruments inserted transanally with the patients in the lithotomy position. They were able to complete the anastomosis in all cases. They had three fistulas at levels of 5 cm and 6 cm and one fatal leak with an anastomosis at 3 cm. The fistulas all occurred among the nine patients with extremely low anastomoses, all of whom would have required abdominoperineal resection but for the instrument. There were three stenoses that readily yielded to digital dilatation. Like Heald, they recommended complementary colostomy in patients with extremely low anastomoses.

Lazorthes and colleagues from Toulouse (Lazorthes, Gadrat, Legrand, Cordova, Monrozies, Fretigny, and Pugnet, 1981), from March, 1978 to May, 1980, performed 60 low EEA™ anastomoses to the rectum or anus. Seven of the anal anastomoses were done by a combined abdominal and transsphincteric approach and seven by a posterior approach and transsphincteric anastomosis. Forty-four of the anastomoses were below the peritoneum, 16 above. Twenty of the anastomoses were 2–3 cm from the mucocutaneous junction, five at 4–5 cm. Like others, they found the pursestring instrument frequently inapplicable to the lower segment. They had three clinically recognizable fistulas in the first nine cases and one in the next 51. There were six wound infections and five cases of minor rectal bleeding. The two deaths were in patients without anastomotic complications.

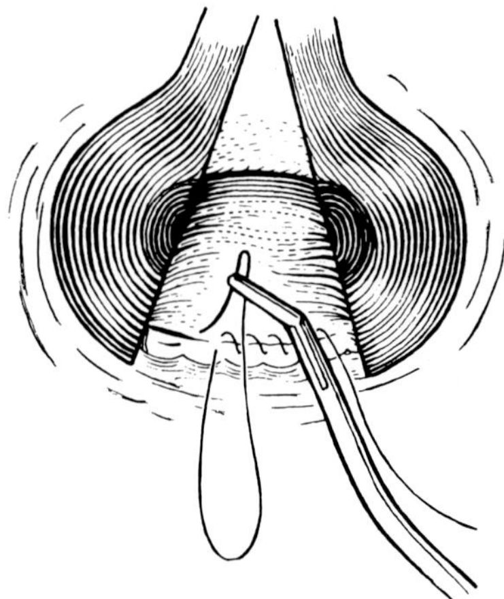

Fig IX–11.—Low colorectal and coloanal EEA™ anastomosis—technique of Polglase, Hughes, and McDermott (1981). With anastomoses made so low as to be to squamous epithelium, the Australian group, like Goligher in England (1979), insert the distal pursestring peranally, developing separate techniques depending on whether the EEA™ instrument is passed downward through a colotomy or upward peranally. (From A.L. Polglase, E.S.R. Hughes, and F.T. McDermott, *Australian and New Zealand Journal of Surgery*, 1981, used by permission.)

Polglase, Hughes, and McDermott from Melbourne, Australia (1981) reported their technique of EEA™ stapling in ultralow anastomoses, placing the distal pursestring transanally (Fig IX–11). They developed two separate techniques. In the first, the EEA™ instrument was inserted orthograde through a colotomy and the distal pursestring was tied from the exterior after the anvil was protruded through the anus. They saw the advantage that the anvil then could be removed to make withdrawal of the instrument effortless. In the second technique, the EEA™ instrument was passed up through the anorectal stump, the upper pursestring was tied, and the EEA™ stapler withdrawn until the cartridge fully emerged from the anus. The lower pursestring then was tied from below. The instrument was operated and removed in the usual way. In their dog experiments, the rectum had been divided from below, 1 cm above the dentate line, and a pursestring inserted from below using a bivalved anal retractor, essentially as Goligher had done. Having perfected the technique on dogs, they then applied it to six patients, in three passing the instrument down from above and in three passing the instrument up from below. In the first three patients, as a precaution, a colostomy was performed and in a fourth because there was a question about the anastomosis. There were no deaths, there was one incomplete lower tissue ring in the patient in whom the colostomy was therefore performed, and this was the single instance of clinically evident leak with fever, purulent anal discharge, and a palpable posterior defect in the anastomosis. Initial incontinence was the rule in these extremely low anastomoses. Two of three patients followed more than six months now are fully continent for solid stool; the third has some seepage. "All six patients have difficulty controlling liquid stool." They indicated that Goligher had used a similar technique with the Soviet stapler.

Probst, Becker, and Ungeheuer (1981) of Frankfurt compared 52 anterior resections performed with the EEA™ instrument and 52 manually between September, 1979 and

August, 1980, performing the manual suture with three rows of sutures, usually without colostomy. The instrument saved some 30 minutes of operating time. There were no deaths with the EEA™ instruments, three anastomotic insufficiencies, and no bleeding. The wound infection rate was 9% in both groups and the length of hospitalization similar. They thought that the instrument should be used only by experienced rectal surgeons.

Smith (1981) of Bethesda, Maryland surveyed 243 members of the American Society of Colon and Rectal Surgeons with respect to their experience with the EEA™ instrument in low rectal anastomoses. The total experience was in 3,594 cases. His Table 1 (our Table IX–2) lists the intraoperative problems reported and Table 2 (our Table IX–3) shows the early postoperative complications. The analysis does not indicate the relationship of the number of cases reported by a surgeon to the number of his complications. Presumably, the eight deaths due to sepsis in the 3,594 cases were due to anastomotic failures. An anastomotic leak ". . . was reported in 352 (9.8 percent) patients. . . ." Smith points out that in the patients who have a Hartmann pouch, "The center rod of the EEA can be introduced via the rectum through a stab wound in the center of the cleared space. . . a 4 cm diameter circle on its anterior wall. . ." and the anvil screwed into place from the abdominal side (Fig IX–12). Smith preferred the manually placed pursestring suture. Like most operators, Smith recommends that the operating surgeon place his left hand on the instrument in the perineum and his right hand on the bowel and remove the instrument himself. He is almost alone in advising inspection of the anastomosis sigmoidoscopically in the operating room. As well, he recommends filling the pelvis with saline and insufflating air per rectum. The final evaluation was that the mortality rate with the EEA™ stapler compared favorably with that of other types of anastomoses and that "The late and postoperative morbidity rate of 17.5 per cent in this series compares favorably with other techniques of anastomosis and offers the possibility of lower anastomoses in less time."

TABLE IX–2.—Intraoperative Complications in 3,594 Stapled Anastomoses (Smith's Table 1)*

	NUMBER OF CASES	PERCENT
Anastomotic leak	352	9.8
Tear during extraction	68	1.9
Anvil not extractable	43	1.2
Complete anastomotic failure (conversion to another technique)	33	0.9
Instrument failure	28	0.8
Knife absent	25	
Teflon ring absent	2	
Staples absent	1	
Bleeding	19	0.5
Total	543	15.1

*From L.E. Smith: Anastomosis with EEA stapler after anterior colonic resection. *Dis. Colon Rectum* 24:236, 1981. Used by permission.

TABLE IX–3.—EARLY POSTOPERATIVE COMPLICATIONS AFTER 3,594 STAPLED ANASTOMOSES (SMITH's TABLE 2)*

	NUMBER OF CASES	PERCENT
Pelvic abscess	90	2.5
Hematoma	27	0.8
Deaths	17	0.5
Sepsis	8	
Myocardial infarction	4	
Pulmonary embolus	2	
Aortic thrombosis	1	
Mesenteric venous thrombosis	1	
Pulmonary failure	1	
	134	3.8

*From L.E. Smith: Anastomosis with EEA stapler after anterior colonic resection. *Dis. Colon Rectum* 24:236, 1981. Used by permission.

In 1980, at the meeting of the Southern Surgical Association, Bricker (Bricker, Johnston, and Patwardhan, 1981) presented his original and highly successful technique for repairing postirradiation damage to the colorectum by doubling a loop of the colorectum on itself, applying the split-open proximal, relatively intact bowel to the split-open distal, diseased and stenotic bowel, then by an ordinary anastomosis attaching the loop thus made to the proximal colon, distal to colostomy. Ravitch at that time suggested that the long and detailed sewing required conceivably might be speeded up by the use of the staplers.

Wheeless of Baltimore (1981) writes, "We have performed this procedure on three occasions. It is an excellent procedure and, in all three cases, the results were very good. Per Doctor Ravitch's comment we used the surgical stapler in all three cases. The TA90 (especially the disposable TA90) is an excellent instrument for making the long suture anastomosis. . . .

"Our opinion concerning the surgical stapler is that it is ideal for tissue in which the blood supply has been compromised. Recently, data from our laboratory indicate that the stapler has a more vascular anastomosis than either the Halsted two-layer classic anastomosis or the Gambee single-layer anastomosis with fine catgut. We have recently measured I^{125} crossing the afferent and efferent vasculature of different anastomoses and by far the stapler remains the most vascular of the available anastomoses."

HARTMANN PROCEDURE

The use of the EEA™ instrument in the reconstruction of patients who have had a Hartmann procedure for the resection of rectal or sigmoidal lesions is an obvious application that undoubtedly has been used by many without being reported, and we have used it with satisfaction on a number of occasions.

Fiala's report from Rohner's clinic in Geneva (Fiala, Marti, Meyer, and Rohner, 1980) of ten EEA™ reconstructions after a Hartmann procedure, which they describe as an indication that they found "particulièrement séduisante," stated that the dissection of the rectum, theretofore often so difficult, had been notably simplified by the EEA™ technique. A year later, their series had reached 12 (Marti, Fiala, and Rohner, 1981).

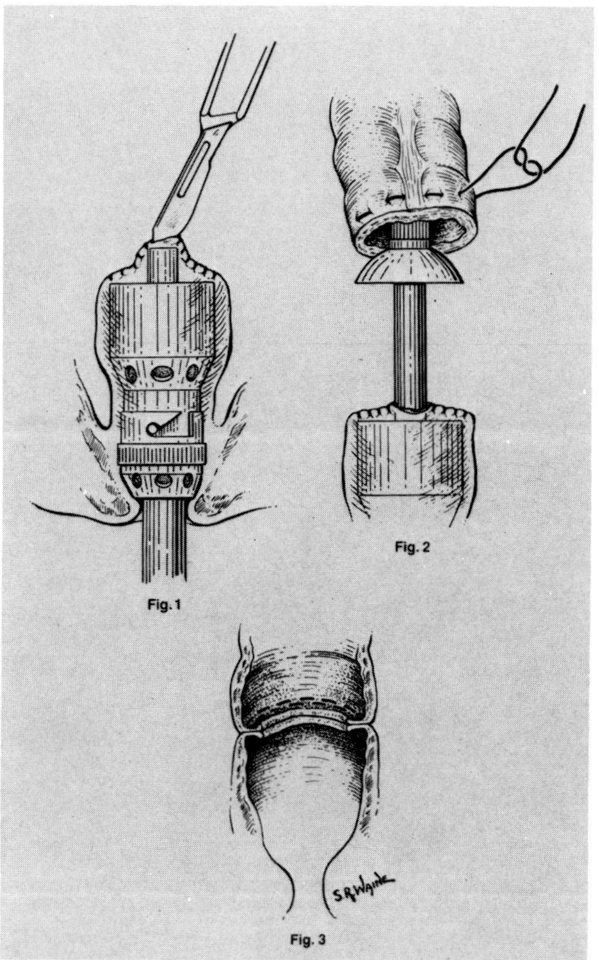

Fig IX–12.—Use of the EEA™ instrument in reconstruction after Hartmann procedure—technique of Robbins, Sohn, Weinstein, and Steichen (1981). The EEA™ instrument is passed up through the anus without the anvil-nose cone until the spindle presses against the upper end of the Hartmann pouch, which need not be dissected except to expose the surface. The spindle is passed through as small an incision as possible, the nose cone applied and slipped into the pursestringed proximal bowel, and the anastomosis performed thereafter as in the other applications of the EEA™ instrument. (From R.D. Robbins, N. Sohn, M.A. Weinstein, and F.M. Steichen, *Colo-Proctology*, 1981, used by permission.)

Robbins, Steichen, and associates (Robbins, Sohn, Weinstein, and Steichen, 1981) from New York illustrate the use of the EEA™ instrument in reconstruction after the Hartmann procedure, without citing their experience (Fig IX–12). Mittal and Cortez from Detroit, in the same year (1981), similarly picture its use without describing their experience. Alexander-Williams (Dorricott, Baddeley, Keighley, Oates, and Alexander-Williams, 1980) and Knight of Shreveport (1982) refer to EEA™ reconstruction after the Hartmann procedure.

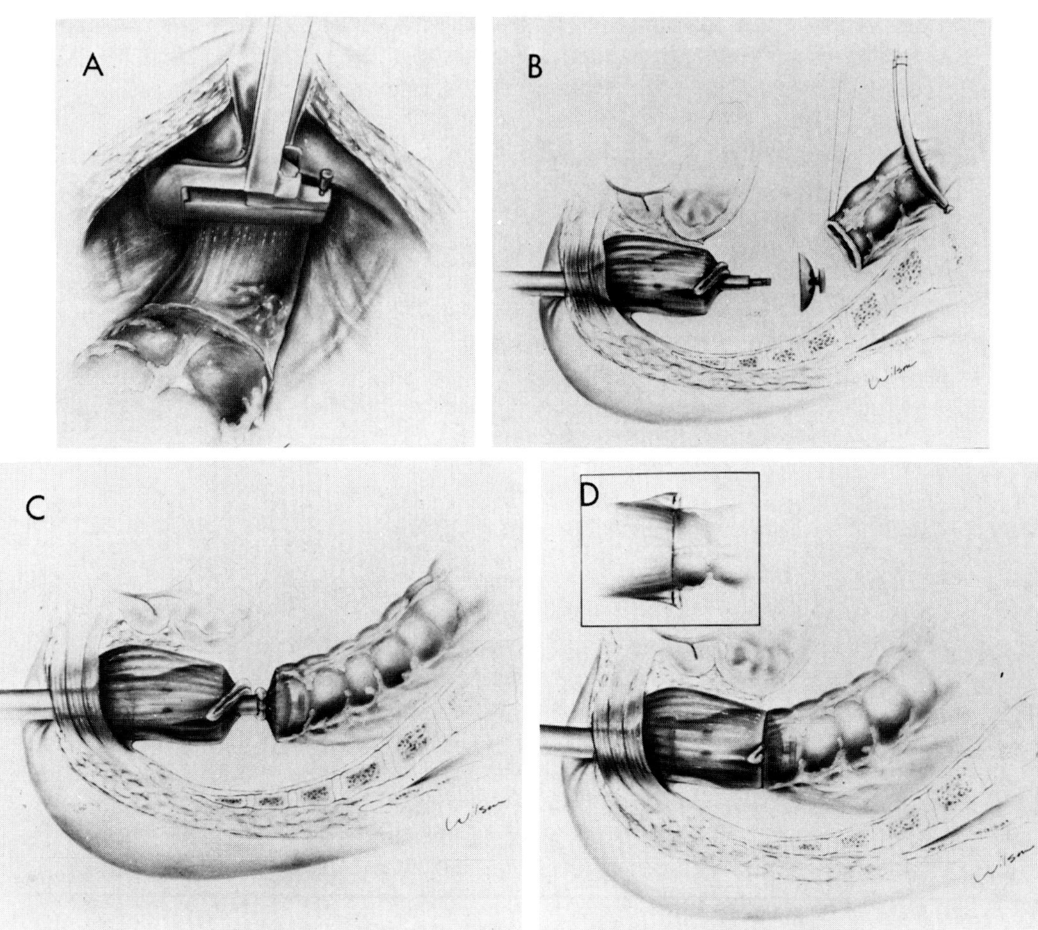

Fig IX–13.—Low anterior resection of the rectum using the EEA™ stapler—technique of Knight and Griffen (1980). **A,** after the rectosigmoid colon has been mobilized, the TA 55™ stapler is applied at the lower limit of the resection, placing a double row of staples. **B,** the EEA™ stapler, with the anvil-nose cone removed, is introduced per anum into the rectal segment. The naked center rod is passed through a stab wound posterior to the staple line and the anvil is fitted to the rod. A noncrushing clamp on the proximal colon prevents spillage. **C,** after the anvil has been attached to the spindle and fitted into the open sigmoid colon, the proximal purse-string is tied and the noncrushing clamp removed. **D,** the EEA™ stapler is closed and activated to make the circular end-to-end inverting anastomosis. In this technique, no attempt is made to include the entire circumference of the rectal segment, and the need for a distal pursestring is obviated. (The *inset* shows the anteroposterior view of the anastomosis.) The EEA™ staple line crosses the TA™ staple line at two points despite which in 40 consecutive cases (Knight, 1983) there have been no leaks. (From C.D. Knight and F.D. Griffen, *Surgery,* 1980, used by permission.)

Somewhat more open to challenge than the use of the EEA[TM] instrument for reconstruction after a Hartmann procedure is the technique of Knight and Griffen of Shreveport, Louisiana (1980) in the performance of a primary low rectal anastomosis (Fig IX–13). They staple off the rectum, pass the EEA[TM] instrument up from the anus, passing the spindle through the posterior wall close to the stapled end, screw on the anvil-nose cone, and complete the anastomosis. The ring of staples of the EEA[TM] instrument necessarily comes across the line of the TA[TM] staples in the rectal end at least once, and perhaps twice. Nevertheless, in his initial report, Knight reported six low anterior resections and reconstructions by this technique with no leaks, no abscesses, no strictures, and no deaths. A more recent communication (1983) brings the total number of operations done by this technique to 40, one-third of the anastomoses below 8 cm, the lowest at 2 cm, still with no clinical leaks, no colostomies. We are becoming encouraged about this technique as a result of our ongoing laboratory studies, and in the clinic of one of us the technique has become routine in the hands of some surgeons.

COLOSTOMY

The instruments have appealed to a number of operators in various applications to the techniques of colostomy formation.

From the Massachusetts General Hospital in Boston, Krause, Freund, and Fischer (1979) demonstrated, in dogs, an ingenious technique for using the EEA[TM] instrument to create an end ileostomy or colostomy. The central rod was passed through a small perforation in the abdominal wall, the anvil-nose cone attached and inserted into the end of the bowel, and the pursestring tied. Operation of the instrument then produced a stapled end colostomy or ileostomy, the knife taking out a full-thickness ring of abdominal wall. Fischer (1982) does not use the procedure clinically. Our own assessment of this technique in the laboratory does not lead us to believe that the truly elegant, although flush, stoma is worth the trouble involved. Nevertheless, at a recent meeting, we were told by several surgeons that they had produced such stapled colostomies with satisfaction.

Brodman and Brodman from the Bronx, New York (1975), to be sure of complete diversion in a loop colostomy, brought out the loop and stapled it with a TA 55[TM] instrument distal to the colotomy.

Photopulos and colleagues (Photopulos, Jones, Walton, and Fowler, 1977), in the performance of temporary diverting colostomies for patients with severe radiation-induced proctosigmoiditis, divided the bowel with the GIA[TM] instrument and brought the two stapled ends out through separate wounds, essentially making a Devine colostomy.

OPERATIONS FOR HIRSCHSPRUNG'S DISEASE

The Duhamel operation (Duhamel, 1956) is one of the technically simplest and most satisfactory of the proposed operations for Hirschsprung's disease, its sole detraction being that if the spur, between the rectum and the colon brought down into the rectum through an extremely low end-to-side anastomosis, was not completely divided, a proximal rectal pouch remained in which a ''fecaloma'' was prone to occur, with resultant complications. The use of the GIA[TM] instrument to staple together the rectum and the colon and divide the spur was an obvious solution, and in 1968 we (Steichen, Talbert, and Ravitch, 1968) reported our animal experiments and an initial clinical experience with the technique (Fig IX–14).

In 1973 we (Talbert, Seashore, and Ravitch, 1974) reported a total of 21 patients operated on by the Duhamel stapler technique since August, 1968, six of them without prior colostomies. In all but one of the 15 patients with prior colostomies, the colostomy was resected at the time of the definitive operation. The only anastomotic complication was in an infant with total aganglionosis of the colon except for the cecum. A limited separation occurred in the anocecal anastomosis, requiring a temporary diverting ileostomy. The stapled colorectal spur division was intact; it was a portion of the hand-sutured anastomosis to the anorectum that broke down. The patient ultimately did well. All children were relieved from their constipation and no child developed a fecaloma. All patients older than three years were continent. There were no instances of postoperative enterocolitis.

Within a year of our original publication, Lister, then of Sheffield (Lister, 1969), stated, "The use of an anastomotic stapling instrument for division of the colorectal spur in the Duhamel procedure was described by Steichen et al. in 1968: the stapling machine provides a method of disposing of the spur more effectively even than our crushing instrument specially designed for the purpose." Lister, at that time, reported two infants with total colonic aganglionosis in whom much of the aganglionic colon was left behind and a Duhamel operation performed with the ileum brought down to an anastomosis just above the anus. The GIA^{TM} instrument was applied twice in one child and three times in the other to produce a long anastomosis between the left colon and the ileum, providing a reservoir capacity and a large absorptive surface. This represented the use of the GIA^{TM} instrument to construct a long side-to-side anastomosis from ileum to rectum and left colon in children with long-segment Hirschsprung's disease, as brilliantly recommended by Martin (1968).

In 1969, at the Symposium of the French Society of Pediatric Surgery, Duhamel still described the use of his two Kocher clamps for spur crushing (Duhamel, 1970). However, at the same meeting, Pagès of Paris (Pagès, 1970), in fact a former pupil and associate of Duhamel's, describing the fecaloma as the single major complication of the Duhamel operation for Hirschsprung's disease, suggested that "primary consideration should be given to using the automatic staplers of the type of that of Ravitch, which would simultaneously produce the enterotomy and avoid the necessity for leaving the crushing clamps in place."

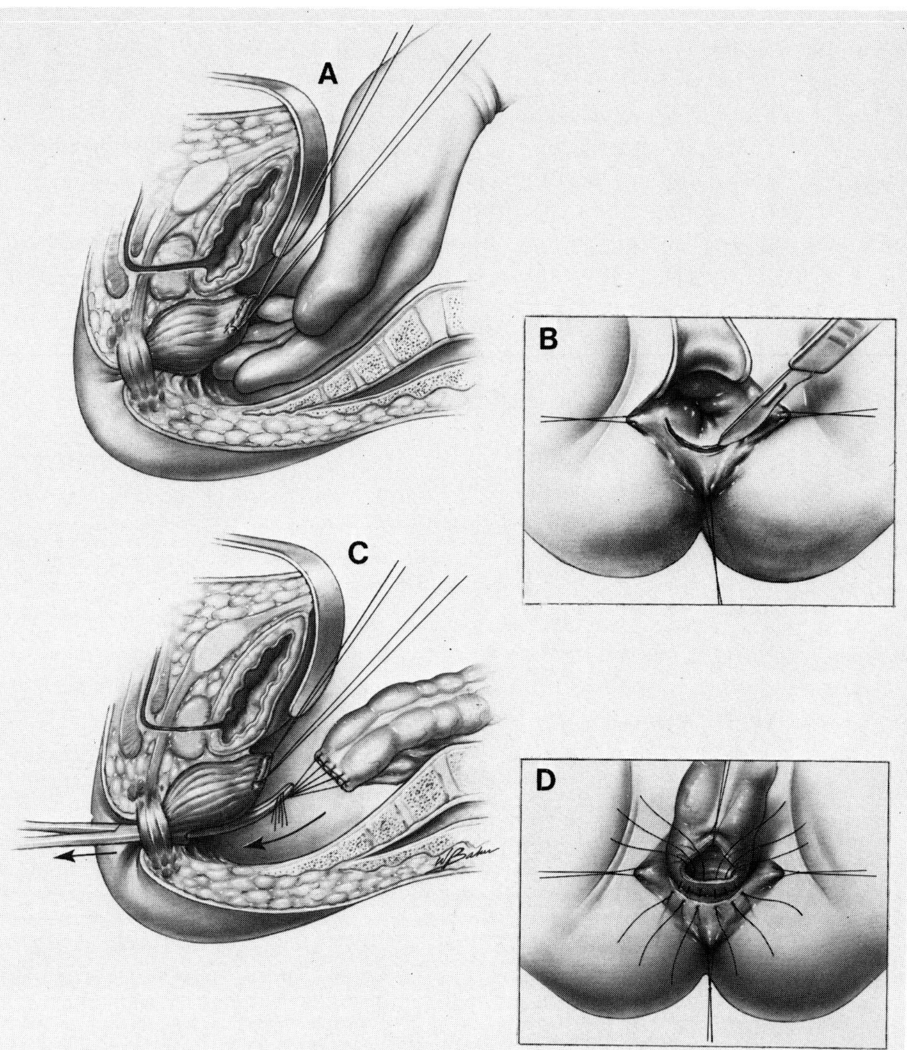

Fig IX–14.—Duhamel operation for Hirschsprung's disease. **A,** the rectum has been stapled and divided below the peritoneal reflexion and the proximal aganglionic bowel resected. Dissection is carried posteriorly close to the bowel. **B,** transverse incision in the rectum just above the sphincter. **C,** that incision having been carried through the bowel transversely, the proximal ganglionated colon is brought down through the incision in the rectum and out the anus. **D,** the proximal bowel is held up over the perineum and a tranverse incision made in its posterior wall. Sutures are being placed between the lower lip of the rectal incision and the lower lip of the colonic incision. The suture is carried around anteriorly, the incision in the wall of the colon being progressively extended around its circumference until the specimen has been liberated and the anastomosis completed.

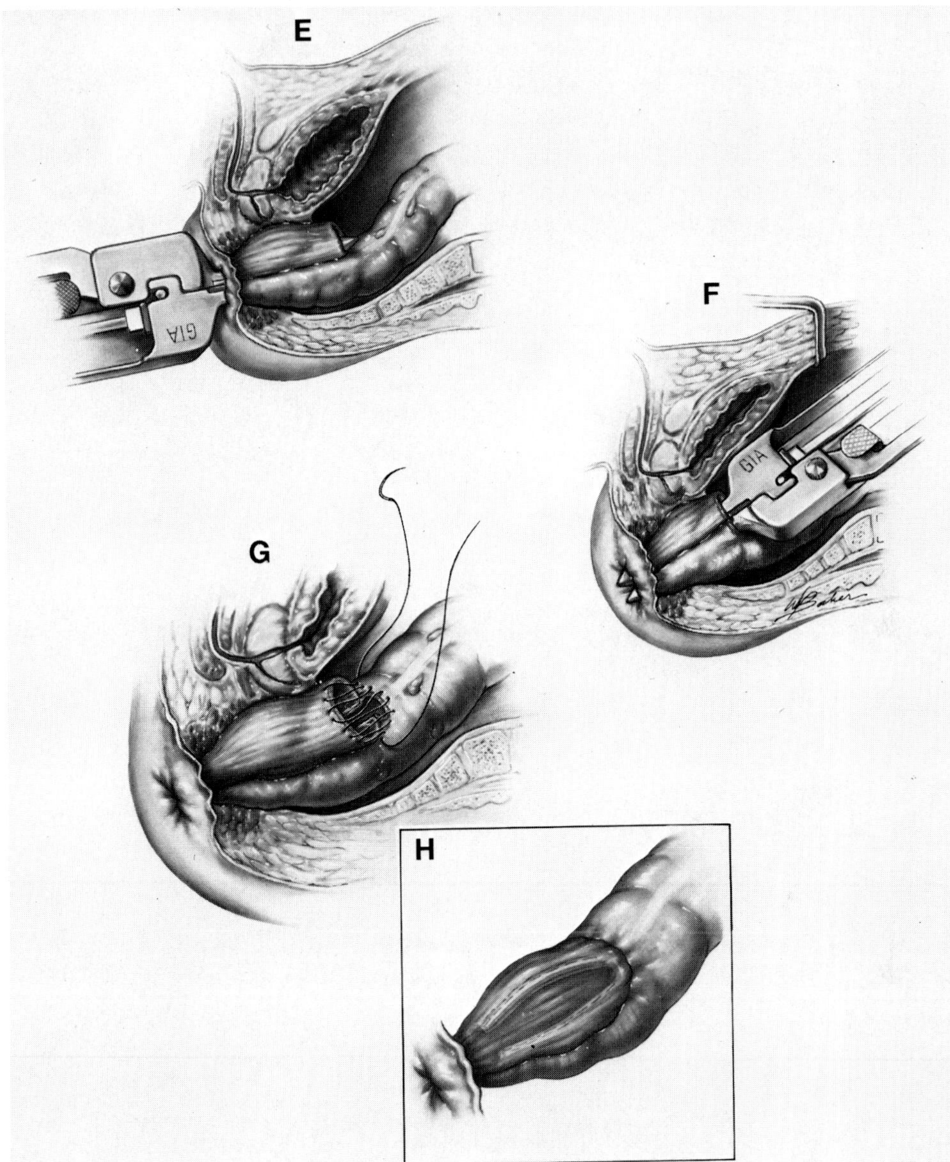

Fig IX–14 (cont.).—E, the GIA™ instrument is inserted, one limb up the rectum and one through the colorectostomy into the colon, the stapled upper end of the rectum having been cut away. In infants, the PGIA™ instrument with its shorter staples should be used. **F,** alternatively, the GIA™ instrument can be inserted from above either through the opened end of the rectum or through the cutaway corner of the stapled closure of the rectum. In older children, sometimes it is necessary to insert the GIA™ instrument both from above and below. **G,** a manual closure of the upper end of the anastomosis is preferred to a stapled closure, to avoid any narrowing of the channel. **H,** the completed anastomosis. (**E–H** from M.M. Ravitch and F.M. Steichen, *Annals of Surgery,* 1972, used by permission.)

NOTES

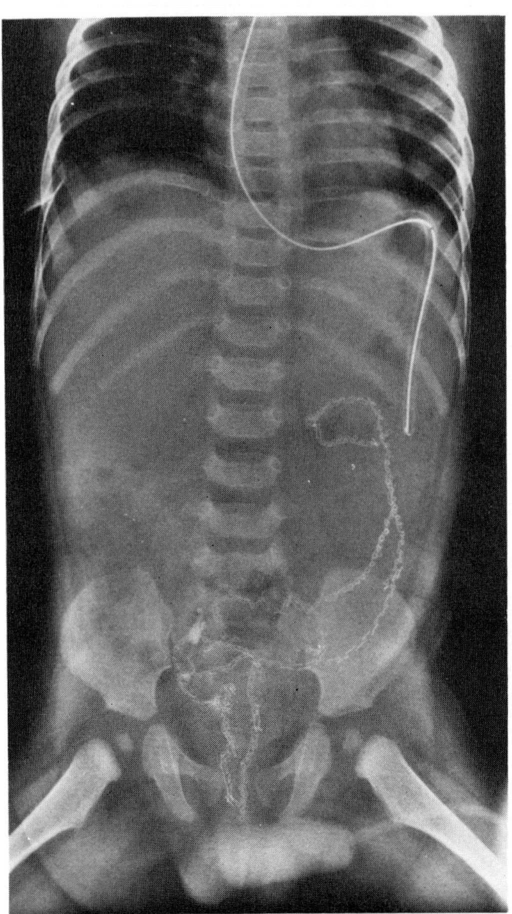

Fig IX–15.—Martin operation for long-segment Hirschsprung's disease. To provide more absorptive surface, the technique of Lester Martin (1968) is used. The bowel is divided high on the descending colon. Any aganglionic bowel remaining proximally is resected and the proximal ganglionated bowel is brought down and anastomosed end-to-side to the rectum as in Figure IX–14**D**. The two loops, the ganglionated bowel that has been anastomosed to the rectum, and the aganglionic left colon then are anastomosed side-to-side by successive applications of the GIA™ instrument introduced repeatedly until there is a common lumen from the proximal end of the descending colon down to the colorectal anastomosis. The GIA™ instrument is serially passed through paired openings, much as shown in Figure V–23**D**. The introduction sites for the GIA™ instrument are closed transversely with the TA™ instruments. The x-ray here reproduced shows the quite long side-to-side anastomosis produced, leaving a long segment of joined bowel, all of which has absorptive function and half of it innervated so as to provide propulsive power. (Courtesy of Dr. Albert Dibbins.)

In 1972, Martin presented his results in nine infants with total colonic aganglionosis (Martin, 1972), in whom he had made a long anastomosis between the ileum brought down to the anus and a significant portion of the retained colon. The technique of the long side-to-side anastomosis was not described except to state that in one child "The septum had initially been divided with an automatic stapling instrument." That child developed protracted diarrhea and was found to have a "regrowth of the septum. . .", which then was divided with relief. In 1979, Martin, writing in the Third Edition of *Pediatric Surgery,* pictured the use of the GIA™ instrument for the rectal portion of the long side-to-side anastomosis in long-segment Hirschsprung's disease, making the remainder manually (Martin, 1979). The GIA™ instrument in fact enormously facilitates this quite long side-to-side anastomosis, which can be made entirely with it (Fig IX–15).

Dudgeon, Coran, and Rosenkrantz (1973) from Los Angeles described another case of ". . .regrowth of the septum. . ." after a stapled division of the septum in the Duhamel operation. That 11-month-old child was discharged apparently well on the fifteenth day. It is not stated whether the stapler was introduced from below or from above. Sometime between the third and fifth week after operation, the child developed vomiting and diarrhea and a septum now could be palpated 2 cm from the mucocutaneous junction. The septum was divided from below, controlled by direct vision through a colotomy and laparotomy. The child did well. It is noteworthy that the child had a colostomy at the time of his Duhamel operation, which was, therefore, carried out on defunctionalized bowel, in which the septum "reformed." As the authors point out, the same thing has occurred with manually sutured anastomoses distal to a defunctionalizing colostomy. The child had not had a rectal examination after operation.

Inasmuch as the GIA^{TM} cut and stapled bowel remains viable out to the cut edge, beyond the staple line, this adhesion of the cut edges is even more likely with staple suture of the bowel than with manual suture closure, but is easily prevented by an occasional digital examination. Parenthetically, it may be pointed out that in Duhamel operations performed by the ordinary technique, in which a spur is found to have been left behind and caused symptoms, we have, as far back as 1968, treated the spur by pulling it down peranally and dividing it with the GIA^{TM} instrument placed on either side of the spur under direct vision.

Burrington and Wayne (1976), at the 1975 meeting of the Surgical Section of the American Academy of Pediatrics, reported their experience with six cases of total colonic aganglionosis. In two of the patients, the GIA^{TM} stapling instrument was used. In the first, a long anastomosis was made and the patient's "protective," proximal, loop ileostomy closed six weeks later and ". . .rectal examination revealed that the septum had partially reformed. . . ." The septum was divided transanally. In the second patient in whom the GIA^{TM} instrument was used, again "protected by proximal loop ileostomy," which was closed five weeks later, the child developed difficulty after five months and it was noted that ". . .a high, short septum still remains. . . ." This may, of course, simply have meant that the septum had not been completely divided initially by what appears to have been a single application of the stapler. On the basis of this experience, Burrington said that he had given up the use of the GIA^{TM} instrument.

From France, Rignault and collaborators (Rignault, Pailler, Berthet, and Tardat, 1976), reporting their overall experience with the staplers, reported satisfactory GIA^{TM} division of the Duhamel spur in three patients.

From the Medical College of Georgia in Augusta, Parrish (1977), in 20 Duhamel operations, crushed the spur with Kocher clamps in the first 13 and, in the last seven patients, used the GIA^{TM} instrument ". . .without any complications and with gratifying results." He pointed out that "This method not only eliminates the incomplete spur problem but also provides for an immediate primary anastomosis, thus eliminating the possibility of accidental clamp dislodgment and all of the nursing problems common to the spur clamp technique. Hospitalization is thus shortened because the long period required for spontaneous slough of the spur-crushing clamps (7 to 15 days) is eliminated."

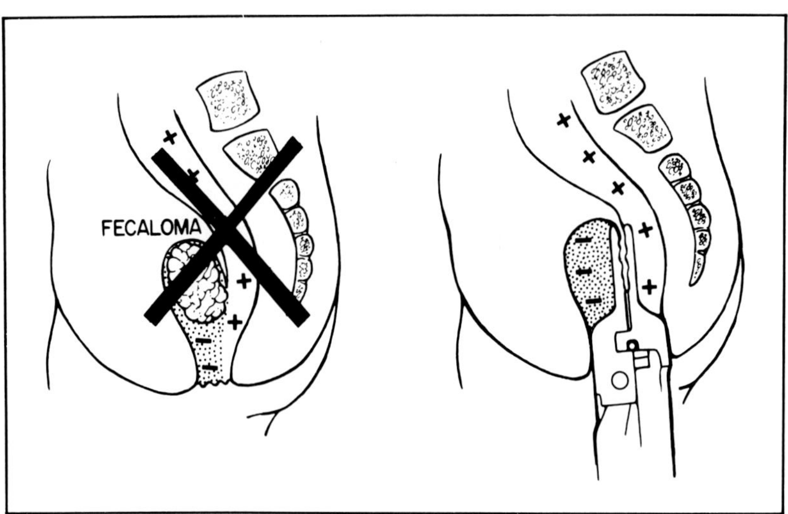

Fig IX–16.—Elimination of spur in Duhamel operation for Hirschsprung's disease. Grosfeld's illustration shows the recess left by incomplete division of the spur with the "conventional" procedure and the formation of a fecal concretion. The GIA™ instrument completely divides the colorectal party wall, leaving a single chamber without a recess for accumulation of a fecal mass. Martin's suggestion, leaving the upper end of the rectum open for manual suture to the colon at the upper end of the septum division (Fig IX–14**G**), is the best insurance against leaving a recess in which a fecaloma can form. (From J.L. Grosfeld, J.N. Ballantine, and J.F. Csicsko, *Archives of Surgery,* 1978, used by permission.)

Grosfeld, Ballantine, and Csicsko (1978), reviewing their experience with 66 Duhamel operations at the James Whitcomb Riley Hospital in Indianapolis, stated that "Division of the spur was usually accomplished by using an autostapling device (Gastro-Intestinal Anastomosis instrument) as advocated by Steichen et al." (Fig IX–16) They state that "In eight of ten patients with classic Duhamel procedures, a fecaloma subsequently developed in the retained aganglionic pouch which is characterized by constipation and soiling. The patients required a transanal division of the persistent colorectal spur. . ." performed by transanal introduction of the GIA™ instrument. They distinguished between "persistence" of the spur after crushing and "regrowth" after division and stapling: "We have not seen reformation of the spur or spur granuloma as described by Dudgeon et al., by Burrington and Wayne, and by Dickinson. . .it is important to carefully separate the two edges of the divided spur at operation so they do not readhere. . .the fecaloma syndrome developed in eight of ten patients on whom classic Duhamel operations were performed and it was successfully relieved by transanal division of the retained colorectal spur by using the autostapling instrument. The need for this reoperative therapy in these cases has led us to abandon the classic [spur crushing] Duhamel operation." They objected, as others had, to the week or more that it required the spur crushers to slough out, to the necessity for immobilization of the baby in Bryant's orthopedic traction or by other techniques, etc. In the discussion of Grosfeld's paper, Soper (1978) of Iowa City said that he now had swung over to the use of the GIA™ staplers in his modification of the Duhamel operation.

From Kuala Lumpur, Malaysia, Somasundaram (1978), discussing pediatric surgery in Malaysia and reporting 33 Duhamel operations, stated, "One significant observation is the low incidence of a rectal pouch, and this is perhaps the single most significant advantage of the GIA stapler. Three children with a persistent rectal pouch required subsequent division of the colorectal septum. In these, the one important technical detail, emphasized by Steichen *et alii*. . .of applying the staples before closing the rectal stump was omitted and may have accounted for this complication.''

Hirai, Miyano, and Kitahara (1979) from the Juntendo University School of Medicine in Tokyo reported their use of the ''Z shaped primary colorectal side-to-side anastomosis using the GIA autosuture surgical stapling instrument. . .'', a modification of the Duhamel operation. In point of fact, the technique is almost precisely that described by us (Steichen, Talbert, and Ravitch, 1968; Talbert, Seashore, and Ravitch, 1974), the entire spur division being with a GIA^{TM} instrument passed from below, and in large children from both above and below. Twenty-five patients had been so operated on between May, 1973 and October, 1977, eight of these without a preliminary colostomy. There was one anastomotic leak producing peritonitis, which was found to be ''. . .leakage at the proximal anastomotic site. . .'', presumably referring to the hand-sutured closure.

Discussion at pediatric surgical meetings the world over would suggest that, in the Duhamel operation, spur division with the GIA^{TM} instrument now is the standard procedure.

We often have been asked whether the EEA^{TM} instrument might not be acceptable for low anastomosis in the treatment of Hirschsprung's disease. Our answer always has been that this would leave an aganglionic segment and, in essence, would be comparable to the old State (1950) and Rehbein (1955) operations, which have largely been abandoned, although they are not totally incompatible with good results. However, Hugh and Ibrahim (1979) from St. Vincent's Medical Center in Darlinghurst, New South Wales report the successful use of the EEA^{TM} instrument for Hirschsprung's disease in an adult male who had had multiple previous operations that had left some aganglionic left colon. The anastomosis was 4 cm above the anal verge and ''When seen one month after discharge from hospital, the patient was well, and had normal bowel actions, with slight incontinence on the one occasion only.'' The aganglionosis had been satisfactorily proved histologically.

In fact, as Swenson said in the original description of his operation, he was using the old Maunsell operation, originally designed to avoid the hazards of an intra-abdominal anastomosis.

OPERATIONS FOR RECTAL PROLAPSE

At the University of Minnesota, Vermeulen, Goldberg, and others (Vermeulen, Nivatvongs, Fang, Balcos, and Goldberg, 1983) have treated rectal prolapse with an extra-abdominal amputation of the redundant bowel and an externally made anastomosis with the EEA^{TM} instrument (Fig IX–17). In essence, this applies modern stapling techniques to the almost-century-old operative principle of Maunsell. The prolapsed bowel having been amputated close to the anus, the ends of the everted anorectum and of the colon passed through it, are pursestringed. The inner segment—colon—is pulled down, the anvil-nose cone inserted, pursestrings tied, and the instrument advanced until the anorectal pursestring can be tied around the shaft. The instrument is operated in the usual fashion, withdrawn, and the everted anastomosis tacked back above the sphincters.

In nine women, average age 79 years, there were no deaths, no recurrences, no

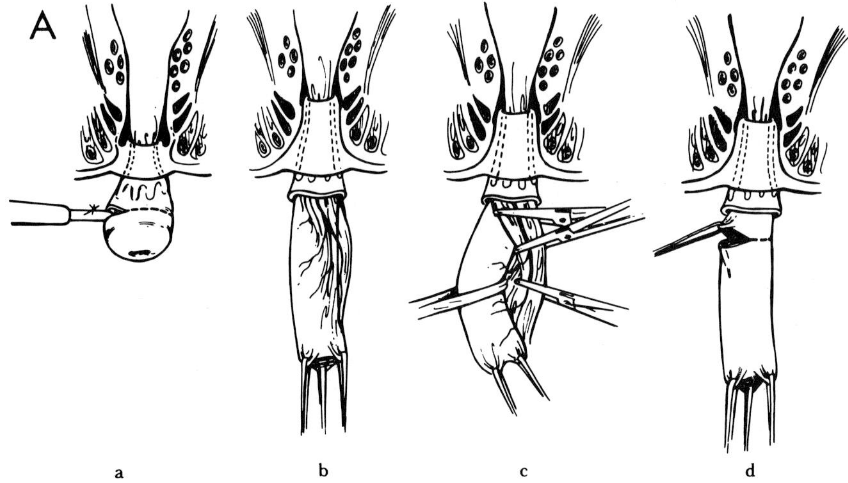

FIG. 1. a, Beginning of incision 1.5 centimeters from dentate line. b, Unfolding of prolapsing segment. c, Division of mesentery. d, Division of inner tube of intestine.

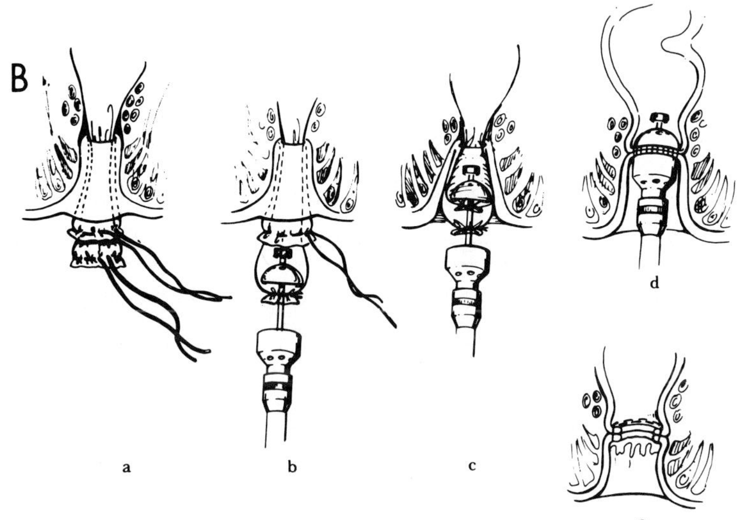

FIG. 2. a, Placement of pursestring sutures. b, Proximal pursestring suture secured around anvil. c, Distal pursestring suture secured. d, Closure of instrument, ready for firing. e, Completed anastomosis.

Fig IX–17.—Extra-abdominal resection of rectum for prolapse. The Minnesota group apply the EEA™ instrument to the Maunsell technique of perineal rectosigmoidectomy for rectal prolapse. In nine female patients of average age 79, operative time varied from 35 to 80 minutes; average blood loss was 120 ml. One patient subsequently bled from the anastomosis and required a single stitch placed per anum. There were no other complications, all patients became continent, and there were no recurrences of prolapse. (From F.D. Vermeulen, S. Nivatvongs, D.T. Fang, E.G. Balcos, and S.M. Goldberg, *SG&O* 156:84, 1983.)

incontinence. One woman required a single stitch to control bleeding from the anastomosis, the only complication.

REFERENCES

Adloff M.: Personal communication, August 16, 1982.

Adloff M., Arnaud J.P., Beeharry S., Turbelin J.M.: Side-to-end anastomosis in low anterior resection with the EEA stapler. *Dis. Colon Rectum* 23:456, 1980.

Athanasiadis S., Barry B.A., Gandji D., Girona J.: Vergleichende Behandlungsergebnisse der maschinellen (EEA und SPTU Staplers) und der manuellen Anastomosetechnik in der Colon- und Rectumchirurgie (abstract). 98th Kongress Deutsche Gesellschaft für Chirurgie, Munich, April 22–25, 1981.

Athanasiadis S., Barry B.A., Girona J.: Vergleich der Behandlungsergebnisse bei Dickdarmanastomosen mit den Klammernahtgeräten EEA und SPTU in einem Kollektiv von 260 Patienten. *Langenbecks Arch. Chir.* 354:111, 1981.

Beart R.W., Kelly K.A.: Randomized prospective evaluation of the EEA stapler for colorectal anastomoses. *Am. J. Surg.* 141:143, 1981.

Becker H., Probst M., Ungeheuer E.: Die maschinelle Anastomose nach anterior Rectumresektion. *Chirurg* 51:341, 1980.

Bérard Ph., Papillon M., Jacquemard R., Labrosse H., Bigay D., Guillemin G.: L'anastomose colo-rectale basse a la pince EEA dans la chirurgie du cancer du rectum. *J. Chir.* (Paris) 118:115, 1981.

Berthold S., Alexander-Williams J., Hänni K., Eckmann L.: Erste Erfahrungen mit einem automatischen Klammernahtgerät für enterale Anastomosen. *Chirurg* 51:671, 1980.

Bolton R.A., Britton D.C.: Restorative surgery of the rectum with a circumferential stapler. *Lancet* 1:850, 1980.

Bricker E.M., Johnston W.D., Patwardhan R.V.: Repair of postirradiation damage to colorectum. *Ann. Surg.* 193:555, 1981.

Brodman R.F., Brodman H.R.: Defunctionalizing a colostomy (Letter to the Editor). *Arch. Surg.* 110:352, 1975.

Brown A.A., Gasson J.E., Brown R.A.: Experience with the EEA stapler in carcinoma of the lower rectum. *S. Afr. Med. J.* 59:258, 1981.

Buchmann P., Uhlschmid G., Hollinger A.: Erfahrungen mit dem EEA-stapler bei Kolonanastomosen. *Helv. Chir. Acta* 47:645, 1980.

Burrington J.D., Wayne E.R.: Modified Duhamel procedure for treatment of total aganglionic colon in childhood. *J. Pediatr. Surg.* 11:391, 1976.

Cade D., Gallagher P., Schofield P.F., Turner L.: Complications of anterior resection of the rectum using the EEA stapling device. *Br. J. Surg.* 68:339, 1981.

Cady J., Godfroy J., Sibaud O., Mercadier M.: La désunion anastomotique en chirurgie colique et rectale. Étude comparative des procédés de suture manuelle et mécanique à propos d'une série de 149 résections. *Ann. Chir.* 34:350, 1980.

Cutait D.E., Cutait R., da Silva J.H., Manzione A., Kiss D.R., Lourencão J.L., Calache J.E.: Stapled anastomosis in colorectal surgery. *Dis. Colon Rectum* 24:155, 1981.

Cutait D.E., Cutait R., da Silva J.H., Manzione A., Lourencão J.L., Calache J.E., Nahas S., Raia A.: Sutura mecânica por grampeamento na anastomose colo ou íleo-retal em ressecções por lesões malignas e benignas do intestino grosso. *Rev. Hosp. Clin. Fac. Med. São Paulo* 35:72, 1980.

Detry R.J., Kestens P.J.: Colorectal anastomoses with the EEA stapler. *World J. Surg.* 5:739, 1981.

Detry R., Otte J.B., Kestens P.J.: Rapport de l'agrafeuse EEA dans la chirurgie colo-rectale. *Acta Chir. Belg.* 1:11, 1981.

Dorricott N.J., Baddeley R.M., Keighley M.R.B., Oates G.D., Alexander-Williams J.: Fifty rectal anastomoses with the EEA stapling instrument: Clinical and radiological leak rates. *Gut* 21:A466, 1980.

Dorsey J.S., Stone R.M.: Low anterior anastomosis with surgical stapler (Letter to the Editor). *Arch. Surg.* 114:639, 1979.

Dudgeon D.L., Coran A.G., Rosenkrantz J.G.: Septum reformation: A complication of the Duhamel procedure. *Surgery* 73:274, 1973.

Duhamel B.: Une nouvelle opération pour le mégacolon congénital: L'abaissement rétro-rectal et trans-anal du colon et son application possible au traitement de quelques autres malformations. *Presse Méd.* 64:2249, 1956.

Duhamel B.: Technique de l'abaissement rétro-rectal et trans-anal. *Ann. Chir. Infant.* 11:88, 1970.

Engelberg M., Reiss R., Saba K.: A simple technique for verification of the competence of gastrointestinal anastomoses with the circular stapling device. *Arch. Surg.* 116:482, 1981.

Fahrenkrug L., Clemmesen T.: Anvendelse af et autosuturinstrument i gastroenterologisk kirurgi. *Ugeskr. Laeger* 143:263, 1981.

Fain S.N.: A new USA stapling apparatus (EEA-31) for a low anterior resection of the rectum. *Am. J. Proctol. Gastroenterol. Colon Rectal Surg.* 37:20, 25–26, 1980.

Fain S.N., Patin C.S., Morgenstern L.: Use of a mechanical suturing apparatus in low colorectal anastomosis. *Arch. Surg.* 110:1079, 1975.

Fasching W., Moritz E.: Zirkuläre Klammeranastomosen im Magen-Darm-Trakt mit den Klammernahtgeräten SPTU und EEA. *Chirurg* 51:644, 1980.

Ferguson E.F. Jr., Houston C.H.: Simplified anterior resection: Use of the TA stapler. *Dis. Colon Rectum* 18:311, 1975.

Fiala J-M., Marti M-C., Meyer P., Rohner A.: L'agrafeuse EEA en chirurgie colique. *Helv. Chir. Acta* 47:639, 1980.

Fischer J.E.: Personal communication, August 2, 1982.

Fratkin L.B.: Personal communication, April 8, 1981.

Goligher J.C.: Recent trends in the practice of sphincter-saving excision for rectal cancer. *Ann. R. Coll. Surg. Engl.* 61:169, 1979.

Goligher J.C.: Use of circular stapling gun with peranal insertion of anorectal purse-string suture for construction of very low colorectal or colo-anal anastomoses. *Br. J. Surg.* 66:501, 1979.

Goligher J.C., Lee P.W.R., Macfie J., Simpkins K.C., Lintott D.J.: Experience with the Russian Model 249 suture gun for anastomosis of the rectum. *Surg. Gynecol. Obstet.* 148:517, 1979.

Graham H.K., Johnston G.W., McKelvey S.T.D., Kennedy T.L.: Five years' experience in stapling the oesophagus and rectum. *Br. J. Surg.* 68:697, 1981.

Grosfeld J.L., Ballantine V.N., Csicsko J.F.: A critical evaluation of the Duhamel operation for Hirschsprung's disease. *Arch. Surg.* 113:454, 1978.

Hänni K., Berthold S., Alexander-Williams J., Eckmann L.: End-zu-End-Anastomose mit dem EEA-Stapler: Himweise zu technischen Details. *Helv. Chir. Acta* 47:651, 1980.

Harford F.J. Jr.: Use of glucagon in conjunction with the end-to-end anastomosis (EEA) stapling device for low anterior anastomoses. *Dis. Colon Rectum* 22:452, 1979.

Heald R.J.: Towards fewer colostomies—the impact of circular stapling devices on the surgery of rectal cancer in a district hospital. *Br. J. Surg.* 67:198, 1980.

Heald R.J., Leicester R.J.: The low stapled anastomosis. *Dis. Colon Rectum* 24:437, 1981.

Hirai Y., Miyano T., Kitahara T.: Z shaped primary colorectal anastomosis using the GIA autosuture for Hirschsprung's disease. *Jpn. J. Surg.* 9:132, 1979.

Hugh T.B., Ibrahim N.: Transanal stapled anastomosis after resection for Hirschsprung's disease. *Med. J. Aust.* 1:578, 1979.

Kalinina T.V.: The use of mechanical suturing for the creation of anastomoses between the rectum and the small or large intestine. *Klin. Khir.* (Kiev) 10:56, 1966.

Kirkegaard P.: A new technique for low anterior resection of the rectum. *Dan. Med. Bull.* 25:235, 1978.

Kirkegaard P., Christiansen J., Hjortrup A.: Anterior resection of mid-rectal cancer with the EEA stapling instrument. *Am. J. Surg.* 140:312, 1980.

Kirkegaard P., Christiansen J., Lauritzen B., Henrichsen S., Jörgensen M.: Primary results after resection and anastomosis for mid-rectal cancer with a new stapling instrument. A primary report. *Acta Chir. Scand.* 145:321, 1979.

Kirwan W.O.: Integrity of low colorectal EEA-stapled anastomosis. *Br. J. Surg.* 68:539, 1981.

Knight C.D.: Personal communication, January 25 and April 23, 1982, and May 20, 1983.

Knight C.D., Griffen F.D.: An improved technique for low anterior resection of the rectum using the EEA stapler. *Surgery* 88:710, 1980.

Krause R., Freund H.R., Fischer J.E.: A new technique for performing end enterostomies using a stapling device. *Am. J. Surg.* 138:461, 1979.

Laitinen S., Huttunen R., Ståhlberg M., Mokka R., Kairaluoma M., Larmi T.K.I.: Experience with the EEA stapling instrument for colorectal anastomosis. *Ann. Chir. Gynaecol.* 69:102, 1980.

Lantin A., Lantin F., Vandeperre J.: Les anastomoses rectales basses à la pince mécanique EEA. Premiers résultats de 24 résections antérieures du rectum. *Acta Chir. Belg.* 1:17, 1981.

Lazorthes F., Gadrat F., Legrand G., Cordova J.A., Monrozies X., Fretigny E., Pugnet G.: Anastomose rectale mécanique a la EEA. Appréciation de soixante cas. *Ann. Chir.* 35:374, 1981.

Ling L., Brommé A., Rydén S.: Low anterior resection using stapling instrument. *Acta Chir. Scand.* 145:487, 1979.

Lister J.: The control of fluid loss in long-segment Hirschsprung's disease. *J. Pediatr. Surg.* 4:657, 1969.

Marti M-C., Fiala J-M., Rohner A.: EEA stapler in large bowel surgery. *World J. Surg.* 5:735, 1981.

Martin L.W.: Surgical management of Hirschsprung's disease involving the small intestine. *Arch. Surg.* 97:183, 1968.

Martin L.W.: Surgical management of total colonic aganglionosis. *Ann. Surg.* 176:343, 1972.

Martin L.W.: In Ravitch M.M., et al. (eds.): *Pediatric Surgery,* 3d ed. Chicago, Year Book Medical Publishers, 1979, pp. 1056–1058.

Mittal V.K., Cortez J.A.: Hartmann procedure reconstruction with EEA stapler. *Dis. Colon Rectum* 24:215, 1981.

Otte J.B., Kestens P.J., Pringot J.: Rétablissement de la continuité colo-rectale, après opération de Hartmann, par anastomose selon la technique de Duhamel simplifiée par l'emploi de l'agrafeuse américaine GIA. *Acta Chir. Belg.* 74:142, 1975.

Pagès R.: Le cul-de-sac de l'opération de Duhamel. *Ann. Chir. Infant.* 11:123, 1970.

Parrish R.A.: Modified Duhamel operation for Hirschsprung's disease. *Am. Surg.* 43:283, 1977.

Photopulos G.J., Jones R.W., Walton L.A., Fowler W.C. Jr.: A simplified method of complete diversionary colostomy for patients with radiation-induced proctosigmoiditis. *Gynecol. Oncol.* 5:180, 1977.

Polglase A.L., Hughes E.S.R., McDermott F.T.: Improved techniques in EEA stapling for ultra low colorectal and colo-anal anastomosis. *Aust. N. Z. J. Surg.* 51:211, 1981.

Probst M., Becker H., Ungeheuer E.: Vergleich der Ergebnisse von konservativer Nahttechnik und maschinelle Anastomosierung bei anteriorer Rektumresektion (abstract). 98th Kongress Deutsche Gesellschaft für Chirurgie, Munich, April 22–25, 1981.

Ravitch M.M.: The use of stapling instruments in surgery of the gastrointestinal tract, with a note on a new instrument for end-to-end low rectal and oesophagojejunal anastomoses. *Aust. N. Z. J. Surg.* 48:444, 1978.

Ravitch M.M., Canalis F., Weinshelbaum A., McCormick J.: Studies in intestinal healing: III. Observations on everting intestinal anastomoses. *Ann. Surg.* 166:670, 1967.

Ravitch M.M., Steichen F.M.: Technics of staple suturing in the gastrointestinal tract. *Ann. Surg.* 175:815, 1972.

Ravitch M.M., Steichen F.M.: A stapling instrument for end-to-end inverting anastomoses in the gastrointestinal tract. *Ann. Surg.* 189:791, 1979.

Rehbein F., Wernicke H.H.: Erfahrungen bei der Operation der Hirschsprungschen Krankheit. *Bruns' Beitr. Klin. Chir.* 191:18, 1955.

Reuter M.J.P.: Les sutures mécaniques en chirurgie digestive et pulmonaire. Thesis, presented in 1982 at Université Louis Pasteur, Faculté de Médecine de Strasbourg, France.

Reynolds W. Jr.: Low anterior resection using an automatic anastomosing instrument. *Am. J. Surg.* 124:433, 1972.

Rignault D., Pailler J-L., Berthet A., Tardat M.: Les sutures mécaniques automatiques en chirurgie digestive. Appréciation de la méthode après 3 ans d'utilisation de l'appareillage américain. *Chirurgie* 102:945, 1976.

Robbins R.D., Sohn N., Weinstein M.A., Steichen F.M.: A simplified technique utilizing the EEA suture device for re-establishing intestinal continuity following Hartmann's operation. *Colo-Proctol.* III:266, 1981.

Schaeffer C.J., Giordano J.M.: Complications associated with EEA stapler in performance of low anterior resections. *Am. Surg.* 47:426, 1981.

Shahinian T.K., Bowen J.R., Dorman B.A., Soderberg C.H. Jr., Thompson W.R.: Experience with the EEA stapling device. *Am. J. Surg.* 139:549, 1980.

Smith L.E.: Anastomosis with EEA stapler after anterior colonic resection. *Dis. Colon Rectum* 24:236, 1981.

Somasundaram K.: The current practice of paediatric surgery in Malaysia. *Aust. N. Z. J. Surg.* 48:356, 1978.

Soper R.T.: In discussion of Grosfeld J.L., Ballantine V.N., Csicsko J.F. *Arch. Surg.* 113:454, 1978.

State D., Rogers W.: The surgical treatment of idiopathic congenital megacolon (Hirschsprung's disease). *Univ. Minn. Med. Bull.* 22:164, 1950.

Steichen F.M., Richards V., Chassin J.L., Weakley F.L., Welter R.: Staplers in intestinal surgery (symposium). *Contemp. Surg.* 14:51, 1979.

Steichen F.M., Talbert J.L., Ravitch M.M.: Primary side-to-side colorectal anastomosis in the Duhamel operation for Hirschsprung's disease. *Surgery* 64:475, 1968.

Stoller J.L., Dowell A.J., Atkinson K.G.: Colorectal anastomosis by transanal end-to-end stapling. *Can. J. Surg.* 23:461, 1980.

Talbert J.L., Seashore J.H., Ravitch M.M.: Evaluation of a modified Duhamel operation for correction of Hirschsprung's disease. *Ann. Surg.* 179:671, 1974.

Thiede A., Jostarndt L., Troidl H., Poser H.L., Bertz U., Hamelmann H.: Der Wert der zirkulären maschinellen Colon- und Rectumananastomose (EEA). *Chirurg* 52:30, 1981.

Thiede A., Jostarndt L., Troidl H., Poser H., Hamelmann H.: Prospektive Studie zum Wert der maschinellen Colon- und Rektum-Anastomosen mit Auto-Suture-Klammernahtgerät EEA (abstract). Münchner Symposium Colo-Rectale Chirurgie im Klinikim Rechts der Isar München, 28 Juni, 1980.

Thiede A., Troidl H., Poser H., Jostarndt L., Hamelmann H.: Prospektive Studie zum Auto-Suture-Klammernahtgerät für Kolon- und Rektumanastomosen. *Zentralbl. Chir.* 105:825, 1980.

Vermeulen F.D., Nivatvongs S., Fang D.T., Balcos E.G., Goldberg S.M.: A technique for perineal rectosigmoidectomy using autosuture devices. *Surg. Gynecol. Obstet.* 156:84, 1983.

Weakley F.L. (Moderator), Beart R.W. Jr., Bubrick M.P., Smith L.E. (Panelists): Symposium: The use and misuse of staples in colonic surgery. *Dis. Colon Rectum* 24:231, 1981.

Wheeless C.R. Jr.: Avoidance of permanent colostomy in pelvic malignancy using the surgical stapler. *Obstet. Gynecol.* 54:501, 1979.

Wheeless C.R. Jr.: Personal communication, July 7, 1981 and July 30, 1982.

CHAPTER X

Urologic and Gynecologic Operations, Skin and Fascia Closure

GENITOURINARY SURGERY

THE CONSTRUCTION OF extrapolated intestinal loops as conduits for urinary diversion procedures is presented in Chapter VIII, "Operations on the Small and Large Bowel," where it would seem most logically to belong, particularly since the stapling techniques are exclusively used to deal with the intestine. Obviously, the TA™ instruments would lend themselves beautifully to segmental resection of the bladder and staple closure were it not for the concern over the likelihood that with these nonabsorbable sutures, stones might form just as they do occasionally in intestinal conduits. However, Healey and Warren (1978) from the University of Texas Medical Branch in Galveston resected the dome of the bladder to the extent of about half of the bladder wall in 12 dogs, closing them with the TA™ staplers. An indwelling Foley urethral catheter was removed the day after operation. The dogs were sacrificed weekly for the first four weeks. No additional sutures were taken in the bladder. Urine cultures were taken at the end of the first week and at the time of sacrifice. The single positive urine culture—*Proteus mirabilis*—was in the dog sacrificed at one week. "Postmortem examination of the urinary bladder showed that the mucosa healed promptly and completely covered the staples by one week. In no case did the staples migrate through the bladder wall into the lumen. By 9 months, the bladder mucosa was grossly normal with no sign of intravesical encroachment."

These results, if confirmed in a larger series of animals, might well justify the use of stapling closures after partial cystectomy. As Healey and Warren state, it is possible that infected urine, or incomplete evacuation of the bladder, which would be expected in many clinical cases, might result in a different outcome. We have the problem under study in the laboratory. It is likely that the use of the staples in closure of the bladder will depend on the development of absorbable staples.

In nephrectomy, we have anecdotal accounts of the use of the LDS™ and TA™ instruments for control of the renal hilus. From the Crimean Medical Institute, Khalid (1981) reports experience with the use of the UKL-60—equivalent to the TA 55™ instrument—in 104 partial nephrectomies in earlier Russian experience. They took care to close the jaws of the instruments slowly so as not to tear the capsule of the kidney. The preservation of intact capsule and suturing through healthy tissues were thought to be of primary importance. Not infrequently, additional sutures were necessary for hemostasis. There were no instances of postoperative bleeding. The complication rate was 3.8% compared to 15.6% in their simultaneous experience with the same operation performed with manual sutures. A specific shortcoming of the stapler was that it could not be applied to portions of the kidney thicker than 2.5 cm or (for the UKL-60) broader than 6 cm. We are aware of no Western reports of partial nephrectomy by staple techniques.

There has been a good deal of interest in the possibility of using the circumferential staplers of the type of the Russian vascular staplers for end-to-end ureteral anastomoses, with reports from Halle in Germany by Panzner (1966), by Klopper of Amsterdam (1967), from Canada, with his own stapler, by Vogelfanger (Vogelfanger, Irvine, and Collins, 1967), from Hungary by Furka (1968), and from the Mayo Clinic by Hacker (Hacker, Wakim, Utz, and Harrison, 1968). Irvine, Leahy, and Vogelfanger (1970), after extensive animal experience, undertook clinical trials with Vogelfanger's vascular stapler and used it in 11 ureteral anastomoses in which they had a single temporary ureteral fistula. There were no obstructions and no urinary tract infection. The experimental results and the preliminary clinical results suggest that staples can be well tolerated in end-to-end, mucosa-to-mucosa, everting ureteral anastomoses, and one would suppose that the adoption of stapling techniques for ureteral anastomosis awaits the development of an instrument whose use is less complicated than that of the vascular-type circular staplers thus far available.

The use of the LDS™ stapler for division and occlusion of the vas deferens in vasectomy, an obvious application (Weiss and Vallejos, 1972), has been popular with some urologists.

GYNECOLOGIC OPERATIONS

We do not ourselves perform elective hysterectomies as a rule, but in the occasional hysterectomy, usually in connection with abdominoperineal resection, we have taken the ovarian vessels with the LDS™ instrument (the uterine vessels are too close to the cervix to permit convenient use of the LDS™ instrument) and generally have stapled (TA 55™) the vaginal vault without any complications in that small experience (20 cases in the 1967–76 series). We also occasionally use the LDS™ instrument to divide and occlude the salpinges for sterilization in the course of laparotomy for other purposes. There is a moderate literature concerned with the use of Auto Suture® instruments in gynecologic surgery, and the probability is that this underrepresents a large volume of gynecologic surgery performed with the staplers.

Kahn from Pietermaritzburg Hospital in South Africa (1968) used the TA™ instruments for suture of the vaginal cuff in 22 patients without difficulty or complication. He thought that one of the advantages might be that there is no decrease in width and no tenting of the vagina as might occur with sutures. There were no complications of any kind and subsequent sexual intercourse was reported to be uneventful.

Albert (1971) from Alice, Texas reported with enthusiasm the use of the GIA™ instrument on the broad ligament ". . .during 11 vaginal hysterectomies and in 13 anterior and posterior repairs, and the TA 30 at the uterine cornua during 13 vaginal hysterectomies." In his technique of vaginal hysterectomy, Albert placed the GIA™ instrument adjacent to the cervix and the uterus on each side, thus freeing the uterus but for its cornual attachments. He comments that "Usually, the uterine arteries will be actively spurting, and figure-eight suture ligature of atraumatic chromic 1, 0 or 00 catgut is applied to control each artery." The TA 30™ instrument then was applied to gather up all of the cornual attachments. The colpoplasties were done by freeing up the vaginal flaps, drawing them between the limbs of the GIA™ instrument, and suturing the flaps together with the GIA™ instrument, simultaneously amputating the excess tissue. Albert went on to say, "Without exception, the postoperative course of these patients has been good, better than that of patients treated by the conventional methods." As for the wire sutures in the colpoplasties, "Most of the wire sutures in the vaginal mucosa remain with the patient. Although they are external when applied, most of them will be buried or internalized in the healing process and will not be a source of trouble. Occasionally, a patient will notice a wire suture appearing on the pad. . . .After two or three weeks, some of the staples will be loose and can be picked out easily in the office. . . .In about six weeks, the patient may again have coitus. None of the patients have had any coital difficulties. Their sexual partners likewise have not complained." Albert (1974) continued to be enthusiastic: "I have used the GIA in the broad ligaments of 36 vaginal hysterectomies and in 42 anterior and posterior repairs, and the TA 30 at the uterine cornua of 33 vaginal hysterectomies. (This does not include the many times I have used the Auto Suture instruments in the broad ligaments or at the cornua during abdominal surgery, where several times I have even been able to apply the TA 90 instrument on each side so that only these two applications sufficed to completely remove the uterus and to close the end of the vagina as well.)" There still were essentially no complications and no complaints.

With respect to hysterectomy, it is obvious that the vessels in the broad ligament can be controlled with the LDS™ instrument, and with less certainty with the TA™ instrument. Albert's technique of vaginal hysterectomy in which the GIA™ instrument is inserted close to the cervix and the uterine wall, and the uterine artery subsequently transfixed in the stapled tissue, will have to be evaluated further before it can be recommended. Stapling of the vaginal vault with the TA™ instrument is expeditious, quick, and secure. Patients should be warned that an occasional staple may have to be removed at the time of speculum examination during the follow-up period, and this appears to be the common resolution of the problem among gynecologists utilizing staple suture of the vaginal vault.

Messitt (1977) reported two patients complaining of dyspareunia after hysterectomies in which the vaginal vault had been closed with staples. In both cases, the dyspareunia was relieved by "removal of the apical vaginal scar." The staples were not exposed to the lumen, and the description of the gross appearance suggests the possibility that there were cysts in the suture line, filled with desquamated epithelium, which could be expressed. No histologic description is given.

We have anecdotal accounts of discomfort to the male during intercourse, with a subsequent finding of open staples in the vaginal suture line, but have seen no published report to this effect.

The drawings of Sedwitz and associates from Raleigh, North Carolina (Sedwitz, Brashear, Tucker, Thomas, and Wilson, 1978) show broad and round ligaments being taken with the TA™ instruments, the uterine vessels and the uterosacral ligaments with hemoclips, and the vagina, distal to the cervix, with the TA™ instrument. This staple-enthusiastic group also use the LDS™ instrument for appendectomy, the fascial staplers for the linea alba, and the skin staplers for the skin. They report an experience with 100 patients. They consider their results better than before they adopted the staplers, and the operating time shorter, but give no analysis of their experience and say nothing about sexual function.

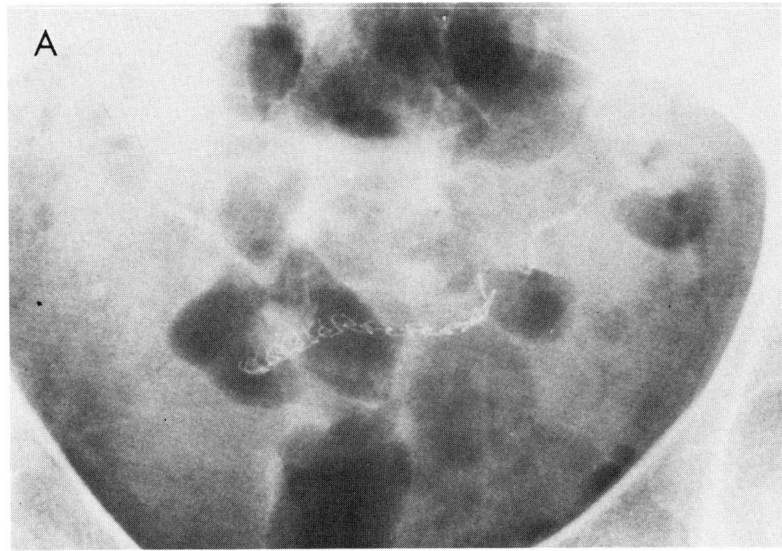

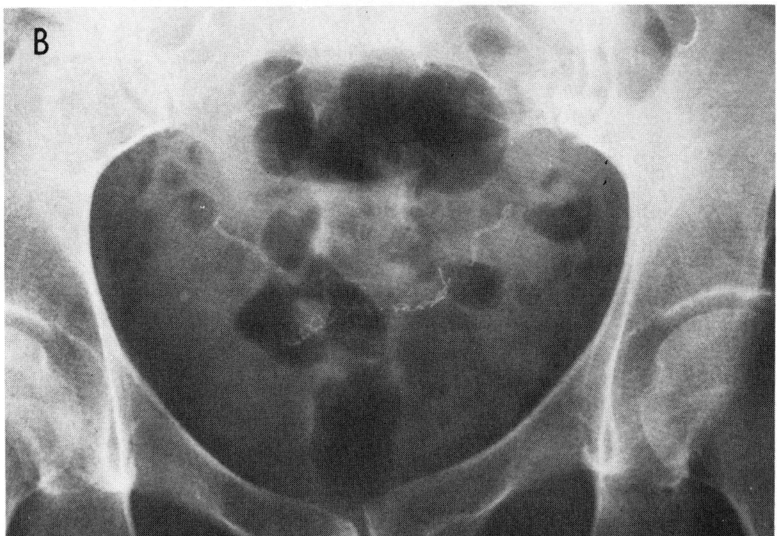

Fig X–1.—Stapling of the vaginal vault in hysterectomy—fate of the staples. A prospective study of the fate of the staples in the vaginal vault being undertaken by clinical examination and by repeated radiography suggests that in sexually active women ". . . the length of the line of staples increases after surgery and this may well be due to restretching of the vaginal vault. During this process, there would appear to be some unfolding of staples but never to the point where they are completely opened." (Photographs and comments from J.M. Beresford, Ottawa, Ontario, 1982.)　　　→

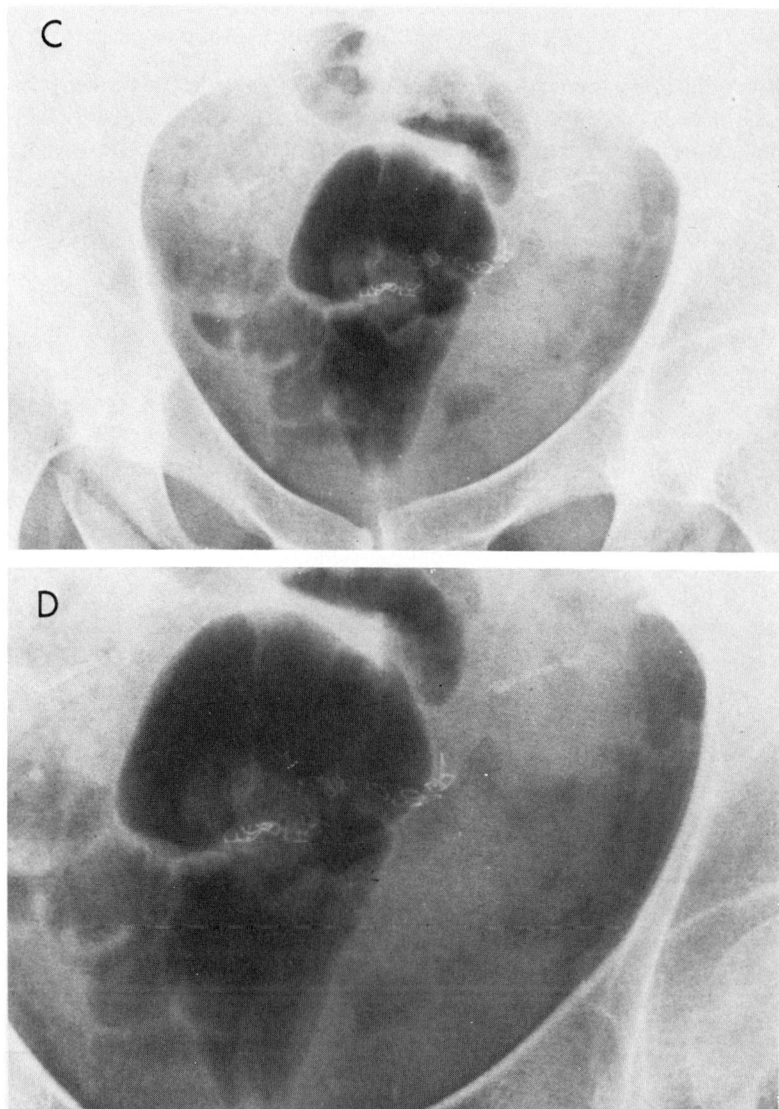

Fig X–1 (cont.) C–D.

There are Russian references both to total hysterectomy and to supravaginal hysterectomy (!) with the staplers.

Beresford in Ottawa (1982) currently is engaged in a prospective study of hysterectomy with stapling techniques (Fig X–1). One of the questions that has been raised is whether, with sexual activity, the staples in the vaginal vault might not open up and gradually become dislodged, as they do in gastric partitioning. The follow-up is too short for evaluation.

SKIN AND FASCIA CLOSURE

Simply on the basis of the numbers of cases in which the instruments are used, certainly the skin stapler in its various forms is the most widely utilized. We, like so many others, use the skin stapler essentially for all skin closures. The advantages are swiftness, precision of application, and ease of removal. If the staples are properly applied with the instrument held lightly against the skin, the bar of the staple will be clear of the skin, and even if the staples are left in for a week there will be no cross-hatching of the skin. We generally use subcutaneous sutures with the staples but others do not.

The staples are conveniently used for tacking down split-thickness skin grafts, spread out on petrolatum gauze to keep the split-thickness skin edges from rolling up. The gauze is patterned to the size of an individual piece of skin and the staples are placed through gauze and skin to attach the graft to the edges of the wound and to anchor gauze and skin to the inside of the fresh wound or granulating tissue of the chronic wound. Ideally, no dressing is required and the grafts can be inspected with ease. The petrolatum gauze backing is peeled off as it separates from the skin graft when it takes and grows into place. The staples will fall out, although occasionally some need to be removed after healing of the graft.

Fascial staples appear to perform satisfactorily, particularly for linea alba closures, and are popular among gynecologists. We are unaware of any prospective trials comparing the security of fascial staples to that of conventional suture techniques of closure of the abdominal wall. Anecdotally, we can report the use of fascial staples without retention sutures in patients with cirrhotic and malignant ascites, for fast midline abdominal closures. Despite early, and at times massive, reaccumulation of ascitic fluid, so far we have not observed any dehiscence. Most of these patients have not survived long enough to permit long-term follow-up with respect to hernia formation. In all patients in whom we plan a staple closure, the linea alba is cleared for 0.75–1 cm on each side of the midline as the incision is made. Facial closure is greatly facilitated by placing several traction sutures and introducing a narrow, malleable retractor behind the fascia to resist the pressure made with the stapler.

For the most part, skin stapling has been enthusiastically accepted and has not been the subject of publications. Farringer's (1973) experience was with an early model of the skin stapler powered by a CO_2 cartridge that was inserted into the sterilized instrument. He analyzed his experience at the Baptist Hospital in Nashville, Tennessee with 100 patients. In ten patients, half of the skin incisions were closed with 4-0 silk and half with stainless steel staples, the patients reporting less discomfort on removal of the staples than from cutting of the silk sutures. In 89 of the patients with laparotomies, the fascial closure was with staples. In these 89, two complications were reported, one disruption in a patient with advanced cirrhosis operated on for an incarcerated incisional hernia and one patient who developed an incisional hernia four months after gastrectomy. The statement is made in both cases that the staples were "intact" at the time of reoperation. Farringer noted that in two patients with perforated appendices and one with perforated diverticulum of the sigmoid and an abscess there was no extrusion of the staples and the wounds healed well.

REFERENCES

Albert R.O.: Automatic staplers for vaginal hysterectomy and colpoplasties. *Obstet. Gynecol.* 37:297, 1971.

Albert R.O.: Use of automatic staplers in vaginal hysterectomy, anterior colpoplasty, and posterior colpoperineoplasty. *Tex. Med.* 70:66, 1974.

Beresford J.M.: Personal communication, February 26, 1982.

Farringer J.L. Jr.: An auto-suture instrument. *Am. J. Surg.* 125:382, 1973.

Furka I.: Ureteral anastomoses made by instrument suturing. *Acta Chir. Acad. Sci. Hung.* 9:53, 1968.

Hacker P.K., Wakim K.G., Utz D.G., Harrison E.G. Jr.: Effect of ureteral reanastomosis by stapling on ureteral and renal function. *J. Urol.* 100:598, 1968.

Healey G.B., Warren M.M.: Experimental closure of urinary bladders with surgical staples. *Invest. Urol.* 16:70, 1978.

Irvine A.H., Leahy C.F., Vogelfanger I.J.: Management of the ureter in renal transplantation. *Br. J. Urol.* 42:402, 1970.

Kahn E.: Auto-suture in abdominal hysterectomy. *Obstet. Gynecol.* 31:852, 1968.

Khalid M.: Mechanical tantalum suture in kidney resection. *Urol. Nephrol.* (Mosk) 3:49, 1981.

Klopper P.J.: Experimental anastomoses of the ureter. *Arch. Chir. Neerl.* 19:319, 1967.

Messitt J.J.: Dyspareunia from auto suture staples. *Obstet. Gynecol.* 49:369, 1977.

Panzer R.: Zur mechanischen End-zu-End-Naht des Ureters. *Chirurg* 37:558, 1966.

Sedwitz J.L., Brashear G.R., Tucker G., Thomas B.D., Wilson B.F.: Simplified technique for abdominal hysterectomy. *Int. Surg.* 63:99, 1978.

Vogelfanger I.J., Irvine A.H., Collins W.E.: Experimental orthotopic kidney transplantation. *Can. J. Surg.* 10:223, 1967.

Weiss F., Vallejos C.F.: Vasectomy technic using an auto-suture. *Int. Surg.* 57:660, 1972.

CHAPTER XI

Operations on the Lung

THE AMERICAN STAPLING INSTRUMENTS, once made available in the United States, were more rapidly adopted by the thoracic surgeons than by the general surgeons. The nature of pulmonary surgery is such that the superiority and safety of a technique is much more immediately demonstrated. The TA^{TM} and GIA^{TM} instruments for transection and stapling of the pulmonary parenchyma, as in wedge resection, excisional biopsies, or completion of fissures in lobectomy, have proved to provide swift, atraumatic, and secure closures without blood loss and with almost no risk of air leaks. It already had been our experience with the Russian instruments, confirmed with further use of the American instruments, that the anatomical dissection type of segmental resection now was obsolete and could be safely abandoned in favor of stapling off any sublobar portion of pulmonary parenchyma that required removal, as demonstrated by Amosov and Berezovsky (1961), who called these ''economical resections.'' If a segment of lung is of significant size, the vessels may be separately ligated and the stapler used on the pulmonary parenchyma and segmental bronchus. For major segments, the bronchus is secured, and ligated or sutured, and the stapler applied at the border of inflated and collapsed lung.

Many thoracic surgeons began with stapling of the pulmonary parenchyma, then cautiously extended to stapling of the bronchi and finally to stapling of the vessels. In point of fact, stapling of the vessels is as secure, or more secure than, careful suturing over the end of the vessels and substantially more secure than any other method of ligation or transfixion. In addition, only as much freeing up of the vessel is required as is necessary to pass the TA 30^{TM} instrument under the vessel whereas substantially more of the vessel needs to be freed for clamping and ligation or manual suturing. By the same token, in pulmonary resection for inflammatory disease, with a mass of glands frozen into the hilus, making the hilar structures difficult to mobilize, if vein, artery, or bronchus can be tunneled under, it can be stapled and divided with a security and safety not seen in the techniques formerly standard, opening up the hilus for easy attack on the remaining structures. As in surgery of the gastrointestinal tract, we stress the point that the stapling instruments must be brought down to the tissues to be stapled, particularly the bronchus and vessels, rather than pulling these structures up into the stapler. We tend to make the analogy with a pin that leaves a minute puncture when thrust through a collapsed rubber balloon but makes a substantial tear when put through a balloon stretched between the fingers. Just as with clamps, so with the stapler, there is some hazard in cracking the brittle main pulmonary artery or main bronchus of an elderly male, but probably somewhat less risk because the TA 30^{TM} instrument is substantially broader and closes more gently and more atraumatically than the narrow jaws of a vascular or bronchial clamp. With the TA^{TM} stapler, the pulmonary veins may be secured intrapericardially with remarkable ease, actually placing the stapler on the atrial wall.

So far as regards the size of the staples to be used, the single, most important point is that for the pulmonary vessels the fine vascular staples—the fine staples in the 30V white cartridge—must be used. For the somewhat thicker atrium, the blue cartridge with the 3.5 mm staples is best used. From our early experience with the Russian staplers in which the degree of compression was not automatically regulated by the thickness of the cartridge but by the degree to which the operator approximated the jaws, so that compression was governed by the feel of the tissues, we became convinced that there is a broad enough range of tolerance of the tissues to stapling so that, except at the extremes of age or size, either of the two American cartridges can be safely utilized for the bronchus. In large males, for the main bronchus, the green cartridge with the 4.8 mm staples is used, and in young women or children, the blue cartridge with the 3.5 mm staples for the bronchus. For moderate thicknesses of pulmonary parenchyma, we use the 3.5 mm staples; for great thicknesses of pulmonary parenchyma, we tend to use the 4.8 mm staples.

Our 1958 observations in Russia impressed us with the advantages and safety of pulmonary resection with the Russian stapling instruments. Our own experiments (Ravitch, Brown, and Daviglus, 1959) were completely supportive. The Western literature on pulmonary resection with staples is otherwise almost entirely clinical. Goldman (1964) (see Fig III–9) did demonstrate the passage of fine vessels in the pulmonary parenchyma, through the B-shaped staple closures.

From the National Heart and Lung Institute and the Surgery Branch of the National Cancer Institute, Scott and associates (Scott, Faraci, Goodman, Militano, Geelhoed, and Chretien, 1975) studied bronchial healing in dogs, after closure with 3-0 silk, 3-0 catgut, and staples. ". . . stumps closed with the automatic stapling device (TA-30) showed the best healing with a minimal degree of inflammation. These findings correlated well with leakage pressures. The average leakage pressure for the silk closed stumps was 139.44 mm Hg $\pm$ 78.9 SD. This was significantly lower ($P < 0.02$) than the average leakage pressure for staple closed stumps (251.25 mm Hg $\pm$ 82.9 SD). It is concluded that the minimal amount of inflammation following staple closure will be associated with improved bronchial stump healing and a lower incidence of bronchopleural fistula." The following year, Scott (Scott, Faraci, Hough, and Chretien, 1976) extended the experiments—this time with 3-0 silk sutures, 3-0 nylon sutures, and staples—to include study of collagen levels. Once more, the staples had the least exudative reaction, the highest collagen levels, and withstood significantly greater pressures before leaking. They concluded that "These results have clinical relevance to the selection of suture materials for stump closures."

Once more, the fundamental principles of surgery are not abrogated for the user of staples. The bronchi should be stapled flush with their parent bronchi—or the trachea, in the case of the main bronchus. Bronchi stapled through diseased portions, as with bronchial tuberculosis or Wegener's granulomatosis, may not heal. One significant disadvantage with stapling the bronchi is that one does not get as good an appreciation of the bronchial mucosa at the level of transection as one does with clamping and suturing. Therefore, if there is any question about tumor margin or the health of the bronchus, it may be necessary to open the bronchus for direct inspection, just distal to the proposed level of transection. A great advantage of bronchial stapling is that granulations around the staples and chronic cough requiring bronchoscopic removal of the staples, common enough when other types of nonabsorbable suture are used, do not occur.

The stapling instruments have completely altered the manner of procuring lung biopsies, excising bullae and blebs, wedging out coin lesions, and have made feasible and reasonable the excision of multiple pulmonary metastases.

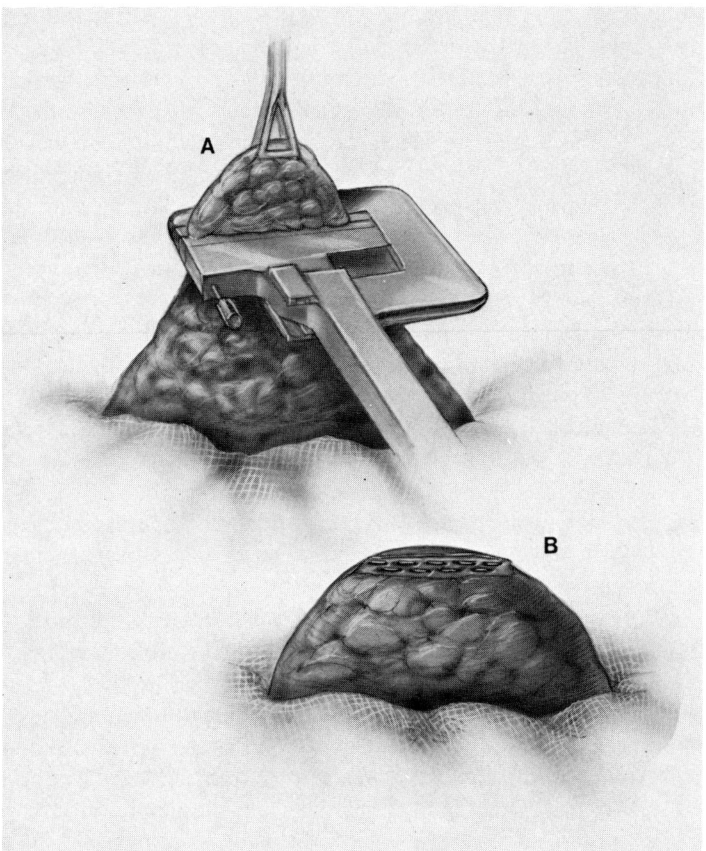

Fig XI–1.—Lung biopsy. **A,** if the situation of the lesion permits, as at the lobar apices, at the tip of the lingula, or sometimes on the convexity of the lobes, the tissue to be biopsied is simply held with the forceps while the TA™ instrument is slid below or behind the lesion until it is clear of the tissue to be excised. The jaws are closed, the staples fired, and the tissue cut away with the scalpel on the edge of the stapler. **B,** the closure is airtight and dry and rarely requires an additional suture.

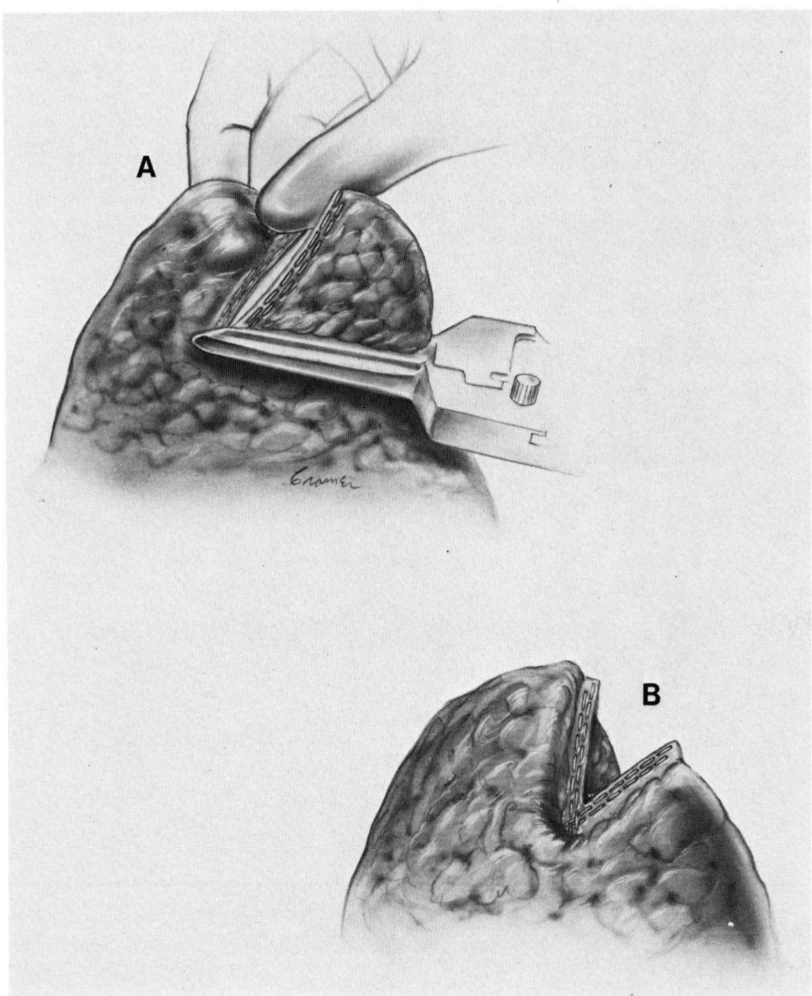

Fig XI–2.—Lung biopsy. Two applications of the GIA™ instrument permit a neat wedge excision. Obviously, the staple suture lines must overlap, but this has caused no problems. This technique is particularly applicable to the excision of lesions on lung surfaces away from the thin edges of the lobes.

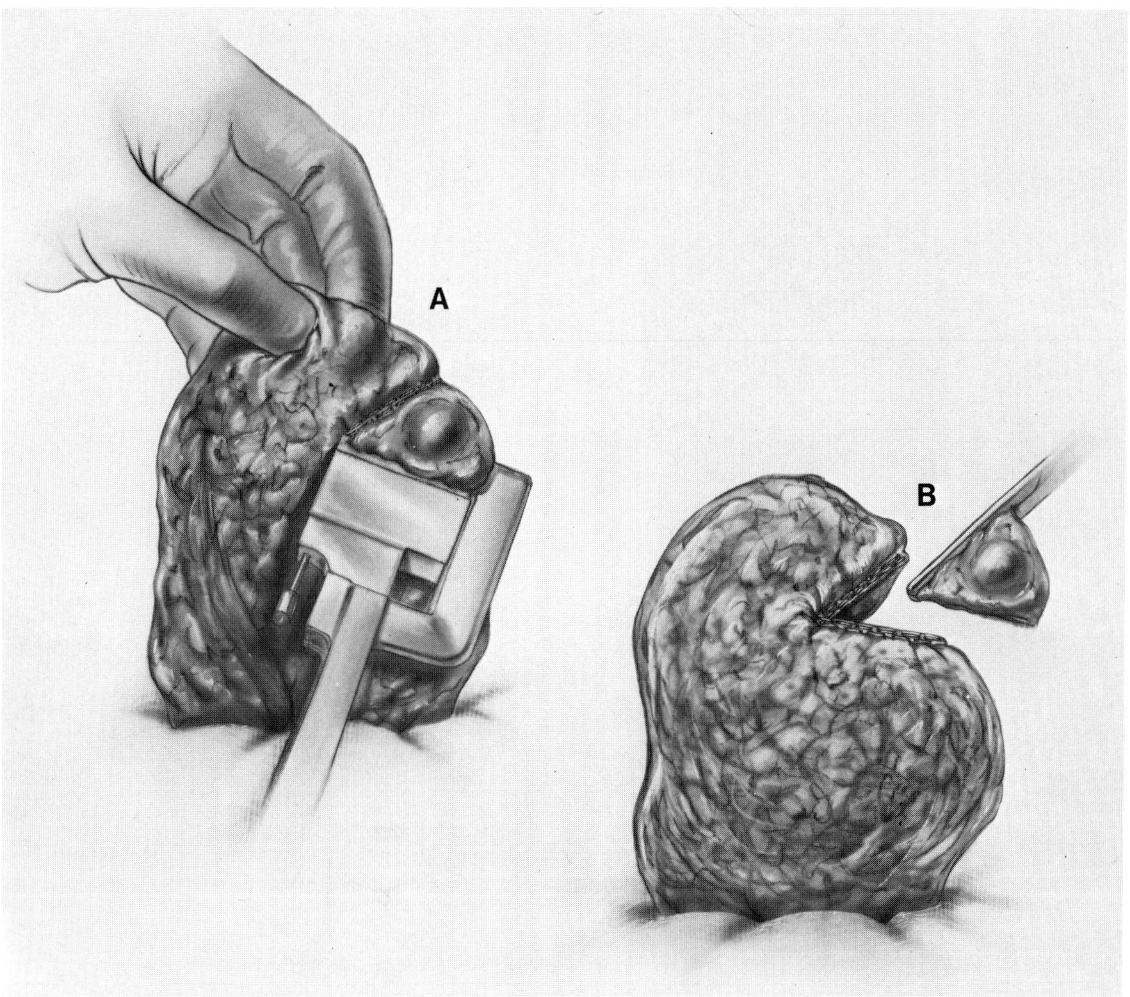

Fig XI–3.—Lung biopsy. Application of the TA™ instrument to a wedge excision of a tumor nodule. One can either press the tissue-retaining pin home into the lower jaw, causing a small hole in the lung, which may require a single suture at the apex of the resection, or simply ignore the pin in this not absolutely critical procedure, due to the fact that the readily compressible pulmonary tissue will not spring the jaws and invite deformation of the staples.

Fig XI–4.—Excision of large emphysematous bulla. A, the TA 90™ instrument is simply slid onto normal lung, immediately at the base of the large bullous sac, and the lung stapled. B, the reconstruction of the pulmonary surface is remarkably even. The ease and dependability of the instruments for this purpose have led us frequently, after resection of apical bullae, to staple off and excise multiple small bullae in the apex of the lower lobe, which we might have foregone in the days of the clamping and sewing technique because of the time, untidiness, the possibility of bleeding or air leak, and the loss of pulmonary parenchyma.　　　→

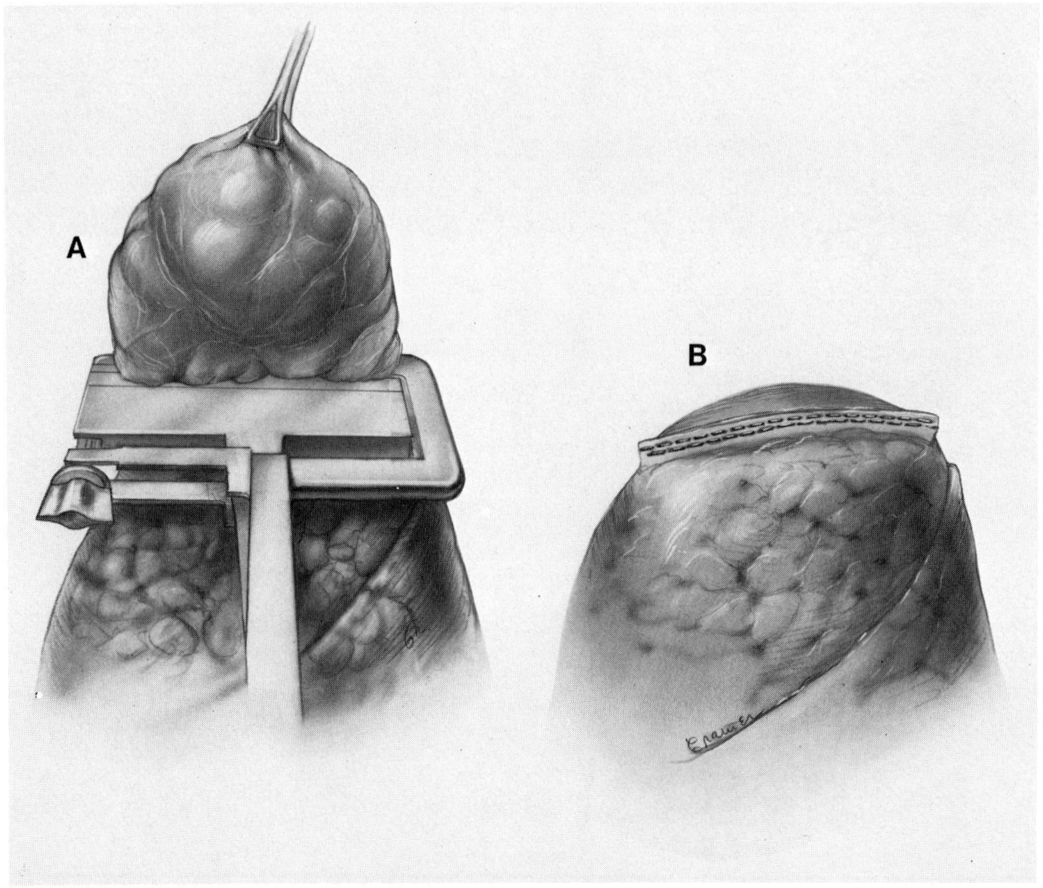

Fig XI–4. See legend on facing page.

Depending on the size of the lesion, lung biopsies and excision of nodules often will extend across one or several segmental planes or across incomplete fissures. Subsegmental resections may complement a lobectomy done for disease that has extended marginally beyond the fissure.

In general, most thoracic surgeons will agree that today the classic segmental dissection in which one separately secured the segmental bronchus and vessels and then dissected out the intersegmental plane has been made obsolete by the staplers. Of course, one still does frequently resect what is in essence a pulmonary segment, such as the lingula, or the apical segment of the right upper lobe, or the superior segment of the right lower lobe, or the apical posterior of the left upper lobe, but there is no need to undertake the frequently bloody, and often untidy, parenchymal dissection. One can secure the segmental artery and, if they are identifiable, the veins, then place the TA 90^{TM} instrument along the edge of the segment to be resected, securing the segmental bronchus and the pulmonary parenchyma with one application of the stapler. Alternatively, and for major segmental resections, one may secure the segmental bronchus and then apply the TA 90^{TM} instrument to the boundary between inflated and collapsed lung.

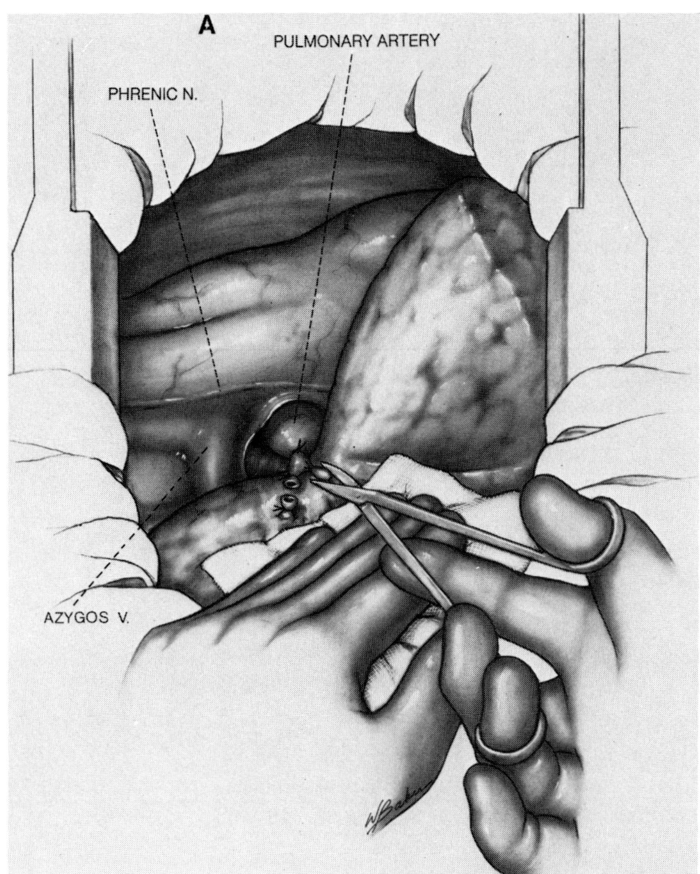

Fig XI–5.—Right upper lobectomy. **A,** individual arteries to the segments of the upper lobes usually are ligated or sutured rather than stapled.

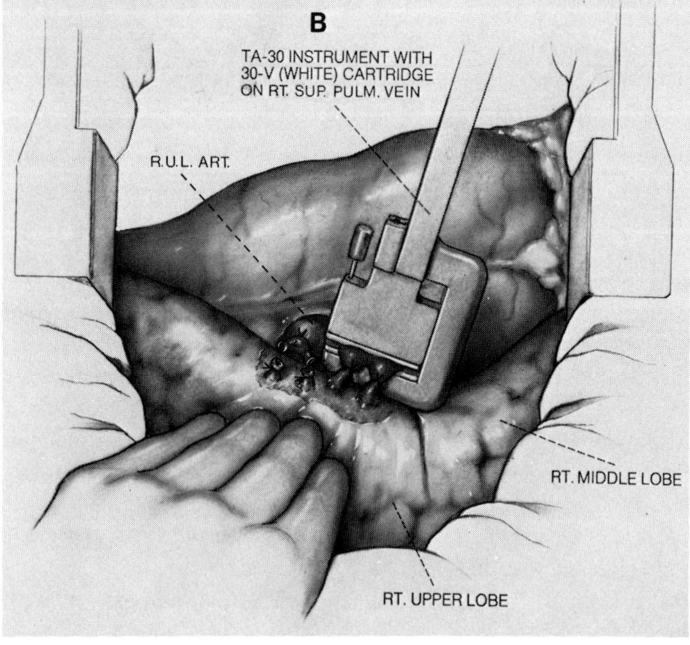

Fig XI–5 (cont.).—**B,** a tunnel having been created under the pulmonary vein to the upper lobe, the lower jaw of the TA 30™ instrument, loaded with the 30V (white) vascular cartridge, is passed under the vein, the tissue-retention pin dropped into place, the instrument closed, and the staples driven home. Stapling the pulmonary vessels is at least as secure as manual suturing and is to be preferred to simple ligation, particularly for the veins or the main arteries.

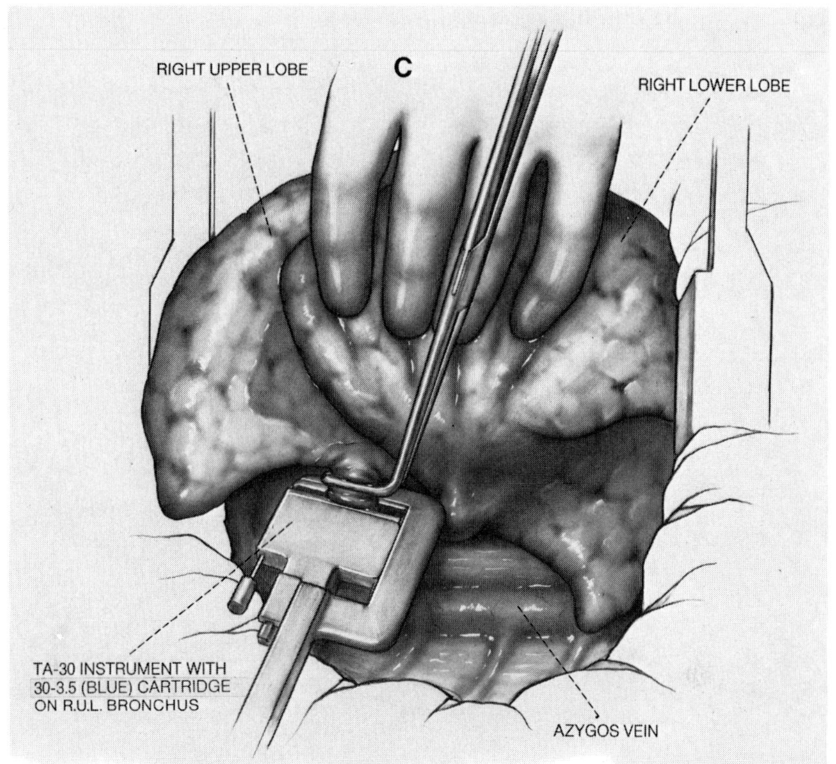

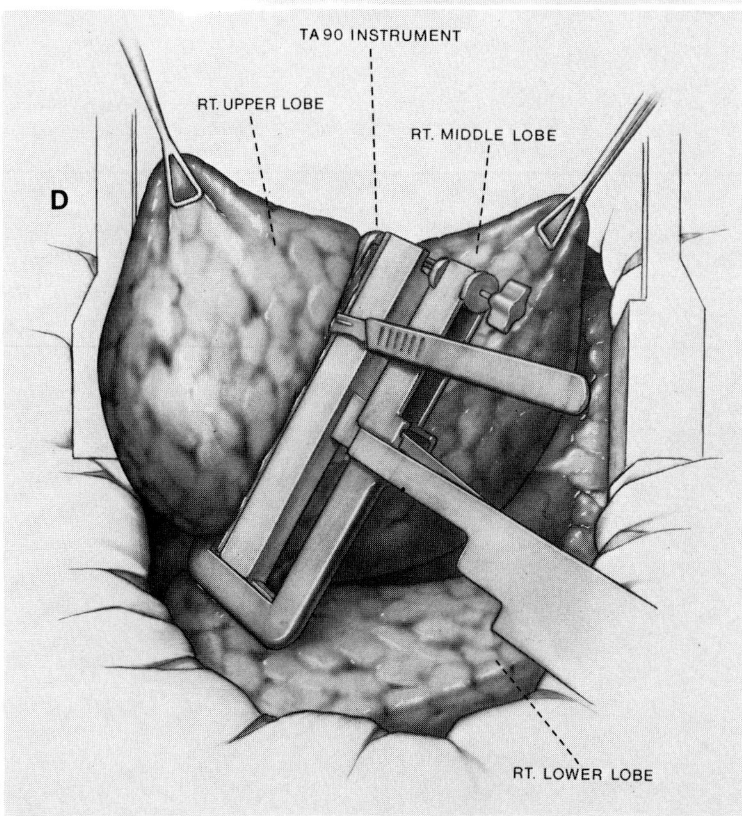

Fig XI–5 (cont.).—C, the upper lobe bronchus has been dissected down to the main bronchus. The TA 30™ instrument, in this case with a blue cartridge with 3.5 mm staples, is passed down alongside and parallel to the main bronchus, so that little or no stump will be left when the bronchus has been stapled and cut away. **D,** in this instance there is not a complete fissure between the upper and middle lobes. The staplers solve this problem easily, and without blood loss or air leak. One simply places the TA 90™ or TA 55™ instrument, as indicated, along the separation between the collapsed lung of the specimen and the inflated lung to be left behind, drives the staples home, and cuts away the specimen on the border of the stapler. *(continued)*

371

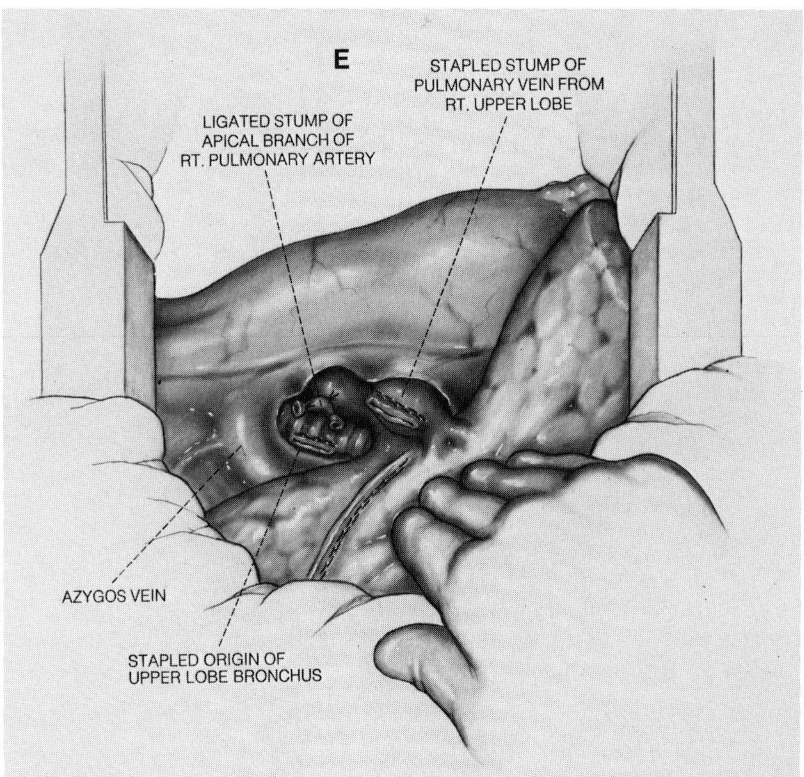

Fig XI–5 (cont.).—E, the lobe having been removed, the bronchus is seen stapled flush with the main bronchus, the pulmonary vein secure, and the stapled surface of the middle lobe a neat, thin line.

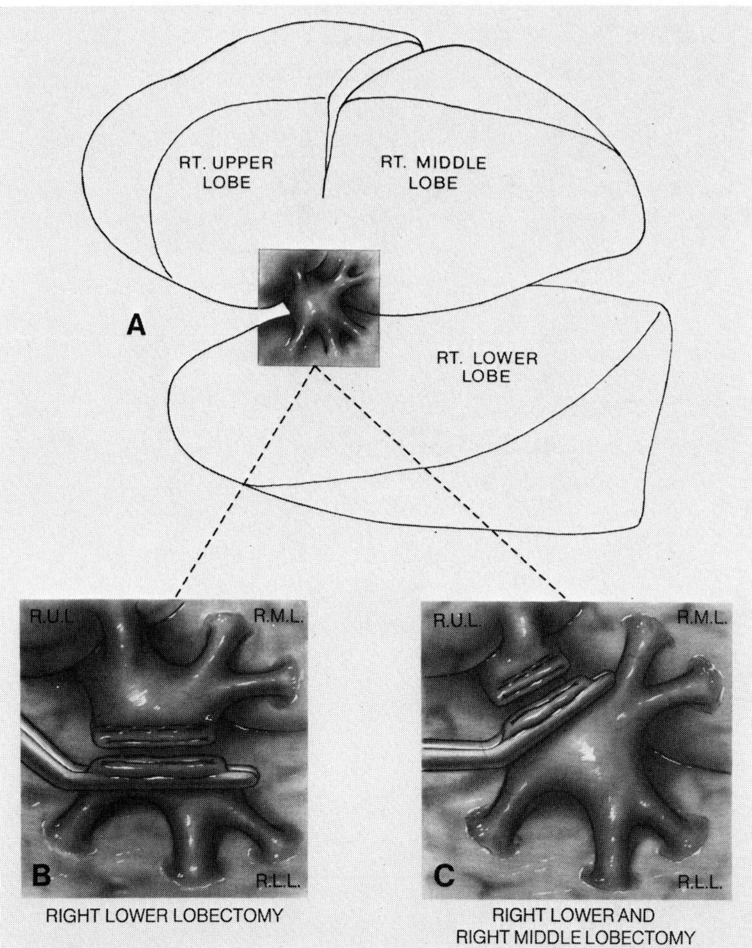

Fig XI–6.—Right lower lobectomy, right bilobectomy. **A,** the right "intermediate" pulmonary artery is shown through the greater fissure. **B,** the proximal arterial stump is shown after the branches to the superior and basilar segments have been taken for a right lower lobectomy. **C,** the proximal arterial stump for a bilobectomy is shown after the arteries to the lower lobe and the middle lobe have been stapled. The TA 30™ instrument with the white cartridge and fine staples is used. Once more, little more dissection is required than will permit the slender lower jaw of the TA 30™ instrument to slip under the vessel and avoid compromise or compression of the branches to the remaining lung. *(continued)*

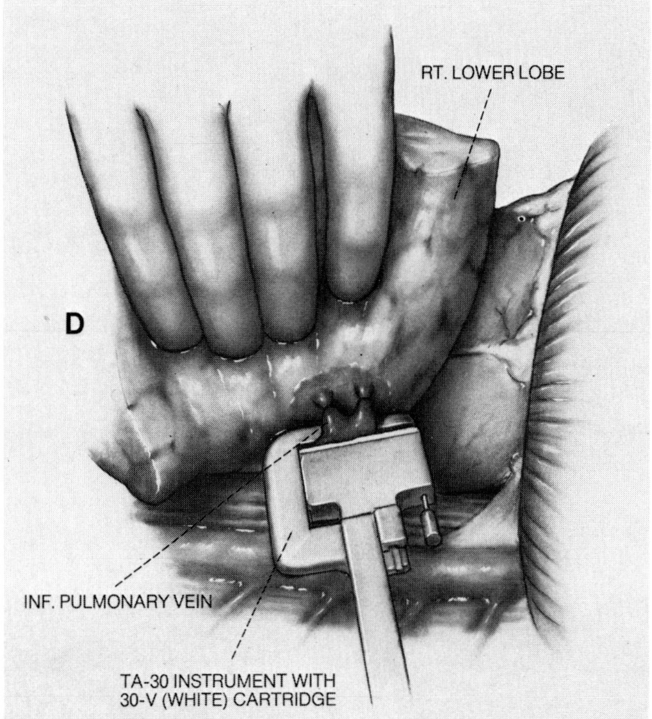

Fig XI–6 (cont.).—D, the inferior pulmonary vein is taken with the TA 30™ instrument. If the middle lobe is being removed, its vein will be taken independently, where it joins the superior pulmonary vein. The stapling of the intermediate bronchus, when the lower and middle lobes are being taken, or the inferior lobe bronchus, for a lower lobectomy, are not shown. Again, the stapler would be laid parallel to and flush with the parent bronchus.

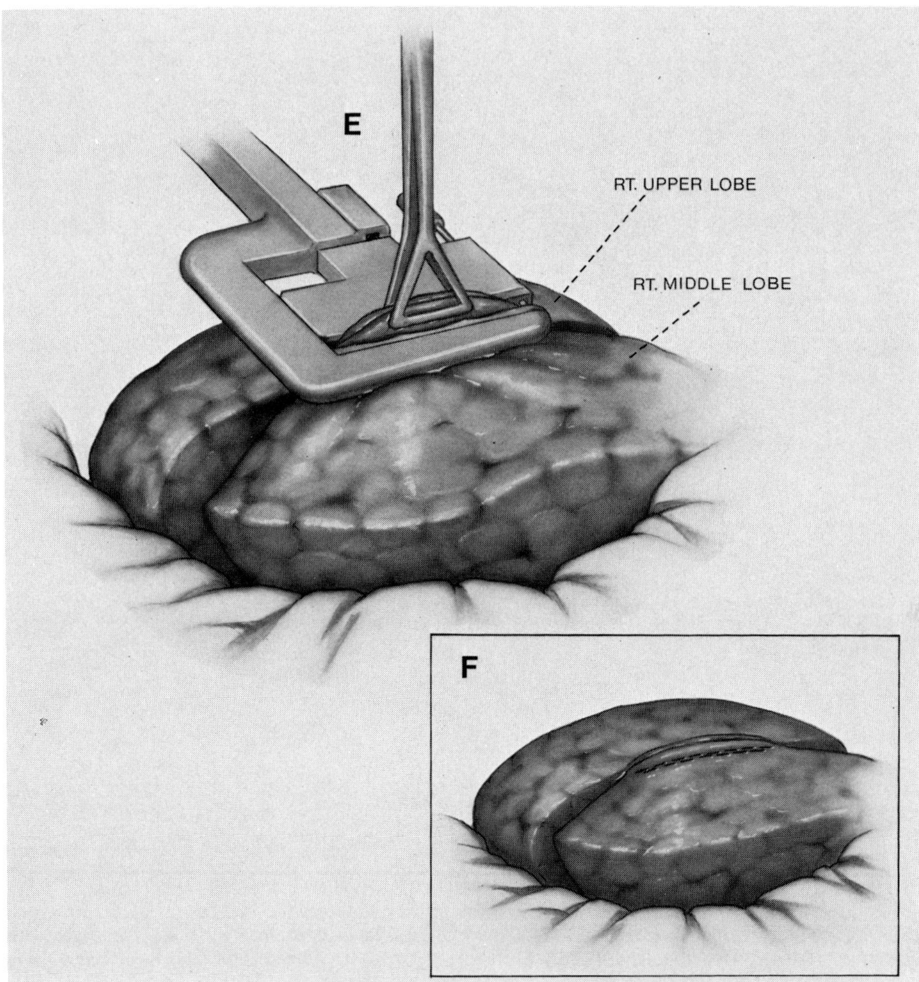

Fig XI–6 (cont.).—E and **F,** after right lower lobectomy, if there is any fear that the middle lobe may twist and strangulate, the edges of the two lobes are grasped across the fissure and readily stapled together, effectively preventing torsion of the middle lobe. Similarly, after right upper lobectomy, the middle lobe may be stapled to the lower lobe.

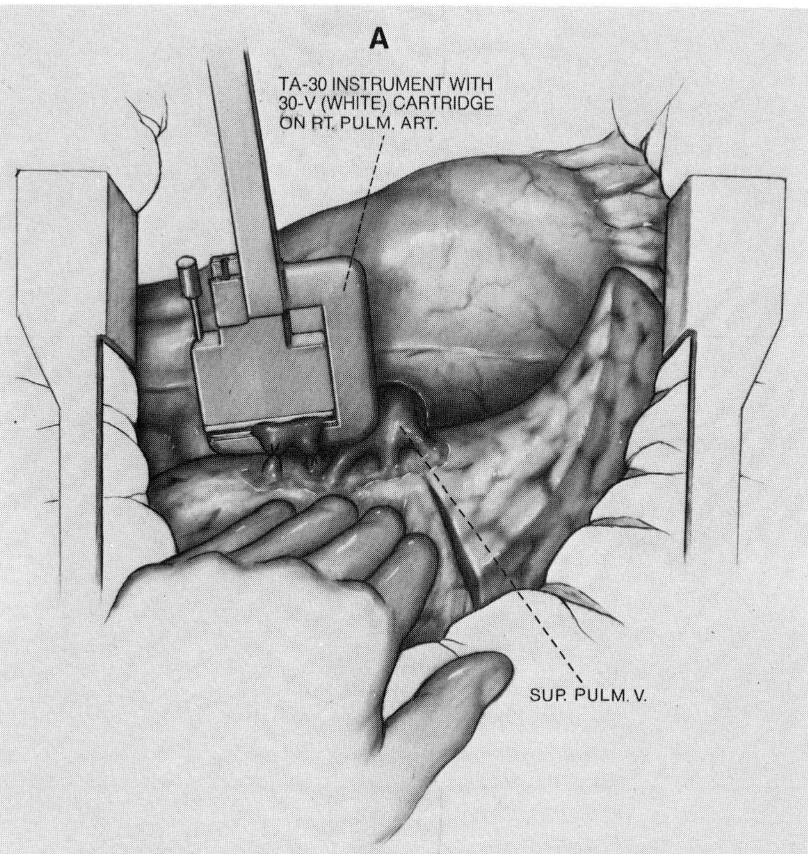

Fig XI–7.—Right pneumonectomy. **A,** a tunnel having been created under the pulmonary artery, and the individual branches ligated peripherally, the lower jaw of the TA 30™ instrument, armed with the white (30V) vascular cartridge, is slipped under the pulmonary artery, which is stapled and cut away on the edge of the TA 30™ instrument. For those who are new to the instrument and not yet confident of it there is no harm in a precautionary placing of the jaws of an open vascular clamp around the artery on the cardiac side of the stapler. In point of fact, there almost never is any bleeding. Occasionally there is enough blood coming between the staples at one or another point to justify a single stitch. It is to be borne in mind that in an elderly patient with a thickened and sclerotic pulmonary artery, the artery can be injured by compression of the stapler, just as it can be by compression between the jaws of an arterial clamp applied in the ordinary procedure of clamping, dividing, and oversewing the artery. **B** and **C,** the superior and inferior veins are taken separately with the vascular stapler, the veins being ligated on the pulmonary side. In either right or left pneumonectomy, if it is necessary to divide the pulmonary veins from within the pericardium, it will be found that the stapler facilitates this to an extraordinary degree. If the staples are to be applied on the veins in the pericardium, the white cartridge is used. If the staplers are to be applied to the atrium, it is preferable to use the blue cartridge with the 3.5 mm staples. In either case, once one has been assured of a free tunnel behind the vein or the atrium, the rather widely opened clamp is slipped around the structure to be stapled and the stapling then done in the ordinary manner. The speed and security with which this can be done as compared to ordinary clamping and suturing will be found to be gratifying.

→

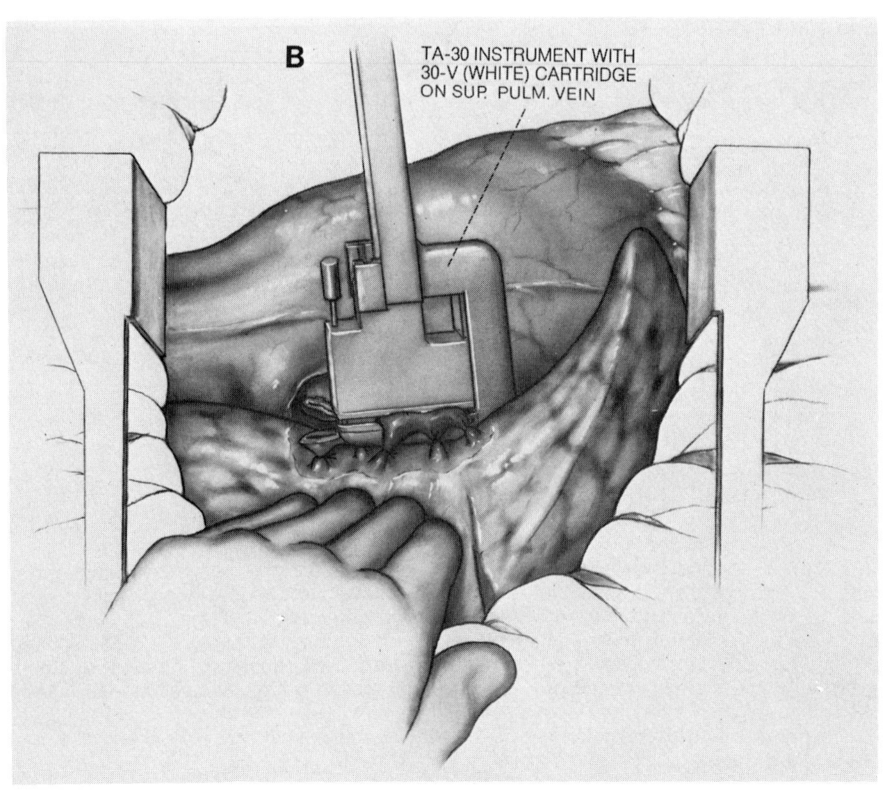

B
TA-30 INSTRUMENT WITH
30-V (WHITE) CARTRIDGE
ON SUP. PULM. VEIN

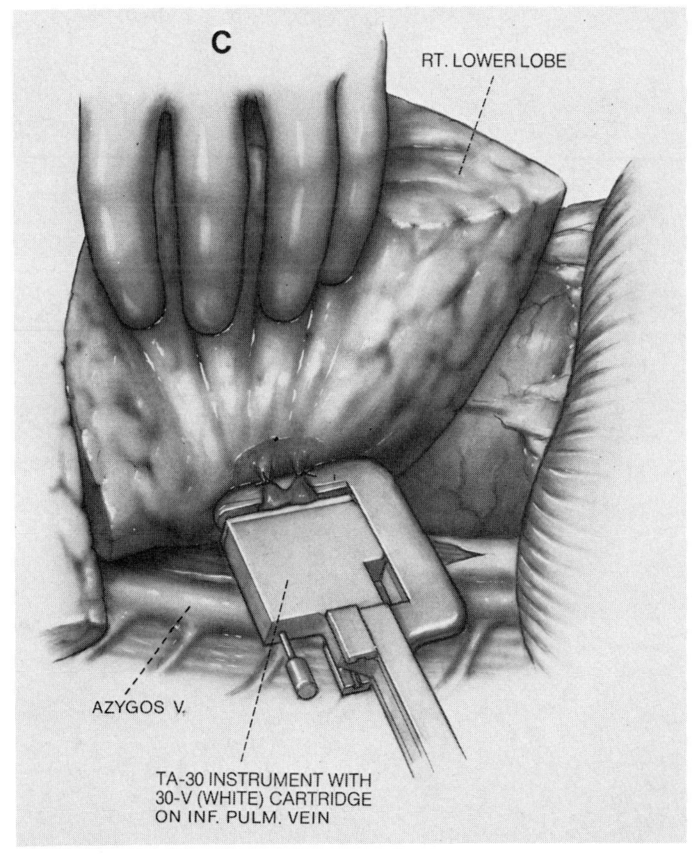

C
RT. LOWER LOBE
AZYGOS V.
TA-30 INSTRUMENT WITH
30-V (WHITE) CARTRIDGE
ON INF. PULM. VEIN

Fig XI–7 (cont.).—D and **E,** the TA 30™ instrument with the 4.8 green cartridge for the large male or the 3.5 blue cartridge for a female or a child, is passed around the main bronchus, then pressed up against the trachea so that there will be essentially no bronchial stump.

There may be momentary air leaks from the staple holes, and we usually place a saline sponge over the bronchus while we proceed with the operation, and within moments the air leak stops. Occasionally, a bronchial artery will escape the staples and require control by a fine silk stitch. Just as with the main pulmonary artery, the main bronchus in an older male may be rigid enough to crack when seized whether with a bronchial clamp or with a stapler and, in both cases, we like to close the clamp, or the stapler, gently and slowly, to minimize this likelihood.　　　　　→

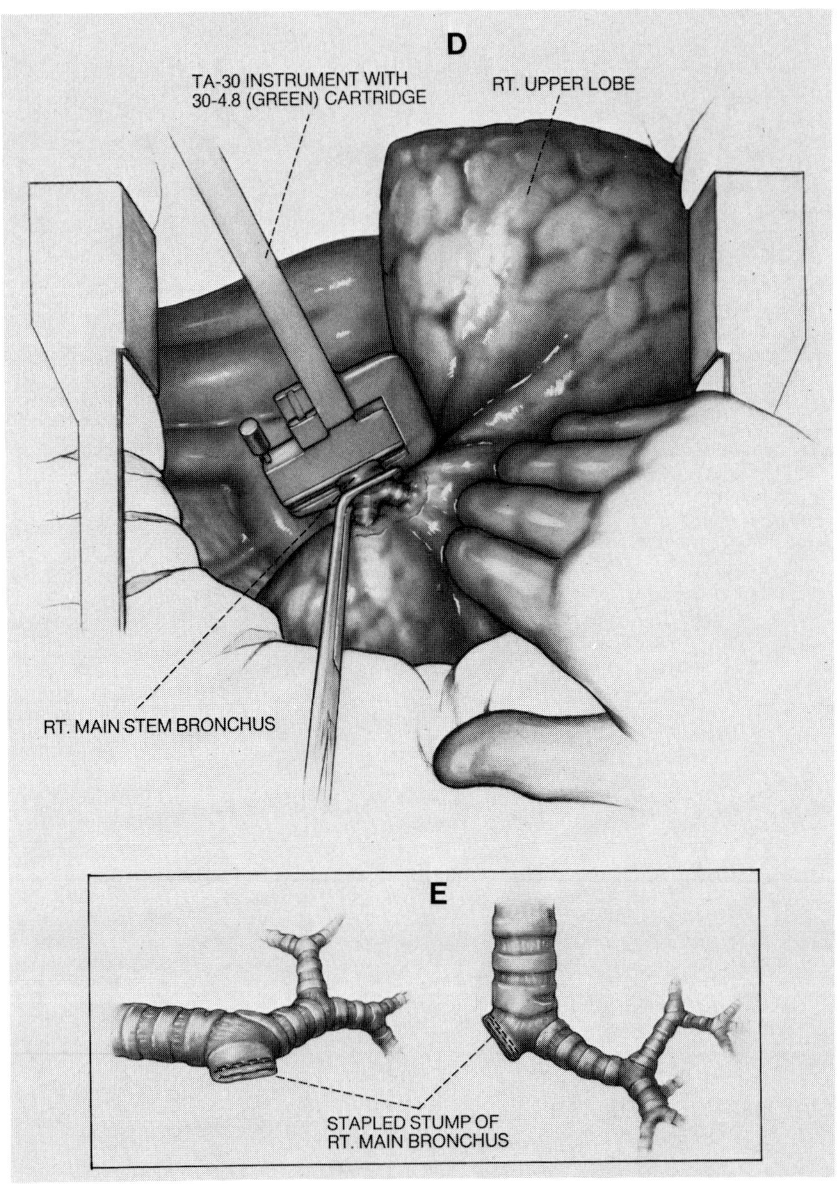
D
TA-30 INSTRUMENT WITH
30-4.8 (GREEN) CARTRIDGE
RT. UPPER LOBE
RT. MAIN STEM BRONCHUS
E
STAPLED STUMP OF
RT. MAIN BRONCHUS

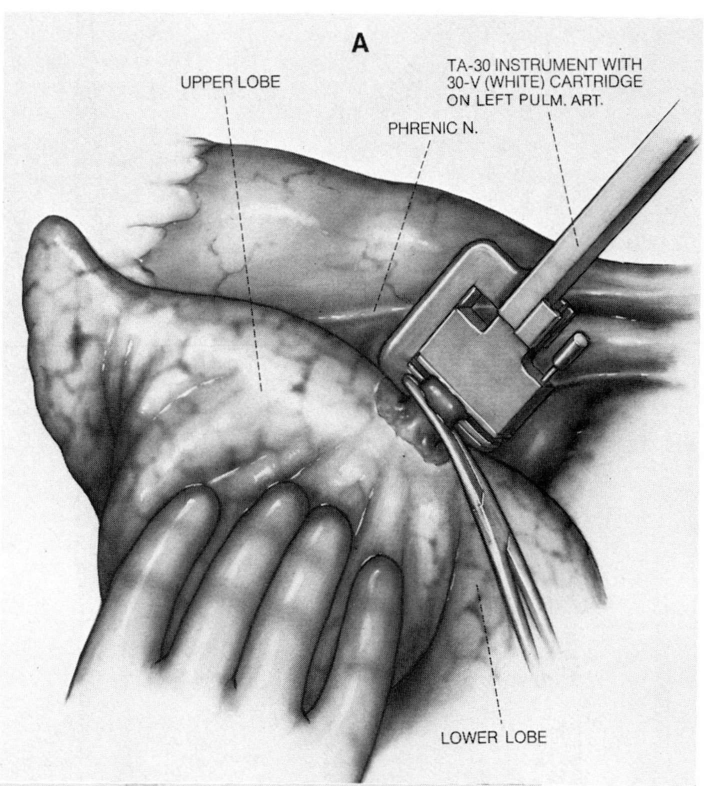

Fig XI–8.—Left pneumonectomy. **A,** the left main pulmonary artery is shown secured with the TA 30™ instrument carrying the white, vascular cartridge. **B,** the superior vein will be ligated peripherally, stapled centrally, and divided on the stapler. The stapler can be applied as close to the mediastinum as a clamp could be, and whereas the sutures in the manual treatment of the vessels would be some distance on the pulmonary side of the clamp, that space is not required with the stapler, since the sutures are placed where the clamp has been applied, a matter of some importance when the local pathologic condition limits the length of vessel that can be mobilized or that is free from disease.

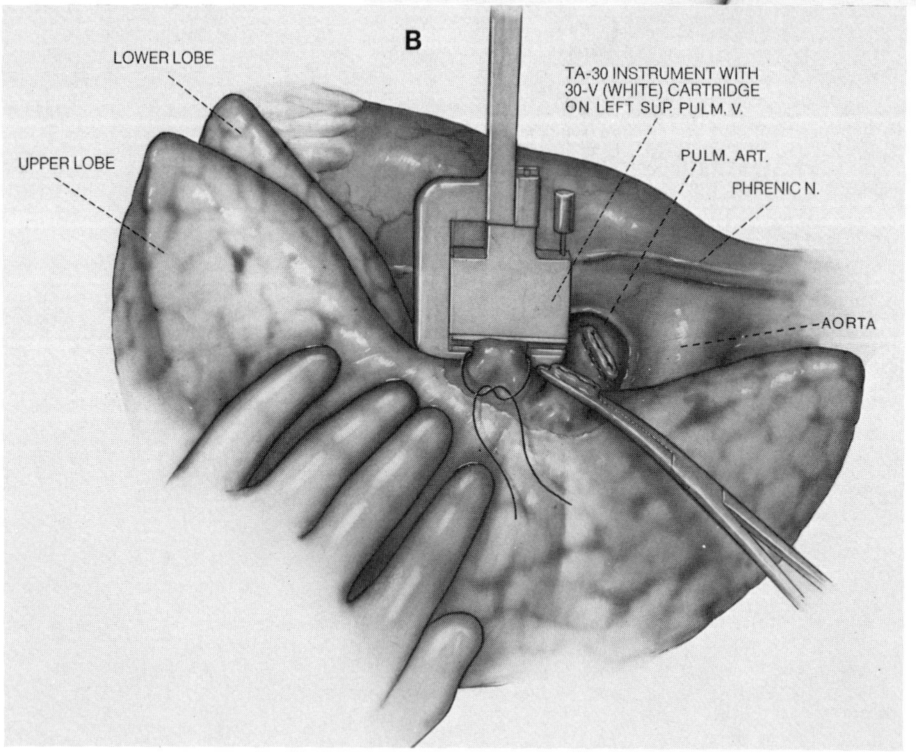

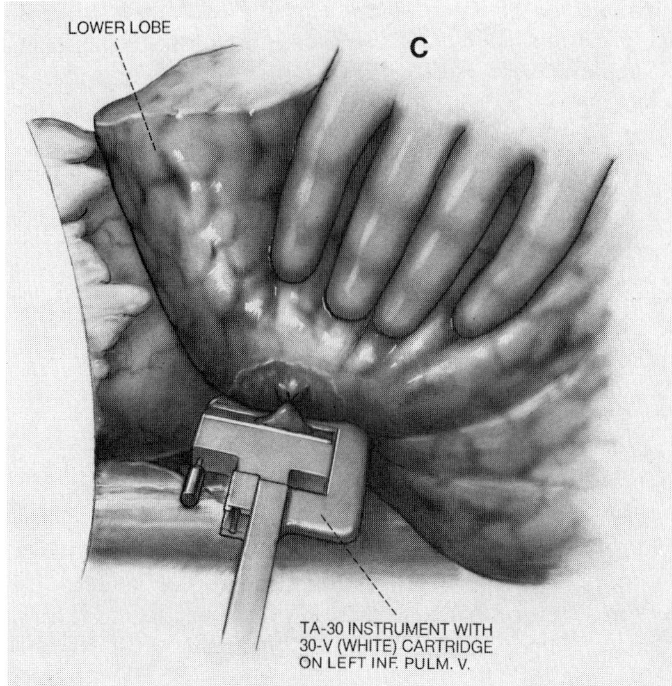

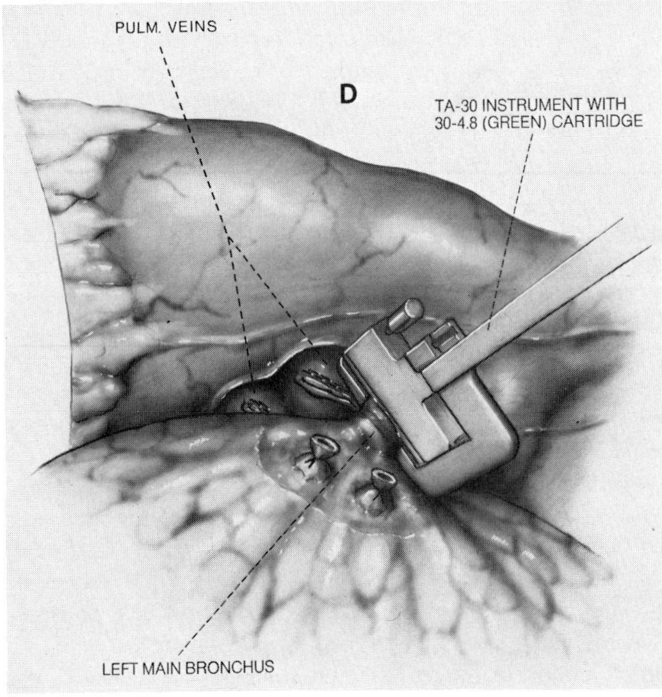

Fig XI–8 (cont.).—C, the inferior pulmonary vein is stapled. **D,** the left main bronchus is being secured. Whereas, on the right, the stapler can fairly readily be placed down against the trachea, on the left the aortic arch and the main pulmonary artery prevent this. For this reason, it is our practice usually to slip the left index finger into the mediastinum on the far side of the trachea to draw the trachea over into the wound. This permits the stapler to be applied directly at the origin of the left main bronchus and avoids the temptation of pulling on the lung to deliver the tracheobronchial junction into the operative site. Stapling tissues under tension invites a tear. One may compare this with putting a needle into the neck of a collapsed balloon, which leaves a minute puncture, whereas if the neck of the balloon is strongly stretched, a pinhole creates a large tear.

In our 1964 report (Ravitch, Steichen, Fishbein, Knowles, and Weil, 1964), still with the Russian UKB 25, which places a single line of staples, the bar of the staples being in line with the long axis of the bronchus, we reported further experience with 139 pulmonary resections—80 lobectomies and bilobectomies, 21 segmentectomies, 13 lobectomies with segmentectomy, and 25 pneumonectomies. In the total of 139 resections there were three bronchopleural fistulas and three empyemas without fistula, one of them quite small. Two of the fistulas occurred in diabetic patients, one of them a tubercular, who was sputum positive at the time of operation. In two of the three patients with leaks accepted as bronchial, the anatomical site of the leak could not be demonstrated to be in the bronchial stump.

Kirksey (Kirksey, Arnold, Calhoon, and Hood, 1970), at the meeting of the Society of Thoracic Surgeons, said that they had begun using the American staplers (TA 55^{TM} and TA 30^{TM}) in February, 1968. In 147 pulmonary resections, 25 pneumonectomies, 54 lobectomies, 25 transsegmental resections, six segmental, and 37 wedge resections, they had one bronchial fistula and empyema, after lobectomy, and two prolonged air leaks after lobectomy, resolving spontaneously. They quoted, for its relevance to the adoption of stapling, Cushing's (1928) comment on acceptance of new techniques by surgeons: "Surgery is a conservative art. It takes to new methods reluctantly as an old dog to new tricks. It was slow to adopt the ligature; slow to adopt the principles of antisepsis; slow to adopt the fastidious technique and painstaking haemostasis that have largely put a stop to operating by the clock. It has been equally slow to adopt the principles of electrosurgery which, from a technical standpoint, are likely to be no less revolutionizing."

At the Oteen, North Carolina Veterans Administration Hospital, Takaro and associates (Dart, Scott, and Takaro, 1970) performed pulmonary resection in 493 patients from December, 1962 to January, 1969, first with the Russian UKL-40. When the Auto Suture® TA 30^{TM} and TA 55^{TM} instruments became available, they performed 13 pneumonectomies and 73 other pulmonary resections with them. Both the Russian and American instruments were used on pulmonary vessels, bronchi, and pulmonary parenchyma. With the Russian instruments, they had eight bronchopleural fistulas and four persistent air leaks, and they stated that with the Russian instruments, improper staple closure ". . .could be attributed to inappropriate size of the staple for the tissue being approximated; or improper manual loading of the individual staples, allowing malposition or premature loss of staples to occur; or defective staples. The American prepackaged, factory-loaded, disposable units, color-coded as to staple length, have helped to eliminate some of these problems. . . .No instances of technical failure and no bronchopleural fistulas were noted following 86 pulmonary resections using the American stapler." They commented further on the lack of uniformity in the Russian staples.

In the discussion that followed this presentation at the meeting of the Society of Thoracic Surgeons, Alfred Goldman of Los Angeles (1970), who earlier had used the Russian instruments, commented on the passage of vessels through the B staples and was enthusiastic about the new American instruments. Richard Overholt of Boston (1970) was able to restrain his enthusiasm for stapling, as was Irving Sarot of New York (1970), both of them on a priori reasoning based on an incorrect understanding of the instruments, suggesting the appropriateness of Kirksey's quotation from Cushing. William Cook of the Bronx, New York (1970) was particularly pleased with the American staplers in pulmonary surgery and stressed the applicability of stapling to the resection of pulmonary bullae, mentioning the applicability to this of the GIA^{TM} instrument.

Konrad and Tarbiat (1971) from Düsseldorf reported pleasure with the occurrence of bronchial fistulas in only four of 80 bronchial closures with the American staplers.

Allen (1971) from the University of Alabama in Birmingham reported his enthusiasm for the use of the American staplers in the resection of large emphysematous bullae.

Hood and associates (Hood, Kirksey, Calhoon, Arnold, and Tate, 1973) from Lubbock, Texas presented before the Society of Thoracic Surgeons their experience in pulmonary resection in 349 consecutive cases. They used the TA 30™ instrument with the 30V cartridge for the pulmonary vessels, including intrapericardial division, the TA 30™ instrument with 4.8 mm staples for the main and lobar bronchi and 30V staples for segmental bronchi, the TA 55™ instrument and 4.8 mm staples for pulmonary parenchyma in most instances, the GIA™ instrument at times to complete an incomplete fissure.

They had two bronchopleural fistulas in their 60 pneumonectomies and none in their 136 lobectomies. There were five prolonged air leaks, three of them requiring further operation, and two empyemas without fistula. They considered the incidence of bronchial and parenchymal leaks to have been lowered by the staples, and said that transsegmental resections were made possible, sparing pulmonary parenchyma that would have been sacrificed by formal segmentectomy, found that less hilar dissection was required and that operating time was shorter.

At that meeting of the Society of Thoracic Surgeons, Kirsh of Ann Arbor (1973) seconded Hood's enthusiasm: "We too have noticed a decreased incidence of complications with the use of these staplers. We have not experienced a single instance of bronchopleural fistula, even in those patients undergoing postoperative mediastinal irradiation. There has also been a decreased incidence of prolonged air leak under circumstances in which one might expect some to occur. . . ." He rightly pointed out the disadvantage that stapling the unopened bronchus prevented inspection of the interior of the bronchus. In the same discussion, Jensik of Chicago (1973) reported 151 patients with pulmonary resection using the staplers in 107 bronchial closures, 17 arterial staplings, and 102 vein staplings, the pulmonary resections including segmental resections and resection of blebs and bullae. They had two fistulas, both in patients with severe, diffuse pulmonary infection, one of them previously irradiated. In resection for carcinoma, they advised frozen section of the bronchial stump of the specimen. In the continued discussion, Harrison of Grand Rapids (1973) reported 199 patients in whom the staplers had been used principally for closure of the bronchus, and on the lung parenchyma. They had had three bronchopleural fistulas and 13 prolonged air leaks that closed spontaneously. They calculated that the average operating time was reduced by 20–30 minutes for each patient. Raymond Read of Little Rock, Arkansas (1973) added to the discussion his experience with 163 pulmonary resections, stating that they had seen a patient ". . . cough up the bronchial suture line as a cast about four or five months after operation," then developing a bronchopleural fistula. They thought that they had compressed the bronchial stump excessively and subsequently used only the green cartridge with the 4.8 mm staples and took care to leave all the adventitia on the main bronchus in lobectomy. In the summation, Kirksey made the useful comment that after right upper lobectomy they stapled the middle lobe to the lower lobe to prevent rotation of the middle lobe, a procedure we have used often (Figs XI–6*E* and *F* show a similar technique after lower lobectomy).

Cook and colleagues (Cook, Lee, You, and Santos, 1974) from the Bronx Municipal Hospital Center reported their results in 150 consecutive pulmonary resections performed using the Auto Suture® staplers. The pulmonary arteries and veins were closed with the TA 30™ instrument and the vascular cartridge. There was one persistent air space after right upper lobectomy, which proved to be from the dissection of the fissure and not from the bronchus; one air leak after right lower lobectomy for carcinoma, successfully treated by closed drainage; one leak from the right upper bronchus requiring a thoracoplasty; and one leak five weeks after right pneumonectomy for tuberculosis and massive hemorrhage.

Wolff (1974), in discussion of Cook, said that he had been using the staplers on the bronchi, had no leaks at all, and found them invaluable for completion of an incomplete fissure or for wedge resection.

In our 1958 visit to Amosov, we had seen him perform pneumonectomy by applying the UKL-60 to the entire pulmonary hilus—bronchus, pulmonary artery, and both pulmonary veins—in a single application. He subsequently modified this to taking the bronchus with one application of the stapler and all of the other hilar attachments to the lung with another application. Gaskin and Bergmann (1975) from the Jewish Hospital of St. Louis undertook to use this latter technique in pneumonectomy for lung cancer. They were able to use the technique in 33 of 41 patients, and intrapericardial stapling and division of the vessels in three more. There were two deaths, one from pulmonary embolism and one from myocardial infarction. They saw minor bleeding from the pulmonary artery in 26 patients, usually stopping spontaneously. Minor air leaks from the bronchi in two patients required one or two sutures. "The majority of the bronchial and vascular leaks occurred when only the UKL-60 with its 4.8 mm staples was available to us. Since we have obtained the American instruments, which can apply smaller staples with tighter compression of tissues, such leaks have become quite infrequent." There were no air leaks, there was one late empyema nine months after operation, and no air leak then.

Vanderhoeft, Rocmans, and Vollinoti (1975) from Brussels reported 76 pulmonary resections with the use of the TA 30™ instrument, 35 pneumonectomies, and 41 lobectomies, with six fistulas. Three of them they thought to be due to bronchial involvement by cancer. In one case, during tracheal aspiration, the aspirator was forced through the suture line and in one case the stapler was known to have been improperly closed.

Lawson, Hutchinson, Longland, and Haque (1977) from the Royal Infirmary, Glasgow, using the American instruments in 58 patients—43 pulmonary resections and 15 excisions of bullae—had no complications and no postoperative deaths.

Hargrove and Harken (1979) from the University of Pennsylvania pointed out the utility, in special instances, of resection of the offending symptomatic carcinomatous lesion, even when a curative operation is impossible. In their patient, who had a right upper lobe carcinoma with serious hemoptysis and unresectable tumor, "A stapler (TA-90) was placed directly across the tumor at the base of the right upper lobe, and the lobe was resected. No bleeding or leakage of air was apparent following removal of the upper lobe. The row of staples was directly through the carcinoma. The patient was discharged two weeks following surgery, with no further hemoptysis." The staples still were visible in the chest film six months later. We have used the same technique for inoperable carcinoma with necrosis and infection, although in that instance we were able to place the stapler beyond the gross tumor, an obviously preferable procedure (Steichen, 1974).

From the Karolinska Hospital in Stockholm, Péterffy and Calabrese (1979) reviewed 298 pulmonary resections performed between 1976 and 1978, 146 with TA 30™ bronchial stapling and 152 with conventional bronchial sutures of chromic catgut. The patients in the two groups were said to be comparable although the study was retrospective. Thirty-five percent of the patients in the TA 30[TM] series had pneumonectomies and 29% in the catgut sutured group. Eighty percent of the operations were performed by nine surgeons who were versed in both techniques. Three patients in each group died within 30 days. There were two bronchial fistulas with the staplers (1%), five with catgut (3%), one empyema without fistula from the stapler, and four with chromic catgut. Prolonged air leaks were the same in both groups. They concluded that closure with the stapler was " . . . simpler and swifter . . . reduces the contamination of the operative field, achieves uniform and tighter closure of the bronchus, leaves a better preserved terminal blood perfusion of the stump and utilizes a more tolerated sewing material with less resultant tissue inflammation."

Forrester-Wood (1980) from Cornwall, England compared two successive groups of pneumonectomies in a total of 450. In the first 225, starting in 1954, the bronchial stump was closed with interrupted sutures of stainless steel or Mersilene. Beginning in 1968, in the second 225 cases, the bronchial stump was closed with the TA 30[TM] instrument. In the manually sutured group there were 18 early and seven late bronchial fistulas, for a total of 25; in the stapled group, five early and one late fistulas, for a total of six. This decrease in the bronchopleural fistula rate from 11% to 2.6% was highly significant; the reduction occurred with resection on either side, the difference being 16% to 5.2% on the right and 6% to 0.8% on the left.

Monod, in his doctoral thesis from the Faculty of Medicine in Brest, Université de Bretagne Occidentale (1980), describes the use of the American stapling instruments in 26 pneumonectomies, 67 lobectomies, eight bilobectomies, 18 segmentectomies and plurisegmentectomies, 88 transsegmentectomies, and 88 cuneiform and superficial resections. For lobectomy and pneumonectomy, staplers were not used on all elements of the hilus and therefore the author gives a list of the individual procedures performed, consisting of: 84 bronchial, 15 pulmonary artery, and 14 pulmonary vein closures; stapling of an incomplete fissure in 61 operations and pulmonary parenchymal resections (wedge, segmental, trans- and multisegmental) on 194 occasions, for a total of 368 procedures. In the 277 patients (some operated on twice) comprising this series there were no deaths due to the use of staples. There was a total of 90 complications, of which two bronchial and nine parenchymal air leaks and two empyemas can be attributed to the use of staples. The remainder, atelectasis in 34 patients, ten interstitial hematomas, hemorrhages requiring reoperation in three patients, 16 residual pleural spaces, and 14 instances of wound infection, were of the type encountered in any postoperative situation following pulmonary surgery. Monod points out, however, that since their use of stapling, pulmonary parenchymal air leaks, persistent oozing of blood, interstitial hematomas, and residual pleural spaces have significantly diminished in frequency and importance.

Irlich, Schulte, and Koch (1981) from the University Department of Surgery, Düsseldorf, at the 98th Kongress of the Deutsche Gesellschaft für Chirurgie, pointed out that up until 1969 with manual closure of the bronchi with wire sutures, and catgut closure of the parenchyma, their incidence of empyema and bronchopleural fistula after pulmonary resection was 4.2%. Beginning in 1969, with the use of the American stapling instruments, this rate fell to 3%. In a series of 332 consecutive pulmonary resections from 1974 to 1979 with bronchus and pulmonary parenchyma both closed with the American stapling instruments there was a 2.1% incidence of empyema and only a single bronchopleural fistula.

From Stanford University, Baumgartner and Mark (1981) reported eight patients out of 180 in whom bronchial suture had been made with a synthetic thread, who had developed new respiratory symptoms that proved to be due to bronchial stump suture granulomas, cured by bronchoscopic extraction of the sutures. Subsequent to that series, the use of the Auto Suture® staplers in more than 100 consecutive pulmonary resections had yielded no bronchopleural fistula and no granuloma.

Reuter's doctoral thesis, Université Louis Pasteur (1982), reports 317 pulmonary stapling procedures performed at the St. Thérèse Clinic in Luxembourg. The instruments were used for the hilar vessels, for the bronchi, and for the pulmonary parenchyma. There were 119 pneumonectomies, 121 lobectomies, 33 bilobectomies, and 34 segmentectomies, the remainder being resections for coin lesions or bullae or closure of traumatic wounds. There were four staple-related deaths, all due to bronchial fistula after pneumonectomy for cancer. In addition to these there were seven leaks that closed with drainage, three after pneumonectomy, three after lobectomy, and one after segmentectomy.

REFERENCES

Allen T.H.: Technic for resection of localized bullous disease of the lung. *Am. Surg.* 37:671, 1971.

Amosov N.M., Berezovsky K.K.: Pulmonary resection with mechanical suture. *J. Thorac. Cardiovasc. Surg.* 41:325, 1961.

Baumgartner W.A., Mark J.B.D.: Bronchoscopic diagnosis and treatment of bronchial stump suture granulomas. *J. Thorac. Cardiovasc. Surg.* 81:553, 1981.

Cook W.A.: In discussion of Dart C.H. Jr., Scott S.M., Takaro T. *Ann. Thorac. Surg.* 9:535, 1970.

Cook W.A., Lee C.W., You K.D., Santos G.H.: Pulmonary resection. Autosuture technique. *N.Y. State J. Med.* 74:967, 1974.

Cushing H., Bovie W.T.: Electro-surgery as an aid in the removal of intracranial tumors. *Surg. Gynecol. Obstet.* 47:751, 1928.

Dart C.H. Jr., Scott S.M., Takaro T.: Six-year clinical experience using automatic stapling devices for lung resections. *Ann. Thorac. Surg.* 9:535, 1970.

Forrester-Wood C.P.: Bronchopleural fistula following pneumonectomy for carcinoma of the bronchus. Mechanical stapling versus hand suturing. *J. Thorac. Cardiovasc. Surg.* 80:406, 1980.

Gaskin R.J., Bergmann M.: Pneumonectomy by "en masse" stapling of hilar vessels. *Ann. Thorac. Surg.* 19:242, 1975.

Goldman A.: An evaluation of automatic suture with UKL-60 and UKL-40 devices by pulmonary resection. *Dis. Chest* 46:29, 1964.

Goldman A.: In discussion of Dart C.H. Jr., Scott S.M., Takaro T. *Ann. Thorac. Surg.* 9:535, 1970.

Hargrove W.C. III, Harken A.H.: Palliation of massive hemoptysis from unresectable carcinoma of the lung. *Chest* 76:234, 1979.

Harrison R.W.: In discussion of Hood R.M., Kirksey T.D., Calhoon J.H., Arnold H.S., Tate R.S. *Ann. Thorac. Surg.* 16:85, 1973.

Hood R.M., Kirksey T.D., Calhoon J.H., Arnold H.S., Tate R.S.: The use of automatic stapling devices in pulmonary resection. *Ann. Thorac. Surg.* 16:85, 1973.

Irlich G., Schulte H.D., Koch J.: Klammernahtgeräte an der Lunge und am Bronchus (abstract). 98th Kongress, Deutsche Gesellschaft für Chirurgie, Munich, April 22–25, 1981.

Jensik R.J.: In discussion of Hood R.M., Kirksey T.D., Calhoon J.H., Arnold H.S., Tate R.S. *Ann. Thorac. Surg.* 16:85, 1973.

Kirksey T.D., Arnold H.S., Calhoon J.H., Hood R.M.: Techniques of pulmonary resection. Tradition and travail. *Ann. Thorac. Surg.* 9:525, 1970.

Kirsh M.M.: In discussion of Hood R.M., Kirksey T.D., Calhoon J.H., Arnold H.S., Tate R.S. *Ann. Thorac. Surg.* 16:85, 1973.

Konrad R.M., Tarbiat S.: Die Insuffizienzquote nach Verwendung des Klammernaht-Gerätes beim Bronchusverschluss. *Thoraxchir. Vask. Chir.* 19:179, 1971.

Lawson W.R., Hutchinson J., Longland C.J., Haque M.A.: Mechanical suture methods in thoracic and abdominal surgery. *Br. J. Surg.* 64:115, 1977.

Monod J.E.: Sutures automatiques et exérèses pulmonaires. Thèse Doctorat en Médecine, Faculté de Médecine de Brest, Université de Bretagne Occidentale, 1980.

Overholt R.: In discussion of Dart C.H. Jr., Scott S.M., Takaro T. *Ann. Thorac. Surg.* 9:535, 1970.

Péterffy A., Calabrese E.: Mechanical and conventional manual sutures of the bronchial stump. *Scand. J. Thorac. Cardiovasc. Surg.* 13:87, 1979.

Ravitch M.M., Brown I.W., Daviglus G.F.: Experimental and clinical use of the Soviet bronchus stapling instrument. *Surgery* 46:97, 1959.

Ravitch M.M., Steichen F.M., Fishbein R.H., Knowles P.W., Weil P.: Clinical experiences with the Soviet mechanical bronchus stapler (UKB-25). *J. Thorac. Cardiovasc. Surg.* 47:446, 1964.

Read R.C.: In discussion of Hood R.M., Kirksey T.D., Calhoon J.H., Arnold H.S., Tate R.S. *Ann. Thorac. Surg.* 16:85, 1973.

Reuter M.J.P.: Les sutures mécaniques en chirurgie digestive et pulmonaire. Thesis, presented in 1982 at Université Louis Pasteur, Faculté de Médecine de Strasbourg, France.

Sabot I.A.: In discussion of Dart C.H. Jr., Scott S.M., Takaro T. *Ann. Thorac. Surg.* 9:535, 1970.

Scott R.N., Faraci R.P., Goodman D.G., Militano T.C., Geelhoed G.W., Chretien P.B.: The role of inflammation in bronchial stump healing. *Ann. Surg.* 181:381, 1975.

Scott R.N., Faraci R.P., Hough A., Chretien P.B.: Bronchial stump closure techniques following pneumonectomy: A serial comparative study. *Ann. Surg.* 184:205, 1976.

Steichen F.M., Benz G.H., Baker L.D.: The use of stapling instruments in pulmonary resection. American College of Surgeons Clinical Congress, 1974. ACS Film Library #960.

Vanderhoeft P., Rocmans P., Vollinoti C.: Les agrafages bronchiques. Bilan de 76 exérèses pulmonaires. *Acta Chir. Belg.* 74:149, 1975.

Wolff W.I.: In discussion of Cook W.A., Lee C.W., You K.D., Santos G.H. *N.Y. State J. Med.* 74:967, 1974.

CHAPTER XII

Operations for Morbid Obesity

OUR OWN EXPERIENCE with jejunoileal shunts and with gastric partitioning for morbid obesity has left us, for the present, disillusioned. The fact that we have not pictured our use of these instruments in these operative procedures reflects our opinion that all of these operations still are to be considered experimental and that none of them has been demonstrated to be both safe enough and effective enough for us, at least, to be willing to continue to perform them. We have referred earlier (see Chapter III and Chapter VIII) to performing, and to dismantling, the jejunoileal shunt, to both of which the instruments lend themselves beautifully by standard Auto Suture® techniques.

The literature of gastric bypass and gastric partitioning for morbid obesity has burgeoned so, with modification following on modification, that we can hardly do justice to it here, despite the fact that stapling has made otherwise difficult and dangerous operations easy—and relatively safe. Suffice it to say that stapling the undivided stomach does not produce a reliably secure closure, and that leaks have been reported from the staple lines and perforations from the small gastric pouch.

Nevertheless, given the wide interest in the subject and the key role of stapling in these operations, we here present the principal gastric stapling operations for morbid obesity, with the original illustrations.

Mason of Iowa was the originator of gastric bypass and partitioning procedures. He performed his first operation, stapled gastric division and manually sutured bypass, in 1966 (Mason and Ito, 1967) (Fig XII–1). In 1973 (Printen and Mason), at the time he reported his second operation, stapling and dividing the stomach but leaving a small greater curvature channel (Fig XII–2), he observed that "The gastric bypass is a lengthy undertaking in the usual obese patient; therefore, a simpler procedure which shortened operating and anesthesia time was developed . . . the gastroplasty. . . ." In his 1975 paper (Mason, Printen, Hartford, and Boyd), he reverted to his original operation, stapled division of the stomach leaving a small proximal gastric pouch, which was anastomosed to a loop of jejunum (Fig XII–3). The short proximal pouch was created ". . . with several applications of the GIA stapler or by cutting between two parallel applications of the TA 90." A gastrojejunostomy was performed manually. He said that their original operation, gastric division and gastrojejunostomy, had seemed a formidable operation and that "The operation had to be simplified if it was to be accepted. We began a series of disappointing attempts to find methods of accomplishing this without compromising effectiveness in weight reduction. The operation now being performed is much like the originally described procedure except that there have been some refinements which have shortened the operating time to 3 hours."

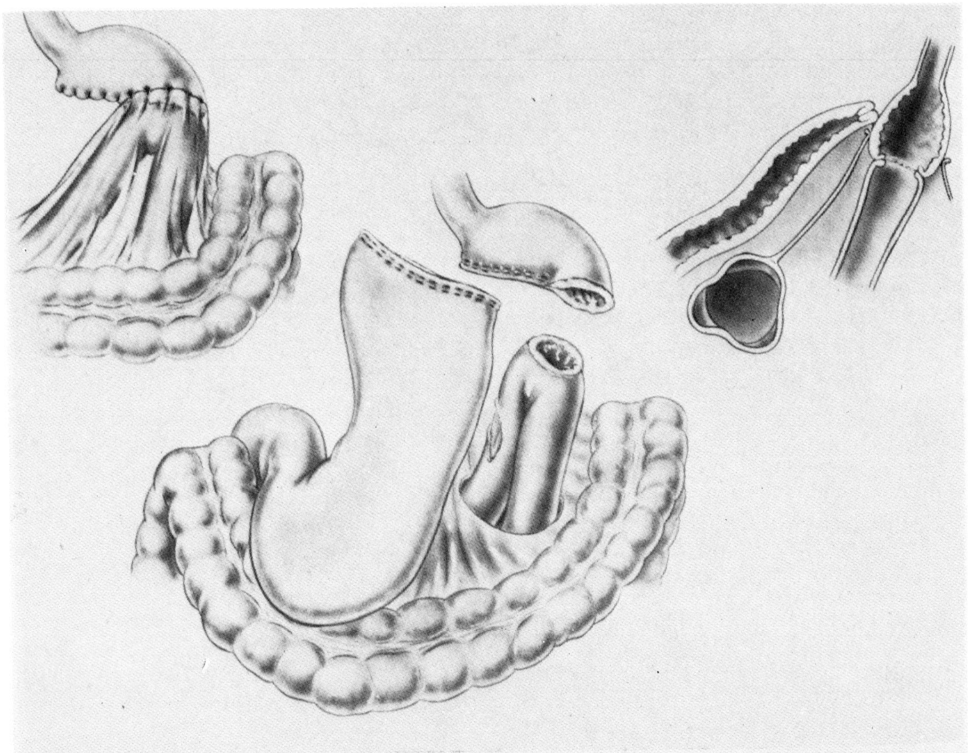

Fig. 1. Illustrates the potentially reversible 90% gastric bypass operation with a short loop, retrocolic gastroenterostomy. The ligament of Treitz is divided. The mesocolon is secured to the 10% stomach pouch and the closed distal 90% of excluded stomach is attached to the anterior wall of the fundic segment. These steps are important in preventing proximal loop stasis.

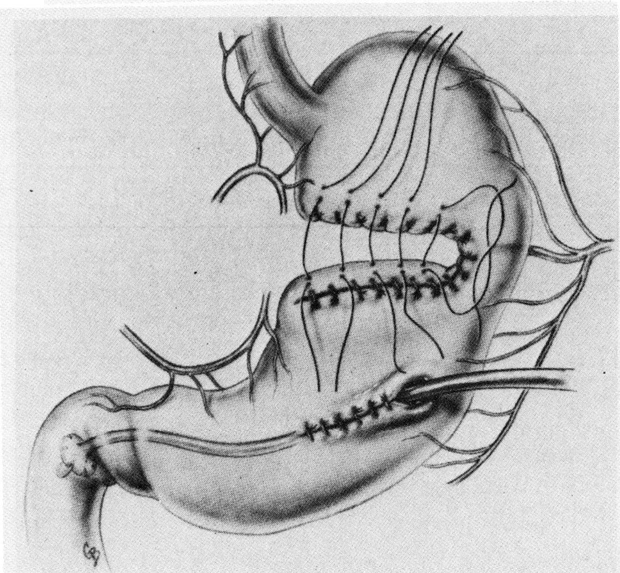

↑ **Fig XII–1.**—Gastric bypass and gastric partitioning for morbid obesity. Mason's (Mason and Ito, 1967) original stapled gastric division and manual gastroenterostomy. (From E.E. Mason and C. Ito, *Annals of Surgery,* 1969, used by permission.)

← **Fig XII–2.**—Mason's gastroplasty, designed to avoid the necessity for complete transection of stomach, and gastroenterostomy. The stomach was stapled to within 15 mm of the greater curvature. (From K.J. Printen and E.E. Mason, *Archives of Surgery,* 1973, used by permission.)

Fig 2.—Gastroplasty furnishes small gastric pouch with 1.5-cm greater curvature channel maintaining gastrointestinal continuity. Distal gastrostomy is mandatory primarily for feeding should channel become obstructed due to postoperative edema.

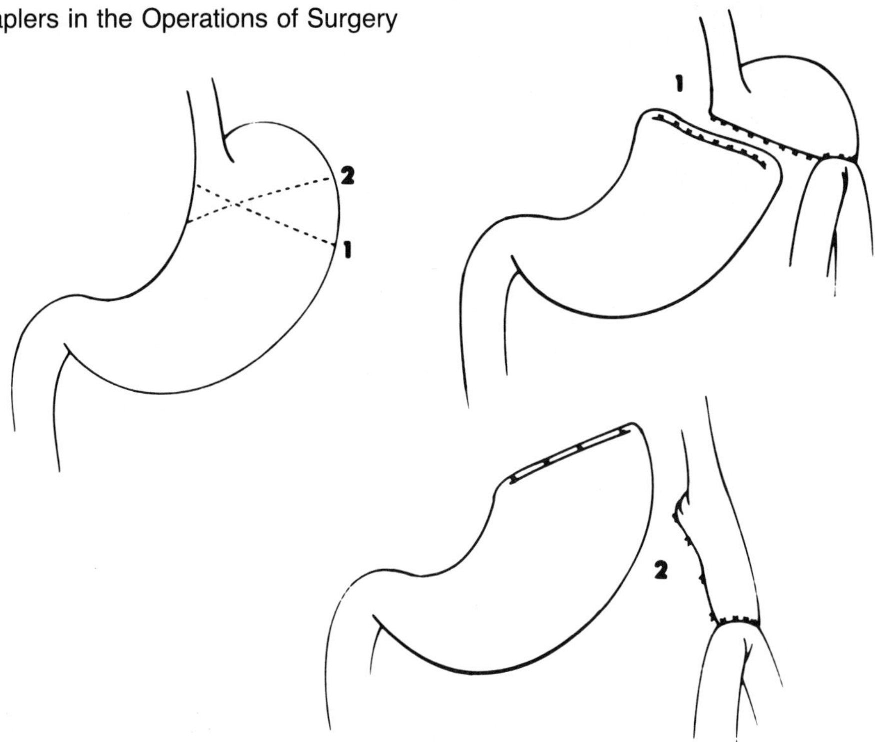

Fig XII–3.—Mason reverted, with minor modifications, to his original operation, stapled, transected stomach, the edges inverted, and a manually made gastroenterostomy. (From E.E. Mason, K.J. Printen, C.E. Hartford, and W.C. Boyd, *Annals of Surgery,* 1975, used by permission.)

It occurred to Alden (1977) of Minneapolis that there was no need to transect the stomach, and that the stomach could be simply stapled in continuity (Fig XII–4). The gastrojejunostomy he performed with the GIA^{TM} instrument, closing the GIA^{TM} introduction site manually. Mason's Figure 2 from his 1979 paper (Mason, Printen, Barron, Lewis, Kealey, and Blommers) (Fig XII–5) shows one of the problems associated with all of these operations, perforations through the suture or staple lines or from either proximal or distal pouch. We pointed out to Alden (Ravitch, 1977) that our animal experiments for gastric bypass, reported in 1967 (Ravitch, Rivarola, and VanGrov), had shown that in the dog, at least, if the stomach was stapled in continuity there would gradually develop gaps in the staple line. Alden found that, in fact, this had developed in some of his patients, but thought that this had not interfered with their weight loss (Alden, 1977).

Pace and Carey and their colleagues (Pace, Martin, Tetirick, Fabri, and Carey, 1979) thought to avoid the need for gastrojejunostomy by leaving a gap in the middle of the staple line (Fig XII–6).

Gomez (1980) of St. Louis, disappointed after his experience with 337 gastroplasties in three years, undertook to modify the operation and in 1980 published a new operative technique (Fig XII–7). He applied the TA 90^{TM} instrument from the *lesser* curvature with a C-clamp to close it near the *greater* curvature, leaving a 12-mm greater-curvature channel. The TA 90^{TM} instrument was applied twice, creating four lines of staples. A "seromuscular suture" of 3-0 Prolene, to prevent the channel from enlarging, was begun at the end of the staple line and carried around the greater curvature and back until it met the staple line.

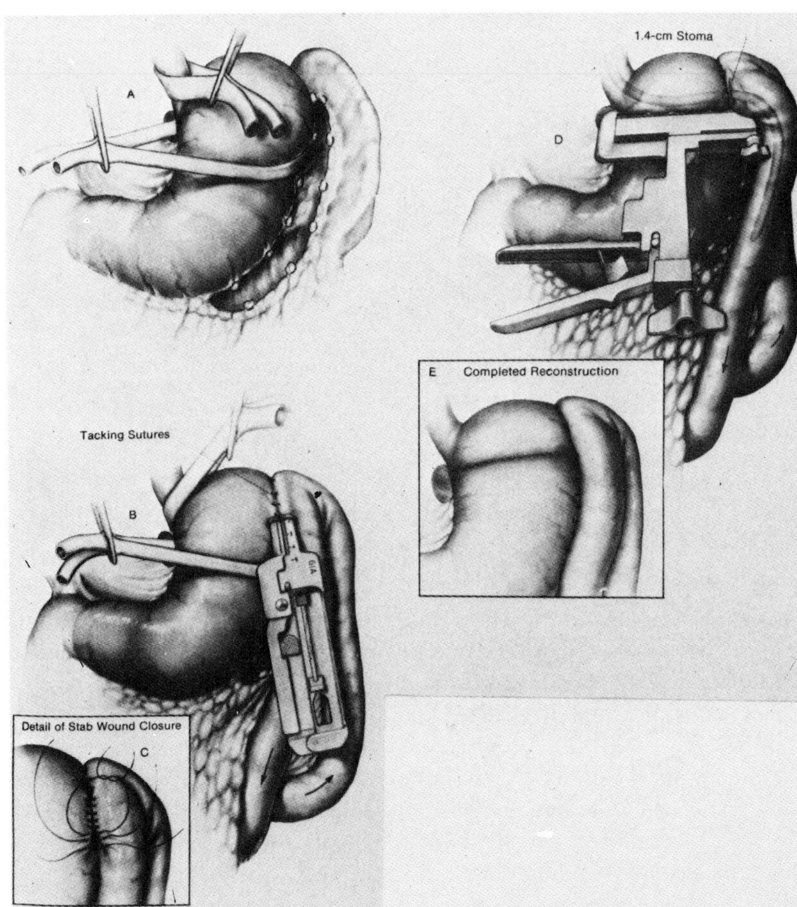

Fig XII–4.—Alden stapled the stomach across in continuity and performed a proximal GIA™ gastrojejunostomy, with manual closure of the GIA™ introduction wound. (From J.F. Alden, *Archives of Surgery,* 1977, used by permission.)

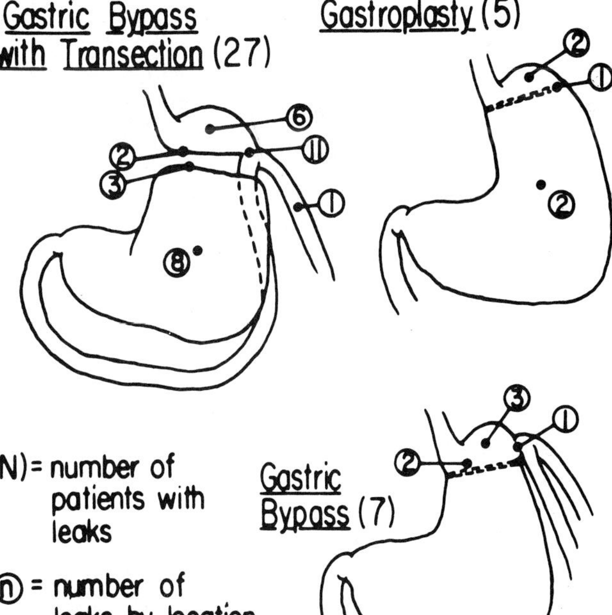

Fig XII–5.—Mason evaluated the problem of leaks and perforations in the Iowa experience. (From E.E. Mason, K.J. Printen, P. Barron, J.W. Lewis, G.P. Kealey, and T.J. Blommers, *Annals of Surgery,* 1979, used by permission.)

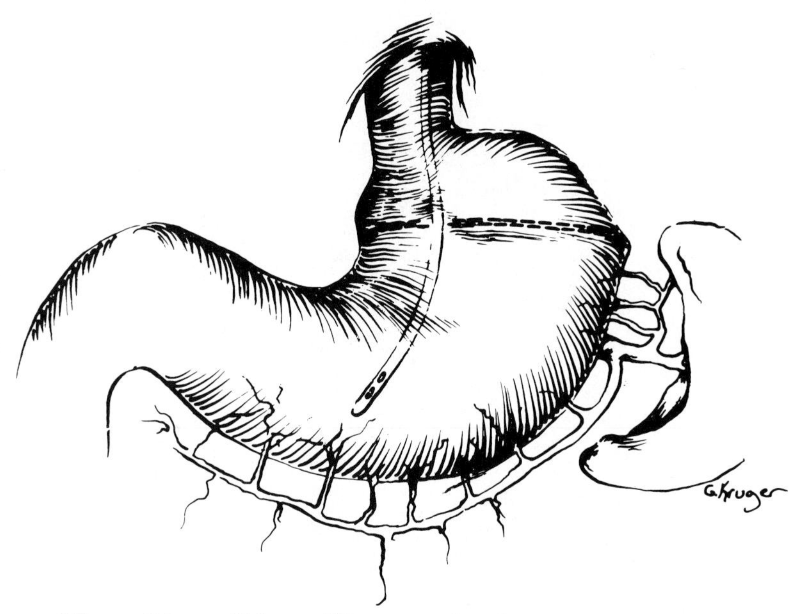

Fig XII–6.—Pace stapled the stomach across in continuity, after removing two staples from the proximal row and one from the distal row, to provide the opening shown, hoping to eliminate the need for a gastroenterostomy. (From W.G. Pace, E.W. Martin Jr., T. Tetirick, P.J. Fabri, and L.C. Carey, *Annals of Surgery,* 1979, used by permission.)

In his 1980 paper, Mason (Mason, Printen, Blommers, Lewis, and Scott) showed the considerable number of variations he had experimented with in his series, including modifications in the size and shape of the pouch, modifications in the site of the gastro-jejunostomy, and use of a Roux-en-Y reconstruction.

With Robert E. Brolin, we (Brolin and Ravitch, 1981) set about to see whether we could prevent the loosening of the staples in gastric partitioning which, in 1967 (Ravitch, Rivarola, and VanGrov), we had demonstrated to occur. We tried a single application of the TA 90^{TM} instrument, leaving a central gap by the Pace technique, and a double application, in either case reinforcing the closure with a strip of Marlex mesh or vascular graft Teflon on the posterior surface of the stomach, or on both surfaces of the stomach (see Fig III–7). As the x-rays show (see Fig III–8), the staples did not so much pull out as gradually open up and slip out. Reinforcing the suture lines with Marlex or Teflon did not prevent the disruption of the suture line and did produce an almost 30% increase in leaks and death due to peritonitis. The staples are made of extremely light metal and, in the dog at least, when applied to the intact stomach, seem gradually to open up and slide out as the stomach attempts to force food through the suture line.

Gomez (1981), continuing his experience with his gastroplasty, reported that "Staple line dehiscence continues to be of concern with stapling in continuity. . . . Twelve percent revision rate included 15 staple line disruptions, 3 enlarged channels. . . ." At this point, he had added to the operation a chromic catgut suture, passing through the stomach at the end of the staple line and tied around a bougie in the greater-curvature channel. This created a sulcus, which made the "seromuscular" suture easier to insert.

Eckhout and Prinzing (1981) from Denver developed what they termed a "vertical stapled gastroplasty." As shown in their illustrations (Fig XII–8), the TA 90^{TM} instrument is applied from a little to the left of the esophagogastric junction, so as to produce a staple line essentially parallel to the lesser curvature of the stomach and leaving a 10 mm channel on the *lesser* curvature, the TA 90^{TM} instrument being applied twice to produce four rows of staples. A bougie is slipped down the lesser curvature through the 10 mm channel, a catgut suture passed through the stomach and tied around the bougie, and then a continuous "seromuscular" 2-0 polypropylene suture passed from the lesser-curvature end of the staple line in front to the lesser-curvature end of the staple line behind.

392

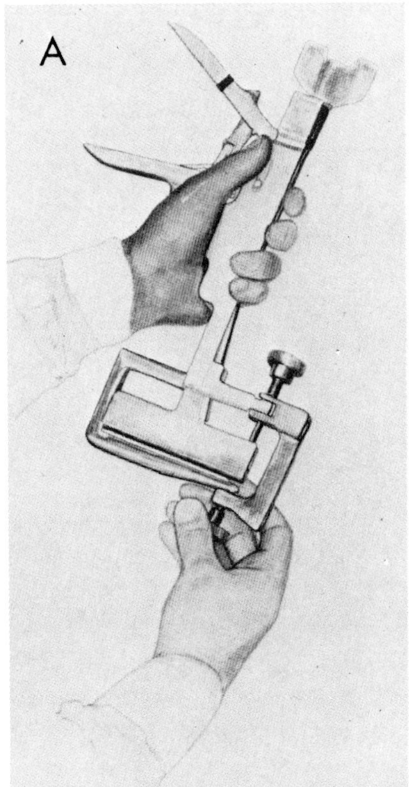

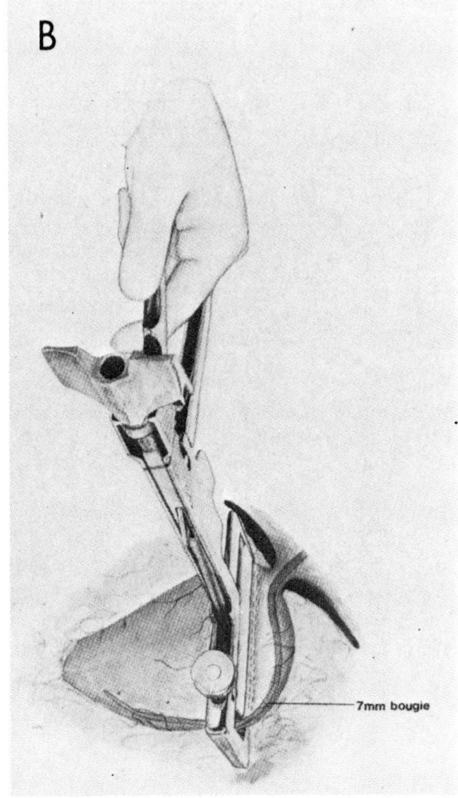

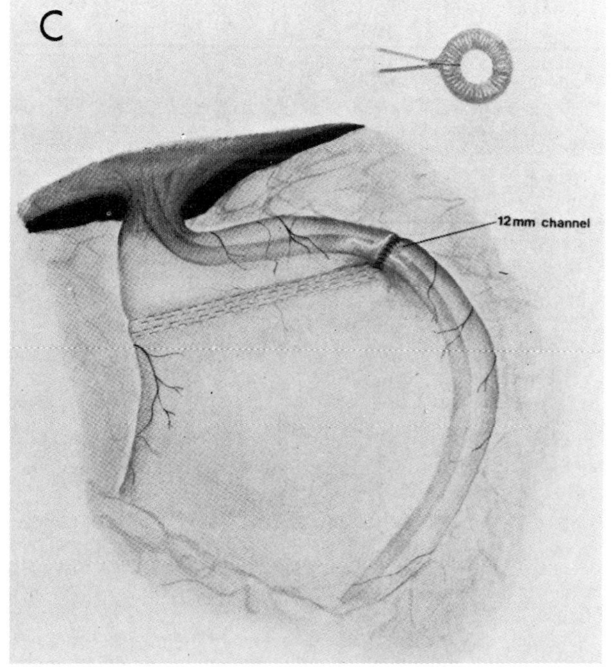

Fig XII–7.—Gomez reverted to Mason's 1973 gastroplasty, but relied on stapling the stomach in continuity rather than almost completely transecting it, leaving a 12-mm greater-curvature channel. The stomach was doubly stapled—producing four lines of staples—a special C-clamp safely locking the nose of the stapler without the need for the tissue-retaining pin. A number of measures have been added with time in the hope of maintaining the channel at its original size, Gomez commenting (1981) that "staple line dehiscence continues to be of concern with stapling in continuity." (From C.A. Gomez, *American Journal of Clinical Nutrition*, 1980, used by permission.)

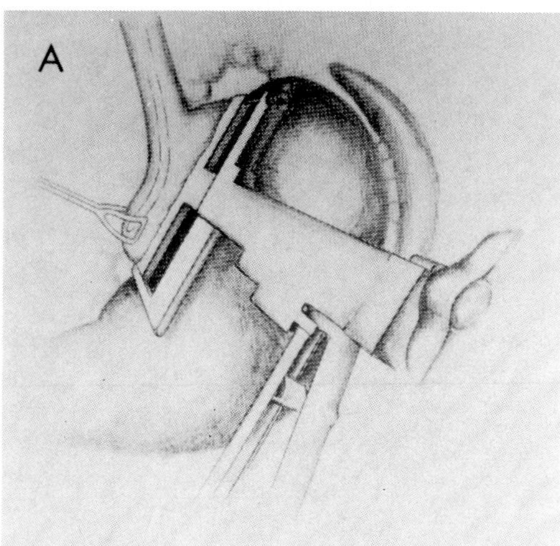

Figure 5. TA 90 stapler applied vertically parallel to the lesser curvature forming a 50 cc pouch. Note NG tube out of harms way. 4.8 mm staples are used in both GB and VSG.

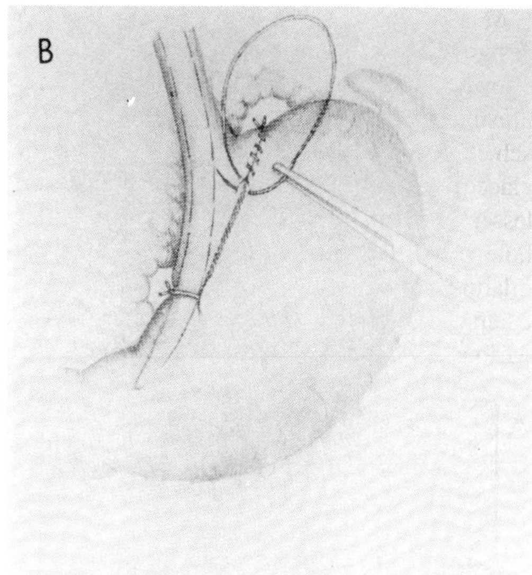

Figure 6. Running 2-0 polypropylene suture encircles all TA 90 staple lines and includes anterior and posterior gastric wall bites. #1 chromic suture tied over #30 dilator.

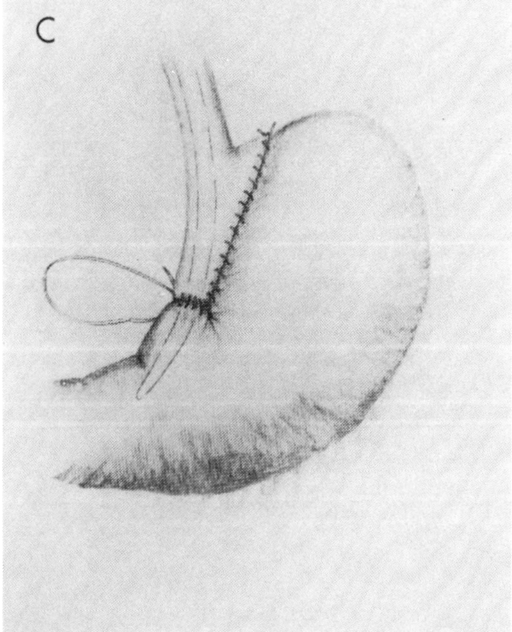

Figure 7. Continuous seromuscular running 2-0 polypropylene suture around channel forms "pseudopylorus."

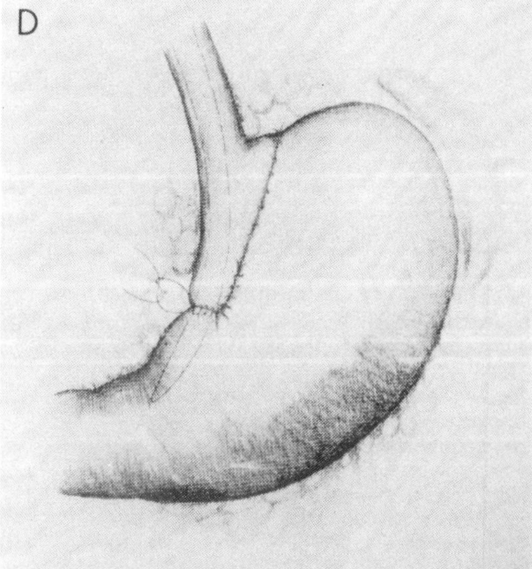

Figure 8. A layer of interrupted nonabsorbable Lembert sutures around channel accentuates "pseudopylorus."

Fig XII–8.—Eckhout and Prinzing hoped that a "vertical stapled gastroplasty," not so directly opposing the propulsive gastric force, might be less liable to disruption than the transversely stapled gastroplasties. Like Gomez (1980), in the effort to maintain the caliber of the channel, now on the lesser curvature, they pass a catgut suture through the stomach and around the bougie, then whip a nonabsorbable suture to approximate the edges of the circular furrow thus created. (From G.V. Eckhout and J.F. Prinzing, *Colorado Medicine,* 1981, used by permission.) →

Mason (1982) stated that in November, 1980 he had adopted ''. . . a modification designed to incorporate the best of what had been learned both at my institution and elsewhere.'' He called this a vertical banded gastroplasty. As will be seen from the illustrations (Fig XII–9), this involves making an EEA™ stapled hole through the stomach, 8–9 cm distal to the esophagogastric junction, just above the crow's-foot and so placed that there is left room for a No. 32 Ewald tube between the stapled hole and the lesser curvature. The TA 90™ instrument then is applied twice from the 2.5 cm EEA™ hole in the stomach up toward the angle of His. To prevent the gastric channel from dilating, a 1.5 cm strip of polypropylene mesh is passed around the lesser-curvature channel and snugly sutured into place. Mason attributes to a number of other surgeons various techniques of vertical gastroplasty.

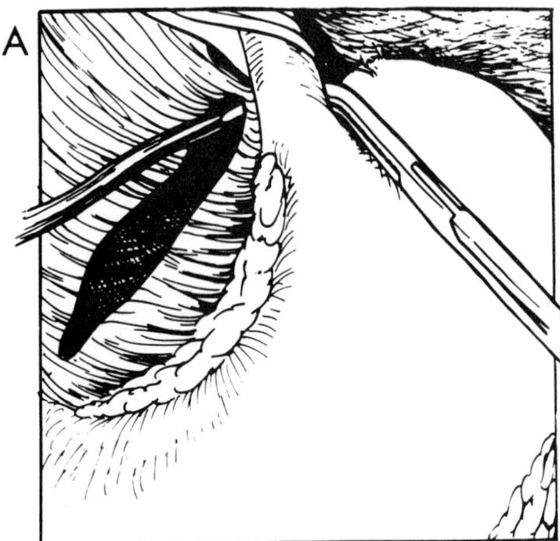

Fig 1.—Penrose drain encircles esophagus and right-angle clamp brings catheter through lesser sac and out esophagogastric angle.

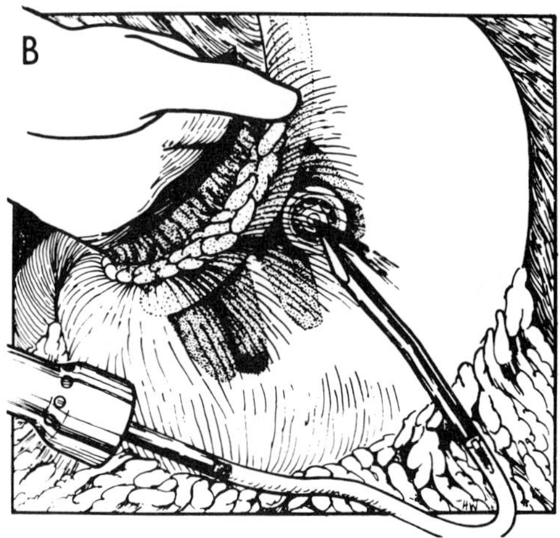

Fig 2.—Trocar is thrust through both walls of stomach and into center of stapler anvil, which is held against posterior stomach wall adjacent to Ewald tube. Attached tubing guides anvil into position.

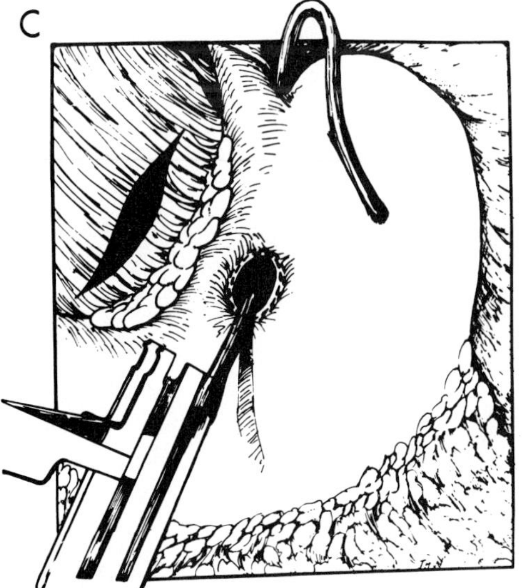

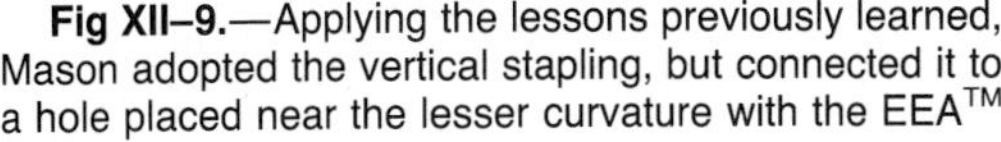

Fig 3.—Catheter placed in lesser sac (Fig 1) has been brought out through window and is used as guide for placement of stapling clamp.

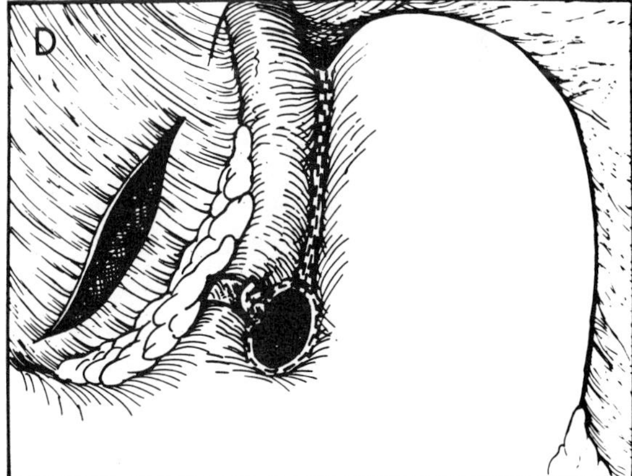

Fig 4.—Completed operation has measured pouch volume of 50 mL or less at pressure of 50 cm. Two sets of staples and polypropylene mesh collar reinforce outlet.

Fig XII–9.—Applying the lessons previously learned, Mason adopted the vertical stapling, but connected it to a hole placed near the lesser curvature with the EEA™ stapler, then wrapping the lesser curvature channel with fabric to prevent dilatation. (From E.E. Mason, *Archives of Surgery,* 1982, used by permission.)

Buckwalter and Herbst of the University of North Carolina (1982) compared proximal gastric stapling and gastrogastrostomy with greater-curvature gastroplasty by the Gomez technique, noting that Gomez "no longer uses a circumferential" ligature, having concluded that this sometimes produces edema and stomal obstruction. Buckwalter, for his gastrogastrostomy technique (Fig XII–10), applied the TA 90™ instrument twice across the stomach, producing four lines of staples, and made a manual 1.0 cm anastomosis between proximal gastric pouch and gastric corpus over the middle of the staple line. They were beginning to use the TA 55™ instrument instead of the TA 90™ instrument.

Remarkably enough, Mason in his invited commentary on the paper by Buckwalter and Herbst, provides as merciless an appraisal of the field of "bariatric" surgery as any offered by its legion of disillusioned critics. "As the authors point out, follow-up data from their gastrogastrostomy patients are incomplete, and they have presented no data regarding the 55 mm staple line and 8 mm stoma. This is, unfortunately, a common pattern in the bariatric surgery literature. Authors tend to present their results, provide some critique, and then introduce another procedure that is as yet untested, but which they feel will be better than the procedure they have just abandoned. The desire to be the first to establish new combinations of variables in gastric reduction operations for treatment of morbid obesity often leads to their premature promotion in anticipation of results that may not be forthcoming."

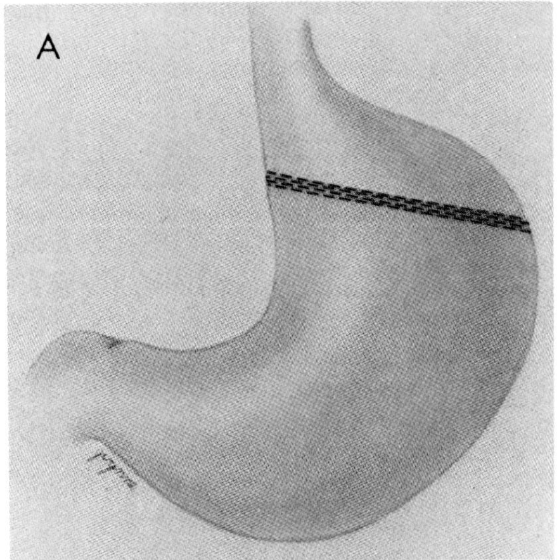

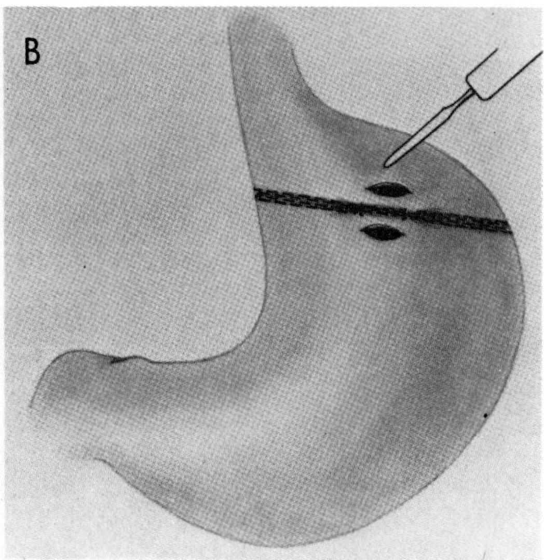

Fig. 6. A 50–60 ml proximal gastric pouch is formed by placing 4 parallel lines of 4.8-mm staples from 2 cartridges.

Fig. 8. Ten-mm openings are made with cautery in the proximal and distal gastric pouches between the 2 silk sutures 2–3 mm above and below the staple line.

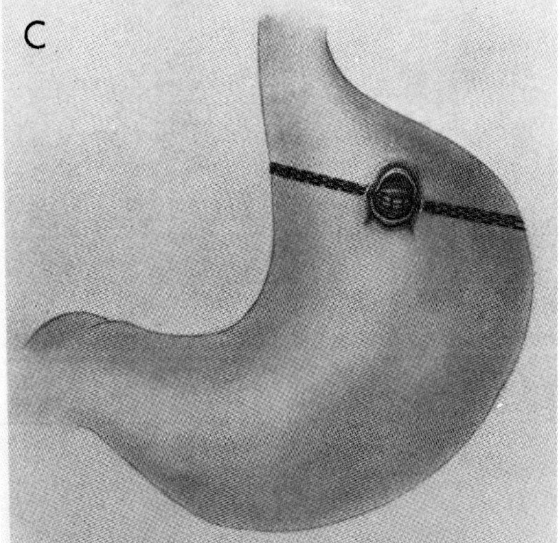

Fig. 9. A continuous Dexon® suture is placed in front o the staple line, establishing the posterior mucosal anasto motic line. The staples form the outer posterior serosa layer of the anastomosis.

Fig XII–10.—Buckwalter and Herbst, like others before them, undertook in-continuity gastric stapling (four lines of staples), restoring alimentary continuity with a small gastrogastrostomy. (From J.A. Buckwalter and C.A. Herbst Jr., *World Journal of Surgery*, 1982, used by permission.)

Martinez (1982) from the Little Company of Mary Hospital in Evergreen Park, Illinois double staples the stomach completely across with a TA 90™ instrument, producing four rows of staples and then performs a bypassing gastrojejunostomy with the 21 mm EEA™ stapler (Fig XII–11). Previously he had used the GIA™ instrument for the 12 mm gastrojejunostomy. No figures are given but it is simply stated that ". . . enlargement of the outflow channel is not anticipated."

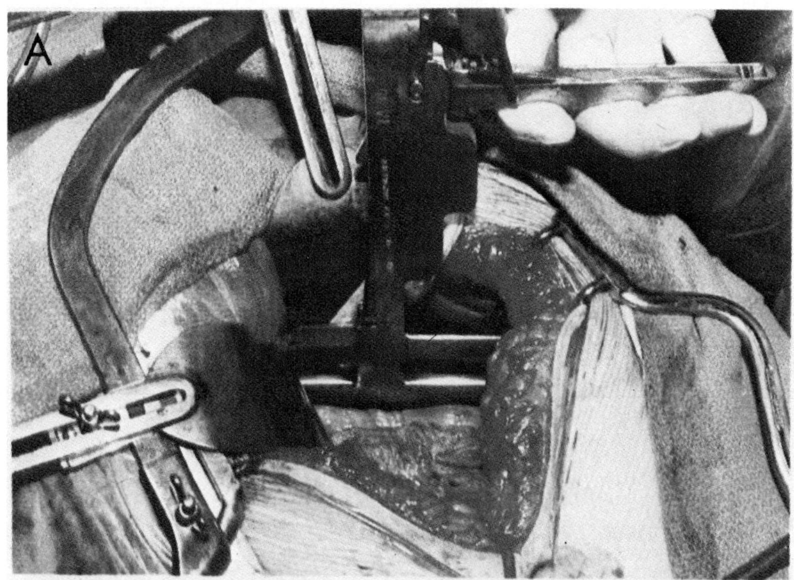

Fig. 6 Gastric partition fashions a proximal gastric reservoir of limited capacity. A second application of a double line of staggered staples is shown.

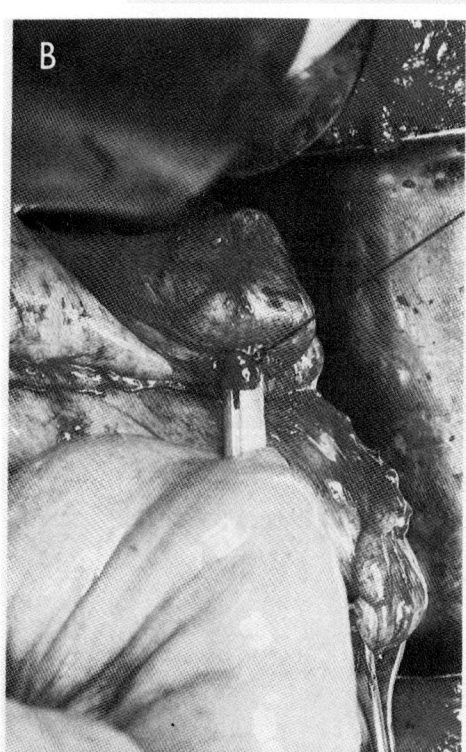

Fig. 11 Adequate overlap of the gastric wall over the anvil of the instrument. Accurate firm tying of the purse string assures fixation of viscus wall to the rod assuring accurate anastomosis.

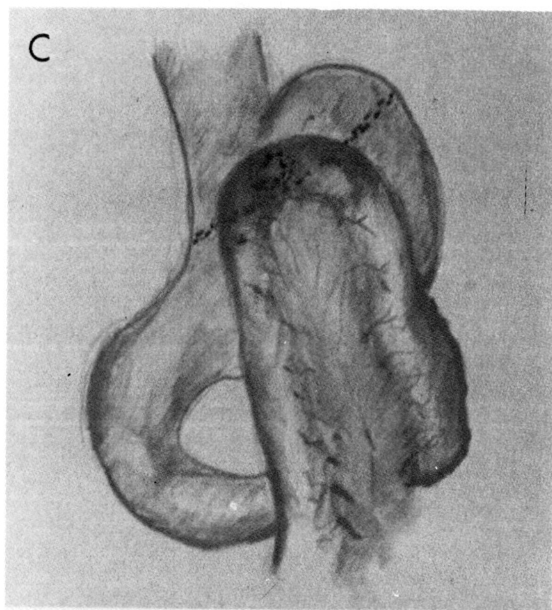

Fig. 14 Drawing of completed antecolic gastrojejunostomy. T colon was omitted for clarity of illustration.

Fig XII–11.—Stapled gastric bypass and gastrojejunostomy—Martinez (1982). The stomach having been stapled with two applications of the TA 90™ instrument—i.e., four rows of staples—the EEA™ instrument without the nose cone is inserted into the jejunum and the central rod out through a stab wound at the proposed site of anastomosis, without a pursestring. The anvil-carrying nose cone is applied and passed into the proximal gastric pouch through a 0 Prolene pursestring suture and the anastomosis performed with the stapler. The enterotomy for introduction of the EEA™ instrument is closed transversely with the TA 55™ instrument. The drawing of the completed reconstruction does not clearly show that there are four lines of staples in the gastric partition. (From L. Martinez, *Contemporary Surgery*, 1982, used by permission.)

This book is devoted to techniques of stapling and not to the advisability of operations with the staplers undertaken for one or another purpose. We do not feel called on to discuss the merits of the various individual operative procedures for weight reduction.

REFERENCES

Alden J.F.: Gastric and jejunoileal bypass. A comparison in the treatment of morbid obesity. *Arch. Surg.* 112:799, 1977.

Alden J.F.: Personal communication, August 9, 1977.

Brolin R.E., Ravitch M.M.: Experimental evaluation of techniques of gastric partitioning for morbid obesity. *Surg. Gynecol. Obstet.* 153:877, 1981.

Buckwalter J.A., Herbst C.A. Jr.: Gastric partition for morbid obesity: Greater curvature gastroplasty or gastrogastrostomy. *World J. Surg.* 6:403, 1982.

Eckhout G.V., Prinzing J.F.: Surgery for morbid obesity. Comparison of gastric bypass with vertically stapled gastroplasty. *Colo. Med.* p. 117, April, 1981.

Gomez C.A.: Gastroplasty in the surgical treatment of morbid obesity. *Am. J. Clin. Nutr.* 33:406, 1980.

Gomez C.A.: Gastroplasty in morbid obesity: A progress report. *World J. Surg.* 5:823, 1981.

Martinez N.S.: Dilemmas of gastric capacity restriction and technical refinements of gastric bypass for morbid obesity. *Contemp. Surg.* 21:17, 1982.

Mason E.E.: Vertical banded gastroplasty for obesity. *Arch. Surg.* 117:701, 1982.

Mason E.E., Ito C.: Gastric bypass in obesity. *Surg. Clin. North Am.* 47:1345, 1967.

Mason E.E., Ito C.: Gastric bypass. *Ann. Surg.* 170:329, 1969.

Mason E.E., Printen K.J., Barron P., Lewis J.W., Kealey G.P., Blommers T.J.: Risk reduction in gastric operations for obesity. *Ann. Surg.* 190:158, 1979.

Mason E.E., Printen K.J., Blommers T.J., Lewis J.W., Scott D.H.: Gastric bypass in morbid obesity. *Am. J. Clin. Nutr.* 33:395, 1980.

Mason E.E., Printen K.J., Hartford C.E., Boyd W.C.: Optimizing results of gastric bypass. *Ann. Surg.* 182:405, 1975.

Pace W.G., Martin E.W. Jr., Tetirick T., Fabri P.J., Carey L.C.: Gastric partitioning for morbid obesity. *Ann. Surg.* 190:392, 1979.

Printen K.J., Mason E.E.: Gastric surgery for relief of morbid obesity. *Arch. Surg.* 106:428, 1973.

Ravitch M.M.: Personal communication, July 18, 1977.

Ravitch M.M., Rivarola A., VanGrov J.: Studies of intestinal healing. I. Preliminary studies of the mechanism of healing of the everting intestinal anastomosis. *Johns Hopkins Med. J.* 121:343, 1967.

Name Index

Subject Index

Page numbers in *italics* indicate figures; page numbers followed by "t" indicate tables.